Preventing Colic in Horses

Written by
Dr. Christine King
BVSc, MACVSc, MVetClinStud

Consulting Editor
Dr. Anthony Blikslager
DVM, PhD, Dip. ACVS

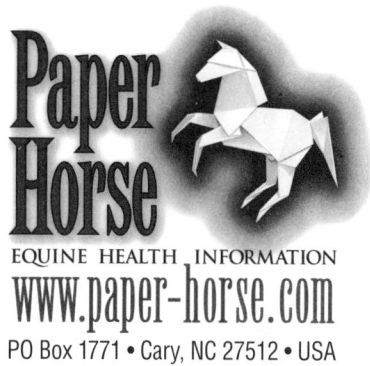

EQUINE HEALTH INFORMATION
www.paper-horse.com
PO Box 1771 • Cary, NC 27512 • USA

Preventing Colic in Horses

ISBN: 0-9674926-0-2

Library of Congress Catalog Card Number: 99-96019

Published by Paper Horse

Post Office Box 1771
Cary, North Carolina, 27512
United States of America

Copyright© 1999 Christine M. King

All rights reserved. No part of this publication may be reproduced, stored in a retrieval system, or transmitted in any form, by any means, without written permission from the publisher.

Illustrations: Copyright© 1999 Robin Peterson

All rights reserved.

Cover Photography: Richard A. Mansmann, VMD, PhD

Cover Design and production: Rich Farrell, *Art Farm inc.,* Apex, NC

Printed by:
Technical Communication Services
North Kansas City, Missouri

Please note...

In writing and producing this book, every effort has been made to provide accurate information and sound advice on preventing colic in horses. But ultimately, it is up to the reader to determine whether and how to use the information contained in this book. We encourage you to discuss management changes that may impact the health and performance of your horse(s) with your regular veterinarian beforehand. As your veterinarian is familiar with your area, the scope and limitations of your facility, and your horse(s), s/he is the best person to consult for advice on horse healthcare. We defer to him/her in all matters discussed in this book.

Please note that neither the publisher, the author, nor the editor: (1) makes any warranty concerning, nor assumes any responsibility for, the results of following the guidelines described in this book; (2) can be held liable to anyone for damages resulting from reliance on any information contained in this book, whether with respect to feeding, care, treatment, patient evaluation, or drug usage, or by reason of any misstatement or inadvertent error; or (3) manufactures any of the drugs, feeds, or other products mentioned in this book, offers any guarantee of any kind on such items, nor will be held responsible for the results that may be obtained from the use of these items. Any trade names used in this book are for example only; their use does not imply endorsement of that product, nor that a similar product with a different trade name is in any way inferior or less effective.

Please read and follow the manufacturer's directions when using any product; and if there is disagreement between those directions and the recommendations contained in this book, discuss the situation with your veterinarian and follow his/her advice.

Thanks to...

Dr. Anthony Blikslager, my consulting editor, for ensuring both the scientific accuracy and practical value of the material in this book. Anthony is a gifted equine surgeon, a noted researcher in the field of gastrointestinal physiology, and, above all, a horseman—a potent combination, to the horse's benefit.

Dr. Richard Mansmann, for taking the time to review the manuscript and make suggestions. Also a born horseman, Dick has spent nigh on 30 years practicing equine medicine, in both private practice and academic settings, so he brings a wealth of experience and good sense to this project. (As with *Equine Lameness,* this book is far better for your contributions, Dick. Thanks, too, for your continued encouragement.)

Linda Mansmann, for acting as my guinea pig. As a horse owner, her perspectives and comments were really valuable; her enthusiasm for this project is also gratefully acknowledged. (Here's to many happy, colic-free years with Louis, aka "Red All Over.")

Dr. Kenneth Kopp, for casting an expert eye over the manuscript and ensuring that the nutritional advice is sound. Dr. Kopp is a consultant in equine nutrition who mixes a background in equine veterinary practice with the science of feeding horses.

Dr. James Kubiak, for agreeing to review the manuscript from yet another perspective. Dr. Kubiak teaches in the Department of Animal Sciences at North Carolina State University, and is the coordinator of REINS—the Regional Equine Information Network System—an organization of volunteers in North Carolina who offer their various skills and expertise (not to mention their time) to horsepeople throughout the state.

Liz Anderson, for her perspectives as both a horse owner and a publisher. Thanks for the pointers, and for not laughing (at least, not out loud) when I said I wanted to publish this book myself.

Dr. Robin Peterson, for the excellent illustrations. Robin trained and worked for some years as an equine surgeon before becoming a medical illustrator, so her drawings have the added dimension of actually having "been there."

*Thanks for so generously giving me your time
and the benefit of your experience.*

Table of Contents

Foreword by Dr. Anthony Blikslager

Chapter 1   What is Colic?   1

Signs of Colic 2
    correlating the signs with a specific problem 5
    correlating signs with severity of the problem 6

The Horse's Digestive System 7
    stomach 8
    small intestine 10
    cecum 12
    large colon 13
    small colon 16
    rectum 17

Incidence of Colic at Specific Sites 18

What Causes Colic? 18
    what is causing the pain? 18
        1. spasms 19
        2. distention 20
        3. traction 22
        4. ischemia (low blood flow) 22

    5. inflammation (with or without ulceration) 25
    how common are these problems? 27

Chapter 2   Risk Factors for Colic   35

Interpreting Study Results 36

Intrinsic (Horse) Factors 38
    breed 38
    gender 42
    age 44
    use/activity 49
    behavior 51
    history 53
    genetics 56

Management Factors 57
    diet 57
    housing 71
    internal parasites 77
    dental care 85
    stress 86
    drugs and chemicals 88

Environmental Factors 93
    geographic location 93
    weather or season 94
    poisonous plants 96

Chapter 3 Strategies for Preventing Colic 105

Simple Management Strategies 106
   1. match the horse's natural diet 107
   2. match the horse's natural feeding schedule 112
   3. match the horse's natural activity pattern 114
   4. minimize changes 115
   5. feed good quality feedstuffs 118
   6. ample access to fresh, clean water 121
   7. deworming program 123
   8. regular dental care 127
   9. environmental management 127
   10. pay attention 128

Preventing Specific Types of Colic 130
   spasmodic or "gas" colic 130
   large colon impactions 131
   avoiding colic at shows and competitions 131
   large colon displacements 132
   ileal impactions 134
   small colon impactions in Miniature Horses 135
   sand colic 136
   enteroliths 137
   gastric ulcers 139
   right dorsal colitis 142
   verminous arteritis *(S. vulgaris* infestation) 142
   meconium impaction in foals 143
   roundworm (ascarid) impactions 143
   colic in older horses 144

Chapter 4   Managing Colic (preventing disasters)   151

Recognizing the Signs 152
Determining the Severity 152
   assessing the horse's physical status 153
      heart rate 154
      gum color 156
      capillary refill time 158
      indicators of hydration status 158
      temperature of the extremities 159
      other physical changes 159
   assessing bowel function 160
      evaluating bowel sounds 160
      manure 162

What To Do with a Colicky Horse 162
   monitoring the situation 163
   drug therapy 164
   things to avoid 167
   recovery 168

Transporting Severely Colicky Horses 170
   the trailer 170
   insurance 171
   during the trip 171
   prior planning 172

Final Word 173

Index   **177**

Foreword

As an equine surgeon, the most common questions I receive following colic surgery on a client's horse are: "What caused my horse's colic?" and "What could I have done to prevent it?" The answer to the first question generally is "I don't know." The answer to the second question is much more difficult, and frequently couched in terms that take into account the tremendous guilt a horse owner feels when their horse has severe colic.

It is true that a number of serious colic episodes are intestinal accidents (similar to a car accident—an 'Act of God'), and there is very little that can be done to prevent an accident. It is also true that only about 5% of colic episodes require surgical intervention. Nevertheless, there is a great deal that can and should be done to reduce the overall occurrence of colic in horses. I am now very happy to report that much of the information I have tried to convey to clients in the middle of the night can now be found in one concise source: Dr. Christine King's *Preventing Colic in Horses*.

The real answer to "What caused my horse's colic?" is mankind's management of the horse. To understand this point, you have to realize that horses have evolved on the American plains as animals that continuously move and graze for most of the day. Knowing this, why would we put a horse in a stall and feed it grain? Because we have adapted the horse's environment to suit our purposes. In fact, some horses are so highly bred for their intended purpose that they cannot live as their ancestors did because of their need for high-energy feed and shelter. But by being aware of what a horse was originally intended to do, we can attempt to simulate its natural feeding and environment as much as possible. This is the major theme of Dr. King's book.

However, the reasons that management and feeding practices trigger colic are complex. As you read this book you will begin to understand why colic develops, and you will begin to develop your own answers as to how to prevent colic in your horses. All of this information was previously available in the veterinary literature, but it has been buried in a great many scientific publications not readily understood by the horse-owning public. Dr. King has done a remarkable job of condensing this information in the context of common sense and practicality. I urge you to read and use this information so that I don't have to talk to you about preventing colic while waiting for your horse to recover from colic surgery.

Anthony T. Blikslager DVM, PhD
Diplomate, American College of Veterinary Surgeons
Assistant Professor, Dept. of Clinical Sciences
College of Veterinary Medicine
North Carolina State University

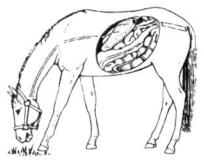

1

What is colic?

Understanding a problem is the first step in preventing it, so before discussing ways of preventing colic, it is worth spending some time reviewing what exactly colic is, and what causes it.

Colic is a sign of abdominal (belly) pain. It is a symptom of disease, rather than a disease in itself. There are dozens of specific conditions that can cause a horse to show signs of abdominal pain. In most cases, colic signs indicate a problem with the digestive system—the focus of this book. Less often, they are caused by a problem with one of the other abdominal organs (liver, kidneys, ovaries, etc.). Occasionally, diseases in the chest cavity cause signs that mimic colic; and some horses with laminitis or muscle cramps can appear colicky. Table 1-1 on page 31 lists conditions that can cause colic-like symptoms, but that do not directly involve the digestive tract.

Signs of Colic

Horses show signs of abdominal pain in a wide variety of ways. Some signs, such as curling the upper lip, are subtle, whereas others, such as repeated or violent rolling, are hard to mistake. Signs of colic include one or more of the following abnormalities.

Abnormal behavior:

- pawing, often with the horse holding the foreleg up for a few moments before pawing
- repeatedly looking at the flank or belly (not necessarily to the side with the problem) and/or biting at the flank
- kicking at the belly
- lying down and either repeatedly getting up and lying down, or remaining down for longer than is normal for that horse at that time of day
- rolling repeatedly, or even just rolling in a place or at a time that is unusual for that horse
  - depending on the degree of pain, the horse may roll either in a distracted, halfhearted way, alternating between flat-out and resting up on its chest, or it may roll more violently, turning from side to side and thrashing its legs
  - horses at pasture often roll without having colic; whereas normal horses usually shake off any dirt as soon as they get up, colicky horses tend not to shake off when they stand
- curling or quivering of the upper lip
  - lip curling in horses with colic is similar to (but usually less pronounced than) the Flehmen response that stallions show around mares, in which the upper lip is curled all the way back, exposing the upper teeth and gums
- grunting or groaning, especially when lying down

- grinding the teeth
  - this is more common in foals than in adult horses, particularly foals with stomach ulcers
- leaving food or being completely disinterested in food
  - some colicky horses refuse grain or hay, but they will nibble at fresh grass
- playing in water with the lips or tongue, or hanging over the water container but not drinking
  - in many cases horses that show this behavior are dehydrated; but not all dehydrated horses do this, and not all horses that do this are dehydrated
- either anxious, restless (and in more severe cases, distressed or violent) behavior, or lethargy and depression

Abnormal posture:

- crouching as if wanting to lie down, but remaining standing; this posture may be repeated several times
- frequently stretching out as if to urinate, or standing stretched out for several minutes
  - this posture can also be seen in some horses with laminitis or exercise-induced muscle damage (myositis, "tying up")
  - it is often mistakenly interpreted as indicating kidney stones (which are *rare* in horses) or some other urinary obstruction, when in most cases it simply indicates abdominal pain
- holding the head in an unusual position, such as with the neck extended and the head rotated to one side
  - this posture is often combined with grimacing, lip curling, or teeth grinding
- lying on the back (more common in young foals)

- ❖ sitting like a dog, on the haunches with the forelegs extended
  - this usually indicates excessive pressure in the stomach
- ❖ standing very still, with the abdomen tensed ("splinted")

Abnormal appearance:

- ❖ abrasions, swellings, or caked dirt on the side of the head, body, and legs as a result of thrashing about on the ground
  - swelling, bruising, and abrasions are common at the side of the eye, making the horse look like a prize-fighter
  - obviously, these signs don't always indicate colic; but they are important when accompanied by other signs of colic
- ❖ bloating (swelling of the abdomen, most obvious in the flank and when looking at the horse from behind)
  - bloating, or abdominal distention, is more easily seen in foals and Miniature Horses because their abdominal walls are much thinner than in adult horses
  - abdominal distention in nonpregnant horses generally indicates gas buildup in the large intestine; in foals, gas buildup in the small intestine can also cause bloating

Abnormalities of bodily functions:

- ❖ inappropriate sweating (i.e. not caused by exercise, overheating, or fever); primarily, it is caused by pain
  - sweating in horses with mild colic tends to be patchy, if present at all; common sites are the base of the ears, the side of the neck, and the lower flank
  - horses with severe colic may be dripping with sweat
- ❖ straining to pass manure (most common in newborn foals with meconium impaction; see page 46)
  - in foals, straining is often accompanied by swishing or "flagging" of the tail

- absence of manure passage for several hours, or finding less manure than normal in the stall for that time of day
  - these signs do not necessarily mean there is a problem, but they can indicate slowed bowel activity
  - another sign of a potential problem is a change in the manure, e.g. loose ("cow pie") or watery manure; hard manure balls coated with whitish-yellow mucus or blood; or manure that has a foul odor

Usually, a horse shows only a handful of these signs during an episode of colic. But seeing *any* of these signs should prompt you to inspect the horse more closely and keep a watchful eye on it. (Managing an episode of colic is discussed in Chapter 4.)

> Horses can show signs of abdominal pain in a variety of ways. If you see any of the signs listed, take a closer look at the horse and keep an eye on it for further changes.

Correlating the signs with a specific problem

For the most part, signs of colic are nonspecific; they simply indicate that the horse is in pain. In very few cases do specific signs signal a particular problem. And even when they do, they are not proof of that problem. For example, teeth grinding is common in foals with stomach ulcers, but it is simply a sign of pain. It does not occur in every foal with ulcers, and foals without ulcers may also grind their teeth. (Frustration, anxiety, neurologic disease, and pain elsewhere in the body are other possible causes.)

Some other specific behaviors or postures that bring to mind particular problems include:

- dog-sitting in horses with excessive pressure in the stomach from buildup of food, fluid, and/or gas
- lying on the back, often with one foreleg drawn forward over the head, in foals with stomach or small intestinal pain

- straining and tail flagging in newborn foals with meconium impaction
- lying on the back in some mares with a large colon volvulus (twist; see page 23); this condition is extremely painful and causes dramatic bloating

The side of the belly at which a horse looks or kicks usually is not significant. Even when it is severe, pain originating in the bowel is not specific for a particular site. All the horse knows, and expresses, is that its belly hurts. This type of pain (visceral; relating to the internal organs, or viscera) is not as easy for the mind to localize as pain arising from a problem with the more superficial structures (skin, muscle, tendon, ligament, joint capsule) or bone.

Correlating signs with severity of the problem

In general, the more obvious the signs of pain, the more serious the problem. For example, horses with mild colic typically show subtle signs, such as curling the lip, holding the head in an abnormal position, or lying down more than usual. Repeated rolling, sweating, and groaning are signs of more severe pain. Also, in horses with serious conditions, the signs tend to be persistent and may become more severe, whereas with mild colic, the signs often are intermittent.

There are two uncommon but important exceptions: (1) intestinal twist or some other problem that has caused a section of the bowel to die, and (2) bowel obstruction which ends in rupture. In each of these cases, the horse passes through a distressed, violently painful stage (which may be missed if it happens overnight or at pasture), but once the bowel has died or ruptured, the horse may not seem very painful. Dead bowel cannot transmit pain signals, and rupture suddenly relieves the pressure of bowel distention.

However, by this time these horses are in shock—circulatory failure from fluid loss into the bowel or abdomen, and absorption of bacterial toxins from the damaged bowel or escaped bowel contents. They tend to stand very still, with the abdomen tensed ("splinted"). They are severely depressed, weak and shaky, and reluctant to move. As shock progresses, the color of their gums changes from dark pink to brick-red, to bluish-purple, to gray (see Chapter 4). Horses at this late stage are very difficult to save; in fact, once the bowel has ruptured, the situation is hopeless. But again, these are *uncommon* scenarios.

Individual response to pain. A final consideration is that each horse responds to pain a little differently. Some are stoic and tough, while others are less tolerant of mild pain. Knowing the horse's tolerance level is useful when interpreting signs of pain. Looking or kicking at the belly takes on far more significance in a horse that normally puts up with minor pain than in a horse that reacts to every little injury. However, *signs of colic should not be ignored in any horse.*

> A specific diagnosis usually cannot be made based on the particular signs. But in most cases, the more obvious the signs of pain, the more serious the problem.

The Horse's Digestive System

The horse's digestive system, from mouth to rectum, is adapted to digest a high-fiber diet that primarily consists of grass and other plant material. In order to break down the plant fiber into digestible substances, horses rely on the large and diverse population of bacteria and other micro-organisms in their digestive tract. This process is called *microbial fermentation* (as opposed to breakdown of feed material exclusively by digestive enzymes).

Cattle, sheep, and goats also rely on microbial fermentation to digest dietary fiber. But in these animals the process occurs in the large, vat-like forestomach (rumen), whereas horses do the bulk of their fiber digesting in their large intestine. Thus, horses are termed *hindgut fermenters,* and ruminants (cattle, sheep, and goats) are called foregut fermenters.

The length and volume of the horse's digestive tract reflect this reliance on hindgut digestion. Horses have a relatively small stomach, a long, narrow small intestine, and a complex and voluminous large intestine, consisting of the cecum and the large and small colons (see Figure 1-1). In the average-size adult horse, the digestive tract is about 100 feet long and holds approximately 210 liters (48 gallons) of water, digestive juices, and food/manure.

Stomach

Horses have a simple stomach: a single chamber in which food is mixed with gastric acid and enzymes (pepsin, which begins protein breakdown), then sent on to the small intestine. A small amount of microbial fermentation also occurs in the stomach. In adult horses, the stomach holds between 8 and 20 liters (2 to 4½ gallons); the average is about 18 liters (4 gallons).

Sphincters

The horse's stomach has two valves, or sphincters, which control the flow of material out of the stomach. The cardiac (or lower esophageal) sphincter, between the esophagus and the stomach, prevents backflow of material into the esophagus. The pyloric sphincter, between the stomach and the duodenum, prevents flow of material into the small intestine until it is well mixed with acid and enzymes, and the larger particles have been broken down.

The cardiac sphincter, and the way in which the esophagus enters the stomach at an angle, forms such a tight seal that it prevents the horse from vomiting or regurgitating material into the esophagus under most circumstances. This puts the stomach at risk of rupturing when it is overfilled with food, fluid, or gas. In most cases, overfilling of the stomach occurs not from excessive food or

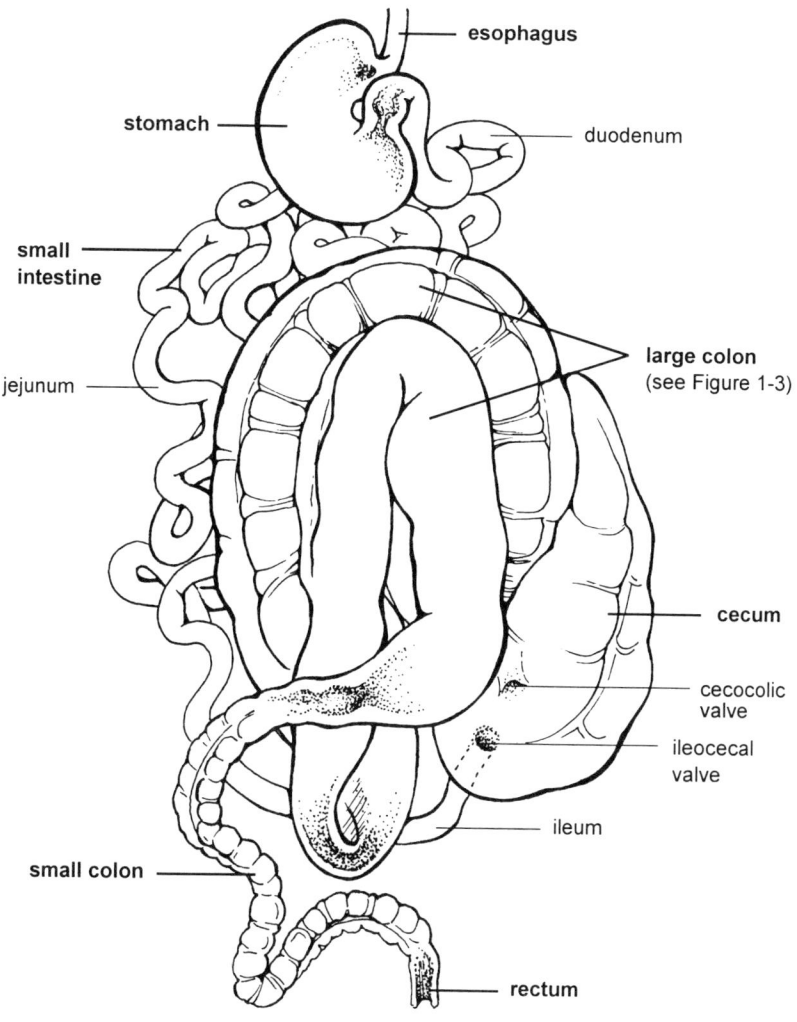

Figure 1-1. The horse's digestive tract.

water intake, but from a problem in the small intestine that slows or prevents emptying of the stomach and/or allows fluid and gas to back-flow into the stomach.

So, food material dribbling from the nostrils in a horse showing signs of colic is an indication that stomach rupture is imminent unless the stomach is immediately decompressed.

One common exception is esophageal obstruction (choke), in which a mass of food becomes lodged in the esophagus. Horses with choke often have saliva containing feed material streaming from their nostrils. They may also seem anxious or distressed, and stand with their head and neck stretched out. But once the obstruction is relieved, most of these horses are fine. Choke can usually be distinguished from colic in two ways: (1) the obstructing mass can often be seen or felt in the jugular groove on the left side of the neck; and (2) horses with choke often make repeated gagging noises and efforts to swallow.

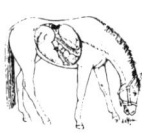

Esophageal obstruction (choke) is fairly common in horses. The feedstuffs most likely to cause choke are hay, pelleted feeds, and solid feeds such as carrots and apples. Sometimes, the horse is able to relieve the obstruction by repeated swallowing. But in other cases, a veterinarian is needed to relieve the obstruction.

Small intestine

The small intestine can be divided into three sections:

- ❖ duodenum, which exits the stomach
- ❖ jejunum, the middle (and longest) segment
- ❖ ileum, which enters the cecum (start of the large intestine)

In all, the small intestine is about 75 feet long (it ranges from 60 to 100 feet, depending on the size of the horse). Most of that length, about 70 feet on average, is jejunum. The entire small intestine accounts for about 75% of the length of the digestive tract, but because of its narrow diameter, it comprises only about 30% of the total capacity of the digestive tract.

Duodenum

The duodenum is the segment into which the stomach empties. It is a major site of digestion for dietary fats and carbohydrates, as bile and pancreatic juices are delivered into the intestine at this point. Protein digestion is also aided by enzymes secreted by the pancreas.

The duodenum is a relatively common site for ulceration in foals. In adult horses, it is one of the bowel segments that becomes inflamed and filled with gas and fluid in cases of proximal or anterior enteritis, also called duodenitis-proximal jejunitis (see below).

Jejunum

Absorption of digested proteins, fats, and carbohydrates takes place in the jejunum. These substances are absorbed as amino acids, mono- and diglycerides, fatty acids, and simple sugars (e.g. glucose). Most vitamins, minerals, electrolytes, and water are also absorbed here.

The jejunum is suspended from the roof of the abdominal cavity by a broad, fan-shaped, translucent sheet called the mesentery. The blood supply to the intestine runs within the mesentery from large vessels at its base (or "root"). The mesentery is fairly long, which allows the 70 feet of jejunum to fold in and out around the rest of the bowel. But because of this mobility, the jejunum is the section of bowel that most often twists on itself (torsion or volvulus) or gets itself trapped in tight places (see pages 23–24).

Duodenitis–proximal jejunitis. This condition involves severe inflammation of the lining of the duodenum and first part (proximal section) of the jejunum. Because the jejunum is so long, large amounts of fluid can be lost from the bloodstream into the bowel with this condition. The result is severe dehydration and shock, and moderate-to-severe pain as the fluid and gas build up in the jejunum and duodenum, and eventually the stomach. Sometimes, horses with proximal enteritis are more depressed than painful. This is probably because of the degree of dehydration and absorption of bacterial toxins from the inflamed bowel, and also because the bowel is less distended than with severely obstructive conditions such as intestinal twists.

Ileum

The ileum is the short, final section of small intestine. Its wall is relatively thick and muscular, so it acts a little like a valve, preventing backflow of cecal material into the small intestine. In fact, the junction between the ileum and the cecum is called the ileocecal valve (see Figure 1-1). The ileum is a fairly common site of obstruction. The two most common causes are impaction with feed material (e.g. poor-quality coastal Bermudagrass hay; see page 65) and intussusception (folding or telescoping of the bowel into itself). The ileum can also be involved in intestinal twists.

Cecum

The cecum is the first part of the large intestine. It is a large, sac-like structure that is roughly triangular or comma-shaped. The base of the cecum, where the ileum enters and the colon exits, is located in the upper, right-hand side of the abdomen (see Figure 1-2). The tip, or apex, of the cecum lies close to the floor of the abdomen, just behind the sternum. The cecum is about 3½ feet long and holds about 33 liters (7–8 gallons), and up to 68 liters (15 gallons), of material.

The cecum's primary role is to thoroughly mix the material exiting the small intestine with bacteria and other microbes that will continue the digestive process, before delivering this mixture to the colon. A significant amount of microbial fermentation of fiber and undigested carbohydrates and proteins occurs in the cecum.

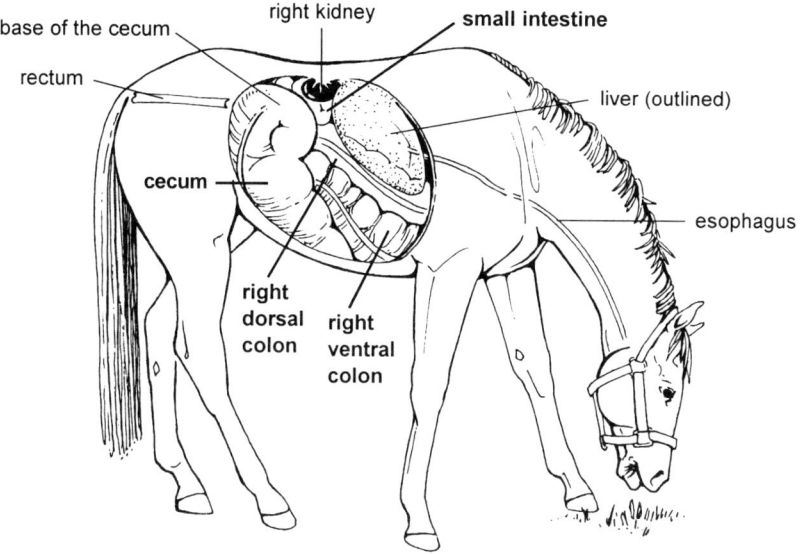

Figure 1-2. Contents of the horse's abdomen from the right side.

Cecal problems, such as impaction, distention with gas (tympany), and parasitic damage, are fairly uncommon. But when they do occur, they can be very difficult to treat successfully. A primary reason is that the signs of cecal problems are not very obvious until the disease is fairly advanced and the cecum is in danger of rupturing—or has already ruptured. Cecal diseases seem to be more common in horses that are hospitalized because of illness or for surgery (see page 86).

Large colon

The large colon is so-named because of its large diameter. It measures only about 11 feet in length but accounts for nearly 40% of the total capacity of the gut (an average of about 80 liters, or 18 gallons). Together, the cecum and large colon fill most of the abdominal cavity in nonpregnant horses.

Configuration

The large colon is arranged in two U-shaped layers—one (dorsal, or upper) stacked on top of the other (ventral, or lower). There is a sharp bend, the pelvic flexure, at the point where upper meets lower (see Figure 1-3). The curve in each U lies close to the liver, which sits up against the diaphragm (the muscular barrier between the abdominal and chest cavities). Beginning at the base of the cecum, in the upper right side of the abdomen, the large colon consists of the following:

- *right ventral colon,* which runs forward and down toward the sternum, curving to the left just behind the liver (at the sternal flexure), before continuing as the…

- *left ventral colon,* which runs toward the pelvis and turns back on itself sharply (at the pelvic flexure) to become the…

- *left dorsal colon,* which runs forward, along the top of the left ventral colon, before curving to the right just behind the liver (at the diaphragmatic flexure) to become the…

- *right dorsal colon,* which runs along the right ventral colon toward the base of the cecum, where it empties into the…

- *transverse colon,* which is a short segment that connects the end of the large colon with the small colon.

The large colon narrows at the pelvic flexure and again where the right dorsal colon meets the much narrower transverse colon. These two points are common sites of obstruction, whether from feed material, sand, enteroliths (see page 67), or foreign objects.

Another feature that contributes to the large colon's common role in colic is its mobility. Although the dorsal and ventral "arms" are connected to each other by a short membrane (which keeps the stacked U's together), the entire large colon is attached at only two points: the beginning (base of the cecum) and end (transverse

1–What is Colic?

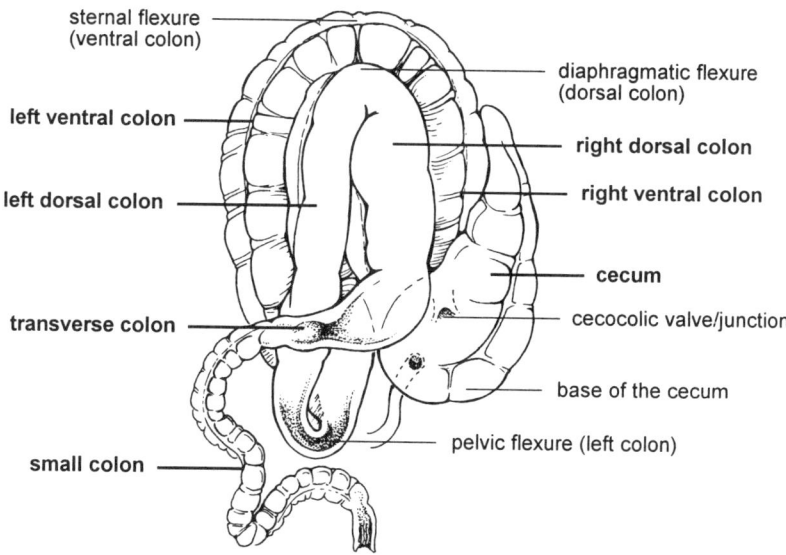

Figure 1-3. The horse's large intestine, viewed from above. (Note that the bowel narrows at the pelvic flexure and the transverse colon.)

colon, which is anchored in place near the roof of the abdomen). Thus, the large colon can: (1) move out of its normal position (displacement), (2) become entrapped, e.g. over the ligament between the spleen and the left kidney (nephrosplenic entrapment), or (3) twist on itself or around its point of attachment (torsion or volvulus). But under normal circumstances, its size when filled with good-quality roughage keeps the large colon in place.

Function

The large colon has two major functions: (1) microbial breakdown of fiber, and (2) absorption of fluids secreted into the digestive system. The bulk of microbial breakdown of fiber, and of any carbohydrates and proteins that escaped digestion and absorption in the small intestine, occurs in the large colon. The major products of this process, volatile fatty acids, are important energy sources.

Microbial fermentation also produces a lot of gas. Ordinarily, this gas is produced at a fairly constant rate. Some is absorbed by the colon; the remainder passes down the digestive tract and is released from the anus. If, for any reason, gas builds up in the colon, colic can result from stretching of the intestinal wall. Gas buildup can also contribute to large colon displacements and twists (see page 52).

The three most common causes of gas buildup in the large colon are: (1) feeding large amounts of grain or other readily digestible carbohydrates, (2) obstruction of either the large or small colon (e.g. impaction with firm, dry feed material), and (3) altered intestinal motility, from a variety of causes. Gas buildup and other abnormalities that can cause colic are discussed later in the chapter.

Small colon

The small colon is the final section of colon before the rectum (see Figure 1-1). It is narrower than the large colon, hence the name, but it is almost as long (average, 10 feet). By this point, the feed material has been as completely digested as possible. The remaining indigestible material (feces, or manure) is formed into balls in the small colon.

As with the jejunum and large colon, the small colon is relatively mobile. But unlike the other two segments, displacements and twists are uncommon in the small colon. The most common problem—obstruction—results from the narrow diameter of the small colon and the efficient way that both the large and small colons extract most of the water from the indigestible remains of a meal. When poor-quality roughage is fed, this process sometimes leaves hard, dry balls of manure that are difficult to pass.

The narrow diameter also makes obstruction with foreign materials and enteroliths more likely in this segment. In newborn foals,

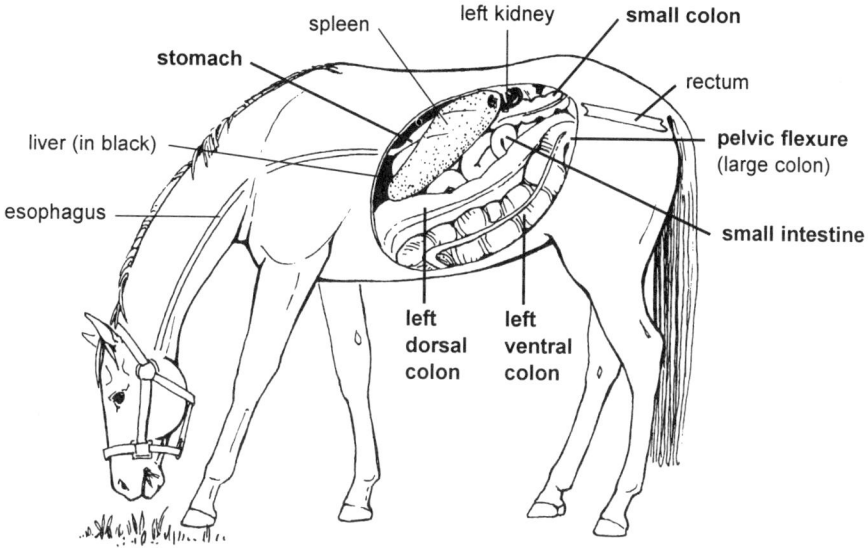

Figure 1-4. Contents of the horse's abdomen from the left side.
(Note: the spleen is drawn smaller than normal to show the colon and small intestine; normally, it partially overlies the colon.)

the small colon is a relatively common site of meconium impaction (see page 46); the rectum is the most common site.

Rectum

The rectum connects the small colon with the anus. It is about 12 inches long and serves as a holding area for manure. Rarely is the rectum the primary site of colic, except in newborn foals with meconium impaction. In adult horses, impactions occur a long way "upstream" from the rectum (e.g. in the large or small colon, or the ileum). So, enemas are of little use in adults, and can even be dangerous when administered incorrectly. Likewise, removing manure from the horse's rectum will not relieve a colon impaction.

Incidence of Colic at Specific Sites

Problems can occur at any point along the digestive tract, but colic most often involves an abnormality in the large colon or small intestine. Below is a breakdown of the incidence of colic associated with specific sections of the digestive tract:

- stomach 4%
- small intestine 33%
- cecum 6%
- large colon 49%
- small colon 7%
- rectum <1%

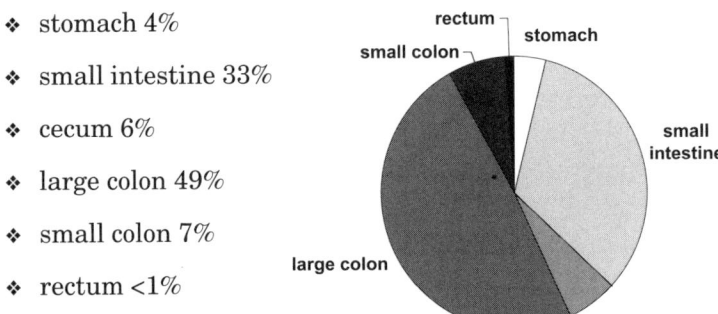

What Causes Colic?

As colic is not a single disease, but rather a manifestation of abdominal pain, answering the question "what causes colic?" is not a simple matter. The pain could be originating anywhere along the 100-or-so feet of digestive tract, and could result from one of several processes.

What is causing the pain?

The pain of colic arises from one or more of the following:

1. *spasms*—sustained or uncoordinated bowel wall contractions

2. *distention*—buildup of food, fluid, and/or gas within the bowel

3. *traction*—pulling on the wall of the bowel (or its mesentery)

4. *ischemia*—reduced blood flow to the bowel

5. *inflammation* of the bowel, with or without ulceration

1. Spasms

Normally, bowel motility consists of a coordinated series of contractions of the muscle layers in the bowel wall. Some of the contractions mix the food, and others move the food downstream in waves. This progressive motility is called peristalsis.

Sustained or uncoordinated contractions of the bowel (spasms or cramps) can occur for a variety of reasons:

- excessive intake of readily digestible carbohydrates, such as grain-based feeds or lush grass (see page 60)
- obstruction by a mass of dry, firm feed material (impaction)
  - the bowel may spasm as it tries to move the material downstream
  - buildup of gas behind the obstruction may also contribute
- internal parasites (worms), especially the larval stages (see Chapter 2)
- irritation or inflammation (e.g. accumulation of sand, enteritis)
- low blood flow (see page 22)

> Spasmodic colic is the most common type of colic. Diets high in carbohydrates (e.g. grain-based feeds, lush pasture) are the most common cause.
>
> Most cases of spasmodic colic are mild and resolve on their own or with simple medical treatment.

Colic that primarily involves this process is called *spasmodic colic*. Overall, it is the most common type of colic. Dietary factors, such as intake of high-carbohydrate meals or poor-quality roughage, are the most common causes. But in many cases, a definite cause cannot be identified. Fortunately, spasmodic colic tends to be mild and usually resolves either on its own or with simple medical treatment.

2. Distention

The bowel has pain receptors that register discomfort when the bowel wall is stretched (distended) from a buildup of food, fluid, and/or gas. There are several possible causes of distention:

- feeding a high-carbohydrate diet
  - this can cause rapid production of large amounts of gas in the cecum and/or large colon (primary tympany; see below)
- simple obstructions—see the next page
- strangulating obstructions, in which both the intestine and its blood supply are obstructed (see page 23)
  - a dramatic example is large colon volvulus (twist); so much gas can build up in the colon that the horse becomes obviously bloated within a matter of hours
- enteritis—e.g. bacterial enteritis in foals and proximal enteritis (duodenitis-proximal jejunitis) in adults
  - in addition to buildup of fluid and gas in the affected segment of bowel, inflammation contributes to the pain
- ileus—marked reduction or absence of peristalsis
  - food, fluid, and gas build up behind the affected segment
  - causes of ileus are listed in Table 1-2 on page 33

The severity of colic signs depends on the amount of bowel wall distention. The more the wall is stretched, the more painful the condition, and the more severe the colic signs.

Primary tympany. Tympany is the term used to describe buildup of gas in a hollow structure, in this case the intestine. Accumulation of gas in an otherwise normal section of intestine is termed *primary* tympany. Gas accumulation as a result of an obstruction or other abnormality is called *secondary* tympany.

1–What is Colic?

The cause of primary tympany is microbial fermentation of carbohydrates, such as concentrates (grain and grain-based "sweet feeds" and pellets) or lush pasture. The result is rapid accumulation of gas in the large intestine, which stretches the wall of the bowel. The products of fermentation may also alter bowel motility, so spasmodic colic can contribute to this situation.

Provided there is no obstruction, the gas is gradually propelled downstream and passed out the anus. This type of colic is sometimes termed *flatulent colic*, for obvious reasons.

Simple obstructions. Simple obstructions are those in which the blood supply to the bowel is not affected to any great degree (unlike strangulating obstructions, which are discussed on page 23). Flow of food, fluids, and gas along the digestive tract can be interrupted by an obstruction at one of three sites:

(1) within the hollow center (lumen) of the bowel—*luminal* obstructions include impaction with firm, dry feed material

(2) the bowel wall itself—*mural* obstructions include thickening of the muscular layer of the wall

(3) outside the bowel—*extramural* obstructions include tumors and abdominal abscesses

> Simple obstructions are the next most common type of colic. Probably the most common cause is impaction of the large colon with fibrous feed material.
>
> Although these obstructions are termed "simple," intensive medical treatment, and sometimes even surgery, may be required to correct the problem.

Simple obstructions can be subdivided into *physical* obstructions, such as impactions, and *functional* obstructions, such as ileus (reduction in progressive bowel motility, or peristalsis). Specific causes are listed in Table 1-2 on page 32. Although these obstructions are termed "simple," intensive medical treatment, and sometimes even surgery, is often required to relieve the obstruction.

3. Traction

Traction on the bowel generally involves one of three structures:

(1) the mesentery—the broad, transparent sheet of tissue that suspends the small intestine

(2) the ligaments that connect two segments of bowel or a section of bowel to another structure

(3) adhesions—fibrous bands that form between two segments of bowel, or between the bowel and another structure

Only a few conditions cause enough tension on the mesentery or an intestinal ligament to produce obvious pain. Displacements and twists are the two most common causes. Entrapment of small intestine is another possible cause (see page 24). But in all of these conditions, the pain is caused not only by tugging on the bowel wall, but also from gaseous distention and reduced blood flow associated with the displacement, twist, or entrapment.

Adhesions. Adhesions result from inflammation of the outer surface of the bowel, most often caused by disease but sometimes by surgical repair. In most cases, colic caused by adhesions is simply a result of pulling or tugging on the surface of the bowel during normal bowel activity. These fibrous bands are inelastic, so when one segment of bowel moves in the normal course of digestion, it can pull on the section of bowel it is adhered to, potentially causing pain. But occasionally, the adhesions are in a location, or are extensive enough, that they partially obstruct the bowel.

4. Ischemia (low blood flow)

The bowel has, and needs, a rich blood supply. Reduction of blood flow (ischemia) can alter bowel motility, and when severe, it may result in tissue damage which can be irreversible. It also causes release of substances which sensitize the nerve endings in that part of the bowel, increasing the intensity of painful impulses.

Blood flow to the bowel can be reduced by three basic processes: (1) compression of the blood vessel, (2) blockage of the blood vessel from within (e.g. by a blood clot), and (3) overall reduction of blood flow to all tissues (e.g. dehydration, shock).

Compression. The classic example of this type of ischemia is strangulating obstruction, in which blood flow to the bowel is severely reduced by compression or twisting (strangulation) of the blood vessels. As the vessels that supply the bowel are intimately associated with the bowel wall and mesentery, conditions that strangulate the bowel's blood supply typically also strangulate the bowel, obstructing the flow of food, fluids, and gas.

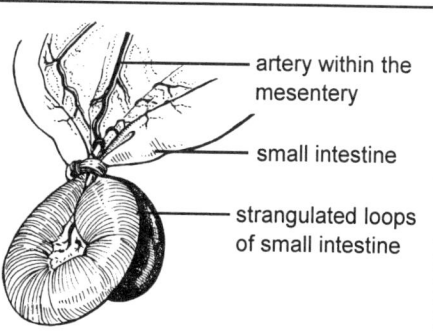

Strangulating obstructions (in this case, a small intestinal volvulus) affect both the bowel and its blood supply. Within a couple of hours, the affected bowel becomes irreparably damaged; toxic shock quickly follows. These cases require immediate surgical correction if the horse is to survive.

— artery within the mesentery
— small intestine
— strangulated loops of small intestine

Strangulating obstructions fall into the following categories:

❖ twisting of the bowel (torsion or volvulus)

• torsion is twisting of the bowel along its length, much like wringing out a wet towel

• volvulus is twisting or knotting of the bowel around itself or its point of attachment (e.g. the mesentery)

• the distinction between these two terms is usually only important to the surgeon who is correcting the problem

✶ **note:** *twisting of the bowel is not caused by rolling*

- intussusception—folding of the bowel into itself, like closing (shortening) the barrel of a telescope
  - not all intussusceptions are strangulating obstructions; some are simple obstructions, but most have at least some compromise of blood flow to the affected bowel
  - the most common site for intussusception is the ileum
- entrapment of bowel within a confined internal space or through a tear in the mesentery
  - the epiploic foramen (a narrow space near the liver and stomach) is one of the more common sites of entrapment
- entrapment of bowel in a hernia or abdominal wall defect
  - hernias can be congenital (present at birth) or acquired (usually resulting from trauma or surgery)
  - bowel can become trapped in an umbilical hernia, the inguinal canal (in the groin), or in a tear or surgical defect in the muscles of the abdominal wall or diaphragm
  - note: umbilical hernias only occasionally cause strangulating obstructions; most do not contain bowel, and in those that do, the bowel does not always become entrapped
- twisting of some other structure around the bowel (or the bowel around that structure)
  - a common example in older horses is strangulation by a pedunculated lipoma, a benign fatty tumor that forms on a thin stalk which lengthens as the tumor enlarges
  - although very uncommon, the small colon in mares can twist around an ovary and become strangulated

Strangulating obstructions are life-threatening conditions that cause severe colic and rapid deterioration in the horse's condition. Without exception, *they require immediate surgical correction.* If surgery is performed within a few hours of the strangulation occurring, the prognosis for survival is reasonable. But the longer the horse must wait before surgery, the poorer the prognosis.

Blockage. The most common cause of blood vessel blockage involving the intestines is damage by the larvae of *Strongylus vulgaris* (redworms or bloodworms; see page 77). These larvae penetrate the bowel wall and make their way into the arteries that supply the bowel. Parasite-induced blood vessel damage is called verminous arteritis. As one of the consequences is obstruction of blood flow by blood clots, this type of colic is sometimes termed *thromboembolic colic*.

> Severe colic caused by the larvae of *Strongylus vulgaris* (redworms or bloodworms) used to be an important disease. But since the introduction of ivermectin, this type of colic (verminous arteritis) has become very uncommon.

Overall reduction of blood flow. Dehydration is common with many conditions in horses. But with the exception of large colon impaction, colic resulting from dehydration alone is very uncommon. Reduction in blood flow severe enough to compromise the bowel usually occurs only with shock, whether from severe infection, endotoxemia (absorption of bacterial toxins), or blood loss.

5. Inflammation (with or without ulceration)

Terms for inflammation of the bowel vary by location: gastritis–stomach, enteritis–small intestine, typhlitis–cecum, colitis–large colon, proctitis–rectum. Ulceration is a severe form of inflammation of the bowel lining (the mucosa), in which erosions or craters develop in the mucosa and may extend into the tissue beneath. Ulceration severe enough to cause signs of colic usually is limited to the stomach (and in foals, the first few inches of the duodenum) and the right dorsal colon.

Causes of inflammation (+/– ulceration) include:

- ❖ internal parasites, especially strongyle larvae (see Chapter 2)
  - internal parasites can also cause spasmodic colic

- ❖ "stress" (a common cause of gastric ulcers in sick foals and young racehorses in training; see page 86)
- ❖ nonsteroidal anti-inflammatory drugs (NSAIDs), especially phenylbutazone ("bute") and flunixin (Banamine®)
  - both gastric ulcers and right dorsal colitis can occur with NSAID use (see page 91)
- ❖ abrasion caused by sand accumulation in the large colon
- ❖ infectious organisms
  - *Salmonella* species
  - *Ehrlichia risticii* (Potomac horse fever)
  - *Clostridium* species (possibly the cause of "colitis X," and incriminated in proximal enteritis and antibiotic-induced colitis in adults, and severe enterocolitis in foals)
- ❖ toxins, e.g. blister beetles, acorns, arsenic (see Chapter 2)

Signs of colic vary with the site and severity of the inflammation. In addition, other problems occur with some of these conditions, such as diarrhea with *Salmonella* infection, laminitis with Potomac horse fever, and kidney damage with blister beetle poisoning. These other problems influence which signs are most obvious in a particular horse. For example, colic may accompany or even precede the diarrhea in a horse with colitis. But it is the diarrhea that is the most serious (potentially life-threatening) problem.

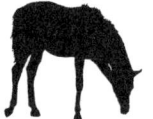

Ulceration severe enough to cause signs of colic is usually limited to the stomach (and in foals, the first few inches of the duodenum) and the right dorsal colon. In most of these cases, there is a history of stress or illness, or of NSAID (nonsteroidal anti-inflammatory drug) use. Stomach ulcers and right dorsal colitis are discussed further in Chapter 2.

How common are these problems?

A landmark study, published in 1986, examined data collected from 4,644 horses with colic that were referred to one of 16 university veterinary hospitals in the United States or England. Of all the horses with colic, surgery was performed in 2,055 (44%). The following statistics were reported from the data collected on all 4,644 horses:

- *simple obstruction* accounted for 34% of the colic cases
  - most cases involved the large colon; the next most common sites were the small colon and the small intestine
- *strangulating obstruction* accounted for 21% of the colic cases
  - most cases involved the small intestine
- *vascular compromise* (reduced blood flow without strangulating obstruction; i.e. ischemia) comprised only 3% of cases
- *enteritis* (inflammation of the small intestine) was diagnosed in 5% of colic cases
- *peritonitis* (inflammation of the abdominal cavity, typically caused by infection) was diagnosed in 4% of colic cases
  - this category included horses with ruptured bowel, so the incidence of primary peritonitis was much lower than 4%
- colic was caused by a problem that *did not involve the digestive tract* in 6% of horses
- the cause of colic was *undiagnosed* in 27% of cases

For the most part, these were horses referred because of severe colic or colic that was not responding to treatment on the farm. In other words, they represent a select population of horses with moderate-to-severe colic.

Statistics from routine veterinary practice

A more recent study, conducted in Texas and published in 1995, compiled the findings from 821 horses with colic that were examined *on the farm* by the regular equine veterinarian. In other words, this study more accurately reflects the incidence of particular colic problems in the horse population at large. In this study, almost one-half (46%) of the horses had spasmodic or "gas" colic (29%), or colic in which a diagnosis was unable to be made (17%), typically because it resolved with medical treatment and needed no further evaluation.

Of the remainder, about 29% of the horses had a simple obstruction, most often a large colon impaction. A little less than 6% had strangulating obstructions, and 8% had enteritis. "Other" causes accounted for 11% of colic cases.

The findings of these two studies are illustrated in the following pie charts. Notice the differences, particularly in the incidence of "surgical" problems such as strangulating obstructions:

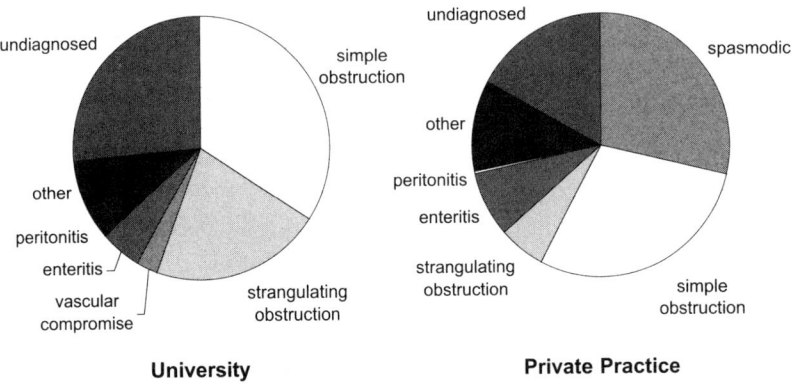

Figure 1-5. The incidence of different types of colic seen in two types of veterinary practice.

Left: A chart of cases referred to university veterinary hospitals.
Right: A chart of cases seen on the farm by the regular veterinarian.

1–What is Colic?

No mention is made of the number of horses that underwent surgery in the Texas study. But as the incidence of strangulating obstructions was only about 6%, and as most other problems can be managed medically, the surgical case rate was probably around 10–15% of all horses seen for colic.

Statistics from an owner/manager survey

An extensive study of colic incidence on horse farms in Virginia and Maryland, in which the incidents were recorded by horse owners or farm managers, provides an even more complete view. Over 1,400 horses were involved in this study, and all incidents of colic, even those not needing veterinary attention, were recorded. In all, there were 104 incidents of colic in 86 horses during the year-long study period. This represents an annual colic incidence of 10.6 cases per 100 horses.

Most (75%) of the colic incidents were mild and resolved either without treatment or with a single medical treatment. In fact, 33% of all colic incidents were so mild or transient that veterinary attention was unnecessary.

Only 9 horses—about 10% of all horses with colic—had severe digestive tract problems. Four of these horses (less than 5% of all colic cases) went to surgery. Three had strangulating obstructions and one had an impaction of the stomach. The five other horses died or were euthanized ("put down") because of serious digestive tract problems that, in other circumstances, may have been amenable to surgery.

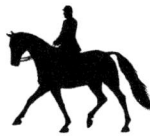

In a recent study in which colic incidents were recorded by horse owners or managers, the following statistics were found:

• about 75% of all colic incidents were mild and resolved either without treatment or with a single medical treatment

– about 33% of all colic incidents were so mild or transient that veterinary attention was not necessary

• only about 10% of all colic incidents were severe enough to warrant surgery

The remainder required more intensive medical treatment.

In summary...

Various other studies show regional differences in the incidence of certain colic conditions (e.g. sand impaction, proximal enteritis, enteroliths; see Chapter 2). But a consistent finding is that *mild, spasmodic colic is by far the most common type of colic.* Typically, it either resolves on its own or readily responds to medical treatment. Another consistent finding is that problems requiring surgery (such as strangulating obstructions and severe impactions or displacements that do not respond to medical therapy) are relatively uncommon, comprising only about 10% of all colic cases.

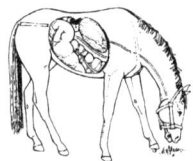

Table 1-1: Causes of colic signs not associated with the digestive tract.

Reproductive System

large follicles or painful ovulation
labor (foaling) or abortion
dystocia (difficulty foaling)
retained placenta
torsion (twisting) of the uterus
ruptured uterine artery (post-foaling)
ruptured uterus (late pregnancy)
ovarian tumor or hematoma (hemorrhage into an ovarian follicle)
lactation tetany (calcium depletion in nursing mares)
vaginal tear during breeding
torsion (twisting) of the testicle

Musculoskeletal System

laminitis ("founder")
"tying up" (exertional rhabdomyolysis, myositis, myopathy)
neck or back injury
hyperkalemic periodic paralysis (HyPP)

Respiratory System

pleuritis (inflammation/infection of the lining of the chest cavity)
pneumothorax (air in the chest cavity, between the lung and chest wall)

Urinary System

bladder or kidney stones, or other causes of urinary obstruction
bladder rupture (newborn foals; see page 47)

Cardiovascular System

pericarditis (inflammation of the thin sac surrounding the heart)
aortic-iliac thrombosis (blood clot in the aorta and/or iliac arteries)

Nervous System

eastern or western equine encephalitis (EEE/WEE)
rabies (colic may be an early sign)
brain or spinal cord injury
tetanus
botulism (colic may be an early sign)

Miscellaneous

peritonitis (inflammation/infection of the abdominal lining)
abdominal (internal) hemorrhage
abdominal abscess or tumor
abscess, tumor, or rupture of the spleen
acute liver damage (hepatitis)
cholelithiasis (obstruction of the bile duct of the liver)
pancreatitis (inflammation of the pancreas with release of digestive enzymes into surrounding tissues)
pheochromocytoma (adrenal gland tumor that secretes adrenaline)
choke (esophageal obstruction; see page 10)

Table 1-2: Specific causes of simple obstruction leading to colic.

Physical Obstruction—foals and young horses

meconium impaction (newborn foals)

atresia (absence or incomplete development of a segment) or other malformation

intussusception* (folding or telescoping of the bowel into itself)

impaction with roundworms *(Parascaris equorum;* ascarids) or tapeworms

foreign material (e.g. hair, rubber fence material, baling twine, rope)

abscess in the wall of the bowel or associated lymph nodes, most often caused by *Streptococcus equi* ("strangles") or *Rhodococcus equi* infection

Physical Obstruction—adult horses

feed impaction (obstruction with firm, dry feed material)

enterolith ("stones"; see page 67)

fecalith (obstruction of the small colon with hard, dry manure balls)

sand impaction (accumulation of sand in the large colon)

stricture (scarring & narrowing of the bowel from prior damage)

adhesions (fibrous bands resulting from inflammation of the bowel; see page 22)

abscess, hematoma, or tumor (within the wall or outside the bowel)

intussusception [see foals and young horses]

ileal hypertrophy (narrowing of the ileum from thickening of its muscular layer)

inflammatory bowel disease (thickening of the bowel wall by inflammatory cells)

strangulating lipoma* (benign fatty tumor that, as it enlarges, develops a long, thin stalk which can wrap around the bowel; most common in old horses)

foreign material (see foals and young horses)

displacement,* especially of the large colon

may also have a strangulating component

continued...

Functional Obstruction

ileus (temporary reduction/absence of bowel activity); causes include:
- dehydration and electrolyte imbalances (especially potassium and calcium)
- drugs, e.g. atropine, Rompun®, Dormosedan®, and morphine
- chemicals such as amitraz (see page 88)
- endotoxin and other bacterial toxins

proximal/anterior enteritis (duodenitis-proximal jejunitis; see page 11)

cecal atony (loss of motility, resulting in gas & fluid buildup in the cecum; the cause is unknown, but may include the items listed for ileus)

peritonitis (reduces bowel motility, and is a source of abdominal pain on its own)

aganglionosis (absence of nerves that control bowel motility) in Paint Horse foals—Lethal White Foal syndrome; see page 56

grass sickness (affects the nerves that control bowel motility; it has not been reported in the U.S.; see page 94)

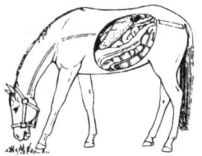

2

Risk Factors for Colic

Effective prevention begins with an understanding of what could be causing the problem or contributing to the situation. In the past 10 years or so, there have been several studies aimed at identifying the factors that contribute to colic. Some of these studies have involved over a thousand horses, which has been important in defining both the overall incidence of colic and the incidence of specific types of colic in the general horse population.

But with respect to factors that increase or decrease the potential for colic to occur (colic risk factors), this research has provided a mixed bag of information: some new perspectives, some affirmation of age-old horsemen's wisdom, and some information whose relevance remains to be fully understood. This chapter discusses what is known about the factors that contribute to colic in horses.

Interpreting Study Results

Even though there have been several studies examining colic risk factors, only a few definite conclusions have been reached. The general trends may be similar among studies, but details regarding specific risk factors often differ.

There are a few possible reasons for differences among studies. One is variation in study design—asking different questions. Another is variation in geographic location—studying horses in different parts of the country (or in another country).

A third reason may be that most types of colic have more than one contributing factor, sometimes several, and many of the colic risk factors (particularly those involving management) are interrelated. For example, to some extent breed, activity, diet, and housing are all interrelated: the horse's breed may dictate its use or activity, which can impact how the horse is fed and housed.

At times it is difficult, if not impossible, to tease apart the specific factors in order to study them individually. Using breed as an example, when breed is analyzed in isolation, with no consideration of the horse's primary use or activity, and therefore the associated management factors, the results can be misleading (see page 38).

Another important consideration is the particular population of horses being studied. Most studies to date have been *hospital-based*, meaning that the data were compiled from horses that were referred to a university veterinary hospital.

The problem here is that most cases of colic are mild and resolve either on their own or with medical treatment on the farm. Relatively few require more intensive medical treatment, and even fewer need surgery. But from looking at the statistics in many hospital-based studies, such as the one discussed on page 27, you could be left with the false and alarming impression that most cases of colic are serious and many require surgical correction.

Manager- and practitioner-based studies

Five important studies have been published in the past 10 years, in which the information was recorded either by owners, trainers, or farm/barn managers (two studies) or by equine veterinarians attending colic cases on the farm (three studies). These are *non-hospital-based* studies that attempt to uncover the actual incidence of colic, including the incidence of specific types of colic, and identify the contributing factors. These studies are outlined in Tables 2–1 to 2–5 on pages 99–102.

The two owner/manager-based studies are particularly important because they include colic cases that were too mild to warrant veterinary attention and that either resolved without treatment or were treated by the owner or manager. These cases would not have made it into a practitioner- or hospital-based study, yet they are essential pieces of the jigsaw puzzle of colic in horses.

In this chapter, colic risk factors are divided into three categories:

❖ intrinsic factors (aspects that are part of that horse)
❖ management factors
❖ environmental factors

Intrinsic (horse) Factors	Management Factors	Environmental Factors
• breed	• diet	• geographic location
• gender	• housing	• weather/season
• age	• water intake	• poisonous plants
• use/activity	• internal parasites	
• behavior (e.g. "vices")	• dental care	
• previous colic or surgery	• stress	
• genetics	• drugs and chemicals	

Intrinsic (Horse) Factors

Breed

The importance of a horse's breed on colic risk is not clear-cut. Results vary among studies, and in some cases one study reports a higher risk for colic in a particular breed while another study reports a lower risk in that breed. One explanation is that different populations of horses are being compared (e.g. hospital-based vs. nonhospital-based studies).

Another likely reason is that the effect of breed is compounded by the horse's use or activity and the associated management factors (especially diet and housing). The range of activities undertaken by a particular breed can be wide. For example, Quarter Horses are used for anything from halter classes to racing; and the list of activities involving Arabians ranges from showing to endurance. So, unless the horse's use is taken into account when analyzing the effect of breed, it is likely that few definite conclusions will be reached. Certain breeds are more prone to particular types of colic, but whether this too is management-related is not yet clear.

Breeds in which colic risk is reported to be different from that in most other breeds, or in which specific types of colic may be more likely, are discussed in the following sections.

Arabians

Findings vary widely among studies. Several studies report a significantly higher incidence of colic in Arabians, others find no difference between Arabians and other breeds, and one study (see below) reports a *lower* colic risk in Arabians.

Manager-based studies. The owner/manager-based study in VA/MD (Table 2-1) found that Arabians had the lowest incidence of colic among the breeds represented in that population of horses.

The annual incidence of colic for all breeds combined was 10.6 cases per 100 horses, but in Arabians it was only 3.2 cases/100 horses—less than one-third of the average for all breeds.

In the owner/manager-based study in MI (Table 2-2), the Arabian breed was not a significant risk factor for colic, although there was a trend toward colic being slightly more likely in Arabians.

Practitioner-based studies. Both practitioner-based studies in TX (Tables 2-3 and 2-4) found that colic was slightly more likely in Arabians than in other breeds. The authors proposed three possible explanations: (1) different management practices compared with other breeds, (2) increased awareness and concern about colic among owners and caretakers of Arabians, or (3) genetic predisposition for gastrointestinal disorders in Arabians. Given that the VA/MD study showed a significantly lower colic risk in Arabians, management factors probably are the key, rather than an inherent predisposition toward colic in Arabians.

> Some studies show an increased incidence of colic in Arabians. Other studies have found no such increase in overall colic risk in this breed. However, colic caused by enteroliths (intestinal "stones") does seem to be more common in Arabians.

Specific conditions. Enteroliths (intestinal "stones"; see page 67) reportedly are more common in Arabians. In a comprehensive study at the University of California at Davis (UC Davis) of colic caused by enteroliths, 39% of the 900 horses with enteroliths were Arabians or Arabian crosses, whereas this breed comprised only 13.5% of the total horse population seen at the veterinary hospital at UC Davis. (Incidentally, Morgans, Saddlebreds, and donkeys also had a higher incidence of enteroliths in that study.)

In a hospital-based study at the University of Georgia, ileal impaction was more common in Arabians than in other breeds. But this has not been the case in other studies. (Diet and tapeworm infestation are the primary factors involved in ileal impaction.)

Thoroughbreds

Some studies report an increased incidence of colic in Thoroughbreds, while others show either no difference or a decreased colic risk in this breed. The horse's use (e.g. racing vs. less demanding activities) probably is the key, in combination with associated management factors, such as diet and housing.

The manager-based study in VA/MD (Table 2-1) found that the colic incidence was higher in Thoroughbreds than in most other breeds. The annual colic incidence in Thoroughbreds was 12.6 cases/100 horses, whereas in all breeds combined it was 10.6 cases/100 horses. By comparison, the annual colic incidence in crossbreds, Quarter Horses, and Arabians was less than 6 cases/100 horses—less than half the rate in Thoroughbreds.

In that study, eventing and training for racing or other strenuous sports were the activities with the highest colic incidence (see page 50). Presumably, Thoroughbreds dominated these groups, which could account for the higher colic incidence in this breed.

In the manager-based study in MI and the practitioner-based studies in TX (Tables 2-2 to 2-4), the colic incidence in Thoroughbreds was similar to that in other breeds.

Standardbreds

Some studies show a significantly lower colic risk in Standardbreds; others show no difference between this and other breeds. The manager-based study in MI (Table 2-2) showed a slightly lower risk for colic in Standardbreds. Only about 3% of the horses with colic were Standardbreds, whereas Standardbreds comprised over 16% of the total horse population studied. However, in the final analysis, the difference was not statistically significant.

Standardbreds appear to be more prone to scrotal or inguinal hernias, in which a section of bowel becomes trapped in the scrotum or inguinal canal (groin; see page 43). And in a recent study at the University of Pennsylvania, intussusception involving the cecum was more common in Standardbreds. In this condition, part of the cecum folds in on itself, or the first part of the large colon telescopes into the cecum.

Miniature Horses

Miniature horses are prone to small colon obstruction, especially impaction with fecaliths (hard masses of manure). Small colon obstruction is more common in young Miniature Horses, probably for two reasons: (1) the narrow diameter of their small colon, and (2) their inquisitive nature, which makes them more likely to swallow foreign materials such as baling twine and plastic that can become lodged in the small colon. (More on small colon obstruction in Minis on page 64.)

> Some studies show a lower incidence of colic in Standardbreds, although scrotal or inguinal hernias (see text) seem to be more common in this breed.

Morgans

In a hospital-based study that used Arabians as the reference group, Morgans tended to be referred for colic more often than Arabians. As a point of comparison, Quarter Horses and crossbreds were admitted significantly less often than Arabians, and therefore Morgans, in that study. And in a recent study at UC Davis, Morgans were one of the breeds in which enteroliths were more common. But in most other studies, Morgans are at no greater risk for colic than are other breeds.

Other breeds

One report suggests an increased incidence of scrotal hernias in Tennessee Walking Horses. In another study, Appaloosas were at slightly higher risk for colic, but this is not supported by other studies. Overo Lethal White Foal syndrome is a fatal condition that causes colic in newborn Paint Horse foals (see page 56).

Gender

The effect of gender is a little more clear; some types of colic are gender-specific (occurring only in one sex) or more common in a particular sex, as discussed below. However, study results differ in the association between gender and overall colic risk.

Studies

The manager-based study in VA/MD (Table 2-1) found no difference in colic risk among the genders (female, male, gelding). But the authors made the comment that some of the broodmares left the farms just before or just after foaling, so they were excluded from the study when their colic risk may have been highest.

In the manager-based study in MI (Table 2-2), mares were at no greater risk for colic than were males, but foaling was a significant risk factor for colic (see Use/Activity on page 51). Geldings were slightly less likely to develop colic than were mares or stallions in that study. In the practitioner-based study in the UK (Table 2-5), there was a significantly lower incidence of colic in stallions than in mares and geldings. But in neither of the two practitioner-based studies in TX (Tables 2-3 and 2-4) was gender found to have a significant effect on colic risk.

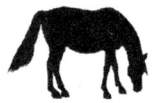
While colic may be no more likely in mares than in stallions or geldings, broodmares are more prone to certain types of colic.

Mares

Specific causes of abdominal pain that are more common in mares, or found only in mares, include:

❖ large colon volvulus (twist)—most common in the first few weeks after foaling

  • this potentially fatal condition also occurs in nonpregnant mares, geldings, and stallions, although much less often

❖ painful ovarian follicles or ovulation

❖ uterine torsion (twisting of the uterus)—an uncommon but important cause of colic in the last 1–2 months of pregnancy

In a hospital-based study at the University of Georgia, 100% of the horses with acute peritonitis (infection of the abdominal cavity) were mares. How many of these mares were broodmares was not reported.

Intact (uncastrated) males

Inguinal or scrotal hernias can cause strangulating obstructions in males. These conditions develop when a section of bowel, usually small intestine, works its way into the inguinal canal, the slit-like opening in the floor of the abdomen through which the testicle and its blood vessels descend into the scrotum. Bowel that enters the inguinal canal can become trapped in the canal (inguinal hernia) or further down, in the scrotum (scrotal hernia).

Most cases of inguinal/scrotal hernia are found in intact males (colts and stallions), although inguinal hernias can also occur after castration in geldings. Scrotal hernias cause obvious swelling on one side of the scrotum or beneath the skin beside the scrotum (most common in young foals). Inguinal hernias usually are much less obvious because the bowel is trapped deep within the groin area. Scrotal and inguinal hernias are much more likely to cause an obstruction and colic in adult horses than in young foals.

Meconium impaction in foals. Meconium impaction is the most common cause of colic in newborn foals (see page 46). It occurs more often in colts than in fillies, possibly because the pelvic canal in males is narrower than in females.

Geldings (castrated males)

An uncommon but potentially serious cause of colic in recently gelded horses is obstruction from adhesions between the bowel, usually small intestine, and the inner opening of the inguinal canal. In effect, a portion of bowel becomes stuck to the opening of the inguinal canal, or to the remnant of the spermatic cord, and the bowel becomes kinked. Colic caused by these adhesions usually develops within a few weeks of castration, but can begin several months later.

Strangulating lipoma. Geldings are also more prone to colic caused by lipomas. These benign, fatty masses within the abdomen can cause strangulating obstructions if the thin stalk they are suspended on stretches and allows the mass to wrap around a section of bowel (like swinging a baseball in the toe of a stocking). This condition, which is called strangulating lipoma, is seen almost exclusively in older horses, most often geldings.

Chronic colic. The principal researcher who conducted the practitioner-based studies in TX, Dr. Noah Cohen, published the findings of a related study involving horses with repeated episodes of colic. He found a significantly higher percentage of geldings in the group with chronic intermittent colic, which implies that geldings may be at higher risk for repeated episodes of colic. But whether this finding is management-related is not clear.

Age

As with gender, certain conditions are more common or are found exclusively in particular age groups. But study findings differ somewhat in the association between age and overall colic risk.

Manager-based studies

In the study in VA/MD (Table 2-1), the incidence of colic was greatest in horses between 2 and 10 years of age. The annual colic incidence in horses less than 2 years old was 4.6 cases/100 horses, and in horses over 10 years old it was 7.4 cases/100 horses. But in horses 2–10 years of age the annual colic incidence was 14.5 cases/100 horses—almost twice the incidence in older horses, and over three times the incidence in the younger horses. However, this finding probably reflects an effect of activity moreso than of age. Eventing and training for racing or other strenuous sports were the activity groups with the highest colic risk in this study (see page 50), and the majority of horses involved in these activities would have been between 2 and 10 years of age.

In the manager-based study in MI (Table 2-2), colic was slightly more likely in older horses.

Practitioner-based studies

The first of the practitioner-based studies in TX (Table 2-3) found no significant effect of age on overall colic incidence. But the second study (Table 2-4) found that the incidence of colic was higher in horses over 10 years of age than in younger horses.

The UK study (Table 2-5) showed no effect of age on overall colic incidence, but spasmodic or undiagnosed colic occurred more often in horses 5–10 years of age. Also in that study, significantly more horses over 15 years of age needed surgery than did younger horses. This finding agrees with a hospital-based study in Minnesota in which horses over 15 years of age required surgery significantly more often than did younger horses. Most of the surgical cases in older horses involved strangulating obstructions (see pages 23–24).

> Some conditions are more likely or occur only in particular age groups. Examples include meconium impaction in newborn foals, roundworm impaction in older foals, and strangulating lipomas in aged horses.

Chronic colic. In a related study by the TX researchers, horses over 8 years of age were significantly more likely to have recurrent or chronic colic than were younger horses. Several other factors were associated with chronic colic, so age alone probably is not a deciding factor in most cases. As the authors suggested, the older the horse, the more opportunities it has to develop colic and so be included in such a study. But it could also reflect an increased incidence of dental problems, tumors, and other causes of colic in older horses.

Age-related conditions

Young foals. The following conditions are more common or found only in foals less than about 3 months of age:

- meconium impaction—inability to pass the material that accumulated in the colon before birth (the "first manure")
  - meconium consists of cells that are shed from the lining of the intestine and a small amount of fluid; foals normally begin passing it within 6–8 hours of birth
  - meconium usually is pasty, but in some foals it forms hard pellets or a large mass that can be difficult to pass
  - straining and tail-flagging are common signs, with bloating sometimes developing after several hours
  - all newborn foals have meconium, but why impaction occurs in some foals and not in others is not known
- enteritis—inflammation of the small intestine, usually caused by bacterial infection
  - diarrhea often becomes the predominant sign in these foals
- atresia (absence or incomplete development of a portion of bowel) and other congenital abnormalities
- stomach ulcers (in sick or stressed foals; see page 86)
- inguinal or scrotal hernia in male foals (see page 43)
  - in many cases the hernia is obvious but it does not cause bowel damage or colic
- umbilical hernia—a gap in the abdominal muscles where the umbilical cord was attached

- the typical umbilical hernia is a small, nonpainful swelling beneath the skin on the underside of the foal's belly
  - most are present at birth or first noticed a day or two later
  - most umbilical hernias do not cause bowel damage or colic
- ruptured bladder or infection in the internal stump of the umbilicus (the urachus, between the bladder and the body wall)
  - these conditions can cause straining and colic-like signs in young foals
  - ruptured bladder and urachal abscess are diagnosed by ultrasound

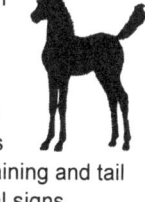

The most common cause of colic in newborn foals is meconium impaction. It is seen more often in colts than in fillies. Straining and tail flagging are typical signs.

Older foals and growing horses. The following conditions are more common between about 3 months and 2 years of age:

- intussusception—folding of the bowel into itself, like closing (shortening) the barrel of a telescope
  - most intussusceptions occur in the ileum or cecum
- impaction with roundworms *(Parascaris equorum;* ascarids)
  - this condition is seen most often in foals that are dewormed for the first time after 3 months of age (see page 84)
- stomach and duodenal ulcers—colic can result from ulceration or from its consequences (scarring and narrowing of the duodenum)
  - narrowing (stricture) of the duodenum can cause either chronic, low-grade colic or severe, obstructive colic
- *Rhodococcus equi* infection—typically causes pneumonia, but enteritis/colitis or abdominal abscesses can develop
  - diarrhea and chronic colic often result
- small colon impaction in Miniature Horses (see page 41)

Foals and young horses are more susceptible to internal parasites than are adult horses. These young horses are naive, in that they do not have the natural resistance to internal parasites that develops with exposure. Also, some studies indicate that anthelmintics (dewormers) may be less effective in foals and yearlings than in adult horses. These factors could predispose young horses to parasite-induced colic in management situations that do not consider young horses in the deworming program.

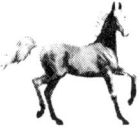

Internal parasites are an important cause of colic in foals & young horses. Deworming programs must take into account two key differences between young and adult horses: young horses are more susceptible to internal parasites, and dewormers may not be as effective.

Young adult horses. Intussusceptions (described above) also occur in young adult horses. In one study in England, tapeworm infestation was more common in horses 3–5 years of age (and in those over 15 years of age) than in middle-aged horses. Incidentally, tapeworm infestation and intussusception are related in some cases.

Older horses. Horses 15 years of age or older are more prone to the following conditions:

- strangulating lipomas (see page 44)

- entrapment of small intestine in the epiploic foramen (a narrow gap between the liver and adjacent structures)

- lymphosarcoma—a malignant tumor of lymph nodes and other lymphoid tissue; it is a rare cause of colic
    - abdominal lymphosarcomas can cause obstruction either from infiltration and thickening of the bowel wall or from compression of the bowel by the tumor mass

- squamous-cell carcinoma of the stomach; rare in horses
    - signs include decreased appetite, mild recurrent colic (may be associated with eating), lethargy, and anemia

- diseases of the cecum, such as impaction
- tapeworm infestation (see Young Adult Horses)

Influence of management factors

Management can play a significant role in the incidence of colic in older horses. In one study, the odds that a horse kept on a dry lot would develop colic increased with age. (A dry lot was defined as any exercise area less than ½ acre that was not grass covered.)

Horses that were 10 years old and kept on a dry lot were almost twice as likely to develop colic as those of the same age that were stabled. And colic was almost 4 times more likely in 15-year-old, and over 7 times more likely in 20-year-old horses kept on dry lots, compared with stabled horses of similar age.

The authors suggested that this might relate to the quality of daily care: older horses may be more likely to develop colic when left outside in dry lots if they have little direct monitoring or care.

Use/Activity

Once again, study results differ somewhat in the association between a horse's use or activity and colic risk. However, most studies support the general conclusion that colic risk tends to be greater in horses in "high-stress occupations" such as athletic competition and showing.

> Colic risk tends to be greater in horses in "high-stress occupations." For example, eventing and training for strenuous activities were the groups with the highest colic incidence in one study.

Manager-based studies

In the VA/MD study (Table 2-1), the incidence of colic was highest in eventers and horses in training for strenuous activities (e.g. racing, steeplechasing, and eventing). Colic incidence was lowest in horses used for lessons and in young horses not yet in use. Following are the annual colic rates for specific activities in that study:

- adults used for lessons—1.6 cases/100 horses
- young horses not yet in use—3.2 cases/100 horses
- hunters—6.6 cases/100 horses
- adults with no specific use—6.7 cases/100 horses
- pleasure horses—10.4 cases/100 horses
- breeding—11.7 cases/100 horses
- dressage—14.0 cases/100 horses
- showing—14.4 cases/100 horses
- racing—15.4 cases/100 horses
- training for strenuous activities—23.6 cases/100 horses
- eventing—24.0 cases/100 horses

In the MI study (Table 2-2), the activities that significantly increased the risk for colic were showing and foaling. (Hunter-jumpers were analyzed separately from the "showing" group, and were not at increased risk for colic.) While not statistically significant, colic also tended to be more prevalent in horses used for dressage, breeding, or training for showing. No racehorses developed colic during the two years of observation in that study. But only about 4% of the population studied (171 of over 3,900 horses) were racehorses.

Practitioner-based studies

In the first TX study (Table 2-3), racing was the only activity significantly associated with colic incidence—and that association was of colic being *less* likely in racehorses. In the second TX study (Table 2-4), use or activity was not significantly associated with colic incidence for any group or type of horse.

Foaling

Mares that foaled during the study period were at increased risk for colic in the MI study. But in the VA/MD and TX studies, foaling was not a significant colic risk. However, in the VA/MD study, the odds of a mare developing colic 60–150 days after foaling were almost 6 times higher than that of other horses. This is the time of peak lactation, and therefore nutritional demand, so the amount of grain fed could have been a key factor (see page 57).

A recent hospital-based study in Germany indicates that mares may be more prone to colic in the post-foaling period than during pregnancy. Mares that had recently foaled were more likely to have colic severe enough to need referral to a veterinary hospital than were mid- or late-pregnant mares. Almost half (46%) of the broodmares referred for colic were mares that had recently foaled. The remainder were equally divided between mares in their second trimester (4–7 months) and mares in their third trimester (8–11 months) of pregnancy.

> Broodmares may be at increased risk for colic after foaling and during peak lactation. When colic occurs in a pregnant or recently foaled mare, both intestinal and uterine problems must be considered.

Three-quarters of the colic cases in these mares involved digestive tract problems, and one-quarter involved the reproductive tract or other internal organs. The most common intestinal causes of colic were large colon impaction and large colon volvulus (twist).

Behavior

Few studies have examined the effect of behavior on colic incidence. Yet many owners and trainers have found that colic is more common in cribbers, horses with a nervous disposition, and those that display other undesirable behaviors of confinement ("stable vices"). In the manager-based study in VA/MD (Table 2-1), there was a tendency for colic to be more likely in horses that crib and in those at the bottom of the "pecking order" (i.e. horses that are not dominant in a herd situation).

Cribbers

It was long thought that colic in cribbers was caused by over-inflation of the stomach with swallowed air. But it has since been proven with radiographic (x-ray) studies that these horses do not swallow air. The air they gulp does not get any further than the first few inches of the esophagus. It is then expelled into the back of the throat, making the grunting or belching noise that is heard when horses crib.

One reason why colic may be more common in cribbers is that they spend much of their time cribbing, rather than grazing or eating hay. Thus, their food intake, when they do stop to eat, is intermittent and their overall roughage intake may be inadequate. And because these horses tend to be light in condition, their ration usually includes grain. As discussed later, colic risk increases as the amount of grain in the diet increases. For the same reasons, horses that compulsively fence-walk, stall-walk, or weave could also be at increased risk for colic.

Rolling and displacements or twists

It is commonly thought that displacements and twists are caused by the horse rolling. This is simply not true; horses roll every day without causing these serious intestinal problems. Although not fully understood, displacements probably begin with altered bowel motility and/or buildup of gas in a particular segment (whether from rapid fermentation of grain or backup behind some fibrous feed material). The gassy segment, being lighter, is more easily moved out of its normal position by bowel activity, which can lead to a displacement, and further gas distention.

But can a horse make a displacement worse, or even cause the displaced bowel to twist, by rolling? It is possible, but extremely unlikely. When a segment of bowel is distended with gas, it tends to fill the abdomen, leaving little room for further displacement. The main reason most veterinarians recommend that you try to keep a colicky horse from rolling by getting it up and walking it around is to prevent the horse from injuring itself. (This is discussed further in Chapter 4.)

Some veterinarians correct certain displacements, in particular nephrosplenic entrapment, by anesthetizing the horse and rolling it. This displacement occurs when the left colon becomes trapped between the body wall and the short ligament that connects the left kidney and the spleen. But rolling doesn't always work; surgery is sometimes necessary to correct this problem.

> Rolling does not cause colic; but colic can cause a horse to roll in pain. It is often best to keep horses with severe colic up and moving, to prevent them from injuring themselves.

History

One consistent finding among studies is that horses that have had colic before are more likely to colic again. In the manager-based study in VA/MD (Table 2-1), colic was almost 4 times more likely in horses that had colic in the past 5 years than in horses with no history of colic. During the study, 16% (or about 1 in 6) of the horses that developed colic had at least one other episode of colic within the year.

In the first practitioner-based study in TX (Table 2-3), colic was almost 6 times more likely in horses with a history of colic than in those with no history of colic. Around 30% of the horses with colic had a history of previous colic.

In the VA/MD study, the information was recorded by owners, trainers, and farm managers, and there was a significant number of colic cases (33%) that were not severe enough to warrant veterinary attention. In contrast, the information in the TX study was reported by veterinarians called out to examine the colicking horses. In other words, the VA/MD study comprised more horses with mild, transient colic. Presumably, the underlying problem was also transient, and it would be reasonable to conclude that these incidents of mild colic do not significantly increase the risk for future colic episodes—unless, of course, any contributing management factors are not changed.

> 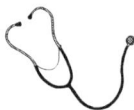 The causes of *recurrent colic* (repeated episodes) vary widely, from mild spasmodic colic caused by a dietary upset, to terminal cancer.
>
> Horses that have the occasional, brief episode of colic (e.g. a couple of times a year) tend to have less serious problems. Horses that have more frequent (e.g. a couple of times a month) or persistent episodes of colic are more likely to have a potentially serious problem, usually of an obstructive nature.
>
> The cause of recurrent colic can be difficult to determine. In some cases, exploratory surgery is necessary to reach a diagnosis—and hopefully a solution.

History of abdominal surgery

In both practitioner-based studies in TX (Tables 2-3 and 2-4), colic was about 5 times more likely in horses with a history of abdominal surgery. And in a related study by the same researchers, a history of abdominal surgery was the risk factor most highly associated with recurrent or chronic intermittent colic.

Adhesions. An important cause of colic following abdominal surgery is the presence of adhesions—fibrous bands that form where the bowel wall has been inflamed (see page 22). When adhesions cause colic, problems usually begin within the first 2 months after surgery. The incidence of adhesions following colic surgery, and the percentage of those adhesions that cause colic, is not known. This is because only a small proportion of horses are reexamined surgically (the only way of identifying adhesions, other than postmortem examination). It is estimated that adhesions will cause a significant problem in about 20% of surgery patients (or 1 in 5). But not all of these animals will need a second surgery.

Other factors. Another possible cause of recurrent colic following surgery is narrowing (stricture) of the inflamed, damaged, or repaired portion of bowel. As with adhesions, the incidence of this problem is difficult to determine, but it probably is quite low. Also a consideration is the persistence of management or environmental factors that caused the initial problem which required surgery. This is unlikely in most cases, as owners and managers tend to be much more careful with horses following colic surgery, at least for the first several months.

Caretaker vs. owner

An intriguing finding in one hospital-based study was that the risk for another episode of colic nearly doubled if the horse was cared for by someone other than the owner (i.e. a trainer or manager). No explanation was obvious from the other data, which leaves two possibilities: (1) owners take better care of their horses than trainers or managers, or (2) nonowners take such good care of the horses that they are more likely than an owner to call a veterinarian when one of the horses in their care develops colic.

Herein lies a common problem with statistics: determining the practical value of the information. The level of management varies widely within the equine industry, and even varies to some extent on an individual farm. And there are just as many conscientious trainers and managers as there are conscientious owners; the same holds true for lax or penny-pinching trainers, managers, and owners.

As a counterpoint, the number and type of caretakers was not significantly associated with colic incidence in the manager-based study in VA/MD (Table 2-1). And in the second TX study (Table 2-4), there was no difference in colic incidence between horses that were boarded and those that were kept on the owner's farm.

Genetics

To date, there is only one confirmed instance in which genetics plays a direct role in colic: Overo Lethal White Foal syndrome, a fatal condition affecting newborn Paint Horse foals. Also called aganglionosis (absence of ganglions), it involves incomplete development of the nerves that supply the muscle in the bowel wall, particularly the ileum and large colon.

Affected segments of bowel are nonfunctional and act like an obstruction. Milk, digestive juices, and gas build up within and behind the paralyzed segment. The result is colic that begins within 12 to 24 hours of birth, worsens despite medical treatment, and cannot be corrected surgically. Affected foals die or must be humanely killed.

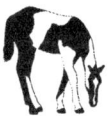

Lethal White Foal syndrome causes fatal colic in newborn Paint Horse foals. Unlike this healthy foal, affected foals are completely white (or almost so), with few or no areas of colored skin or hair, and blue eyes.

This condition is an inherited trait that most often occurs in foals born to matings between two overos of the "frame" color type. (Frame overos have continuous color along the topline from withers to tail [i.e. white does not cross the back], and the colored areas "frame" the white areas.) Affected foals are born white, or almost so, with few or no areas of colored skin or hair, and blue eyes.

Possible genetic links

Several specific conditions tend to be more common in certain breeds, which could indicate a genetic factor. Examples include inguinal/scrotal hernias in Standardbreds and Tennessee Walking Horses; cecal intussusception in Standardbreds; and enteroliths in Arabians (and in one study Morgans, Saddlebreds, and donkeys). However, management factors probably play as much of a role, particularly with cecal problems and enteroliths. Umbilical hernias are more common in certain Thoroughbred lines, although a direct genetic link has yet to be proven.

Management Factors

Diet

As with many of the factors discussed earlier, study findings regarding diet and colic incidence sometimes are inconclusive or contradictory. One possible reason is that, even within the U.S., feeds and feeding practices vary widely among geographic areas. Also, the effects of diet and feeding schedule often cannot be separated from other management practices, and may also depend on the horse's use.

Amount and type of grain & other concentrates

Colic tends to be less common in horses fed roughage-only diets (pasture and/or hay), and colic risk increases as the amount of grain or other concentrates (grain-based pellets, "sweet feed," etc.) increases. In the VA/MD study (Table 2-1), significant findings related to diet included the following:

1. Colic incidence was low in horses on pasture (i.e. those receiving no grain).

2. Colic incidence increased as the amount of concentrates fed increased.

    → horses receiving up to 2.5 kg (5½ lb) of concentrates per day were only slightly more likely to develop colic than horses receiving no concentrates

    → horses receiving 2.5–5 kg (5½–11 lb) of concentrates per day were *almost 5 times more likely to develop colic* than horses receiving no concentrates

    → horses receiving more than 5 kg (11 lb) of concentrates per day were *over 6 times more likely to develop colic* than horses receiving no concentrates

3. Feeding the more processed types of concentrate, such as pellets, rather than simple grains, increased the colic risk.

→ horses fed either whole grain or a mix that included whole grains were only slightly more likely to develop colic than horses fed no concentrates

→ horses fed sweet feed were 4½ times more likely to develop colic than horses fed no concentrates

→ horse fed pellets were over 6 times more likely to develop colic than horses fed no concentrates

The explanation given for point 3 was that processed feeds are more easily digested than whole grains, and therefore may alter conditions within the colon more dramatically. (This concept is discussed on page 60, in the section "What is the big deal with concentrates?")

The Texas study. However, the second practitioner-based study in TX (Table 2-4) found that neither the amount nor the type of concentrates fed was significantly associated with colic risk. The amount of concentrates fed ranged from less than 100 grams (less than ½ a cup) to over 11 kg (24 lb) per day. The average was 2–3 kg/day, which, in the VA/MD study, carried only a slightly higher colic risk than feeding no concentrates. So, perhaps there were too few horses in the TX study that were receiving large amounts of grain for an effect of grain feeding to be significant.

Another possible reason for the discrepancy between studies is a difference in other dietary or management factors between the mid-Atlantic states and Texas. As discussed later, hay was the key dietary factor in the TX study; both the type of hay fed and recent changes in hay feeding were associated with colic risk.

Corn. In a study involving several university veterinary hospitals in the northeastern U.S. and Ontario Canada, feeding whole-grain corn increased the risk for colic. For each kilogram (2.2 lb)

of corn fed, the colic risk was increased over 3 times. However, this finding should not be interpreted to mean that feeding corn causes colic. Corn is simply another grain, and when incorporated into a balanced ration, it has many nutritional benefits. But like any grain or grain-based (i.e. high-carbohydrate) feedstuff, colic risk increases with the amount fed.

Frequency of concentrate feeding

The VA/MD study also found that dividing the daily concentrate ration into two or more meals did not reduce the colic risk when feeding large amounts of concentrates. Horses fed concentrates twice a day were 4½ times more likely to develop colic, and those fed concentrates three or more times a day were over 5 times more likely to develop colic, than horses fed no concentrates.

As the horses being fed grain two or more times a day were probably being fed more grain per day than horses receiving grain only once a day, these results support the following conclusions: (1) horses fed large amounts of concentrates are more likely to develop colic than horses fed small amounts or no concentrates, and (2) dividing the concentrate ration into two or more meals does not reduce the colic risk when feeding large amounts of concentrates.

> Colic risk increases with the amount of concentrates fed, over about 5 lb/day. Dividing the concentrate ration into two or more smaller meals does not lessen the colic risk when large amounts of concentrates are fed.

What is the big deal with concentrates?

The horse's digestive system is adapted to handle fairly continuous input of high-fiber food. The easily digestible components (sugars, starch, fats, proteins) are broken down and absorbed in the small intestine. Bacteria and other microbes in the cecum and large colon handle the overflow (any undigested carbohydrates and protein) and break down the less digestible plant fiber.

When large amounts of readily digestible carbohydrates (e.g. grain and grain-based sweet feed or pellets) are fed in a single meal, the small intestine cannot digest and absorb it all. As a result, larger than usual amounts of carbohydrate reach the cecum and large colon.

Simple sugars and starch are quickly fermented by the resident microbes, which causes rapid increases in acidity and gas production within the bowel. These changes are the same as those that occur with grain overload (which can lead to colic and laminitis), but on a smaller scale. In fact, one researcher referred to this dietary effect as "subclinical grain overload."

Rapid fermentation of carbohydrates also draws water from the bloodstream into the large intestine, causing a temporary state of mild dehydration. For the first 8 hours after grain feeding, the body adds fluid from the bloodstream into the bowel contents (a process called secretion). Most of the fluid is then absorbed back into the bloodstream over the next few hours as digested material moves down the colon.

Association with colic. When large amounts of grain are fed twice a day (i.e. every 8–12 hours), a cycle of rapid fermentation and fluid secretion/absorption develops which can easily be upset. Just as balance is being restored after the last meal, another load of carbohydrate is dumped into the large intestine, and the cycle must begin again.

Possible consequences of an upset in this cycle include:

- spasmodic or "gas" colic from rapid gas buildup in the colon
  - the products of carbohydrate fermentation can alter bowel motility, which could also contribute to spasmodic colic
- feed impaction from dehydration of bowel contents further downstream, such as at the pelvic flexure of the large colon, the transverse colon, or the small colon (see Figure 1-3)

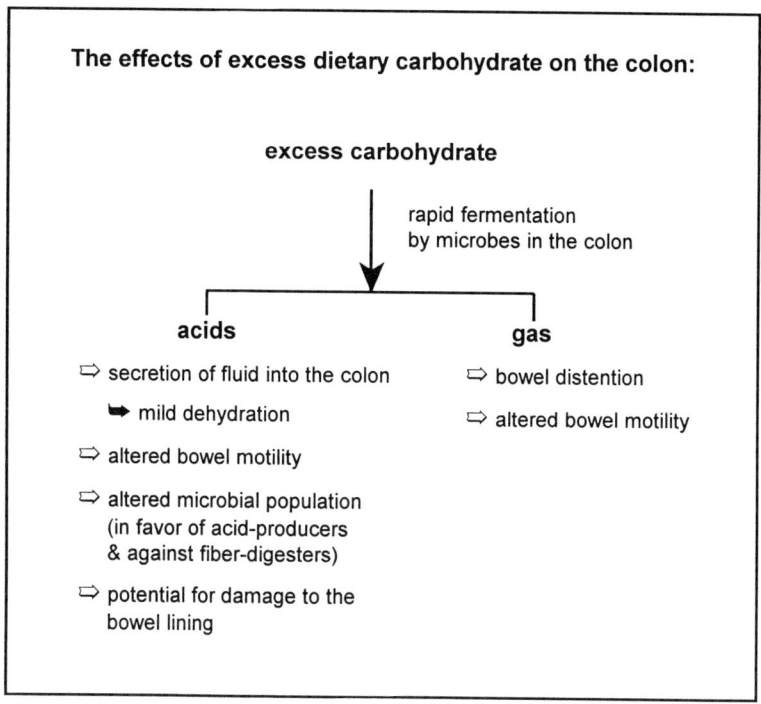

- ❖ large colon displacement from fluctuations in the amount of colon gas (especially rapid increases) and alterations in bowel motility
  - • large colon displacement was significantly associated with feeding pelleted grain in a study at the University of Georgia (note: this probably does not apply to complete pelleted feeds, which contain a significant amount of roughage)
- ❖ proximal enteritis? (duodenitis–proximal jejunitis; page 11)
  - • some fermentation of carbohydrates occurs in the small intestine and, under certain circumstances, it may contribute to this serious condition
  - • most horses with proximal enteritis are on high-grain diets

Frequent grain feeding. It is easy to see why, in the VA/MD study, feeding grain more often than twice a day did not decrease the risk associated with feeding large amounts of grain. The colon would have little time to restore its balance when carbohydrates are being delivered more often than every 8–12 hours.

"Although horses can be maintained indefinitely with twice-daily feedings, one should recognize that a delicate balance has been achieved in the cycling of certain physiologic systems. Disruption of this balance may result from insidious disease conditions, such as internal parasitism, or from subtle changes in management, such as altered feeding intervals or temporary lapses in water or salt availability."

'Feeding and digestive problems in horses.' LL Clarke, MC Roberts, and RA Argenzio. *Veterinary Clinics of North America: Equine Practice—Clinical Nutrition,* 1990; 6:433–450.

But what is a "large" amount? There is little published data on just how much carbohydrate it takes to overwhelm the ability of the small intestine to digest and absorb it, and therefore to upset the balance in the large intestine.

No doubt it depends on the horse's size. It may also depend on the horse's diet. To some extent, the microbial population in the large intestine adapts to the materials that are supplied (see page 116). Nevertheless, the changes in acidity, gas production, and fluid balance discussed earlier do occur in horses that are adapted to a high-grain diet; just not to the same extent.

In the VA/MD study, the colic risk became significant when more than 2.5 kg (5½ lb) of concentrates were fed per day. Whether this is the case for other types of horses (e.g. ponies and draft breeds) and horses in other parts of the country remains to be seen. It would be useless to set an arbitrary figure, given the wide variation in horse types, diets, activities, and environments, but this study finding is a good start.

Feeding more than 2.5 kg (5½ lb) of grain or other concentrates per day may not *cause* colic, but it could increase the potential for colic to develop, especially if other risk factors are present.

Roughage

Horses' digestive systems are designed to process high-fiber diets. So, it is not surprising that the VA/MD study showed a lower incidence of colic in horses fed roughage diets (pasture and/or hay).

One hospital-based study showed a slightly lower incidence of colic in horses fed some concentrates, compared with horses on roughage-only diets. But management factors likely played a role with this finding. Many of the horses fed only roughage were kept on pasture, and, according to the authors, may have been less well-managed in other respects than stabled horses.

Fresh grass. Although considered roughage, fresh grass is high in readily digestible carbohydrates when young and rapidly growing (e.g. in the spring, after a drought, and sometimes in the fall if the weather is mild and wet). So, lush pasture can cause colic by the same means as grain: an excess of readily digestible carbohydrate reaching the large intestine. Mild spasmodic or "gas" colic is the most common type of colic caused by lush pasture.

In the practitioner-based study in the UK (Table 2-5), a recent change in management was blamed for at least 43% of the cases of spasmodic or mild, undiagnosed colic. The most common management change was turnout onto lush pasture in the spring.

In most parts of this country, fresh grass is a potential colic risk for only a few weeks of the year. Preventing this type of colic is discussed in Chapter 3.

Hay quality

In the second practitioner-based study in TX (Table 2-4), feeding hay other than coastal/Bermuda or alfalfa significantly increased the colic risk. Hay quality and digestibility appeared to be the key. Hays listed as "other" included haygrazer, peanut, red-top cane, sorghum, and Sudan grass, all of which are harvested at a fairly mature stage of growth and tend to be less digestible than coastal/Bermuda and alfalfa hays.

Other types of hay included prairie grass (average to poor in quality), Bahia grass (which is susceptible to mold and mildew), and Kleingrass (which many horses do not find very palatable). Of the 35 horses in the study that were fed one of these other hays, 29 (83%) were in the colic group.

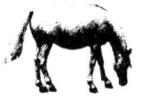

Although colic tends to be less common in horses on roughage-only diets (pasture and/or hay), hay quality appears to be important in minimizing the colic risk. The lower the hay quality, the higher the colic risk.

Also in this study, a recent change in hay feeding significantly increased the colic risk (see page 68). Changes included switching to a different type of hay, and even feeding a new batch of the same type of hay (e.g. a different cutting or another source). The authors suggested that changes in digestibility may be involved. For example, changing to poorer quality hay may predispose the horse to large colon impaction (the second-most common type of colic in this study).

Roughage quality and Minis. Miniature Horses are susceptible to small colon obstruction. In many cases (73% of surgical cases in one study), the obstruction is composed of dry, firm, fibrous feed material. It has been suggested that hay of a quality that is adequate for larger horses may be too coarse for Minis. Another consideration is that dental problems, which are fairly common in this breed, could interfere with proper chewing of an otherwise acceptable foodstuff. (Preventing colic in Miniature Horses is discussed in Chapter 3.)

Coastal Bermudagrass hay

Dr. Parks, from the University of Georgia, recently conducted a survey of equine surgeons in the southern U.S., in which he asked their opinions of a possible link between ileal impaction (obstruction in the last part of the small intestine) and feeding of coastal Bermudagrass hay. From their answers, he compiled the following statistics:

- 58% (21 of 36 surgeons) considered coastal Bermuda hay to be a contributing factor in ileal impaction

- 36% of the surgeons felt that horses recently moved to the southern U.S. were more likely to develop ileal impaction than those raised in that part of the country

- 64% reported an association between ileal impaction and changing to coastal hay from pasture or another type of hay

- 39% had observed repeated episodes of ileal impaction, which were often associated with continued feeding of coastal hay

This was simply an opinion-based survey. No "hard data" (numbers of cases) were collected. But a recent report from Auburn University in Alabama supports the opinion that coastal Bermuda hay does play a role in ileal impaction. Of 28 horses requiring surgery for ileal impaction, 27 were fed coastal Bermuda hay as the primary hay source. However, coastal Bermuda hay is commonly fed in the southern U.S., which partially accounts for the high percentage of cases fed this hay.

In a related study by the principal author of the two TX studies, coastal Bermuda hay was found to be a significant cause of recurrent colic and chronic, intermittent colic.

But many equine nutritionists feel that coastal hay is unfairly maligned. In a paper titled *"Myths and wives' tales of feeding horses: some truth, some fiction,"* Dr. Stephen Jackson, an equine nutritionist in Kentucky, had this to say about coastal hay:

> "I have fed coastal hay all of my life with no increase in the amount of gastrointestinal upset over that experienced by horse owners that do not choose to feed coastal Bermuda hay. My family raises coastal Bermuda hay in Texas and are able to harvest more nutrients per acre using this hay than for any other appropriate forage crop that they could raise. Coastal Bermuda grass is very responsive to the application of nitrogen fertilizer and this is reflected in the variability one sees in looking at the composition of coastal hay grown in different parts of the country, or indeed within a given state."
>
> Proceedings of the 18th Bain-Fallon Memorial Lectures, Australian Equine Veterinary Association, 1996; page 174.

According to nutritionists at the North Carolina Cooperative Extension Service, "plant maturity is probably the single most important factor influencing [the] nutrient content and quality of hay." The bottom line seems to be that *good quality* coastal hay is a good feed source for horses and is no more likely to cause impaction colic than any other hay. But *poor quality* coastal hay, which is very stemmy and poorly digestible, can cause impactions, both in the ileum and in the large colon. (Evaluating hay quality is discussed on page 119.)

Alfalfa hay

There is a reported association between feeding alfalfa hay and colic caused by enteroliths. Enteroliths can occur in any part of the country, but they tend to be more common in the western U.S., where alfalfa is often used as the major roughage source.

Alfalfa is implicated because of its high magnesium and protein content. Protein may be as important as the mineral content because protein digestion in the large colon releases ammonium, which is then free to form complexes with available magnesium and phosphorus. Enteroliths tend to form when the contents of the colon are less acidic than normal, so alfalfa may further contribute by reducing the acidity of the colon contents.

Studies. Surgeons at the University of California at Davis (UC Davis) compared bowel contents from two groups of horses that underwent colic surgery: those with enteroliths, and those with other simple large colon obstructions. They found that the bowel contents from horses with enteroliths were less acidic and had higher levels of calcium, magnesium, phosphorus, sodium, potassium, and nitrogen than horses that did not have enteroliths.

When feeding practices were compared, horses with enteroliths were fed a diet that contained an average of 87% alfalfa, whereas the other horses were fed a diet that comprised about 60% alfalfa. In another study from researchers at UC Davis, two-thirds of the horses with enteroliths were fed a diet that consisted exclusively of alfalfa hay.

Alfalfa and ulcers. In alfalfa's favor, researchers at the University of Tennessee reported that fewer and smaller stomach ulcers were found in horses fed a diet consisting of alfalfa hay and grain than in those fed only bromegrass hay. Apparently, because of its high protein and calcium content, alfalfa may act as a natural antacid, which could help protect the stomach lining from ulceration. (But whether this diet is of use in preventing colic caused by gastric ulcers, or in healing existing ulcers, remains to be seen.)

Enteroliths

Enteroliths are rock-hard masses of accumulated *struvite,* which is a crystal formed mostly of magnesium, ammonium, and phosphorus.

These "stones" form in the large colon, around some sort of foreign material (e.g. a piece of wire, a pebble, baling twine) or fibrous feed material, much like an oyster forms a pearl around a grain of sand or other irritant. The stone enlarges over time as more struvite is laid down around the outer surface.

Most small enteroliths are passed in the manure. Those that remain in the colon, gradually enlarging, may be "silent" for years. But eventually, most cause an obstruction (with chronic, intermittent colic or persistent colic) and must be surgically removed.

Feeding changes

The colic risk tends to increase when the horse's diet is changed. In the manager-based study in VA/MD (Table 2-1), changing the amount or type of concentrates fed during the year increased the colic risk by almost 4 times. And more than one change per year in hay feeding doubled the colic risk.

In the first practitioner-based TX study (Table 2-3), a recent change of diet significantly increased the colic risk. Colic was over 3 times more likely in the 1–2 weeks after a dietary change, and 5 times more likely in the 48 hours after a diet change. But to put things into perspective, 80% of the horses in the colic group had not had any recent changes in their diet.

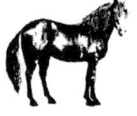

The colic risk increases whenever the horse's diet is changed. As much as possible, dietary changes should be made gradually (see Chapter 3).

A recent change of diet also significantly increased the colic risk in the second TX study (Table 2-4). Of the changes evaluated, a change in hay feeding was the one most highly correlated with colic risk. In fact, a change in hay feeding carried the highest colic risk of all the dietary and management factors evaluated. The odds of a horse developing colic within 2 weeks of a change in hay were almost 10 times greater than if the horse had no change in hay. (By comparison, previous colic surgery increased the colic risk by only 5 times.)

While the researchers did not analyze the specific changes in hay feeding, even using a new batch or source of the same type of hay was recorded as a change in hay feeding. As mentioned earlier, a decrease in hay quality was probably a key factor.

Colic associated with eating

In some horses with recurrent or chronic colic, the colic episodes begin during a meal or shortly afterward. Three general conditions are more likely to have this association:

- stomach ulcers, especially when the horses are fed grain
  - colic after nursing or eating is also common in foals with duodenal ulcers, especially if the duodenum has become narrowed (strictured)
  - although rare, squamous-cell carcinoma of the stomach creates erosions that may cause colic associated with eating
- adhesions (see page 22)
- partial ileal obstruction
  - narrowing of the ileum can cause colic associated with movement of food, especially hay, down the small intestine
  - examples include tapeworm infestation and thickening of the muscular layer of the ileal wall (ileal hypertrophy; cause unknown)

Unusual feed materials

Acorns can cause colic in horses, although many horses eat the occasional acorn without any ill effects. Apples, other sweet fruits, and bread, in large quantities, can cause spasmodic or gas colic because they are high in readily digestible carbohydrates. Grass clippings often cause colic for the same reason; they can also cause choke (esophageal obstruction) or obstruction further down the digestive tract. When eaten in large quantities, persimmons (a type of fruit) can cause stomach impaction.

Feed contaminants

Objects such as wood, plastic, rubber, or baling twine, can cause colic by obstructing the bowel or by stimulating formation of an enterolith (described on page 67).

Blister beetles. Blister beetles are small insects that infest alfalfa fields. They are most prevalent in the central and western U.S. When the hay is cut and baled, the blister beetles are killed and baled with the hay. These insects contain a highly irritant toxin, cantharidin, which causes severe ulceration of the digestive tract, and kidney damage. Colic and severe diarrhea are typical findings in horses with blister beetle toxicity.

This problem is more likely in infested alfalfa that has been crimped or otherwise "conditioned" during cutting and baling, because these processes crush the beetles, potentially exposing the horse to more of the toxin.

Mycotoxin. Moldy hay or grain can also cause colic. In most cases, the culprit is a fungal toxin, or mycotoxin. In a study at North Carolina State University, a correlation was found between the incidence of colic and the presence of mycotoxins in grain and hay. Liver damage, which is an uncommon cause of colic, can also be caused by certain mycotoxins in grain or hay.

Mycotoxins

Ideally, all horse feeds should be free of mycotoxins. But as this goal is not always attainable, the North Carolina Cooperative Extension Service lists the following *maximum acceptable levels* of specific mycotoxins in horse feeds:

aflatoxin: *50 ppb* (parts per billion)

T_2 toxin: *50 ppb*

deoxynivalenol (DON): *400 ppb*

zearalenone (F_2): *100 ppb*

fumonisin (FB_1): *zero*

In terms of colic risk, T_2, F_2, and DON may be the most important mycotoxins, particularly when they are present in combination. To have your horse feeds analyzed for mycotoxins, contact your county Extension Service agent.

Housing

Study results concerning housing and the horse's environment are perhaps the least conclusive. It makes sense to presume that confining an animal which, in its natural state, spends most of the day and night roaming around and grazing, would have some impact on its health and well-being.

Add to the mix a diet that is substantially different from what the horse's system is designed to handle, and it is no surprise that various conditions, including lung diseases and exercise-related muscle disorders, not to mention undesirable behaviors, are more common in horses that are kept in stalls most or all of the time. So why not digestive problems, too?

One explanation for the inconclusive results is that several factors related to housing are interconnected. "Housing" incorporates the horse's environment, feeding and turnout/exercise schedules, water sources, and even social interactions (from the need for company to competition for food). In fact, the first practitioner-based study in TX (Table 2-3) showed that changes in activity level, diet, and stabling conditions are all significantly associated with one another. So, it can be difficult, if not impossible, to study the effects of individual factors, such as housing, independently.

Inside vs. outside

Another reason why there is little conclusive evidence for an effect of housing on colic risk is flawed study design—not asking the right questions. For example, the manager-based study in MI (Table 2-2) merely compared access to indoor housing with access to outdoor housing. Time spent indoors versus outdoors (i.e. how much access) was not reported. Not surprisingly, they found no significant difference in colic incidence between the two housing situations: access to indoor vs. access to outdoor housing.

The manager-based study in VA/MD (Table 2-1) also found no significant effect of housing on colic risk, although colic incidence was slightly higher in horses stalled for 9–24 hours/day (i.e. confined for more than 8 hours/day). The authors did note, however, that colic incidence was low in horses kept at pasture.

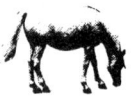
Horses are grazing animals, so it makes sense that confining them could have an impact on their health. One study showed that colic risk is slightly increased in horses that are stabled for more than 50% of the time (i.e. more than 12 hours/day).

The first practitioner-based study in TX (Table 2-3) showed no significant effect of housing on colic incidence. But most of the horses were kept outside for at least 50% of the day. In the second TX study (Table 2-4), colic was slightly more likely in horses that were stalled for more than 50% of the day (i.e. confined for more than 12 hours/day).

Large colon impaction. A British study of horses with chronic colic (defined as signs of colic that persisted for 3 days or more) produced some interesting results. Large colon impaction was the most common cause of chronic colic, and it was far more common in horses that were stabled full-time:

Housing	All horses with chronic colic	Horses with large colon impaction
stabled full-time	36%	69%
stabled part-time	52%	28%
on pasture full-time	12%	3%

Of all the horses with chronic colic, only about one-third (36%) were stabled full-time, yet the majority (69%) of large colon impactions occurred in these horses. The implication here is that regular turnout is important in preventing large colon impactions. Notice, too, that the incidence of chronic colic was lowest (by 3–4 times) in horses kept on pasture full-time.

Changes in housing

The incidence of colic tends to increase when changes are made in a horse's routine, activity level, and/or environment. In the manager-based study in VA/MD (Table 2-1), colic risk was slightly increased in horses that had more than 4 changes in housing during the study year.

Practitioner-based studies. In both of the practitioner-based studies in TX (Tables 2-3 and 2-4), a change in stabling conditions within the past 2 weeks increased the colic risk. Details were not provided, but the authors did note in the first study that changes in housing were more common during the early summer and fall, which could reflect a change in pasture access or turnout time.

Also in the TX studies, colic was more likely in horses that had a change in activity level in the past 1–2 weeks. Details were not reported. Nevertheless, this finding highlights the importance of consistency in a horse's routine.

In the practitioner-based study in the UK (Table 2-5), a recent management change was a possible cause of spasmodic or mild, undiagnosed colic in at least 43% of cases. The most common change was turnout onto lush spring pasture, which reflects a dietary change as much as a housing change. This is consistent with the findings of the TX studies: changes in activity level, diet, and stabling conditions were all significantly associated with one another, but of these factors, recent dietary change carried the highest risk for colic.

> Changes in diet, activity level, and housing are all potential risk factors for colic. Of the three, a change of diet carries the highest risk for colic.

Bedding type

The type of stall bedding was not significantly associated with colic risk in either the manager-based study in VA/MD or in the first practitioner-based study in TX.

Pasture access and rotation

A hospital-based study in the northeastern U.S. and Ontario Canada found that horses with access to three pastures in the past month were about half as likely to develop colic as were horses with access to only one pasture. The number of horses with access to three pastures was small (15 horses), so this result must not be overinterpreted. But it does raise the possibility that roughage intake or quality was greater in the horses with access to more than one pasture.

Pasture rotation. However, also in that study, horses with access to four pastures in the past month were twice as likely to develop colic as those with access to one pasture. This result is not easy to explain. The authors noted that most of the horses with access to four pastures were on a paddock rotation system, as opposed to a less structured grazing system. If the routine was that the horses were not moved to a fresh pasture until the one they were on was eaten down, roughage intake and quality may not have been as high as horses grazing fewer pastures in a less structured system. Also, internal parasites and intake of sand could become a problem in such a rotational grazing system.

Farm size and stocking rate

The second practitioner-based study in TX (Table 2-4) found that colic was slightly more likely on farms smaller than 25 acres and on those with more than 0.25 horses/acre (i.e. more than 1 horse per 4 acres). Also in that study, horses receiving no exercise other than pasture turnout were significantly less likely to develop colic than horses that were exercised at least once a week. In addition, each of these factors (farm size, stocking rate, and activity level), as well as housing and water source, were all interrelated. The authors interpreted these findings to indicate that horses kept at pasture—which generally are from the larger farms with the lower stocking rates—are at decreased risk for colic (or, at least, less likely to be observed to have colic).

Water

The study that reported on pasture rotation also found that horses in outside enclosures (pasture or drylot) without constant access to water were more than twice as likely to develop colic as horses that had an ample supply of water. Typically, owners or trainers put the horses outside without water for "just an hour or two." But it is easy to imagine how that hour or two could have stretched into a whole morning or afternoon in some cases.

In the manager-based study in MI (Table 2-2), horses that were provided with group drinking water from a source other than a bucket, tank, or automatic waterer were almost 7 times *less* likely to develop colic than horses provided with one of these water

---

Basic Water Requirements

0.03 x body weight (kg) = liters per day*

The minimum water requirement for mature, nonlactating horses under comfortable environmental conditions is 30 ml of water per kilogram of body weight per day (30 ml/kg/day).

For a 500-kg (1100-lb) horse, that's at least 15 liters (3½ gallons) of water per day. Water requirements substantially increase with exercise, lactation, increases in environmental temperature and humidity, and the amount of roughage in the diet (see page 122).

* (to convert pounds to kilograms, divide the body weight in pounds by 2.2; to calculate gallons per day, divide liters per day by 4.4)

sources. The researchers noted that on farms listing "other" for group water source, most horses were provided with water from more than one source. So, the type of water source probably is not as important as ready access and a plentiful supply of water. Another key factor may be that the horses provided with more than one group water source were kept at pasture, and were therefore at less risk for colic.

In the second TX study, horses with access to a pond were significantly less likely to develop colic than horses provided with other water sources. Also in that study, stalled horses provided with water from a bucket were at slightly increased risk for colic.

Heating drinking water in winter. In the MI study, heating the water in freezing weather had no significant effect on colic incidence. Nevertheless, this practice is important at times when water sources are likely to freeze because inadequate water intake is often a contributing factor in large colon impactions.

Heating the drinking water

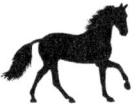

A study at the University of Pennsylvania showed that ponies kept in an unheated barn in winter and offered unheated (near-freezing) water drank 40% less than when they were offered heated water.

Two methods of providing heated water were studied:
- keeping the water warm using a bucket heater
- filling the buckets with hot tap water at 46–49° C (115–120° F) twice a day, at meal times

Water intake was similar for both methods. In all ponies, water intake was greatest within 3 hours of feeding or refill, by which time the hot tap water had cooled to about 21° C (70° F).

The authors concluded that providing hot tap water twice a day is a simple and effective way of ensuring adequate water intake during the winter months.

Internal Parasites

Internal parasites remain an important cause of colic in horses. Before the arrival of anthelmintics (dewormers) that are highly effective against the larval (immature) stages, severe colic caused by large strongyles was relatively common and had a fairly high mortality rate. Nowadays, this type of colic is very uncommon and the focus of internal parasite control has shifted from the large strongyles to the small strongyles (cyathostomes) and tapeworms. In young horses, roundworms are also a consideration.

Large strongyles

Large strongyles *(Strongylus vulgaris, S. edentatus,* and *S. equinus)* are an important cause of colic where deworming programs are inadequate. *Strongylus vulgaris* ("redworm" or "bloodworm") has the potential to cause the most damage. During this parasite's lifecycle, larvae on the pasture are swallowed, penetrate the bowel lining, and migrate along the blood vessels in the bowel wall. Eventually, some of the larvae migrate as far as the cranial mesenteric artery, which is the major vessel that branches off the aorta and supplies most of the bowel with blood.

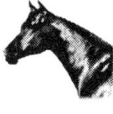

In terms of colic risk, the major internal parasites (worms) are:
- large strongyles ("redworms" or "bloodworms")
- small strongyles (also called cyathostomes)
- tapeworms
- roundworms (in young horses)

With the large strongyles now readily controllable with dewormers such as ivermectin and moxidectin, effective deworming programs now target the small strongyles and tapeworms.

These parasites can cause colic by two mechanisms:

1. Penetration of the bowel lining and migration into the small vessels within the bowel wall causes inflammation, blood vessel constriction, and altered bowel motility.

    • These changes can result in mild, spasmodic colic within a few days of the horse grazing infected pasture. Spasmodic colic may also occur several months later, when maturing larvae return to the interior of the bowel to become adults.

2. Larval migration within the arteries narrows the vessels by causing constriction, inflammation and thickening of the vessel wall, and sometimes blood clots within the vessels.

• These changes reduce blood flow to the affected bowel, which can alter bowel motility and cause spasmodic colic.

When large numbers of larvae migrate into the cranial mesenteric artery or its branches, the damage they cause can severely reduce blood flow through the affected artery. As a result, the section of bowel wall supplied by that artery may die, causing severe and sometimes fatal colic. Fortunately, this type of colic—verminous arteritis or thromboembolic colic—is now very uncommon (less than 1% of cases in the MI study), owing to the widespread use of highly effective anthelmintics such as ivermectin.

Small strongyles (cyathostomes)

Small strongyles (*Cyathostomum, Cylicocylus, Cylicostephanus,* and others) were originally considered to be of only minor importance. But now that the large strongyles are readily controllable, it has become clear that small strongyles are important internal parasites in horses, even though their effects on the horse may not be as dramatic.

The impact of the small strongyles is two-fold: (1) their ability to be present in large numbers without causing severe disease, and (2) their resistance to most anthelmintics during certain stages of their lifecycle. Heavy loads of small strongyles can cause weight loss, lethargy, poor coat condition, slowed growth, colic, and diarrhea. This condition is termed larval cyathostomiasis. Lighter infestations are not obvious, although it is common for a horse's general health and performance to improve after larvicidal treatment (discussed in Chapter 3).

2–Risk Factors for Colic

Unlike large strongyles, the larvae of small strongyles do not migrate through the bowel wall. Instead, they burrow into the lining and become dormant (encysted) for part of their lifecycle. These encysted, or hypobiotic, larvae are resistant to most anthelmintics. They remain encysted for months (sometimes for more than 2 years) before "hatching" or emerging into the interior of the bowel and maturing into adults.

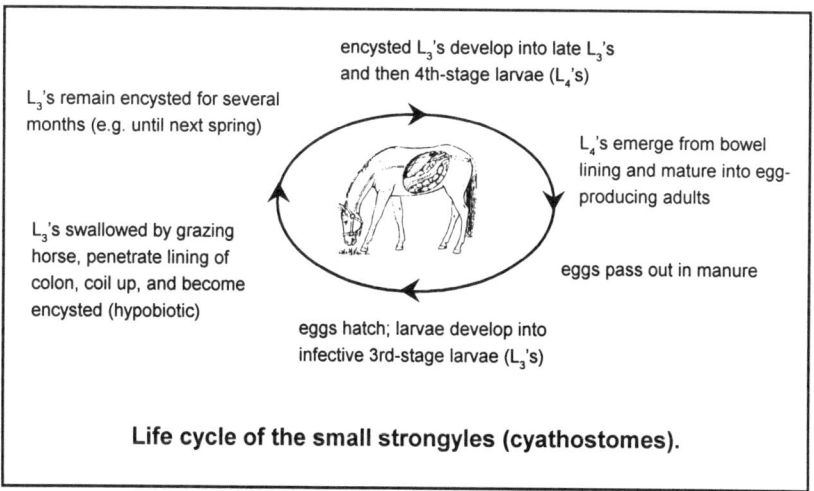

Life cycle of the small strongyles (cyathostomes).

Colic associated with small strongyle infestation is caused by inflammation of the bowel lining and altered bowel motility. The mere presence of strongyle larvae in the intestine can alter bowel motility, potentially leading to colic. But penetration of the bowel lining by the larvae, and later, the emergence of many larvae at once, cause more pronounced inflammation and motility changes.

What triggers the hypobiotic larvae to resume their development and emerge into the bowel interior all at once is not yet known. But it is probably some type of environmental factor. In temperate climates, the larvae tend to emerge in the late winter or early spring, whereas in warmer areas, the larvae may emerge in the late summer or fall.

"Effects of three anthelmintic schedules on colic incidence." Proof that small strongyles are a significant cause of colic was provided by this study, published in 1990 by Dr. Christine Uhlinger. Four groups of horses in southeastern Pennsylvania were followed for 5 years. The herds consisted mostly of adult performance horses, and averaged 30–40 horses each.

Even though the horses had been dewormed with non-ivermectin products every two months for at least two years before the study began, average fecal egg counts were 900 to 2,200 eggs per gram of manure. (Effective deworming programs should keep fecal egg counts below 200 eggs/gram.) Culture of the manure showed these eggs to be from small strongyles.

Three anthelmintic programs were evaluated during the study: (1) a non-ivermectin product, such as pyrantel, thiabendazole, or piperazine, every two months; (2) a non-ivermectin product every month; and (3) ivermectin every two months.

With the first protocol (a non-ivermectin dewormer every two months), the annual colic incidence was 24–46 cases/100 horses, depending on the herd. Using a non-ivermectin product once a month, instead of every two months, reduced the annual colic incidence to 2–5 cases/100 horses—one-tenth the rate of program one! However, the drop in the number of colic cases was gradual, not reaching its lowest point until 2 to 3 years after the new program had begun. The ivermectin program also reduced the annual colic incidence to 2–3 cases/100 horses after 2 to 3 years.

Dr. Uhlinger's conclusions were as follows: (1) a high proportion of the colic cases in these herds were parasite-related, and small strongyles (cyathostomes) were the primary cause; and (2) treatment with non-ivermectin anthelmintics every two months may not maximize horse health in all management systems.

Other studies. Few recent studies are as clear in the association between colic incidence and strongyle infection (whether large or small strongyles) as the study by Dr. Uhlinger. One explanation is that worm burdens, as indicated by fecal egg counts, in her study were unusually high for well-managed adult horses.

In a recent study at the University of Liverpool, England, there was no correlation between the number of strongyle eggs in manure and the incidence of spasmodic colic. However, the average fecal egg count was only 131 eggs/gram, which indicates that the deworming programs used on those horses were fairly effective. And in the manager-based study in VA/MD (Table 2-1), no association was found between colic incidence and the presence of strongyle eggs in manure.

> Internal parasites, in particular large and small strongyles, remain a significant cause of colic on farms where they are not adequately controlled.

So, it could be concluded that on farms where strongyles are not adequately controlled, these parasites account for a significant proportion of colic cases. But on farms in which an effective deworming program is in place, strongyle infestation is not a major cause of colic.

Tapeworms

There has long been debate as to whether tapeworms (especially *Anoplocephala perfoliata*) are a significant problem in horses. These parasites do not migrate from the bowel during their life-cycle, nor do they "hibernate" in the bowel wall; they simply remain attached to the lining of the bowel.

In many cases, perhaps even in the majority of horses, tapeworms can be present without causing any obvious problems. But tapeworms damage the lining of the bowel, and in large numbers they have been known to cause obstruction, particularly in the ileum, cecum, and the start of the large colon, where they tend to gather.

Ileal obstruction may simply be a physical effect of many tapeworms in an anatomically narrow portion of the bowel, with the result that food can become slowed or stopped at that site (ileal impaction). But these parasites also alter bowel motility, which can lead to spasmodic colic, impaction, and sometimes even intussusception (telescoping of the bowel into itself) at the ileum or cecum. Although rare, tapeworm infestation has also resulted in perforation of the cecum and subsequent peritonitis (infection of the abdominal cavity, which can be fatal).

Studies. In a recent study at the University of Liverpool in England, tapeworm infestation increased the risk for ileal impaction by up to 44 times and the risk for spasmodic colic by up to 8 times. From examination of manure for tapeworm eggs and measurement of serum antibodies against tapeworms, it was calculated that these parasites accounted for 22% of the spasmodic colic cases and 81% of the ileal impaction cases seen in these horses.

> Tapeworm infestation can be difficult to detect by routine fecal-egg-count methods. Special procedures must be used; and even then, tapeworm infestation may go undetected or its severity underestimated.
>
> Recently, a blood test has been developed which measures specific antibodies produced by the horse in response to tapeworms. Preliminary studies are promising in terms of accurately detecting tapeworm infestation and determining its severity.

In a recent study at the University of Pennsylvania, tapeworms were found in 52% of horses that had cecal intussusception (diagnosed during surgery or at post-mortem examination). This condition occurs when a portion of the cecum folds in on itself or the first part of the large colon telescopes into the cecum. The authors commented that the incidence of tapeworm infestation could have been even higher than 52%, as the bowel was not opened (and therefore its lining was not examined) in every case.

However, there could be a regional effect here. In a recent study of horses with ileal impaction that required surgery at Auburn University in Alabama, tapeworms were not identified as a significant cause of ileal impaction. (Coastal Bermuda hay was awarded that honor; see page 65.)

Deworming program and colic incidence

In none of the four manager- or practitioner-based studies (VA/MD, MI, UK, and the first TX study) were parasites found to be a significant cause of colic. This is probably because most of the horses in those studies were regularly dewormed. For example, in the first TX study (Table 2-3), only 34 out of more than 1600 horses were never dewormed or had an unknown deworming history. The rest of the horses were regularly dewormed, most commonly with ivermectin.

So although fecal egg counts were not reported, it could be concluded that most of the horses in these studies were on an adequate deworming program, at least in terms of colic risk.

The second practitioner-based study in TX (Table 2-4) supports the conclusion that regular deworming decreases the colic risk. In that study, horses that were not on a regular deworming program (defined as deworming at least once every 12 weeks) were more than twice as likely to develop colic as horses that were regularly dewormed.

Deworming program details. The first TX study provided the most detailed information on anthelmintic use. No significant associations were found between colic incidence and the following: frequency of deworming; number of anthelmintics used in the deworming program; whether or not anthelmintics were used on a rotating basis; and use of a particular anthelmintic. Nor was there any significant association between the type of colic and the anthelmintic used most recently.

> In terms of colic risk, the specific dewormer used, or the deworming program chosen, may not be as important as regular use of an effective product.

These results suggest that the specific anthelmintic used, or the particular deworming program chosen, may not be as important as regular use of an effective product.

Strongid C. Neither of the TX studies found a significant effect of feeding pyrantel tartrate (Strongid C® or its generic equivalent) daily on colic incidence. However, this finding should not be interpreted to mean that Strongid C is ineffective in preventing colic. It simply indicates that daily pyrantel tartrate was as effective as other deworming programs used on the horses in these studies. (Also, parasites are only one possible cause of colic in horses.)

Recent deworming and colic

Occasionally, horses develop mild colic within a couple of days of being dewormed. In the second practitioner-based study in TX (Table 2-4), deworming in the past 7 days slightly increased the risk for colic. And in the practitioner-based study in the UK (Table 2-5), recent anthelmintic administration was a possible contributing factor in horses with spasmodic or mild, undiagnosed colic. But to put things into perspective, in each of these studies, less than 10% of horses with colic had recently been dewormed.

In most cases, colic that occurs within a few days of deworming is mild and resolves on its own or with minor medical treatment.

A possible explanation for this association is altered bowel motility, either in response to dead or dying parasites or from the drug itself. At least one benzimidazole anthelmintic (mebendazole) has been shown to disrupt intestinal motility in the presence of strongyle infection. In support of the altered motility theory, a hospital-based study at the University of Georgia found a significant association between recent deworming and colic caused by large colon displacement. But with one exception (roundworms), colic following deworming usually is mild and resolves either on its own or with minor medical treatment.

Roundworms. A more serious problem occurs in foals and young horses that are heavily infested with roundworms (*Parascaris equorum*, or ascarids). Adult roundworms are large, being about half the diameter of a pencil and several inches long. It doesn't take very many roundworms to cause an obstruction when the worms are paralyzed or killed (depending on the product) all at once. In some cases, impaction with roundworms can rupture the intestine, which is fatal.

Foals dewormed for the first time after 3 months of age are most susceptible to roundworm impaction because it takes 3–4 months from the time the eggs are swallowed for these parasites to reach mature size in the intestine. Starting a foal's deworming program at 6–8 weeks of age prevents this problem.

Dental Care

Adult horses have 24 large "cheek" teeth (premolars and molars); 6 each, upper and lower, left and right. On the surface that faces the matching tooth, each cheek tooth has a broad, rectangular, roughened surface that is designed to grind fibrous plant material into fine particles.

By breaking up the otherwise poorly digestible leaves, stems, and seeds, effective chewing ensures proper digestion by exposing the more digestible inner parts of the plant to digestive enzymes. It could also reduce the potential for long or large particles of plant material to obstruct the intestine.

Studies. While it therefore makes sense that dental problems could increase the risk for certain types of colic, especially impactions, to date this association has not been proven. In the first practitioner-based study in TX (Table 2-3), there was no significant association between the frequency of dental care and the incidence of colic. However, most of the horses had routine dental care at least once a year; only about 5% had never had dental care. So, there were too few horses that did not receive regular dental care to draw any definite conclusions. In the second TX study (Table 2-4), dental care at least once a year slightly decreased the colic risk, but the difference was small.

Stress

Stress is a difficult concept to define in people, and even more difficult in animals. Our notion of what stresses a horse is based on an understanding of normal horse behavior and observation of a horse's behavior in "stressful" situations. Researchers have attempted to measure stress based on increases in blood cortisol levels (a hormone released during stress) and changes in the white blood cell count. But as each individual's tolerance for, and response to, stressful situations is a little different, stress is virtually impossible to measure in horses. Thus, any link between stress and colic is based on assumption.

In humans, there is plenty of evidence that stress increases the incidence of gastrointestinal complaints, and it could reasonably be assumed that the same holds true for horses.

Stomach (gastric) ulcers

Gastric ulceration is one cause of colic that seems to have a stress component. It is fairly common in young foals that are stressed by illness and, presumably, the extra handling that is required for treatment. And in adult horses, ulcers are common in horses performing strenuous activities. However, gastric ulcers usually do not cause obvious signs of colic in adult horses. Instead, the signs typically are vague: poor appetite (particularly for grain), loss of condition, reduced performance, and attitude changes.

Cecal impaction

Cecal impaction (obstruction of the cecum with feed material) also may have a stress component. This problem is more common in horses with chronic pain (e.g. painful eye conditions, laminitis) and those that are hospitalized for illness or surgery. Presumably, the biochemical processes triggered by pain, illness, or anesthesia and surgery alter bowel motility, leading to cecal atony (loss of tone and motility) and impaction. In a small percentage of cases, cecal impaction terminates in rupture of the cecum, which is fatal.

Salmonella infection

Hospitalization for illness or surgery also increases the incidence of colitis caused by *Salmonella* bacteria. However, diarrhea is the main feature of this condition. Colic may precede or accompany the diarrhea (which typically is profuse and watery), but it is not the primary complaint.

Transport/shipping

Long-distance transport may increase the potential for colic, particularly large colon impaction. But in the majority of cases, the cause is probably inadequate water intake and altered feeding and exercise schedules, rather than stress. In the VA/MD study, recent transport (travel in the past two weeks) increased the colic

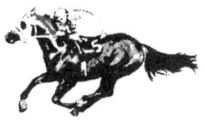

Gastric ulcers reportedly occur in 80–100% of racehorses in active training and in about 75% of 3-day-event horses. Possible factors include:

- *stress*—confinement, excitement in anticipation of fast work or competition, frequent transport, strange surroundings, etc.
- *high-intensity exercise*—reduces blood flow to the stomach and increases the contact of gastric acid with the less protected parts of the stomach (squamous mucosa; see page 139)
- *high-grain diets*—fermentation of carbohydrates in the stomach increases gastric acidity (a key factor in ulcer formation)
- *intermittent feeding* or withholding feed for several hours before fast work or competition—fasting causes gastric ulcers in horses

But the effects of ulceration in adult horses tend to be insidious: decreased appetite, coat and body condition, and performance.

risk by about three times. Two possible reasons were proposed: (1) transport causes a physiological response that alters gastrointestinal function, or (2) transport interrupts feeding or exercise routines and/or affects water intake. But in the second TX study (Table 2-4), neither recent transport nor the distance traveled had any significant effect on colic risk.

Illness

Also in the VA/MD study, recent illness involving a fever was found to significantly increase the colic risk. Horses that had a fever in the past two weeks were 11 times more likely to develop colic than were healthy horses. The reasons proposed for why transport may increase colic risk are good initial explanations.

Although the second TX study did not specifically evaluate fever or other illness, medical or surgical treatment in the past 7 days had no significant effect on colic risk in that study.

Certain infectious conditions, in particular strangles *(Streptococcus equi* infection) and *Rhodococcus* pneumonia, can lead to "seeding" of the abdomen with bacteria. Abscessation of the bowel wall or associated lymph nodes may result and can cause chronic colic. But abdominal abscesses are uncommon complications of these common respiratory infections.

Drugs and Chemicals

The following drugs and chemicals have been associated with colic in horses, although colic usually is only one of the signs, and may not be the most obvious abnormality.

Amitraz

Amitraz is an acaricide (a product that kills ticks and mites) that is used in cattle. It is highly toxic to horses and causes severe, often fatal impaction colic. *Amitraz should <u>never</u> be used in horses.*

Antibiotics

Certain antibiotics alter the normal balance of micro-organisms in the bowel, which can lead to enterocolitis (inflammation of the small and large intestines). The most obvious signs are depression, disinterest in food, and diarrhea, which can be severe and life-threatening. Colic may precede or accompany the diarrhea.

This problem can occur with any antibiotic, whether given orally or by injection, although *it is very uncommon*. It is more likely in stressed horses on high-grain diets (e.g. young racehorses), and with the following drugs: trimethoprim–sulfonamides (TMPS), ceftiofur (Naxcel®), and some forms of erythromycin and tetracycline. Lincomycin often causes potentially fatal colitis in horses.

Arsenic-containing products

Acute overdose of arsenic (as distinct from small amounts taken over a long period of time) can cause severe inflammation of the digestive tract, which can be fatal. One oral source of arsenic is Fowler's Solution, a tonic used to stimulate a horse's appetite and improve its coat condition. (Legend has it that accidental overdose of arsenic is what killed Phar Lap, the Australian racehorse who raced in the U.S. in the 1930's.)

> Atropine was originally discovered as an extract from the plant *Atropa belladonna*. Products containing belladonna extract were once popular as colic remedies (e.g. Dr. Bell's). These products were effective for mild, spasmodic colic because they reduced bowel motility (and hence the spasms). But overuse of these products or use in horses with more serious types of colic can be disastrous.

Atropine and opiates

Atropine is often prescribed by veterinarians to treat a variety of eye problems in horses. It is used to keep the pupil dilated, and thus reduce pain and prevent adhesions within the eye. But when using atropine, it is important to follow the dosing instructions carefully. Even when used topically, atropine is absorbed into the system and can slow bowel motility, which may lead to impaction colic. Opiate pain-relievers such as morphine also slow intestinal motility, and can cause impaction colic when overused.

Castor oil

Castor oil is sometimes used as a purgative in people. However, in horses it can cause painful colitis (inflammation of the colon) which can be fatal. Profuse, watery diarrhea and toxic shock can readily be induced by giving a horse castor oil.

DSS

DSS (dioctyl sodium sulfosuccinate) is a laxative that is sometimes given orally to adult horses with impactions, and either orally or as an enema to young foals with meconium impaction. Overuse can cause cramping, colic, and diarrhea.

Levamisole

Levamisole is a dewormer that is used in cattle, sheep, and goats. It is sometimes used in horses as an immune system stimulant, although more specific products are now available for this purpose. Levamisole has a narrow safety margin in horses. Overdose can cause colic, sweating, hypersensitivity to sound, and head-pressing (pressing the head against a solid object).

Monensin

Monensin is a feed additive sometimes used in poultry and cattle rations. It is highly toxic to horses. Toxicity has occurred when feeds containing or contaminated with monensin have been fed to horses. Weakness and collapse, with abnormalities in heart rate and rhythm, are the most prominent signs of monensin toxicity; mild colic may also be seen. Salinomycin is a related compound that is also used as a feed additive and can cause similar signs. To avoid toxicity with either of these compounds, *feeds formulated for poultry or cattle should not be fed to horses.*

Nonsteroidal anti-inflammatory drugs (NSAIDs)

This class of drugs includes phenylbutazone ("bute," PBZ, BTZ), flunixin (Banamine®), ketoprofen (Ketofen®), naproxen, indomethacin, diclofenac, meclofenamic acid, and aspirin. Any NSAID can cause colic by creating ulceration in the stomach or the right dorsal colon (right dorsal colitis). NSAIDs have also been associated with an increased incidence of large colon impaction, apparently by altering bowel motility.

Signs of ulceration. Stomach ulcers do not always cause obvious symptoms in adult horses, although they are a possible cause of colic associated with eating. The more common signs of gastric ulceration are mentioned on page 86.

Right dorsal colitis typically causes mild-to-moderate colic, sometimes with diarrhea. Ulceration may be extensive enough that protein is lost from the bloodstream through the damaged bowel. When large amounts of protein are lost, edema (fluid accumulation in the tissues) develops in the legs and along the underside of the belly and chest. Horses in this condition can be difficult to save. In those that survive, the right dorsal colon may become permanently narrowed by scar tissue (strictured), which can be a cause of chronic recurrent colic.

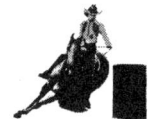

Given the frequency with which NSAIDs are used in horses, it is fair to say that these are very safe drugs. However, it is best to keep in mind that adverse effects (stomach ulcers, right dorsal colitis, and kidney damage) can occur in any horse given NSAIDs.

The risk increases when high doses are given for several days, two NSAIDs are used together, or the horse is dehydrated.

Circumstances of NSAID-induced ulceration. In most cases, stomach ulcers form only after high doses of NSAIDs are given for several days, although they can develop in young foals even at normal dosages. Stress, intermittent feeding, and dehydration make ulceration more likely in both foals and adult horses.

Right dorsal colitis can occur with even normal doses of NSAIDs. It is thought that certain horses are peculiarly sensitive to these drugs, or the mechanisms that normally protect against ulceration are impaired in these horses. The same factors that increase the risk for stomach ulcers (stress, dehydration, etc.) may increase the potential for right dorsal colitis to develop in susceptible horses.

Organophosphates

Organophosphates, or OPs, are relatively common topical insecticides, applied on the skin as powders or rinses. Examples include diazinon, malathion, ronnel, and chlorpyrofos. Some OPs, such as trichlorfon and dichlorvos, are used orally as boticides (dewormers that target stomach bots), although ivermectin and moxidectin are much safer and are now the most commonly used boticides.

OPs have a narrow safety margin, so accurate dosing based on the horse's body weight is important. Toxicity can occur with overdosing, frequent use, or accidental ingestion (by eating or drinking). Signs of toxicity include anxiety, salivation, sweating, trembling, colic, and diarrhea. Acepromazine, a common sedative, increases the potential for OP toxicity when used at the same time. These insecticides should not be used in young foals.

Prostaglandins

Prostaglandin $F_{2\alpha}$ (Lutalyse®, Estrumate®, etc.) is often used in broodmares to short-cycle or synchronize estrus (heat). Even at routine dosages, it can cause cramping, sweating, and other signs of colic which can last from a few minutes to a couple of hours.

Vaccines

In the manager-based study in VA/MD (Table 2-1), recent vaccination increased the colic risk by a little over three times. No single type of vaccine was found to carry a higher risk than any other.

Basically, colic risk was slightly increased in the two weeks following vaccination, regardless of the type of vaccine given. But in the first practitioner-based study in TX (Table 2-3), recent vaccination did not increase the incidence of colic.

The VA/MD study also found that horses vaccinated against Potomac horse fever (PHF) during the study year were twice as likely to develop colic as horses that were not vaccinated against this disease. But rather than the vaccine causing colic, the authors concluded that vaccination against PHF was simply an indicator of the level of preventive healthcare on a farm. For example, farms with a history of PHF had a slightly higher incidence of colic, and managers on those farms may therefore have been more likely to vaccinate against the disease. This gives the impression that vaccination against PHF increases the colic risk, when vaccination could simply have been implemented *in response to* an episode or history of the disease.

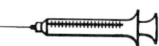

In one study, colic incidence was slightly increased in the 14 days following vaccination. This is in keeping with what some veterinarians and horse owners have observed: mild, transient colic is occasionally seen shortly after vaccination (sometimes the same day). But why this occurs in some horses is not known.

Environmental Factors

Geographic location

There is no evidence that the overall colic risk is affected by the region or state (or even country) in which a horse lives. But location can be important with specific types of colic. The following geographic associations have been reported in the United States:

- enteroliths—most common in California, but an increased incidence has also been reported in Florida and Indiana

- sand colic—most common in desert areas, Florida, and coastal areas of the mid-Atlantic states
- ileal impaction—southeastern states
- proximal (anterior) enteritis—southeastern states
- Potomac horse fever—mid-Atlantic states, northeastern states, and the Midwest
  - as the carrier appears to be an aquatic snail, PHF is most likely to occur in horses that have access to natural water courses, such as rivers and streams

Note: These conditions can occur anywhere in the U.S.; they are simply more common in the areas listed. For example, sand colic can occur on any farm with sandy soil, especially when the pasture quality is relatively poor.

Grass sickness is a foreign example of a specific type of colic with a regional incidence. To date, grass sickness has been reported only in the United Kingdom and certain European countries (typically in horses imported from the U.K.), although a similar disease has been reported in South America. This debilitating and sometimes fatal disease involves degeneration of the nerves that regulate bowel motility. It is most common in pastured horses, which has lead to speculation that an environmental toxin (possibly a fungal toxin) is involved.

Weather or Season

Most equine veterinarians agree that colic caused by large colon impaction is more common in very hot, dry weather and in very cold weather (cold enough to freeze outside water sources). And more than one study has reported an increased incidence of ileal or small colon impaction in the fall, possibly as the amount and quality of pasture grass decreases or the roughage source changes from pasture to hay. But there does not appear to be a consistent effect of season or weather on the overall incidence of colic.

Manager- and practitioner-based studies

In the VA/MD study (Table 2-1), most cases of colic occurred in March, August, and December, with a steady increase in colic incidence between April and August. The first TX study (Table 2-3) found no significant association between colic incidence and season. But a recent change in housing increased the risk for colic, and these housing changes were more common in the early summer and in the fall.

The seasonal incidence of colic in the UK study (Table 2-5) varied widely in the two-year study period. However, in both years there were two major peaks: in the spring (April/May) and in the fall (September). The monthly colic incidence was compared with the average monthly rainfall and temperature, but no significant correlations were found.

> In some studies, colic was more likely in the spring and late summer/fall, and just after a weather change. Any effect of season or the weather on colic incidence most likely relates to changes in water intake, exercise level, and/or roughage intake.

Weather changes

In the second practitioner-based study in TX (Table 2-4), a substantial change in the weather in the past 3 days significantly increased the colic risk. However, the authors cautioned that the association was not strong, details were often inadequate, and recall by owners and managers could have been biased because of the common belief that weather influences colic risk.

They summed up by saying, "although clinical experience would suggest that weather-related factors are associated with development of colic in horses, the precise conditions that predispose to colic remain ill-defined." But it is tempting to speculate that the key factors probably are changes in water intake, activity level, and roughage intake, especially in hot, dry weather and when horses are kept inside because of inclement weather.

The manager-based study in VA/MD (Table 2-1) did not find a strong association between weather and colic incidence, but the colic risk was slightly higher on the days on which it snowed and when the humidity was low (less than 50%) on the previous day.

Internal parasites

Climate and season have considerable influence on the lifecycles of internal parasites, which could cause regional and seasonal differences in the incidence of parasite-induced colic. For example, the number of infective strongyle larvae on the pasture varies with region and season. Strongyle eggs hatch at temperatures between 45° F and 100° F. Infective larvae can survive freezing, but they are very susceptible to heat, especially if the environment is very dry. According to one authority, temperatures above 85° F can kill strongyle larvae.

So in warmer regions, the number of infective strongyle larvae on the pasture may be lowest in the summer months and higher in the fall and spring. But in cooler climates, larval numbers on the pasture may peak in the summer and early fall. Given that colic is more common in the spring and fall in some studies, perhaps parasites should be added to the list of possible causes.

Poisonous Plants

Several species of plants can cause colic in horses, but usually in association with other signs. With one or two exceptions, grazing horses avoid poisonous plants unless they are very hungry, so toxicity is usually restricted to horses grazing poor quality pasture. Toxicity can also occur in horses fed poor quality hay that contains a lot of weeds.

The plants most likely to cause colic are briefly discussed below. Your county extension agent should be able to help with identification of the poisonous plants that grow in your area.

Black locust *(Robinia pseudoacacia)*

The highest concentration of toxin is found in the bark of the black locust tree. Only a very small amount is needed to cause signs of toxicity, which include colic and diarrhea, often accompanied by depression, weakness, pale gums, and irregular heartbeat.

Castor bean *(Ricinus communis)*

Castor beans contain substances that are extremely irritating to the horse's digestive tract. They cause painful colitis (inflammation of the colon) which can be fatal. But signs of toxicity may not be apparent for several hours. Accidental poisoning has been reported in horses that were permitted to graze around castor plants (which are sometimes used ornamentally in garden landscapes) or that ate lawn clippings containing castor beans.

Nightshades *(Solanum* species)

Common names in this group include climbing, silver-leaf, cut-leafed, black, and deadly nightshades; European bittersweet; white horsenettle; and Buffalo burr. Central nervous system abnormalities (e.g. depression, weakness, collapse) are usually more obvious than digestive system signs (salivation, spasmodic colic, and diarrhea).

Oak *(Quercus* species)

Oak or acorn toxicity occasionally occurs in horses that eat large quantities of oak buds, leaves (either fresh or dried), or acorns. The signs appear suddenly and include colic, straining, and bloody diarrhea. Loud intestinal sounds may be heard, and acorn husks are sometimes found in the manure. The horse's urine may be discolored red or brown as a result of kidney damage. Sudden death has also been reported. However, horses can eat small quantities of oak leaves and acorns without ill effects.

Oleander *(Nerium oleander)*

The lethal dose of oleander in horses is 30–40 dried leaves, but as few as 10 leaves are deadly in some cases. The toxin primarily affects the heart, but profuse diarrhea and colic may also be seen. The plant has a very bitter taste, but poisoning has occurred when horses were fed grass clippings containing oleander leaves. In at least one case, poisoning occurred when the horse was tied near an oleander bush and it nibbled the leaves out of boredom.

Pokeweed *(Phytolacca americana)*

Gastrointestinal irritation, manifest as colic and diarrhea, is the predominant sign of pokeweed poisoning. Other signs include oral ulceration and anemia from red blood cell damage. Death can occur from respiratory failure. All parts of the plant contain the toxin, but the roots are most toxic, the berries least toxic.

Tobacco *(Nicotiona* species)

Nicotine is the principal toxin in this group of plants. Eating tobacco leaves or the bark or leaves from wild tree tobacco causes salivation, intestinal cramping, and diarrhea. Muscle tremors, weakness, collapse, and respiratory failure can also develop.

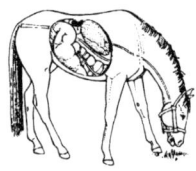

Table 2-1: Manager-based study of colic incidence and risk factors in Virginia and Maryland (VA/MD).

This study was conducted between November 1990 and January 1991:

- farms with >20 horses were randomly selected in two neighboring counties in VA and MD, just west of Washington, DC; a total of 31 farms participated
- detailed records were kept on 1427 horses during the study year
- *all colic incidents were recorded by the owner/manager,* regardless of whether a veterinarian was called—even minor colics needing no treatment (or treated by the owner or manager) were recorded
- >170 farm and horse variables were analyzed for their possible role in colic
- farm-level factors were divided into the following categories
  - farm (e.g. major use of horses, length of time farm owned by current owner)
  - horses (e.g. number of resident and visiting horses)
  - employees (e.g. number, proportion of part-time employees)
  - feedstuffs (e.g. sources, feeding frequency, use of supplements, storage)
  - water (e.g. source, delivery system in stable and pasture)
  - habitat (e.g. bedding type, frequency of stall cleaning and bedding changes)
  - pasture (e.g. forage and soil types, rotation, manure removal)
  - health (e.g. disease history, parasite control program)
- horse-level factors were divided into the following categories
  - horse (e.g. age, breed, gender, vices, residence time on farm)
  - housing (e.g. time spent stalled or pastured, stall bedding, pasture size)
  - use (predominant use, work schedule)
  - nutrition (specifics of diet and feeding schedule)
  - health history for year before study (e.g. past illness, preventive programs)
  - events during the study year (e.g. breeding, transport, illness, deworming)
  - changes during the study year (e.g. housing, nutrition, exercise)

'Prospective study of equine colic incidence and mortality.' MK Tinker, NA White, P Lessard, *et al. Equine Veterinary Journal,* 1997; 29(6):448–453.

'Prospective study of equine colic risk factors.' MK Tinker, NA White, P Lessard, *et al. Equine Veterinary Journal,* 1997; 29(6):454–458.

'Assessment of risk associated with events in a prospective study of equine colic.' MK Tinker, NA White, P Lessard, *et al. Proceedings of the 42nd Annual Convention of the American Association of Equine Practitioners,* 1996; 42:332–333.

Table 2-2: Manager-based study of colic risk factors in Michigan (MI).

This study used data from the Michigan Equine Monitoring System (a project designed to monitor health and economic activity on equine farms in Michigan, USA), collected between February 1992 and April 1994:

- each month, data on all types of equine health and activity on the farms were *recorded by the owner, trainer, or farm/barn manager*
- records were collected for a total of 3,925 horses on 138 farms
- risk factors evaluated at the farm level included the following
  - year (1992–93 or 1993–94)
  - geographic region (northern, central, southwestern, or southeastern MI)
  - average number of horses on the farm during the study period
  - individual and group grain-feeding methods (loose on ground, in container on ground, in raised container, other)
  - individual and group forage-feeding methods (as above for grain feeding)
  - individual and group watering methods (bucket, automatic, tank, other)
  - water heated in freezing weather (yes/no)
- risk factors evaluated at the horse level included the following
  - age
  - breed
  - gender (mare, stallion, gelding)
  - housing (access to indoor housing, access to outdoor housing)
  - activity (breeding, training, draft, dressage, racing, hunter/jumper, etc.)
  - reproductive status and activity (breeding, foaling) during the study period
  - deworming (number of dewormings during the study period)
  - health events during the study period (preventive programs, illness, injuries)

'Risk factors for colic in the Michigan (USA) equine population.' JB Kaneene, R Miller, WA Ross, *et al. Preventive Veterinary Medicine,* 1997; 30:23–36.

Table 2-3: The first of two practitioner-based studies of management factors associated with colic in Texas (TX).

This study comprised data collected by equine veterinarians working in private practice in Texas, between October 1991 and December 1992:

- 82 participating veterinarians kept records of the first colic case they were called to treat each month, and the next non-colic emergency case
- 821 horses were examined for colic, and 821 horses were examined for other medical emergencies (e.g. skin lacerations, musculoskeletal disorders, acute respiratory disease)
- data compared for each colic case and the next non-colic emergency included the following
  - age, breed, gender
  - farm acreage, number of horses at the farm
  - conditions under which the horse was kept, type of stall bedding
  - recent change in housing or stabling conditions (within the past 2 weeks)
  - feeding practices, feed offered
  - recent change in diet (within the past 2 weeks)
  - performance level (type of activity)
  - recent change in activity level
  - recent transport
  - frequency of dental care
  - parasite control program, including when the horse was last dewormed
  - immunization program, including when the horse was last vaccinated
  - any previous episodes of colic

'Case-control study of the association between various management factors and development of colic in horses.' ND Cohen, PL Matejka, CM Honnas, and RN Hooper (The Texas Equine Colic Study Group). *Journal of the American Veterinary Medical Association,* 1995; 206(5):667–673.

Table 2-4: The second of two practitioner-based studies of management factors associated with colic in Texas (TX).

> This study comprised data collected by 145 equine veterinarians working in private practice in Texas, between March 1997 and February 1998. Details are as described for the earlier study (Table 2-3), except that this study involved 1030 horses with colic and 1030 horses with non-colic medical emergencies, and the various dietary and management factors were recorded in more detail.
>
> 'Dietary and other management factors associated with colic in horses.' ND Cohen, PG Gibbs, and AM Woods. *Journal of the American Veterinary Medical Association,* 1999; 215(1):53–60.

Table 2-5: Practitioner-based study of colic types and management factors in England (UK).

> This study involved data collected by 7 equine veterinarians in a private practice in Buckinghamshire, England, between January 1989 and December 1990:
>
> - information was recorded for 200 colic episodes in 179 horses, and from 100 horses without colic that were attended for routine healthcare or non-digestive system problems during the study period
> - data from the horses with colic included the following
>   - age, breed, and gender (also recorded for the 100 horses without colic)
>   - recent changes in management and diet (within the past 24 hours)
>   - recent drug administration
>   - any previous colic episodes
>   - findings of clinical examination
>   - type of colic (spasmodic/undiagnosed, flatulent, pelvic flexure impaction, other impactions, "surgical" colic, and colitis)
>   - method of treatment
> - average monthly temperature and rainfall were also recorded
>
> 'A two year, prospective survey of equine colic in general practice.' CJ Proudman. *Equine Veterinary Journal,* 1991; 24(2):90–93.

2–Risk Factors for Colic

Summary of the various factors associated with colic in horses:

Intrinsic (horse) Factors	Management Factors	Environmental Factors
• breed	• diet	• geographic location
• gender	• housing	• weather/season
• age	• water intake	• poisonous plants
• use/activity	• internal parasites	
• behavior (e.g. "vices")	• dental care	
• previous colic or surgery	• stress	
• genetics	• drugs and chemicals	

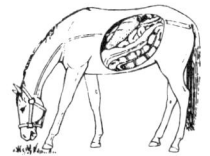

3

Strategies for Preventing Colic

So, *can* colic be prevented? The short answer is *Yes, sometimes.* Of course, many of the risk factors identified in the previous chapter are outside our control, particularly the intrinsic (horse) factors such as age, breed, and gender. But most, if not all, of the *management* factors can be modified in some way to reduce the incidence of colic both in an individual horse and in an entire group of horses. The anthelmintic study outlined on page 80 is an excellent example: the annual incidence of colic was reduced from 24–46 cases/100 horses to less than 5 cases/100 horses (a decrease of 80–90%!), just by introducing an effective deworming program.

Simple Management Strategies

In that anthelmintic study, the incidence of colic was substantially reduced by altering one management factor, but those farms still reported 2 to 5 cases of colic per 100 horses per year. This highlights an important point: colic has numerous possible causes or contributing factors, so altering one key factor can decrease the colic incidence, but it may not prevent every case of colic.

Because colic is a multifactorial problem, *colic prevention requires a multifactorial approach.* As most cases of colic have at least one management component, and management is the one area we can influence to any great degree, *prevention focuses on management.* Below is a list of ten management strategies that can reduce the incidence of colic in an individual horse and in groups of horses.

Management Strategies for Preventing Colic

1. Match the horse's natural diet as closely as possible.
2. Match the horse's natural feeding schedule as closely as possible.
3. Match the horse's natural activity pattern as closely as possible.
4. Minimize changes in diet, housing, and activity level.
5. Feed only good quality feedstuffs.
6. Ensure ample access to fresh, clean water.
7. Maintain a good deworming program.
8. Maintain a regular schedule of dental care.
9. Maintain good environmental management.
10. Pay attention to your horse(s).

These are all basic things, many of which most horse owners are already doing, to some degree. But often the success or failure of a program lies in the details. In the following sections I'll explain why the individual strategies are important, and provide practical suggestions for implementing them. Management changes sometimes require a few tough decisions, changes in old habits, and, probably most important, commitment—a willingness to make it happen and stick with it. It may also take some creative thinking to find modifications that will work in your situation.

Aside from reducing the incidence of colic, these strategies are worth implementing for another reason: they can decrease the incidence and severity of lung diseases, such as chronic obstructive pulmonary disease (COPD), and exercise-related muscle problems ("tying up," myositis, exertional rhabdomyolysis). And some can even help with behavioral problems.

1. Match the Horse's Natural Diet

The equine digestive system is designed to extract the bulk of the horse's nutritional requirements from forage—grass and other high-fiber plant materials (also termed roughage). In the natural state, very little of the horse's nutritional needs are met by grain (i.e. grass seed heads) or other feeds that are rich in readily digestible carbohydrates. Instead, the horse relies on microbial breakdown of plant fiber in the large intestine to supply the bulk of its energy needs.

Domesticated horses are no different in this respect from their wild counterparts. Regardless of whether it's a child's pony, an Olympic-level dressage horse, or a racehorse, optimal digestive health and function requires that the bulk of the horse's diet be roughage (pasture and/or hay). Nutritionists often put it this way: *horses have an absolute need for roughage.*

Meeting the horse's roughage requirements

Following are some guidelines for feeding horses, provided by the National Research Council, in their publication *'Nutrient Requirements of Horses'*:

❖ horses should be fed *1–2% of their body weight per day* of good quality roughage (pasture* or hay)

• for a 450-kg (1000-lb) horse with no access to pasture, feeding 1% of the horse's body weight equals 4.5 kg (10 lb) of hay per day; this is the recommended *minimum* amount

• this recommendation applies across the board in horses older than 12 months, regardless of what else they are fed

• another way of putting it is to feed *at least 1 kg of roughage per 100 kg of body weight* (or 1 lb per 100 lb body weight)

---

*Calculating Pasture Intake

The roughage requirement (1–2% of body weight per day) is for *dry matter*. Well cured hay is almost 100% dry matter. But fresh grass can be as little as 20% dry matter, so the water content must be factored in when calculating the contribution of pasture to a horse's roughage intake. When the water content of the pasture is not known, follow these general guidelines:

• multiply the roughage requirement by 3 to estimate the amount of fresh grass needed to supply this amount of dry matter (averaged-out across the growing season, fresh grass is about 30% dry matter and 70% water)

• figure that the average adult horse eats about 1.6 kg (3.5 lb) of grass per hour of grazing (although this is *highly* variable)

So, to provide even 1% of body weight as dry matter, a 450-kg horse would need to graze steadily for at least 8 hours:

1% x 450 kg = 4.5 kg (the minimum roughage requirement, as dry matter)

4.5 kg x 3 = 13.5 kg (the amount of grass needed to meet the requirement)

13.5 kg ÷ 1.6 kg/hr = 8.4 hrs (grazing time needed to eat 13.5 kg of grass)

❖ when grain must be fed to meet the horse's energy needs, *at least 50% of the total ration should be roughage*
  • this means that for every pound of grain fed, *at least* one pound of hay must be fed
  • specific exceptions are horses performing intense work and rapidly growing horses; but even in these cases, *at least 1% of the body weight should be fed as roughage*
  • the proportions of roughage to grain for different types of horses are listed in Table 3-1 on page 146

"Since the advent of modern anthelmintics, the most important cause of colic in horses is nutritional mismanagement. Nutritionally induced colic can be grouped into two categories:

1. Improper forage:grain ratios, or inadequate amounts of forage.

2. Use of tainted feedstuffs.

[By far] the more important of these two is inadequate fibre intake."

...

"There are few, if any, instances when overfeeding hay can lead to a problem, but there are numerous problems that can develop if hay is limited."

'Nutrition and productivity: practical problems related to nutrition.' SG Jackson and JD Pagan. *Proceedings of the 18th Bain-Fallon Memorial Lectures, Australian Equine Veterinary Assocation,* 1996; pages 139–140.

Feeding for energy needs

Energy is the most crucial nutritional component; not protein or calcium, or any other nutrient. Each of the bodily functions requires energy, so insufficient dietary energy can have profound effects on many systems. And an excess of dietary energy can have such diverse effects as colic, diarrhea, laminitis, exercise-related muscle problems, developmental orthopedic problems (e.g. physitis/epiphysitis, osteochondrosis, flexural limb deformities), and reproductive failure.

Thus, formulating a ration should begin with assessing the horse's energy requirements, based on its body weight and activity level. Table 3-2 on page 147 lists some daily nutrient requirements for adult horses of different sizes, performing various levels of work.

Overfeeding. One of the most common feeding errors, and one that predisposes horses to colic, is overfeeding grain or other concentrates (grain-based sweet feeds and pellets). These feedstuffs contain high levels of readily digestible carbohydrates which, when fed in large amounts, can alter conditions within the large intestine. As discussed in Chapter 2, the colic risk increases as the amount of concentrates increases. Thus, concentrates should be fed *only as supplements* when the horse's energy requirements for work, growth, pregnancy, or lactation cannot be fully met by roughage alone.

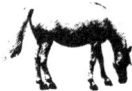
The maintenance energy needs of an adult horse can be met by roughage (pasture and/or hay) alone. Grain should be fed only as a supplement.

The micro-organisms in the horse's large intestine break down most types of plant fiber into substances that can be absorbed by the horse and used to produce energy. Thus, *hay or pasture is an energy source.* In fact, the maintenance energy requirements of an adult horse can usually be fully met by hay or pasture alone (see Box 3-1 on page 150). Provided the hay/pasture is of good quality, the maintenance requirements for protein, calcium, and phosphorus are also met.

However, two points about roughage-only diets are worth making: (1) The diet may be deficient in certain vitamins and minerals, so salt and a balanced mineral supplement may need to be provided. (2) Lush spring grass can be very high in digestible energy, far in excess of the adult horse's maintenance needs. So, pasture access may need to be limited in overweight and laminitis-prone horses, and the roughage requirement (1–2% of body weight per day) met with good quality hay until the pasture matures.

How much is too much? In the Virginia-Maryland study discussed in Chapter 2, the colic risk became significant when more than 2.5 kg (5½ lb) of concentrates were fed per day. Whether this applies across the board, to all types of horses in various management situations, awaits further study. But for now, it is as good a guidepost as we have. Feeding more than 2.5 kg of grain per day may not *cause* colic, but it could increase the risk for colic to develop. Strategies for feeding concentrates when a high-energy diet is required are discussed on page 113.

Dietary fat. Adding fat to the ration is an excellent way of reducing the amount of grain when a horse's energy needs demand a high-energy diet. The average equine diet contains very little fat (usually around 2–3%). But unlike grains, increasing the amount of fat above that normally found in the diet does not cause digestive problems.

> Adding fat to the diet is an excellent way of reducing the amount of grain when the horse's energy needs demand a high-energy diet.
>
> High-fat diets in horses do not carry the same health risks as they do in people. A "high-fat" diet in a horse seldom exceeds 15% fat (and often is less than 10% fat)—far less than the average "low-fat" human diet!

The aim is to meet part of the horse's energy needs with fat, thereby allowing the amount of grain to be decreased. Fat can be added in several forms (e.g. vegetable oil, rice bran, animal fat), but the commercial high-fat balanced rations are best because they ensure that the horse's diet contains sufficient vitamins and minerals. Before feeding a high-fat diet, it is a good idea to consult with an equine nutritionist to ensure that the final ration is balanced and meets the individual horse's needs.

2. Match the Horse's Natural Feeding Schedule

Horses kept on pasture graze for most of the day and much of the night. When grass is all they have to eat, it is necessary during much of the year for them to graze for this long simply to supply their energy needs. Confined horses do not need to eat all day and night to supply their energy needs which, although not ideal, can be met in a couple of concentrated meals. However, their digestive systems function best when there is fairly continuous intake of high-fiber food throughout the day and night.

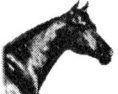

The easiest way to match the natural feeding schedule in horses confined to a stall or paddock is to make hay available at all times. If weight gain is a problem, calculate the horse's daily roughage requirement and feed that amount, divided into at least two meals.

In horses that are kept in stalls, pens, or small paddocks, matching the natural feeding schedule is easily accomplished by making sure the horse has hay at all times. With this approach, the horse can "graze" throughout the day and night as it would at pasture.

Exception. Some overweight horses and ponies gain weight when hay is available at all times, especially if they get little or no regular exercise. (Paddock or dry lot turnout does not count as exercise in these inactive horses.) In such cases, the hay ration—at least 1% of the body weight per day—should be divided into two or three portions and fed at intervals (e.g. morning and evening, or morning, afternoon, and night).

Once-a-day feeding, with no access to roughage in between feedings, is not a good idea. Studies on the development and healing of stomach ulcers have shown that the concentrations of acid and bile in the stomach can reach levels capable of causing ulceration within 14 hours of fasting. So if confined horses are not provided with hay throughout the day and night, they should be given hay at least twice a day.

3–Strategies for Preventing Colic

Feeding grain and other concentrates

As discussed in Chapter 2, it takes 8–12 hours for balance in the large intestine to be restored after a large carbohydrate meal. So, feeding large amounts of concentrates more often than every 8–12 hours can upset the balance and increase the potential for colic. And as one study showed, dividing the daily concentrate ration into two or more meals does not reduce the colic risk associated with feeding large amounts of grain.

So, how can you minimize the risk for colic when concentrates (grain or grain-based sweet feeds or pellets) must be fed to meet the horse's energy needs? There are two alternatives:

1. Divide the daily concentrate ration into several (6–8) small meals and feed them every few hours.

    • the objective is to feed amounts that the small intestine is able to digest and absorb, so that little or no readily fermentable carbohydrate reaches the large intestine

    • but obviously, this strategy is impractical in most settings

2. Divide the daily concentrate ration into two meals, and feed them at least 8 (and preferably 12) hours apart.

    • with this strategy, colic risk will be minimized *only if the total amount of concentrates fed is kept to a minimum*

    • studies are lacking on how much carbohydrate it takes to overwhelm the small intestine's ability to digest and absorb it, but it is probably best to limit the amount of concentrates fed in a single meal to less than 1.5 kg (about 3 lb)

    • note: there are certain instances in which this strategy is not ideal (see Exceptions, on the next page)

With either alternative, roughage should be available at all times. This may be even more important in horses on high-energy diets than in those on maintenance diets. For one thing, horses on high-energy diets still need to eat at least 1% of body weight per day as roughage. And for another, feeding roughage with each concentrate meal may slow emptying of the stomach and, therefore, delivery of carbohydrates to the small intestine. Chopped roughage (e.g. chopped hay, alfalfa cubes) or beet pulp may be more effective in this regard than hay because it can be fed mixed with the concentrates. (An alternative is to feed some hay before the grain meal.) Ample and regular intake of roughage may also moderate the swings in fluid and acidity in the colon.

Exceptions. There are three groups of horses for which the twice-daily grain feeding strategy is not ideal: (1) horses with stomach ulcers whose work level requires a high-energy diet, (2) horses that have had large amounts of small intestine removed during surgery, and (3) horses performing intensive power work (e.g. racing, 3-day-eventing, polo). The first strategy (small, nutrient-rich meals several times a day) is preferable in these horses; in fact, complete balanced rations may be useful in such instances. Managing horses with gastric ulcers is discussed further on page 139.

3. Match the Horse's Natural Activity Pattern

In a natural setting, a horse's normal activity pattern consists of grazing for most of the day and much of the night, gradually moving from one area to another in search of good grass. Grazing is interspersed with rest periods, trips to the nearest water source, and short bursts of activity (e.g. play, running from danger).

As discussed in Chapter 2, the colic risk is lower in horses on pasture than in those confined to stalls. Diet, water intake, and the horse's occupation probably have as much to do with this as the daily activity pattern. Nevertheless, pasture turnout is ideal for most horses, provided safety (good fencing, compatible company, etc.) is kept in mind.

3–Strategies for Preventing Colic

When pasturing is not an option, stabled horses should be turned out for as long as possible every day (unless the horse has a medical condition for which activity is inadvisable). When turnout in a pasture or dry lot is not an option, the horse should be exercised (ridden, driven, or longed) every day and, if possible, hand-walked or hand-grazed for as long as is practical at least once a day. This is a poor substitute for pasture turnout, but it is a vast improvement on spending all day and night confined to a stall or yard.

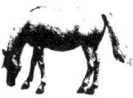

In one recent study, the colic incidence was lower in horses that were turned out for more than 50% of the day (i.e. for more than 12 hours/day) than in horses that were stalled for more than 50% of the day.

Cold weather

Horses are well adapted to coping with cold weather, so unless the horse is sick, very thin, or body clipped, or wind chill factors are well into the negative figures, cold weather is no excuse for not turning a horse out for at least a few hours each day. Horses are also well designed to cope with rain.

4. Minimize Changes

Several studies have shown that changes in the horse's diet, housing, and activity level increase the risk for colic. Of these three factors, dietary changes carry the most risk for colic. So, keep the horse's digestive system running like clockwork by following these guidelines:

❖ make any dietary changes slowly, over a period of 1–2 weeks (see Adaptability, on the next page)

• it is usually safe to suddenly *decrease* the amount of grain, but it can be harmful to suddenly begin feeding large amounts or rapidly increase the amount of grain fed

• when increasing the amount of concentrates, it is usually safe to increase the amount fed by ½ lb per day

- when making changes in hay feeding, start feeding the new hay, mixed with the old, before running out of the old batch
- try to buy hay of similar quality each time, preferably from the same source
❖ keep feeding times regular, even on weekends
❖ follow the suggestions for feeding concentrates on page 113 (the object being to minimize fluctuations within the colon)

When injury or illness requires that a horse be confined, even for only a few days, immediately decreasing or cutting out the grain is not a problem. In fact, it is the best strategy for avoiding digestive upsets, muscle problems (e.g. "tying up"), and behavioral problems associated with confinement. When the horse resumes training, grain can be gradually reintroduced, if needed.

 In horses with a history of colic, especially those that have had colic surgery, it is particularly important to avoid surprising the digestive system with sudden dietary changes.

Adaptability

The horse's digestive system is quite adaptable, when given sufficient time. The large and diverse population of micro-organisms in the cecum and colon responds to changes in the diet by adjusting the relative proportions of carbohydrate-fermenting and fiber-digesting microbes. This is a good strategy for ensuring digestive efficiency under a variety of feeding conditions.

But if the diet is changed too quickly, especially if the amount of carbohydrates is suddenly increased, an imbalance in the microbial population occurs which can be harmful. Colic is one potential consequence; laminitis (founder) is another.

However, not all horses that experience dietary changes or inconsistencies develop colic. For example, colic is uncommon in horses that are kept on pasture year-round, despite the fact that forage quality can change dramatically from one season to the next.

There is considerable variation in nutrient content (not to mention water content and digestibility) between lush spring grass and the mature, almost woody stalks of late summer.

The key here is that the nutrient composition changes gradually, over weeks or months. When sudden changes do occur, such as with the first spring flush or a greening-up after rain in the summer or early fall, horses on pasture sometimes develop mild spasmodic or "gas" colic from the sudden increase in readily digestible carbohydrates.

Studies have shown that the microbial population in the large intestine takes at least 2 weeks (and probably much longer) to adjust to the sudden introduction of carbohydrates. So when changing a horse's diet, do it gradually, giving the microbes time to make the necessary adjustments.

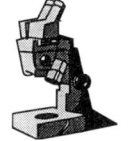

A recent study in ponies showed that suddenly adding grain to a hay-only diet dramatically alters the ratio of carbohydrate-fermenting and fiber-digesting microbes in the colon.

Three diets were compared: 100% grass hay; 70% hay and 30% rolled barley; and 50% hay and 50% barley.

Microbial adaptation to the 50% grain diet was incomplete, and fiber digestibility with both the 30% and the 50% grain diets was significantly depressed, even after 2 weeks on the new diet.

'Effect of the hay:grain ratio on digestive physiology and microbial ecosystem in ponies.' A de Fombelle, E Jacotot, C Drogoul, et al. Proceedings of the 16th Equine Nutrition and Physiology Symposium, 1999; pages 151–154.

Changes in housing and activity

A change in housing refers to changing from pasture turnout to confinement (or vice versa), or substantially changing the amount of turnout each day; not moving the horse to a different barn. (Although moving the horse to another barn may involve management or environmental factors that could increase the colic risk.) The changes most likely to increase the colic risk are those that decrease the amount of turnout time. The most likely factors involved are roughage availability, type, and quality, and the amount of daily activity. Psychological factors (lack of compatible company, a change in surroundings and routine, restriction, etc.) could also be involved in some situations.

Making housing changes. Changes in housing often are inevitable with changes in the season, with illness or injury, and when boarding a horse at a barn with limited turnout facilities. In these instances, pay particular attention to roughage and water intake and quality, provide daily exercise (if appropriate), and wherever possible, make any changes gradually.

Making changes in activity level. Changes in a horse's activity level are also inevitable from time to time. A *decrease* in activity is likely to affect the colic risk only if the horse is confined (e.g. stabled because of injury) but the amount of concentrates fed is not reduced. Turning a horse out at the end of the competition season is unlikely to increase the colic risk. An *increase* in activity could affect the colic risk if the diet is also changed (e.g. the amount of concentrates is increased) or if the horse finds the new workload stressful. Again, making any changes as gradually as possible minimizes the colic risk.

5. Feed Good Quality Feedstuffs

This strategy involves identifying and avoiding: (1) poor quality feeds and (2) spoiled or contaminated feeds.

Avoid poor quality feeds

To minimize the colic risk, feedstuffs of the best possible quality should be fed. Even if the horse in question is an overweight pony that no-one rides any more, and its propensity toward laminitis requires that it be confined to a dry lot and fed only grass hay, that hay should be of the best quality available. Poor quality hay not only has low nutritional value, it may cause impaction colic. It can be false economy to feed a poor quality hay as a way of controlling the horse's energy intake. It is often far better, both nutritionally and financially, to feed less of a good quality hay.

Hay quality. Good quality grass hay is leafy and soft, with relatively narrow, flexible stems; it should have few or no seed heads, and be free of weeds. A definite green color usually indicates high vitamin and protein content, whereas browning indicates a loss of nutrients. The North Carolina Cooperative Extension Service lists the following favorable characteristics of some legume hays:

- alfalfa—pale or bright green; small stems with abundant leaves; harvested in bud or when only 10% of the stems have flowers

- red clover—light or dark brown in color; 25–50% of the stems have flowers

- lespedeza—usually bright green; ideally, cut in early bloom

Forage testing is the most objective way of evaluating hay quality. In general, high-quality grass hays and grass/legume hay mixes have a total digestible nutrient (TDN) content of at least 57%. High-quality legume hays contain over 60% TDN.

Hay belly

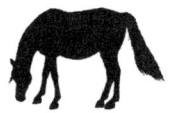

Some people are concerned that their horse will get a "hay belly" (a large abdomen) on a hay-only diet. But hay belly results from *feeding poor-quality roughage* and *lack of regular exercise*, not simply from feeding hay.*

The same is true for "grass belly." Typically, the roughage source is very fibrous and has a low protein content and digestibility, so the horse must eat more to supply its nutritional needs. Combine a colon filled with poorly digestible fibrous material, and poor muscle tone along the topline and in the abdominal muscles, and you get a flabby horse with a big belly.

(* When the deworming history is suspect, internal parasites should also be considered, particularly in immature horses.)

Unusual feed sources. Nontraditional feed sources (e.g. cottonseed, peanut, or rice hulls; food industry by-products) should not be fed to horses without first consulting an equine nutritionist. Just because a feedstuff is fed to cattle or other livestock does not mean it is suitable for feeding to horses. When using these materials, it is important to ensure adequate digestibility in horses, and that the final ration is balanced.

Avoid spoiled or contaminated feeds

Spoiled or contaminated feed should not be fed, regardless of whether the horse is willing to eat it. Certain micro-organisms found in these feeds produce toxins that can cause serious illness (including colic) and even death. Examples include botulism and mycotoxins (see page 70).

Identifying spoiled feed. Spoilage from improper harvesting or storage usually involves excessive moisture. Moldy feed typically has a musty smell and may seem dusty (the dust is actually a cloud of fungal spores). Moldy feed may also have tiny black spots (mildew), and improperly cured hay may feel quite warm and damp. However, feeds contaminated with botulism organisms or their toxins are impossible to identify without laboratory testing.

Botulism. Specific foodstuffs incriminated in botulism outbreaks in horses include silage (fermented forage usually fed to cattle); grass hay stored as large round bales; hay in which a dead pasture animal (e.g. mouse, bird, snake) has been baled; and grain in which a mouse, bird, or other small animal has died. Hay or grain in which an animal carcass is found should be thrown out.

Blister beetles. Another feed contaminant that causes colic, and sometimes even death, is blister beetles in alfalfa hay. As few as 2 or 3 beetles can cause severe colitis (see page 69). When feeding alfalfa hay, it is best to buy it from areas in which blister beetle infestation is unlikely (ask your local dealer where the hay came from) or from growers or dealers who can certify that the crop is beetle-free. It is worth inspecting each batch of alfalfa hay before feeding it. However, the distribution of beetles in infested alfalfa can be very patchy, so these small insects are easily missed.

Feeds formulated for other animals. Do not feed horses rations that are formulated for cattle, pigs, or poultry. For one thing, the nutritional needs of the various species are different. And for another, certain feed additives used in rations for other species can be harmful to horses; some are potentially fatal. The most striking example is monensin (and the related product, salinomycin; see page 90). When buying premixed feeds, it is best to choose rations that are specifically formulated for horses.

> Spoiled/contaminated feed should not be fed, regardless of whether the horse will eat it. Discard the feed if any of the following apply:
> - musty or moldy smell, or obvious mold or mildew
> - excessive moisture or heat (particularly with hay)
> - an animal carcass or animal part is found in the feed
> - blister beetles are found
>
> It is not worth risking the horse's health just to save a few dollars.

6. Ample Access to Fresh, Clean Water

Always make sure the horse has fresh water available, even if turning the horse out for just an hour or two. That hour or two can easily stretch into the whole morning or afternoon if you are held up or get busy with something else. As one study showed, the colic risk was increased in horses turned out, even for just a few hours, without water (see page 75).

Water intake during transport and exercise. Ensuring ample water intake during long-distance transport or exercise that lasts for several hours (e.g. trail riding, endurance events) can take a little planning. Stopping every few hours and offering the horse some water is worthwhile during long-distance transport, although it can be impractical when transporting several horses.

So, ensuring that the horse has free access to fresh, clean water on arrival is essential. Giving the horse mineral oil by stomach tube before a long trip is of doubtful value in preventing impaction colic; what the horse needs is water.

Adequate water intake is even more important in horses exercising for several hours, because the horse is losing body water and electrolytes in the form of sweat. Dehydration predisposes to large colon impaction, and loss or redistribution of electrolytes (especially potassium and calcium) adds to the colic risk by altering bowel motility. Adding electrolytes to the ration or administering an electrolyte-rich oral paste increases the horse's water intake, but it is very important that the horse be given access to plenty of fresh (i.e. electrolyte-free) water after such treatment.

Importance of clean water. Ensuring that the water is fresh and clean is important for at least two reasons:

❖ stale, tainted, or contaminated water is unpalatable, which reduces the horse's water intake
  • water with a high salt content can also be unpalatable

Water Requirements

The basic water requirement for a mature, nonlactating horse is about 15 liters, or 3½ gallons, per day (see page 75). But horses on hay-only diets often need more:

• the National Research Council (NRC) recommends supplying *2–3 liters of water per kilogram of dry matter fed,* per day
  – a 500-kg (1100-lb) horse fed 2% of its body weight (i.e. 10 kg) in dry matter needs 20–30 liters (4½–7 gallons) of water per day

• in hot weather, horses may require up to 8 liters/kg dry matter/day
  – that's up to 80 liters (18 gallons) per day for a 500-kg horse

Exercise further increases the water requirement by up to 300%.

- certain algae that multiply in stagnant water (e.g. ponds) during warm weather can cause serious illness
  - "blue-green" algae have been responsible for sudden death in whole groups of livestock

Heating the drinking water in winter. Some horses drink less when the water temperature is near-freezing. Even though a study in Michigan found that heating the drinking water in winter did not affect the colic risk, it is probably worth ensuring adequate water intake during the winter months by making warm water available. Suitable methods include using a bucket heater and providing hot water twice a day (see page 76).

7. Deworming Program

No single deworming program fits all horses. The ideal program depends on the type, number, and ages of the horses, the pasture management system, and the geographic location (i.e. environmental conditions throughout the year). It is best to work out an appropriate deworming program with your local veterinarian.

Efficacy of deworming products and programs

No deworming product is 100% effective in ridding every horse of all internal parasites. However, it is not necessary for a product to kill every worm in order to minimize the incidence of colic, optimize health and feed efficiency, and reduce pasture contamination with parasite eggs and larvae. As discussed in Chapter 2, the particular deworming product or schedule used may not be very important on its own—in terms of colic risk—provided the horse is regularly dewormed with an effective product.

Fecal egg counts. Whichever product and program is chosen (daily vs. monthly, 2-monthly, or 3-monthly; single product vs. rotation of products, etc.), it is worth having your veterinarian

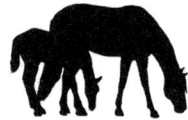

The fecal egg count is a measure of the number of parasite eggs per gram (epg) of manure. Aim to keep the herd's average fecal egg count below 100 epg.

perform fecal egg counts once or twice a year, to make sure the program is effective. However, it is important to realize that the standard method of performing fecal egg counts can be quite inaccurate in detecting tapeworms and encysted small strongyles. These two parasites require special consideration when designing a deworming program.

Tapeworms

Tapeworms are not eliminated by most dewormers. Products that are effective for treating tapeworm infestation in horses include:

- pyrantel pamoate (Strongid P®), given *once* at 2–3 times the standard dose, and repeated every 8 weeks if necessary
- daily pyrantel tartrate (Strongid C®) at the recommended dose for at least 2 weeks
- praziquantel (Droncit®), a tapeworm treatment used in dogs
  - currently, praziquantel is not approved for use in horses, although numerous equine veterinarians have found it safe and effective against tapeworms in horses
  - use this product only under veterinary advice

The tapeworm lifecycle involves a tiny mite that is active on the pasture only during the warmer months. Once the mite has eaten the tapeworm egg, it takes 2–4 months for the egg to develop into an infective stage. It then takes a couple more months for the infective stage that is swallowed with the mite by the grazing horse to mature into an adult tapeworm.

So, in temperate climates, it is usually recommended that treatment be given in the fall (after the first frost). In warmer areas, where the mites may remain active on the pasture well into the fall, treatment may be worthwhile throughout the fall and winter.

Is treatment for tapeworms really necessary? As discussed in Chapter 2, tapeworms do not cause obvious problems in most horses. However, they increase the risk for ileal impaction, intussusception involving the ileum and cecum, and spasmodic colic. So, deciding whether or not to treat for tapeworms may involve weighing the cost of treatment (which is quite low) against the potential for serious problems (also low; but when they do occur, problems such as ileal impaction and intussusception can require costly surgery). Occasionally, horses with heavy tapeworm burdens colic after treatment; however, serious problems are rare.

Two other points may aid in decision-making: (1) young horses (less than about 6 years of age) may be most at risk for tapeworm-related problems; and (2) horses with no pasture access do not need treatment, unless they have been on pasture in recent years.

Small strongyles

Small strongyles (cyathostomes) are among the most problematic internal parasites in horses. For part of their lifecycle, larvae are encysted in the bowel wall, insusceptible to most dewormers. The encysted stage typically lasts a few months (e.g. over winter), but it can persist for more than 2 years. A further problem is that infestation with encysted small strongyles is undetectable by fecal egg count. (Encysted larvae do not produce eggs.)

Ivermectin and most other dewormers* are effective against the adult worms. But only two currently available dewormers claim to be effective against the encysted stages:

* moxidectin (Quest®), at the recommended dose and schedule
* fenbendazole (Panacur®), when twice the standard dose is given each day for 5 days

These products are often referred to as *larvicidal* treatments, because they are targeted against the larvae. According to some studies, moxidectin is less effective against the *early* encysted stages (early third-stage larvae, or EL_3's) than the 5-day course of double-dose fenbendazole. And as the majority of encysted larvae are EL_3's, rather than late L_3's or L_4's, the fenbendazole program may be more effective than moxidectin.

(* It is now fairly common for adult small strongyles to be resistant to standard doses of pyrantel pamoate and to several of the benzimidazole anthelmintics (mebendazole, oxfendazole, thiabendazole, fenbendazole, etc.). However, it seems that the 5-day double-dose fenbendazole program is effective against both adult strongyles and encysted larvae.)

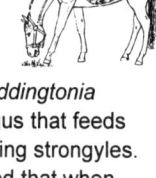

Biological control of cyathostomes was the subject of a recent study in Louisiana. *Duddingtonia flagrans* is a fungus that feeds on worms, including strongyles. This study showed that when horses were fed the harmless fungal spores, the number of strongyle larvae on the pasture around the manure piles was reduced an average of 80%.

When to treat. When to use the larvicidal treatment depends on geographic location, time of year, pasture management, and the deworming program. As infective larvae are picked up while the horse is grazing, a common recommendation for horses in cooler climates is to use the larvicidal treatment in the fall, after the grazing season has ended.

In areas of the country in which horses may graze year-round, where in the deworming program to include the larvicidal treatment should be a decision for you and your veterinarian to make together. Hoechst-Roussel, the manufacturer of Panacur, recommends using the larvicidal treatment in July for horses in the south-central states or southwest, and in May and again in November for horses in the deep south. They also recommend giving every newly introduced horse the larvicidal treatment on arrival—a very good strategy.

Strongid C. Daily pyrantel tartrate (Strongid C® or its generic equivalent) is not effective against encysted small strongyles. But when used consistently, it effectively prevents new infections, and thus invasion of the bowel wall with incoming larvae. However, before beginning the Strongid C program, adult horses should be given a larvicidal treatment (either moxidectin or fenbendazole) to remove any encysted larvae already present.

8. Regular Dental Care

Regular dental care means having the horse's teeth examined every 6–12 months by an equine veterinarian or reputable equine dentist. Whether or not the teeth need floating (or more involved procedures) this frequently will depend on the horse's age, head/jaw conformation, and diet. Regular dental examination is particularly important in old horses.

9. Environmental Management

In terms of colic incidence, good environmental management includes minimizing the following:

- ❖ opportunities for intake of "foreign" materials (baling twine, rope, sand, etc.)
    - inspect hay for baling twine, sticks, and other foreign materials before feeding it
    - do not leave baling twine lying around where curious horses can nibble on it, and possibly swallow it
    - avoid using rubber fencing, particularly with young horses; swallowed pieces of rubber can cause an obstruction
    - see page 136 for recommendations on reducing sand intake
- ❖ the incentive for behavioral problems ("vices")
    - turn horses out for as much of the day as possible, preferably with compatible company

- make sure that stalled horses always have hay and can see other horses nearby; provide stall toys if necessary
- ❖ exposure to poisonous plants and chemicals
  - inspect the pasture for poisonous plants; contact your county extension agent for help in identifying suspect plants
  - do not overgraze pastures; well-fed horses usually avoid poisonous plants
  - follow the label instructions when using insecticides, and store all harmful chemicals away from feed storage areas
  - do not administer any prescription drugs (including anti-inflammatory drugs) without or against veterinary advice

10. Pay Attention

This strategy is not intended to point the finger at people whose horses have colicked. Horses can and do colic under the best of management situations and with the most caring and diligent of owners. The following is not an exhaustive list, but is simply meant as a reminder of some common sources of problems:

- ❖ check feeders before each meal to see that the horse is eating all its feed
- ❖ if the horse is leaving feed, check the feed quality before investigating a problem with the horse (unless, of course, the horse appears to be sick)
  - moist feed additives can quickly turn any leftover feed sour in warm weather, and high-fat products may become rancid
  - check each new batch of hay for foreign material, mold, and overall quality (see pages 119–120)
- ❖ note the amount, color, and consistency of the horse's manure when cleaning stalls or paddocks

- monitor the amount horses are drinking if water is provided in a bucket or trough
  - this is particularly important in very hot and very cold weather
  - check automatic waterers daily, especially in the winter (when water pipes can freeze)
- when horses are fed in groups, watch to make sure each horse gets its share of feed
  - add an extra pile of hay to prevent fighting and ensure that every horse gets enough
  - when feeding grain or supplements, feed each horse separately
- monitor each horse's body weight regularly, and keep records throughout the year
- check pastured horses at least once a day to make sure they are well and have plenty of water

> Horses can colic under the best of management situations. But good management minimizes the incidence of most types of colic.

  - check broodmares at least twice a day during the last few months of pregnancy and the first few months after foaling
- regularly inspect pastures by walking through them
  - what may seem like a reasonable amount of grass from a distance can be meager up close, or consist mostly of weeds
  - horses are selective grazers, often leaving grass that seems fine to us; don't assume that what they've left they'll eat later
  - inspect pastures frequently toward the end of the grazing season as the grass matures and becomes very dry
  - provide good quality hay if the amount of palatable grass in the pasture declines significantly

Preventing Specific Types of Colic

Most of the following recommendations for preventing specific types of colic, or preventing colic in particular types of horses or situations, are based more on practical experience and extrapolation from clinical studies than on "hard data" from scientific research. Hopefully, in the next few years studies into particular types of colic will allow more specific recommendations.

Spasmodic or "Gas" Colic

Spasmodic colic is the most common type of colic in adult horses. Probably the two most frequently incriminated factors are high-carbohydrate diets (e.g. grain, lush pasture) and internal parasites. Implementing the 10 management strategies discussed in the first part of the chapter can substantially reduce the incidence of spasmodic colic. The following recommendations are especially important:

- ❖ keep the amount of concentrates (grain and grain-based sweet feed and pellets) to a minimum
    - limit the total amount fed in each meal, and feed roughage (e.g. chopped or cubed hay, beet pulp) with the concentrates
- ❖ do not suddenly turn horses out onto lush spring pasture; instead, gradually increase the grazing time over 1–2 weeks
- ❖ feed hay to pastured horses during the spring flush, even though there may be plenty of grass
    - most horses on lush pasture will eat a surprising amount of hay; in fact, they may need it to meet their roughage requirements (see page 108)
    - if necessary, limit the time spent on lush pasture until the grass matures a little

- provide daily exercise—every day, in some form
- maintain a regular deworming program
  - in some horses, daily Strongid C® can reduce the incidence of repeated bouts of colic

Large Colon Impactions

Most large colon impactions can be prevented by following the 10 strategies discussed earlier. Particularly important are providing:

- good quality roughage, especially hay that is not too mature
  - poor-quality roughage is one of the key factors in most impactions, whether of the large colon, small colon, or ileum
  - selecting good quality hay is discussed further on page 119
- access to fresh, clean water at all times
  - many large colon impactions occur when water intake is reduced for any reason
  - if necessary, add salt to the diet or provide a salt block to encourage the horse to drink more
- daily exercise
- as much pasture turnout as possible

Avoiding Colic at Shows and Competitions

The most common types of colic in horses at shows or other competitions away from home are spasmodic colic and large colon impaction. The most likely factors are the stress of transport and strange surroundings, a change of water and routine (feeding, exercise, and turnout schedules), and in some cases, a change of bedding. Thus, the most effective preventive strategy involves minimizing changes:

- ❖ feed the same ration as fed at home, including hay, and keep to the horse's regular feeding schedule
- ❖ make sure the horse has good quality hay at all times
- ❖ make sure the horse has fresh, clean water at all times
  - with horses that are reluctant to drink "strange" water, take water from home or flavor the water with something the horse likes (e.g. molasses, peppermint)
  - add salt or electrolytes to the ration or provide a salt block to encourage the horse to drink

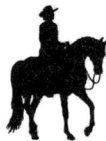

The incidence of colic at shows and other competitions at which the horse must be boarded can be reduced by *minimizing change.*

- ❖ exercise the horse each day; longe, ride, or drive the horse on days when you are not competing
- ❖ hand-graze the horse for at least 30 minutes every day, if there is a suitable area; otherwise, hand-walk the horse
- ❖ if possible, use the same type of bedding used at home
  - horses bedded on shavings at home will often eat straw bedding if there is insufficient hay available
  - to avoid impaction colic in horses that must be bedded on straw, feed plenty of good quality hay
- ❖ if possible, see that the horse has compatible company

Large Colon Displacements

Most large colon displacements can be prevented by following the 10 strategies discussed earlier. Of particular importance are:

- ❖ keeping the amount of concentrates to a minimum
  - feeding high-grain rations is a common factor in horses with large colon displacements

- feeding plenty of high-quality roughage
- providing regular exercise and as much turnout as possible
- maintaining an effective deworming program

Large colon twists in broodmares

The reason large colon twists (volvulus) are most common in broodmares, especially after foaling, is not known. But it is conceivable that in recently foaled mares it is a combination of two factors: abdominal fill and altered bowel motility.

Abdominal fill. During pregnancy, the growing fetus occupies progressively more of the abdomen, such that in late pregnancy, much of the abdomen is taken up by the fetus. After the mare has foaled, but before the abdominal wall has regained its nonpregnant tone, there is suddenly a lot of extra room in the abdomen.

Altered bowel motility. With the large colon so mobile, it is perhaps surprising that displacements and twists are not more common after foaling. This suggests that abnormal bowel motility is a key player. The energy requirements in late pregnancy and in the first few weeks of lactation are high, and most often are met by increasing the amount of concentrates fed. This is an appropriate nutritional strategy. However, as discussed in Chapter 2, large carbohydrate meals cause an increase in colon gas, and a cycle of rapid inflation and gradual deflation may be set up in the colons of horses fed large amounts of grain.

> Feeding plenty of good quality roughage is important for preventing large colon displacements and twists, particularly in the first few weeks after foaling.

This effect, together with altered bowel motility caused by the products of carbohydrate fermentation, could make displacement more likely. It also explains how displacements and twists can occur before foaling and in nonpregnant mares and male horses.

There has also been some suggestion that marginally low calcium levels (which can affect bowel motility) could be involved in the first few weeks after foaling, when milk production is high.

Recommendations. Based on these theories, recommendations for preventing large colon twists in broodmares include:

- feeding plenty of good quality roughage, particularly in the first few weeks after foaling
  - in late-pregnant mares, roughage intake may be limited by the size of the fetus, so forage quality is very important
- feeding a high-fat balanced ration, in place of traditional concentrates, to meet the mare's increased energy needs
  - a mare's nutritional needs increase in late pregnancy and are highest during the first 2–3 months of lactation
- ensuring adequate calcium intake in recently foaled mares

Ileal Impactions

Ileal impactions can occur for a variety of reasons, although the big two are tapeworms and poor-quality hay, especially coastal Bermudagrass hay. Treating for tapeworms is discussed on page 124. Given that there is some evidence of an association between ileal impaction and feeding coastal Bermuda hay, at least in the southeastern U.S., it may be wise for owners in this part of the country to do one or other of the following:

- if the coastal hay that is available is not of good quality (green, soft, and fragrant), buy another type of hay instead
- if lower-quality coastal hay must be fed, mix it with *good quality* hay of another type (either a grass or a legume hay)
  - the goal is to feed less of the coastal hay without reducing the horse's overall roughage intake

Mixing coastal hay with a legume hay, such as alfalfa, clover, or lespedeza, is a good strategy. Legume hays are a little higher in digestible energy and other nutrients than grass hays, which could make up for the lower quality of the coastal hay. The average nutrient composition for commonly fed hays is listed in Table 3-3 on page 148.

(Note: Ileal impaction does not appear to be a problem when horses graze coastal Bermuda grass pasture.)

> When feeding any type of hay, buy the best quality hay available, preferably hay cut early in the season. Digestibility declines the later in the growth cycle the plant is cut.
>
> If nutritional analysis is available, choose a hay that looks good and has a total digestible nutrient (TDN) content of >55%.

Small Colon Impactions in Miniature Horses

Three factors appear to be important in preventing small colon and other impactions in Miniature Horses:

- ❖ feed only high-quality roughage
  - when buying hay, choose the leafiest, least stemmy hay available
- ❖ continue regular dental care
  - because of the shape of their heads, Minis are prone to dental problems throughout their lives
  - dental care is particularly important in young Minis
- ❖ keep the environment free of swallowable foreign materials, especially when raising young Minis

Miniature Horses are also susceptible to the various types of colic that occur in larger horses, so the 10 management strategies discussed earlier in the chapter are worthwhile when raising these little horses.

Sand Colic

The most common means of preventing sand colic is by regularly feeding psyllium (Metamucil® or its equine or generic equivalent). However, veterinary opinions are divided on the effectiveness of psyllium in ridding the large colon of sand. A couple of well constructed studies have shown that adding psyllium to the diet, or even directly into the digestive tract during surgery, does not increase sand removal from the horse's large colon. But some veterinarians firmly believe that feeding psyllium or administering it by stomach tube does aid in elimination of sand from the bowel and in prevention of sand colic.

Researchers at the University of Florida recently conducted a study on sand intake and removal in horses, with the following results:

- significant amounts of sand may be consumed when grain is fed in contact with sand, or when horses retrieve grain dropped onto sand

- very little sand is consumed when grass hay is fed on sand
  - but because of its small leaf size and high palatability, more sand may be taken in when alfalfa hay is fed on sand

- feeding grass hay at 1.5% of body weight per day was just as effective in ridding the bowel of sand as was feeding psyllium (either in a single dose or twice daily in feed)
  - grass hay at 2.5% of body weight was even more effective

The authors concluded that "hay may be primarily responsible for movement of sand through the gut and that the larger the hay intake (2.5% vs. 1.5%) the quicker the sand moves through."

'A group of experiments on the management of sand intake and removal in equine.' (sic) S Lieb and J Weise. *Proceedings of the 16th Equine Nutrition and Physiology Symposium*, 1999; page 257.

Some veterinarians recommend feeding psyllium on a daily basis to horses on sandy pastures. Others suggest periodic treatments (e.g. once or twice a month). Mineral oil and bran are of little or no benefit in ridding the bowel of accumulated sand. Mineral oil may, however, be of some use when treating sand impactions. (Although if the impaction is not relieved and the horse must go to surgery, mineral oil in the colon can make the surgery more difficult and compromise bowel healing.)

Management. Regardless of whether psyllium is used, *it is important to minimize the horse's opportunity to eat more sand:*

- when feeding horses outside, minimize sand intake with one of the following methods
  - raise outside feeders off the ground and feed hay in a hay net or rack
  - use feeders and hay nets/racks that minimize spillage
  - lay a large sheet of plywood, carpet, or rubber matting beneath the feeder and keep it swept clean of sand
  - feed the horses inside, then turn them out later
- practice good pasture management to minimize sand intake during grazing
  - avoid overstocking and overgrazing
  - improve the pastures, where appropriate
  - provide good quality hay when the pasture quality declines

Enteroliths

Recommendations for preventing enteroliths in at-risk horses center on limiting the amount of protein, magnesium, and phosphorus in the diet. At-risk horses include Arabians in "enterolith territory" (see page 93) and horses that have had enteroliths removed or have been seen to pass small stones in their manure.

Mineral intake

Enteroliths are primarily composed of magnesium, ammonium, and phosphorus. Horses with enteroliths reportedly have higher concentrations of these (and other) minerals in their colons. So, it may be worth having the mineral content of the horse's diet (grain, hay, pasture, and supplements) and water analyzed.

Dietary adjustments can then be made to reduce the horse's intake of magnesium, protein, and phosphorus to levels more in line with the NRC recommendations for that horse's age, size, and activity level. Daily protein and phosphorus requirements for adult horses are listed in Table 3-2, on page 147; daily magnesium requirements are given below.

Recommended dietary levels of magnesium

Body Weight	Maintenance (grams of Mg/day)	Working Horses (grams of Mg/day)
200 kg (440 lb)	3.0	4.3 - 6.8
400 kg (880 lb)	6.0	7.7 - 12.3
500 kg (1100 lb)	7.5	9.4 - 15.1
600 kg (1320 lb)	9.0	11.2 - 17.8

Common feeding recommendations include:

- ❖ eliminating alfalfa from the diet or feeding it "diluted" with some other roughage source (e.g. grass hay)
  - note: the horse's overall roughage intake should not be decreased in the process
- ❖ limiting the amount of grain and bran in the diet
  - compared with most forages, grains are high in phosphorus (see Table 3-3, on page 148)
  - as it is a grain by-product, bran is also high in phosphorus

Nidus

Most enteroliths form around a central core, or nidus, most often some type of foreign material such as a piece of wire, a pebble, or baling twine. So, keeping the horse's feed and environment clean and free of "potential niduses" may be important in preventing enterolith formation. Fibrous plant material can also act as a nidus, so once again, roughage quality is important.

Acidifiers

Enteroliths form more readily when the contents of the colon are less acidic than normal. In fact, outside the body the outer few millimeters of an enterolith can be dissolved by placing the stone in a mildly acidic solution such as vinegar. This fact has led some people to recommend feeding cider vinegar (e.g. 1 cup twice a day, mixed in feed) to at-risk horses.

But although one study showed that feeding cider vinegar twice daily to ponies increased the acidity in the colon, existing enteroliths are dissolved extremely slowly and only partially. This strategy is not effective with large enteroliths, and there is no evidence that feeding cider vinegar prevents enteroliths from forming.

Gastric Ulcers

There are two separate regions in the lining, or mucosa, of the horse's stomach where ulcers can form: the glandular mucosa and the squamous mucosa. The glandular mucosa is in the lower part of the stomach and is the "active" area; it is the site of acid and enzyme production. Protective substances such as bicarbonate and mucus are also secreted by the glandular mucosa. The squamous mucosa is in the upper part of the stomach; it does not secrete acid, enzymes, or protective substances.

Although gastric ulcer disease is not fully understood in horses, it is known that the site of ulceration (glandular vs. squamous mucosa) depends on the cause. NSAID-induced ulcers occur in the glandular mucosa. These drugs cause ulceration by inhibiting production of prostaglandins—substances that have a role in protecting the mucosa from erosion by gastric acid. Stress-induced ulcers occur in the "unprotected" squamous mucosa.

Preventing NSAID-induced ulcers

As discussed in Chapter 2, any nonsteroidal anti-inflammatory drug (NSAID) can cause ulceration, although phenylbutazone ("bute") and flunixin (Banamine®) are most often incriminated. Preventing NSAID-induced ulcers involves:

- using these drugs only when necessary
- keeping the dosage and frequency as low as possible and the duration of treatment as short as possible
  - do not combine two or more NSAIDs (e.g. do not give bute and Banamine together)
- making sure the horse always has plenty of fresh water

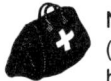

New-generation NSAIDs (COX-2 inhibitors) that have few gastrointestinal side effects are being developed and tested. But studies investigating their effectiveness and safety in horses are not yet completed.

Corn oil. Vegetable oils, particularly corn oil, are relatively high in linoleic acid, which the body can use to produce the prostaglandins that help protect the mucosa from acid damage. It has been suggested that adding ½ to 1 cup of corn oil to the feed twice a day may help protect the stomach from ulceration. Whether or not this strategy is effective remains to be seen, but it does little harm.

Preventing stress-induced ulcers

Most horses with stress-induced ulcers respond to the 10 simple management strategies discussed earlier in the chapter. Of most importance are the following:

- ❖ make sure the horse has good quality roughage at all times
  - food buffers the gastric acid, so keeping food in the stomach helps protect the mucosa from acid damage
  - unlike grains and processed feeds, hay remains in the stomach for several hours, which may help limit acid damage
- ❖ minimize the amount of concentrates in the diet, and feed the concentrates mixed with roughage
  - some fermentation of carbohydrates occurs in the stomach, so feeding grain may add to the acid load in the stomach
  - when a high-energy diet must be fed, use a high-fat balanced ration and feed it in several small meals per day
- ❖ provide as much pasture turnout as possible, for exercise, grazing, and social interaction
- ❖ keep to regular feeding and exercise schedules

As suggested by one recent study, feeding alfalfa may reduce the incidence and severity of gastric ulcers (see page 67). Adding corn oil to the diet may also be of benefit, both to help prevent ulcers and as a supplemental energy source.

Acid suppressors. Histamine type 2 (H-2) blockers, such as cimetidine (Tagamet®) and ranitidine (Zantac®), are the mainstay of ulcer therapy in foals and adult horses. But whether they are effective for ulcer prevention is not clear.

Recently, omeprazole, a potent acid suppressor used to treat gastric ulcers in humans, has become available in paste-form for use in horses (Gastrogard®). Studies indicate that this drug speeds ulcer healing and can prevent new ulcers from forming in horses in high-stress occupations (e.g. race training). But whether this strategy will be cost-effective and safe long-term needs further evaluation.

Right Dorsal Colitis

Inflammation and ulceration of the right dorsal colon is most often associated with NSAID use (particularly phenylbutazone and flunixin [Banamine]). Thus, preventing right dorsal colitis involves avoiding NSAID use unless absolutely necessary; keeping the dose, frequency, and duration of treatment low when these drugs are needed; and making sure the horse has access to fresh, clean water at all times. The harmful effects of NSAIDs are more likely in horses that become even mildly dehydrated.

Other less common causes of right dorsal colitis are Potomac horse fever and internal parasites. Vaccinating against Potomac horse fever, preventing access to natural water courses (rivers, streams) in areas where the disease is common, and using an effective deworming program help prevent colitis from these agents.

Dietary management. Horses recovering from right dorsal colitis are often kept on diets low in long-stem roughage (i.e. hay). Complete pelleted feeds are recommended, both in the recovery period and long-term. However, good quality hay may actually be beneficial in these horses because the proportion of volatile fatty acids produced during its microbial digestion in the large colon favors repair of ulcerated areas.

Verminous Arteritis *(S. vulgaris* Infestation)

Preventing colic caused by *Strongylus vulgaris* (redworms or bloodworms) is a simple matter of regularly using a dewormer that is effective against the larval stages of this parasite. Suitable products include ivermectin, moxidectin (Quest®), fenbendazole (Panacur® at double the standard dose, daily for five days), and pyrantel tartrate (Strongid C®, daily). Consult with your veterinarian to devise a suitable deworming program for your horses. Good pasture management is also important, regardless of how effective a particular product or program claims to be.

Meconium Impaction in Foals

Some breeders and veterinarians give enemas to all newborn foals, simply to prevent meconium impaction. This approach has merit in that the foals that may have developed meconium impaction have been spared the stress and pain of impaction. However, some people feel this is excessive and prefer simply to observe all newborn foals closely, giving enemas only to those having difficulty passing their meconium. In most foals, nursing from the mare and moving around are sufficient to stimulate bowel activity for meconium passage.

All foals strain a little when passing their meconium; this is normal. If the foal has been straining for more than an hour without passing anything, it is usually safe to give it a mild enema. But if the foal still does not pass its meconium or continues to strain after passing some meconium, call a veterinarian rather than giving another enema.

Roundworm (Ascarid) Impactions

The horses most at risk for roundworm impaction are foals, weanlings, or yearlings that:

- ❖ have never been dewormed or that have an unknown or questionable deworming history,
- ❖ look obviously parasitized (e.g. pot-bellied with a long, scruffy, dull haircoat), even if they have been dewormed, or
- ❖ have large, white worms in their manure or protruding from their anus

To prevent roundworm impaction in heavily parasitized foals, it is best to deworm the foal with a moderately effective product, such as fenbendazole (Panacur®) or thiabendazole at the standard dosage. This approach reduces worm numbers without killing all the adult worms at once and creating an obstruction. After 1–2 weeks, the foal can be dewormed at a higher dosage or with a more effective product, such as ivermectin. Some veterinarians administer mineral oil by stomach tube to prevent roundworm impaction after deworming in these foals.

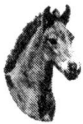

Most veterinarians recommend starting a foal's deworming program at 6–8 weeks of age. When deworming older foals (over about 3 months of age) for the first time, it may be best to use a dewormer that is only moderately effective against roundworms, such as the standard dosage of fenbendazole or thiabendazole.

Treatement at a higher dosage or with a more effective product (e.g. ivermectin) can be repeated 1–2 weeks later.

The most effective way of preventing roundworm impaction is by preventing roundworm infestation. This is as simple as maintaining an effective deworming program for all horses on the farm, especially broodmares and foals, and maintaining good pasture management. Roundworm eggs are particularly resilient, so each new foal crop is at risk. Most veterinarians recommend beginning the foal's deworming program at 6–8 weeks of age, with deworming every 2 months or daily Strongid C®.

Colic in Older Horses

Horses older than about 15 years of age are prone to certain types of colic that are not preventable (e.g. strangulating lipoma, epiploic foramen entrapment, tumors; see page 48). But like any other adult horse, older horses are also prone to spasmodic colic, large colon impactions, sand colic, etc.

The 10 strategies outlined earlier in the chapter should minimize the incidence and impact of these preventable types of colic in aged horses. Of particular importance are:

❖ feeding plenty of high-quality roughage

❖ feeding a high-fat balanced ration if the horse's weight cannot be maintained on roughage alone

- feed a ration that is specifically formulated for older horses
- old horses may be less competitive in a group-feeding situation, so it is best to feed them separately

❖ dental examination every 6 months (or as recommended by a veterinarian or equine dentist)

❖ monitoring pastured horses at least once a day

It is often said that old age is not a disease. With good management (and a little luck), it is possible to keep most horses healthy and active well into their 20's.

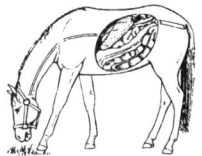

Table 3-1: Dietary proportions for specific types of horse or activity.

Type of Horse & Activity Level	Roughage (% of diet)	Concentrates (% of diet)
Maintenance*	100%	0%
Working horses:**		
light work	65%	35%
moderate work	50%	50%
intense work	35%	65%
Breeding:		
breeding stallion	70%	30%
pregnant mare (9–10 mths)	80%	20%
pregnant mare (11 mths)	70%	30%
lactating mare (first 3 mths)	50%	50%
lactating mare (4+ mths)	65%	35%
Growing horses:		
weanling	30%	70%
yearling	40%	60%
2-year-old (not in training)	65%	35%
2-year-old (in training)	50%	50%

* *maintenance* requirements are those needed to maintain body weight in an adult horse that does little or no regular work

** *light work* is that performed by a show horse training for and participating in English or Western Pleasure classes, equitation, etc.

moderate work is that performed by a working ranch horse, or a horse performing more athletic activities than showing (roping, cutting, barrel racing, jumping, etc.)

intense work includes race training, polo, and 3-day-eventing

Note: regardless of the ratio of hay to grain, all horses should be fed at least 1% of their body weight per day of good quality roughage (pasture and/or hay).

(From *Nutrient Requirements of Horses*, 5th edition, National Research Council, National Academy Press, Washington, DC, 1989.)

3–Strategies for Preventing Colic

Table 3-2: Daily nutrient requirements for adult horses of various sizes and activity levels.

Body Weight & Activity Level	Dig. Energy (Mcal/day)	Crude Protein (grams/day)	Calcium (grams/day)	Phosphorus (grams/day)
200 kg (440 lb)				
maintenance	7.4	296	8	6
light work	9.3	370	11	8
moderate work	11.1	444	14	10
intense work	14.8	592	18	13
400 kg (880 lb)				
maintenance	13.4	536	16	11
light work	16.8	670	20	15
moderate work	20.1	804	25	17
intense work	26.8	1072	33	23
500 kg (1100 lb)				
maintenance	16.4	656	20	14
light work	20.5	820	25	18
moderate work	24.6	984	30	21
intense work	32.8	1312	40	29
600 kg (1320 lb)				
maintenance	19.4	776	24	17
light work	24.3	970	30	21
moderate work	29.1	1164	36	25
intense work	38.8	1552	47	34

Dig. Energy = digestible energy, measured in megacalories per day (Mcal/day)

for explanations of maintenance and the various levels of work, see Table 3-1

(From *Nutrient Requirements of Horses*, 5th edition, National Research Council, National Academy Press, Washington, DC, 1989.)

Table 3-3: Nutrient composition of some common feedstuffs.

Feed	Digestible Energy (Mcal/kg of feed)	Crude Protein (%)	Calcium (%)	Phosphorus (%)
Forages				
alfalfa hay				
early bloom	2.24 - 2.48	18.0 - 19.9	1.28 - 1.41	0.19 - 0.21
midbloom	2.07 - 2.28	17.0 - 18.7	1.24 - 1.37	0.22 - 0.24
full bloom	1.97 - 2.17	15.5 - 17.0	1.08 - 1.19	0.22 - 0.24
bromegrass				
hay (mid)	1.87 - 2.13	12.6 - 14.4	0.25 - 0.29	0.25 - 0.28
hay (mature)	1.57 - 1.69	5.6 - 6.0	0.24 - 0.26	0.20 - 0.22
clover hay				
alsike	1.71 - 1.95	12.4 - 14.2	1.14 - 1.30	0.22 - 0.25
red	1.96 - 2.22	13.2 - 15.0	1.22 - 1.38	0.22 - 0.24
coastal Bermuda				
fresh grass	0.72 - 2.38	3.8 - 12.6	0.15 - 0.49	0.08 - 0.27
hay (early)	1.92 - 2.17	10.6 - 12.0	0.35 - 0.40	0.24 - 0.27
hay (midbloom)	1.96 - 2.10	10.9 - 12.0	0.30 - 0.32	0.19 - 0.20
hay (late bloom)	1.74 - 1.87	7.3 - 7.8	0.24 - 0.26	0.17 - 0.18
fescue				
fresh grass	0.70 - 2.22	4.7 - 15.0	0.16 - 0.51	0.12 - 0.37
hay (full bloom)	1.89 - 2.06	11.8 - 12.9	0.40 - 0.43	0.29 - 0.32
hay (mature)	1.76 - 1.95	9.8 - 10.8	0.37 - 0.41	0.27 - 0.30
Johnson grass				
hay	1.50 - 1.66	6.7 - 7.5	0.80 - 0.89	0.27 - 0.30
Kentucky bluegrass				
fresh grass	0.64 - 2.09	5.4 - 17.4	0.15 - 0.50	0.14 - 0.44
hay (full bloom)	1.58 - 1.71	8.2 - 8.9	0.24 - 0.26	0.25 - 0.27
lespedeza hay				
common	1.93 - 2.13	11.4 - 12.6	1.07 - 1.18	0.17 - 0.19
kobe	1.96 - 2.08	10.0 - 10.6	1.11 - 1.18	0.32 - 0.34
orchard grass				
fresh grass	0.54 - 2.29	2.8 - 12.8	0.06 - 0.25	0.05 - 0.39
hay (early)	1.94 - 2.17	11.4 - 12.8	0.24 - 0.27	0.30 - 0.34
hay (late bloom)	1.72 - 1.90	7.6 - 8.4	0.24 - 0.26	0.27 - 0.30
pangola grass				
fresh grass	0.39 - 1.95	1.8 - 9.1	0.08 - 0.38	0.04 - 0.22
hay (early)	1.72 - 1.89	9.2 - 10.1	0.53 - 0.58	0.19 - 0.21
hay (midbloom)	1.62 - 1.78	6.7 - 7.4	0.42 - 0.46	0.21 - 0.23
hay (full/late bloom)	1.41 - 1.55	5.7 - 6.3	0.35 - 0.38	0.16 - 0.18

Feed	Digestible Energy (Mcal/kg of feed)	Crude Protein (%)	Calcium (%)	Phosphorus (%)
Forages, cont'd				
ryegrass				
fresh grass	0.51 - 2.20	4.0 - 17.9	0.15 - 0.65	0.09 - 0.41
hay (late bloom)	1.57 - 1.84	8.8 - 10.3	0.53 - 0.62	0.29 - 0.34
timothy hay				
early bloom	1.83 - 2.06	9.6 - 10.8	0.45 - 0.51	0.25 - 0.29
midbloom	1.77 - 1.99	8.6 - 9.7	0.43 - 0.48	0.20 - 0.23
full bloom	1.73 - 1.94	7.2 - 8.1	0.38 - 0.43	0.18 - 0.20
Grains				
barley	3.17 - 3.68	11.0 - 14.0	0.05	0.34 - 0.38
corn	3.38 - 3.84	9.1 - 10.4	0.05	0.27 - 0.31
oats	2.85 - 3.36	9.1 - 14.0	0.05 - 0.11	0.31 - 0.38
wheat				
red	3.41 - 3.86	11.4 - 14.6	0.03 - 0.05	0.36 - 0.42
white	3.54 - 3.92	10.6 - 11.8	0.06 - 0.07	0.30 - 0.33

1 kg (1000 grams) = 2.2 lb   1 lb = 0.45 kg (454 grams)

To convert Mcal/kg to Mcal/lb, divide by 2.2
   e.g. 3.5 Mcal/kg ÷ 2.2 = 1.6 Mcal/lb

To convert % to grams per kilogram, move the decimal point one place to the right
   e.g. 11.8 % crude protein = 118 grams of protein per kilogram (g/kg) of feed

Note: Growing conditions can dramatically affect the nutrient content of feedstuffs; the values in these tables are guidelines only. Feed analysis is recommended to determine the exact nutrient content of a particular batch of feed.

(From *Nutrient Requirements of Horses,* 5th edition, National Research Council, National Academy Press, Washington, DC, 1989.)

Box 3-1: An example of ration formulation for an adult horse.

This example uses an adult horse weighing 500 kg (1100 lb) and performing little regular work:

- the digestible energy (DE) requirement is 16.4 Mcal/day [Table 3-2]
- good quality timothy hay, cut midbloom, contains an average of 1.9 Mcal of DE per kilogram [Table 3-3]
- if the horse has no access to pasture, its energy requirements can be met by feeding 8.6 kg (19 lb) of hay per day (16.4 Mcal ÷ 1.9 Mcal/kg = 8.6 kg)
- this amount of hay also meets the horse's roughage requirement (1–2% of body weight per day); 8.6 kg of hay is 1.7% of this horse's body weight
- and it meets the horse's crude protein, calcium, and phosphorus needs
  - the crude protein requirement for this horse is 656 grams/day; 8.6 kg of this hay provides 774 grams of protein
  - the calcium requirement is 20 grams/day; this amount of hay provides 38.7 grams of calcium
  - the phosphorus requirement is 14 grams/day; this amount of hay provides 18 grams of phosphorus

---

Once this horse begins regular light exercise, its additional energy requirements could be met by adding grain to the diet:

- the horse's DE requirement is now 20.5 Mcal/day [Table 3-2]
  - feeding 8.6 kg/day of timothy hay supplies only 16.4 Mcal/day, leaving a deficit of 4.1 Mcal/day
- adding 1.3 kg (2.9 lb) of oats *or* 1.1 kg (2.5 lb) of corn *per day* makes up the deficit in DE
- the roughage requirement (1–2% of body weight) is met with this ration, and the diet is at least 65% roughage [Table 3-1]
- this ration also meets the horse's new crude protein, calcium, and phosphorus requirements
  - the crude protein requirement for this horse is now 820 grams/day; this ration provides 924 grams (oats) or 881 grams (corn) of protein
  - the calcium requirement is now 25 grams/day; this ration provides 39.7 grams (oats) or 39.3 grams (corn) of calcium
  - the phosphorus requirement is now 18 grams/day; this ration provides 22.5 grams (oats) or 21.2 grams (corn) of phosphorus

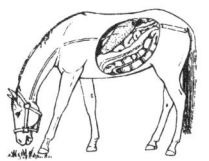

4

Managing Colic

(preventing disasters)

Not all cases of colic can be prevented. But a disastrous outcome (death or permanent disability) often *can be prevented* by monitoring the situation closely and knowing when to involve a veterinarian. Surgical techniques and survival rates have dramatically improved over the past two decades. But even so, the outcome generally is dictated by how long the condition was present without appropriate treatment. This chapter discusses ways that owners, trainers, and farm/barn managers can prevent disasters when managing an episode of colic in one of the horses in their care.

Recognizing the Signs

Successful management of a colic episode begins with early recognition and close monitoring. The signs of colic are listed on pages 2 to 5. In most cases, the first signs of colic are subtle behavioral changes, such as lying down more than usual or curling the upper lip, and disinterest in food. These signs are easily missed or disregarded, especially if the person in charge of the horse is unfamiliar with the particular horse's normal behavior patterns.

It is fairly common with simple obstructions (impactions, enteroliths, etc.) for colic signs to wax and wane—appearing and disappearing, or increasing and decreasing in severity—for several hours (or even days) before worsening. Consider this situation a warning sign that something other than mild spasmodic colic is present. In most of these cases, veterinary attention is necessary. Even if surgery is not needed, fluid therapy (either intravenously or by stomach tube) usually is required in horses that have been colicking for more than a few hours.

Determining the Severity

A good outcome—a healthy horse in as short a time as possible, with as little intervention and expense as possible—depends on someone determining early whether the colic bout is one of the mild types or is potentially serious. This involves assessing the horse's physical status and bowel function, and monitoring these aspects for improvement or deterioration.

Horses with colic that requires surgical correction typically make up only about 10% of all colic cases. But when the problem is severe enough to warrant surgery, the sooner it is recognized and surgery is performed, the better for all concerned—most importantly, the horse. In general, survival rates are highest and the incidence of complications is lowest when surgery is performed early. Also, the total hospitalization time (and therefore the bill) tends to be shorter (and lower) when surgery is performed early.

Assessing the Horse's Physical Status

In general, the more obvious the behavioral abnormalities, the more serious the colic episode. For example, a horse that is rolling and thrashing about, unresponsive to the handler's attempts to get the horse up, is in real trouble. But as discussed in Chapter 1, relying solely on the apparent degree of pain can be misleading.

The conclusions you reach from observing the horse's behavior should be backed up by assessing the horse's physical status; in particular, how its *cardiovascular system* is coping. Serious problems with the digestive tract cause dehydration, and absorption of bacterial toxins from inflamed or damaged bowel can compromise cardiovascular function. As a result, circulation to the tissues may be substantially decreased. These changes are manifested by the following abnormalities:

> **Assessing Physical Status**
>
> Assessing the horse's physical status is an important part of determining whether veterinary attention is needed. With a little know-how, any owner, trainer, or farm/barn manager can make the following assessments:
> - heart rate
> - gum color & capillary refill time
> - hydration status (body fluid balance), as indicated by gum moisture and skin elasticity
> - other signs of shock, such as cool extremities and weakness

- ❖ increased heart rate
- ❖ changes in gum color (pale, red, purple, or grey)
- ❖ increased capillary refill time (explained on page 158)
- ❖ tacky or dry gums, and prolonged tenting of the skin
- ❖ cool extremities (e.g. lower legs, ears)

Veterinarians use these observations to assess the seriousness of the situation. But they are simple things any owner, trainer, or manager can assess and monitor, without any special equipment.

Heart rate

A horse's heart rate can be measured a couple of ways. The easiest is to listen with a stethoscope over the horse's girth area, just behind or above the point of its left elbow, and count the heart beats over one minute. In young, very thin, or very fit horses, it is sometimes possible to feel the heart beat with your hand.

If the heartbeat cannot be heard or felt, you'll need to find a pulse. Three places at which a pulse can be felt on most horses are:

1. the side of the face, at the lower end of the facial crest (the bony ridge that runs from just below the eye to midway between eye and nostril)

    – a branch of the facial artery crosses the face just in front of the point where the facial crest ends

2. the side or lower edge of the lower jaw, just in front of the large cheek muscle (masseter muscle)

    – the facial artery and vein cross the underside of the jaw and run up the side of the face at this location

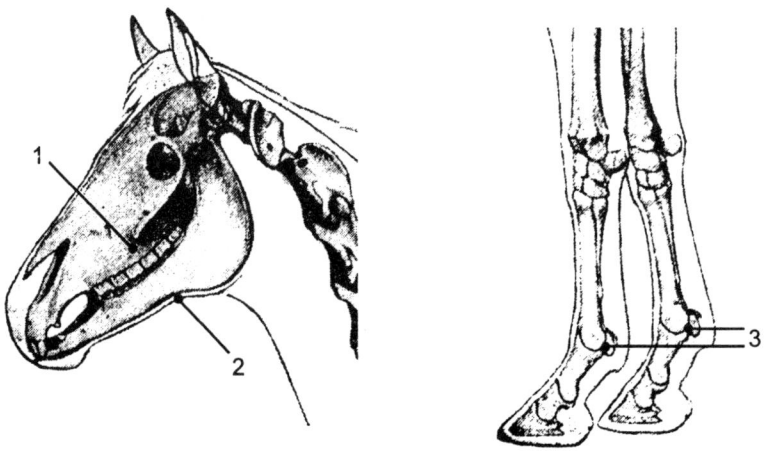

Figure 4-1: Locations at which the pulse rate may be measured.

3. both sides of the fetlock, toward the back of the leg
   - the digital arteries run down the outer edges of the sesamoid bones

Regardless of how or where the heart/pulse rate is measured, either count the number of beats over a full minute or count the number of beats over 30 seconds and double it. (If the horse is moving around too much, count the heart/pulse rate over 15 seconds and multiply by 4 to get the number of beats per minute.)

Normal heart rate. The normal resting heart rate for an average-size adult horse is in the range of 30–40 beats/minute. The rate tends to be a little higher, usually by 10–20 beats/minute, in smaller horses (e.g. young horses, ponies). In very young foals, the heart rate is normally in the range of 70–100 beats/minute.

Heart rate and colic severity. Pain alone can cause a moderate increase in heart rate, often into the 50–60 beats/minute range (adults). However, it is fairly common for horses with mild-to-moderate colic to have heart rates of less than 50 beats/minute. Dehydration can also cause a modest increase in heart rate.

Bowel wall inflammation or damage severe enough to allow absorption of toxins into the bloodstream causes a significant increase in heart rate. In general, the higher the heart rate, the more serious the problem. With very few exceptions, the prognosis worsens as the heart rate increases:

- ❖ horses with heart rates less than 60 beats/min usually have a good prognosis for recovery, with appropriate treatment
  - two important exceptions are discussed on the next page
- ❖ horses with heart rates between 60 and 100 beats/min have a guarded prognosis, and are more likely to need surgery
  - one exception is proximal enteritis (see page 11); heart rates can be quite high, but with prompt and intensive medical therapy, the prognosis is reasonably good

- ❖ horses with heart rates over 100 beats/min have a poor prognosis for survival, even with surgery
  - such high heart rates indicate severe circulatory compromise (shock); these horses do not tolerate general anesthesia well, and they often have inoperable problems

There are two conditions in which heart rate can be an unreliable indicator of the severity of the problem: large colon volvulus (twist) and late-stage endotoxemia (absorption of bacterial toxins into the bloodstream). With each of these conditions, the heart rate may be much lower than expected. However, there are other signs that indicate a major problem is present. Such signs include bloating and severe, unrelenting pain with large colon volvulus; and severe depression, weakness, cold extremities, and purple-gray gums in horses dying of endotoxemia.

Monitoring the heart rate. In the majority of cases, heart rate is a reliable indicator of the seriousness of the problem, and it is a useful means of monitoring recovery or deterioration in the horse's condition. If the heart rate is 50 beats/minute or lower, and signs of colic are mild, monitor the heart rate every 15–30 minutes until the horse's condition changes.

If the heart rate remains elevated* above 50 beats/minute, call a veterinarian. Heart rates of 50–60 beats/minute in an adult horse do not necessarily indicate a serious problem, but they can signal pain or dehydration, each of which should be addressed by a veterinarian. (* Excitement or fear temporarily increases the heart rate. In horses that are unused to handling or are in a strange environment, retake the heart rate once the horse has relaxed.)

Gum color

In healthy horses, the gums are light pink, about the color of canned salmon. With intestinal conditions that result in endotoxemia and circulatory compromise, gum color may progress through the following stages:

- ❖ pale—in the early stages of endotoxemia or shock, the gums may be paler than normal
  - (blood loss and other types of anemia can also cause pale gums, as can severe pain without circulatory compromise)
- ❖ dark pink, then brick-red
  - this is a pivotal stage; horses at this point can usually be "turned around" with appropriate treatment, but beyond this point it can be very difficult to save the horse
  - with most simple obstructions (e.g. impaction, enteroliths), gum color does not progress beyond this point, *unless* the bowel wall becomes compromised by persistent obstruction
- ❖ bluish-purple—indicates advanced endotoxemia, such as occurs with strangulating obstructions that have been present for several hours, or bowel rupture
  - sometimes the earliest indication of toxemia is purplish discoloration of the gum just around the tooth margin (a "toxic line")
- ❖ gray—indicates utter cardiovascular collapse and signals a very poor prognosis; death is imminent
  - even with intensive therapy, it is generally impossible to save horses at this late stage

> **Checklist of Physical Status**
>
> Call a veterinarian immediately if any of the following is found in a horse showing signs of colic:
>
> ❏ moderate or severe pain
> ❏ the heart rate remains at over 50 beats/minute (adult horse)
> ❏ the gums are dark pink, red, or bluish-purple in color
> ❏ the capillary refill time is more than 2 seconds
> ❏ the gums are tacky or dry, and the skin remains tented when gently pinched
> ❏ the extremities are cold (yet the weather is mild)

Monitoring gum color. Horses with mild colic (e.g. spasmodic colic) usually have normal gum color. This is a positive sign. Horses with more serious types of colic may have normal gum color initially, but as the condition persists or worsens, the gums become darker pink or red. This is an important change and one that should prompt you to call a veterinarian immediately. Fluid therapy is necessary in these horses, regardless of whether they have a problem that requires surgery.

Capillary refill time

When you briefly press a healthy horse's gum with your thumb, color should return to the blanched area (the pale area created by thumb pressure) within 1–2 seconds. This is termed the capillary refill time: the time it takes for the tiny blood vessels nearest the surface to refill after the blood has been pressed out of them.

With circulatory compromise, the capillary refill time lengthens. At the same time, gum color is changing, so these assessments are made together. If the gums are light pink and the capillary refill time is less than 2 seconds, the horse's circulation is adequate at present. If either the gum color or the capillary refill time changes, call a veterinarian immediately.

Indicators of hydration status

Potentially serious colic problems typically result in dehydration, whether or not toxemia also develops. Fluid does not need to be lost from the body to cause dehydration; it just needs to be redistributed from the tissues and bloodstream into another location, such as an obstructed portion of bowel or the abdominal cavity.

In addition to an elevated heart rate, moderate-to-severe dehydration causes two other observable changes: tacky or dry gums (indicates reduced saliva production), and a tendency for the skin to stay tented when pinched up (indicates dehydrated skin and subcutaneous tissues).

Skin tenting. In a well-hydrated adult horse, the skin should spring back into position within 1 second of being gently pinched up. With moderate-to-severe dehydration, the skin remains tented for several seconds.

Two notes: (1) In young foals and old horses, the skin tends to stay tented for longer than in younger adult horses; this is normal. (2) Skin tenting on the side of the neck (the most common site for testing) can be inaccurate. If the skin springs back in place quickly, the horse's hydration status is good. But if the skin remains tented for a few seconds, double-check the result by testing a more reliable area, such as the skin over the point of the shoulder or the bony ridge above the eye.

Temperature of the extremities

When the circulation is severely compromised, blood flow is diverted from "non-essential" areas, such as the skin, to the essential organs. The first areas in which reduced blood flow is evident are the extremities, especially the lower legs and the ears. In severely dehydrated horses and those in shock, the lower legs and the tips of the ears may feel cold.

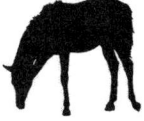

As most cases of colic are mild, *most horses with colic have:*
• normal or only slightly elevated heart rate
• light-pink, moist gums with a normal capillary refill time
• normal skin tenting and appropriately warm or cool extremities

It is important to factor-in environmental conditions when making this assessment. The extremities normally feel cold in cold weather or when the skin is wet; and even in a severely shocky horse, the extremities may not feel very cold in hot weather. But poor circulation is easily recognized by other indicators, such as high heart rate and changes in gum color and capillary refill time.

Other physical changes

In most horses with colic, the body temperature (measured with a rectal thermometer) is normal. If the temperature is elevated above 101.5° F (38.6° C), call a veterinarian.

The respiratory rate may be elevated because of pain, anxiety, alterations in blood acidity, or pressure on the diaphragm from large colon distention. But in most cases, the respiratory rate is not very useful in determining the severity of a colic episode.

Assessing Bowel Function

One of the primary ways veterinarians evaluate bowel function in horses is by listening to the bowel sounds with a stethoscope placed on the horse's abdomen (belly). This is something owners, trainers, and managers can also do to assess and monitor colic episodes. If you don't have a stethoscope, bowel sounds can be heard by placing your ear against the horse's flank; just be careful not to get kicked.

Evaluating bowel sounds

To thoroughly evaluate bowel sounds, listen over the upper and lower parts of the abdomen, on both sides of the horse. Interpreting bowel sounds takes practice. But in a pinch, it is enough to tell whether bowel sounds are present or not. Bowel sounds are described as being:

- ❖ normal—quiet gurgling or squelching (mixing) and occasional loud rumbling (propulsive) sounds are heard soon after you begin listening

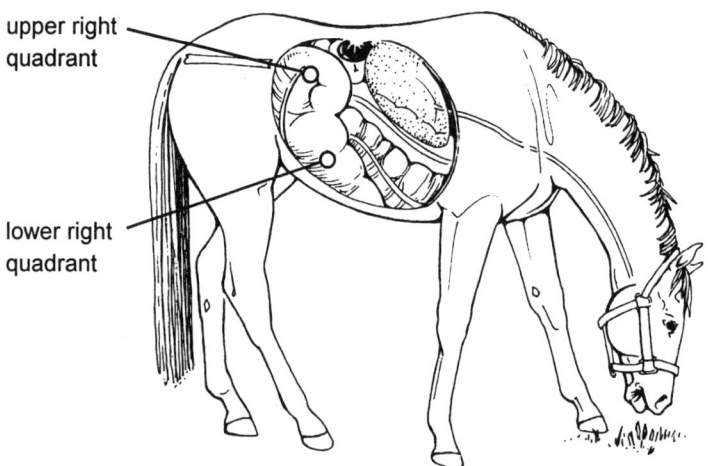

Figure 4-2: Listening to the abdomen on the right side of the horse.

4–Managing Colic

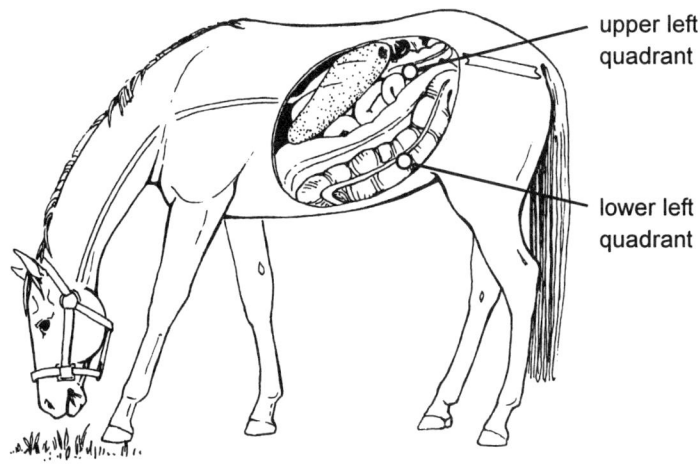

Figure 4-3: Listening to the abdomen on the left side of the horse.

* increased—squelching or rumbling sounds are louder and/or more frequent than normal (common with spasmodic colic)
* decreased—squelching or rumbling sounds are heard, but they are not as loud or as frequent as normal, and you may have to listen for several seconds before hearing anything
* absent—few or no sounds are heard in any quadrant, after listening for at least 1 minute

When evaluating the bowel sounds, it is important to take into consideration when the horse was last fed and exercised. Feeding stimulates bowel activity and increases both the frequency and intensity of bowel sounds for a few hours. Exercise, particularly if strenuous, tends to decrease bowel sounds for an hour or two.

Reduced or absent bowel sounds. Absence of bowel sounds in a horse showing moderate to severe signs of colic usually indicates an obstruction of some sort. However, reduced or absent bowel sounds are simply a nonspecific indication that bowel motility is decreased; they are not absolute proof of an obstruction. For example, sick horses that are not eating have decreased bowel sounds. As with every other assessment, *bowel sounds should be interpreted in light of other findings*, such as severity of the colic signs and changes in the horse's physical status.

Manure

Passage of manure is an unreliable indicator of the severity of the problem. Many of the conditions that cause colic alter bowel motility and reduce either the amount or frequency of manure passage. Yet even with complete obstructions, the horse may continue to pass small amounts of manure for several hours. (Manure "downstream" from the obstruction may be passed until the small colon is empty.) However, passage of manure is a positive sign in a horse that is recovering from colic.

Don't rely on manure passage to determine how serious the problem is, but consider it a positive sign when a horse that is recovering from a bout of colic begins passing manure again.

Manure consistency. When bowel motility is slowed or the horse is dehydrated, the manure balls may become dry and firm, with a thick, stringy, creamy-yellow coating of mucus. Some form of fluid therapy may be needed in these horses. If a horse with signs of colic begins passing loose or watery manure (i.e. diarrhea), call a veterinarian immediately.

What To Do With a Colicky Horse

Most cases of colic (as many as 75% in one comprehensive study) are mild and resolve either on their own or with medical treatment. If the signs of colic are mild and the heart rate and other assessments are normal, it is usually safe to monitor the horse for an hour or so and see if the condition improves. But if the heart rate is over 50 beats/minute, if the horse is showing any abnormalities of circulatory function, or if the colic pain is moderate to severe, don't wait—call a veterinarian immediately.

Monitoring the Situation

When waiting it out, or while you're waiting for the veterinarian to arrive, there are several things you should be doing:

- monitor the horse's physical status every 15 minutes
  - if nothing else, take the horse's heart rate, check its gum color, and listen to its bowel sounds
  - write down your findings (e.g. make a chart similar to the one on page 176)
  - if any of these things change for the worse, call the veterinarian immediately (unless s/he is already on the way)
- move the horse to a small area (e.g. a stall or small yard) where you can watch it closely and see any manure it passes
- take away any grain and hay, but leave the water
  - if the horse has an impaction, allowing the horse to eat is simply adding more material to the obstruction
- if it is dark or if nightfall is approaching, arrange for some lighting so that you (and, if necessary, the veterinarian) can examine the horse properly
- walk the horse around if it is continually rolling or thrashing
  - walking can be an effective way of calming the horse and preventing it from injuring itself
  - walking can even help resolve mild, spasmodic colic
  - but don't exhaust the horse by relentlessly walking it for hours; if the horse just wants to lie quietly, let it be
- keep the horse under close observation, and *reevaluate, reevaluate, reevaluate!*

- if signs persist or worsen, call a veterinarian without delay
- if the horse seems more comfortable, keep checking it every 15 minutes for the next hour, then hourly for the next few hours (see Recovery on page 168)

Some veterinarians recommend a short, brisk trot (e.g. 50–100 yards, on a lead) for horses with mild colic. And numerous owners have found that a short trailer ride is also effective at relieving mild colic. But these activities have little effect on, and in some cases can delay appropriate treatment of, more serious types of colic. Accurate assessment is the key to determining the best way of managing a particular case of colic.

Drug Therapy

This section is written for owners, trainers, and managers who, whether of necessity or preference, are in the habit of using injectable drugs on the horses in their care. Regardless of your situation, or the reason why you are not involving a veterinarian, if you are administering drugs to a colicky horse without first discussing the horse's condition with a veterinarian, *please* read and follow these guidelines.

1. Evaluate the horse's physical status *first*

Before giving any drugs, thoroughly evaluate the horse's physical status. Record your findings (see the chart on page 176), noting the time you made your observations and when you gave the drug. Also record how much of the drug you gave the horse. This information is very important if the horse's condition deteriorates and a veterinarian must examine the horse.

Banamine® (flunixin), in particular, can mask signs of deterioration in the horse's condition. The seriousness of the situation may not be obvious if use of this drug is not factored in when the horse is reexamined. This can have potentially disastrous consequences if treatment is delayed because Banamine was masking the horse's true status.

Before using Banamine, it is also important to take the horse's rectal temperature and make a note of it. This drug can lower the body temperature in a horse with a fever. Fever is uncommon in horses with colic, but when present, it usually signals a problem that needs veterinary attention.

2. Circulatory compromise *needs* veterinary attention

If there is any indication of circulatory compromise (e.g. high heart rate, discolored gums, slow capillary refill time), talk to a veterinarian *before* giving any drugs. These horses need more than a shot of pain-killer, and certain drugs should be avoided or reduced dosages used in such cases.

Most of the commonly used sedatives, including Rompun® (xylazine), Dormosedan® (detomidine), and acepromazine ("ace"), cause a drop in blood pressure which can be harmful in a horse with compromised circulation. So, call a veterinarian if there are signs of circulatory compromise. S/he may still have you give the drug, but leave the decision, and the dosage, to him/her.

> The goal of drug therapy in horses with colic is to relieve pain while monitoring the condition for improvement or deterioration. Be very cautious about giving drugs that may affect your or the veterinarian's ability to accurately assess the horse's condition.

3. Use only recommended drugs and dosages

Give only the recommended drugs and dosages. With most "colic" drugs, including Banamine, Rompun, and Dormosedan, colic pain can often be controlled with a much lower dose than is used for relief of other types of pain (Banamine) or for sedation (Rompun, Dormosedan). For example, the standard 10-ml dose of Banamine is excessive and unnecessary for relief of colic pain; 3 to 5 ml is sufficient. In fact, horses in which 5 ml of Banamine is ineffective need immediate veterinary attention, not more Banamine.

Recommended dosages for the commonly used colic drugs are given in Table 4-1 on page 174.

4. Do not combine drugs

Giving two or more drugs together does not necessarily enhance their effects, and it makes side effects more likely. In particular, do not give Rompun and Dormosedan together. These drugs are in the same class and have similar actions, including lowering the horse's blood pressure. Giving both together can have disastrous effects in horses with already compromised circulation.

Some veterinarians often give low doses of Banamine and Rompun together. But leave drug mixing to the veterinarian. Horses with colic that do not respond to Banamine or Rompun alone need veterinary attention, not another drug.

5. Do not give repeated doses

If the first injection was ineffective or signs of colic return, call a veterinarian rather than giving a second dose. The veterinarian may recommend a second dose after reviewing the case with you, but leave that decision to him/her. There are way too many stories of disastrous outcomes when horses were treated for days with repeated injections of Banamine, rather than being examined by a veterinarian and treated appropriately. It may be that all that's needed is some fluid therapy, but call the veterinarian and let him or her determine what is best for the horse.

(Incidentally, Banamine can slow bowel healing, which is another reason for not overusing this drug in horses with colic.)

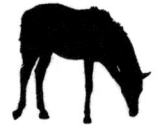
How well, and for how long, a drug relieves colic pain can be useful in determining how serious the situation is: If the pain persists or returns within about 30 minutes, call a veterinarian.

6. Learn about the drug

Familiarize yourself with the indications and contraindications—when to use it and when *not* to use it—for every drug in your equine medicine cabinet. Also be aware of the potential side effects for each drug; what would you do if the horse had an adverse reaction to the drug? A veterinarian is the best person to ask for this type of information.

Things to Avoid

Unless you have the necessary training, equipment, and experience, do not attempt to:

- pass any kind of tube into the horse's esophagus or stomach
  - it is very easy to damage the horse's nasal passages, throat, larynx, and/or esophagus with improper technique
  - if the tube goes into the trachea (windpipe) rather than the esophagus, any fluid passed down the tube will flow straight into the horse's lungs

- insert anything into the horse's rectum; this includes your hand, a hose, and any other kind of tube or device
  - the rectum is easily damaged, even when taking due care, and full-thickness rectal tears can result in fatal peritonitis
  - impactions in adult horses generally cannot be relieved by removing manure from the rectum or giving an enema; these procedures are a waste of time and can be harmful

- give any intravenous injections; even with practice, *every* intravenous injection carries the following risks
  - injection into the carotid artery, which lies directly beneath the jugular vein; carotid injection can cause immediate seizures (convulsions), collapse, blindness, and even death

- injection of some of the drug outside the vein, which can cause tissue damage, sometimes severe
- inflammation of the vein (phlebitis), which can result in obstruction of the vein with a blood clot (thrombophlebitis); infection of the clot (septic thrombophlebitis) may develop and can be very serious
- missing the vein entirely and injecting the drug into the surrounding tissue, thus slowing the drug's delivery into the bloodstream and the onset of its effects

❖ give the horse any fluids or mineral oil by mouth (i.e. do not pour any liquid into the horse's mouth)
- most horses resist oral administration of fluids, and in the struggle it is easy for some of the liquid that doesn't land on your clothes to be inhaled instead of swallowed
- too little fluid or mineral oil can be given by mouth to be effective in rehydrating the horse or relieving an impaction
- mineral oil in the lung can cause a particularly nasty pneumonia, so it should be given only by stomach tube
- castor oil, kerosene, turpentine, and any such "home remedies" are useless and dangerous, and should never be given orally to horses

Recovery

All going well, the colic episode will have resolved completely with minimal intervention. (Those cases that do not resolve with treatment on the farm are discussed in the next section.) If a veterinarian was called to examine and treat the horse, follow his/her advice on returning the horse to its normal feeding and activity schedules once all signs of colic have abated. If the colic episode resolved on its own or with a single injection of analgesic, follow these guidelines:

4–Managing Colic

- ❖ once the horse seems comfortable, see if it is interested in eating by taking it to a grassy area and letting it graze for a few minutes
    - then return the horse to the stall or pen and keep an eye on it for the next 30–60 minutes
    - note: wait an hour or so after giving a pain-reliever before seeing if the horse is interested in food
- ❖ if the horse readily ate grass and shows no signs of pain over the next hour, give it some hay
    - continue to observe it closely for signs of colic
    - also monitor the horse's water intake during this time
- ❖ provided the horse has been comfortable, alert, and interested in eating hay for several hours, give half of its usual ration at the next scheduled feeding
    - if the horse is normally kept at pasture, turn it out, but keep an eye on it over the next 12–24 hours

At some point, it is worth giving some thought to what factors could have contributed to the colic incident:
- Have there been any recent dietary changes or changes in housing or activity level?
- Is the horse on an adequate deworming program?
- Does the horse have plenty of fresh, clean water available?

Horses that have colicked once are more likely to colic again, so try to identify any management changes that could reduce the risk for repeated bouts of colic.

As long as the horse remains pain-free, alert, and interested in food, the normal feeding schedule can be resumed—unless its diet may have contributed to the colic episode (e.g. a high-grain ration, lush pasture, change in hay), in which case it is worth reviewing the diet and making appropriate changes. Regular exercise can be resumed once the horse is back to its normal feeding schedule.

If, at any time, colic signs return, it is best to consult a veterinarian. The horse needs further evaluation, and it may also require fluid therapy or some other medical treatment.

Transporting Severely Colicky Horses

In the few cases that need immediate surgery, it is important to get the horse to a veterinary hospital as quickly and as safely as possible. Following are some suggestions for safe transport of severely colicky horses to a surgical facility.

The Trailer

If possible, use a truck or trailer in which it would be relatively easy to extract the horse if it goes down during the trip. This may involve using a truck or trailer with a wide fold-down ramp, and removing any partitions before loading the horse. Provided horses have plenty of room to position themselves, most do not need partitions to maintain their balance while traveling. However, the partition may be necessary when transporting horses in shock and mares with foals; nonslip flooring is also important for these horses. Be sure to tie the lead rope long enough that if the horse goes down, its head won't be caught at an abnormal angle.

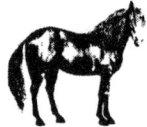

Even if it's not clear whether the horse needs surgery (or the decision for surgery has not yet been made) transporting the horse to a surgical facility sooner rather than later is a good idea. The horse is "on the spot" if things worsen, and in the meantime it can be receiving more intensive medical care (e.g. intravenous fluids) and observation than is sometimes possible on the farm.

But if it will take a couple of hours to organize the ideal truck or trailer, and there is another vehicle immediately available, use the one at hand (provided it is safe) and get the horse to the hospital as quickly as possible. Time is of the essence when dealing with serious intestinal problems, particularly those that compromise circulatory function.

It is a good idea for every horse owner to have an emergency plan in which a truck or trailer is available, or can be borrowed from a friend or neighbor, at any time for situations such as this.

Insurance

If the horse is insured (either mortality or major medical/surgical coverage), let the veterinarian know and contact the insurance company as soon as possible when it looks like surgery may be necessary. But rather than spending valuable time on the phone now, put your insurance papers in the truck, get the horse to the veterinary hospital, and call the insurance company from there.

During the Trip

It is unsafe for any person to ride in the trailer with the horse, even if in a separate compartment. It is better for you to pull over and check on the horse during the trip, rather than having someone ride in the trailer with the horse. When you pull over, reassure the horse, check any equipment the veterinarian may have inserted (e.g. stomach tube, intravenous fluid system), and, if necessary, administer any drugs the veterinarian sent with the horse. If there are no stomach tubes or fluids to check on, don't stop; get the horse to the hospital as soon as possible.

Stomach tube

If, during the initial examination, the veterinarian finds significant gas or fluid accumulation in the horse's stomach, s/he may decide to leave the stomach tube in place, taping it to the horse's halter for security. Check on the tube at least once during a long trip. The veterinarian will instruct you on what to do.

Intravenous fluids

Other than the time factor, one thing that significantly increases the survival rate in horses with serious colic is administration of intravenous (IV) fluids before surgery. Ideally, this begins on the farm, as soon as the attending veterinarian has examined the horse and determined that it needs surgery.

Moderately-to-severely dehydrated horses and those in shock often need 20–30 liters of fluid, sometimes more. This volume is best given IV, as soon and as rapidly as possible. So, before loading the horse onto the trailer, the veterinarian may insert an IV catheter and begin fluid therapy. Provided there is a place to hang the fluid bags in the trailer, the horse can be receiving fluids during the trip. The veterinarian will advise you on what to look for and how to change the fluid bags, if necessary, during the trip.

Sedatives or analgesics

The veterinarian may also send some sedatives or analgesics with the horse, with instructions on when and how to give them. It is important to advise the veterinarian on arrival what and how much was given, and when, if it was necessary to give any drugs during the trip. This is especially important when the attending veterinarian is referring the case to another veterinarian (e.g. an equine surgeon), and will not be present when the horse arrives at the hospital.

Prior Planning

Prior planning makes all the difference in an emergency. When boarding your horse or going away and leaving your horse in the care of someone else, make sure that you are readily contactable in an emergency. Give the caretaker written authority to make certain medical decisions on your behalf in an emergency, if you cannot be contacted.

Discuss with the caretaker, and *state in writing*, where you "draw the line." For example, you will agree to medical therapy and hospitalization, up to a certain monetary limit, but will not agree to surgery without discussion with the attending veterinarian. If you want all reasonable measures taken to save your horse, including surgery, make that clear and put it in writing.

The sooner surgery is performed, the better the horse's chances of recovery, so eliminate as many obstacles as possible by making your wishes known. It is also a good idea to discuss this scenario with your regular veterinarian, and put your decision in writing.

If you would consider colic surgery for your horse, be prepared to spend $3,000–$5,000 on the surgery and aftercare, depending on the condition needing treatment. It can cost more if postoperative complications are significant. So, consider major medical/surgical insurance coverage for valuable or much loved horses.

Final Word

Although this chapter ended discussing crisis situations, it is worth restating that most cases of colic are mild and resolve quickly, with minimal intervention. And a significant proportion of the remaining cases can be managed either on the farm or at a veterinary hospital with fluid therapy, analgesics, mineral oil, or other specific medical therapies. Only about 10% of horses with colic (i.e. 1 in 10 colic cases) have a problem that requires surgery.

Regardless of the type of colic, the best chance for a satisfactory outcome is achieved with early recognition, accurate assessment, close monitoring, and involvement of a veterinarian if the condition is severe or has not resolved within an hour or so.

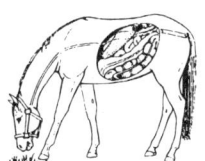

Table 4-1: Recommended drug dosages for treating colic in horses. *Please see text for precautions.*

Drug: Trade name (drug name)	Recommended Dosage & Route*	Amount for an Average Horse⁺	Comments
Rompun (xylazine)	0.4–0.7 mg/kg (0.2–0.3 mg/lb) IV or IM	2–3 ml of the large animal formulation (100 mg/ml) IV	if giving IM, double the dosage
Banamine (flunixin)	0.3–0.5 mg/kg (0.14–0.22 mg/lb) IV	3–5 ml (50 mg/ml) **Note:** 10 ml is *excessive*	can be given IM, but may cause muscle damage (sometimes severe)
Dormosedan (detomidine)	5–10 µg/kg# (2.3–4.5 µg/lb) IV or IM	¼–½ ml (10 mg/ml) IV	only for severe pain, and not without veterinary advice
Torbugesic (butorphanol)	0.02–0.05 mg/kg (0.01–0.02 mg/lb) IV or IM	1–2½ ml (10 mg/ml) IV	if giving IM, double the dosage

* IV: intravenously   IM: intramuscularly   1 ml = 1 cc
  (Note: IM injections take longer to work than IV injections)

+ an adult horse weighing 450–500 kg (1000–1100 lb)
  see Box 4-1 for an example of how these calculations were made

µg is microgram, or one-thousandth of a milligram (0.001 mg)

Dipyrone is currently unavailable, and is only useful for mild colic. Phenylbutazone ("bute," PBZ, BTZ) is relatively ineffective for most types of colic; and acepromazine ("ace") has no effect on colic pain and it lowers the blood pressure.

4–Managing Colic

Box 4-1: An example of how to calculate drug dosages.

This example uses Banamine to demonstrate the simple calculations:

1. Determine the weight of the horse, using either livestock scales or a weight tape, or estimate its weight.
   – for ease of calculations, I'm using a 500-kg horse

2. Check the recommended dosage for the drug, which is usually given in milligrams per kilogram (mg/kg).
   – for this example, I'm using a dosage of 0.5 mg/kg [Table 4-1]

3. Multiply the horse's body weight by the mg/kg dosage.
   – 500 kg x 0.5 mg/kg = 250 mg, the total *dose* of drug to be given

4. Check the bottle label for the concentration of the solution, which is usually given in milligrams per milliliter (mg/ml).
   – for Banamine, the concentration is 50 mg/ml

5. Divide the total dose of drug to be given by the concentration.
   – 250 mg ÷ 50 mg/ml = 5 ml, the total *volume* of drug to be given

If you're used to thinking of body weights in pounds rather than kilograms:

1. Use the drug dosage in mg/lb
   – if the drug dosage is given in mg/kg, divide it by 2.2 to get mg/lb

2. Body weight x drug dosage = total dose of drug to be given
   – for an 1100-lb horse, 1100 lb x 0.22 mg/lb [Table 4-1] = 242 mg

3. Divide the total dose of drug by the concentration of the solution
   – 242 mg ÷ 50 mg/ml = 4.84 ml (5 ml is close enough)

Chart for monitoring horses with colic

Time	Heart Rate (beats/min.)	Gum Color (light pink, dark pink-red, purple)	Capillary Refill Time (seconds)	Hydration Status (gum moisture, skin tenting & temp.)	Bowel Activity (bowel sounds, manure)	Treatment

Index

A

activity/use and colic risk   49–51
adhesions   **22**, 54, 69
age and colic risk   44–49
alfalfa
   and blister beetles   69–70
   and enteroliths   66–67
   and gastric ulcers   67
anterior enteritis
   see proximal enteritis
ascarid impaction
   see roundworm impaction

B

bedding and colic risk   74
behavior and colic risk   51–53
Bermuda/coastal grass hay
   65–66, **134–135**
blister beetles   69–70, 120–121
bowel function (assessing)
   bowel sounds   160–162
   manure   162
breed and colic risk   38–41
   Arabians   38–39
   Thoroughbreds   40
   Standardbreds   40–41
   Miniature Horses   41
   Morgans   41
   other breeds   41
broodmares
   colic in broodmares   51
   preventing large colon twists
   133–134

C

capillary refill time   158
cecum   9, **12–13**, 15
choke/esophageal obstruction   10
chronic colic   44, 45, 54
coastal Bermudagrass hay
   65–66, **134–135**
colic assoc. with eating   68–69
colic at shows and competitions
   131–132
colic in older horses   144–145
colic signs   2–5
concentrates and colic risk   57–63
   amount and type   57–59
   frequency   59
   what is the big deal?   59–60
   association with colic   60–61
   what is a large amount?   62–63
concentrates (feeding)   113–114
cribbing and colic risk   52
cyathostomes
   see small strongyles

D

dental care   **85**, 127
deworming program   83, **123–127**
diet and colic risk   57–70
   concentrates   57–63
   roughage   63–67
   feeding changes   68
   colic assoc. with eating   68–69
   unusual feed materials   69

diet and colic risk (cont.)
   feed contaminants 69–70
dietary changes 115–116
digestive system 7–17
   stomach 8–10
   small intestine 10–12
   cecum 12–13
   large colon 13–16
   small colon 16–17
   rectum 17
drugs and chemicals 88–93
   amitraz 88
   antibiotics 89
   arsenic 89
   atropine & opiates 89
   castor oil 90
   DSS 90
   levamisole 90
   monensin 90
   NSAIDs 91–92
   organophosphates 92
   prostaglandins 92
   vaccines 92–93
drug therapy 164–167, 174(T)
duodenitis–proximal jejunitis 11
duodenum 9, 11

E

energy (dietary)
   feeding for needs 109–110
   overfeeding 110
   dietary fat 111
   feeding concentrates 113–114
enteroliths **67**
   and alfalfa 66–67
   and Arabians 39
   geographic distribution 93
   prevention 137–139
esophageal obstruction/choke 10

F

fecal egg counts 123–124

feed contaminants
   blister beetles 69–70, 120–121
   botulism 120
   monensin 90, 121
   mycotoxins 70
flatulent colic 21
foaling and colic risk 51

G

"gas" colic 20–21, 60, 63, **130**
   (often used interchangeably with spasmodic colic)
gastric (stomach) ulcers
   and alfalfa 67
   stress-induced ulcers 86, 87
   NSAID-induced ulcers 91–92
   prevention 139–141
gender and colic risk 42–44
   mares 42–43
   intact males 43
   geldings 43–44
genetics and colic risk 56
geographic location 93–94
gum color 156–158

H

"hay belly" 119
hay quality 64, 68, **119**, 134–135
heart rate 154–156
hernias 24
history and colic risk 53–55
   previous colic 53–54
   abdominal surgery 54–55
housing and colic risk 71–75
   inside vs. outside 71–73
   changes in housing 73
   bedding type 74
   pasture access and rotation 74
   farm size & stocking rate 74–75
housing changes 117–118

hydration status 158–159

I, J

ileal obstruction/impaction 65, 69, 81, 94, **134–135**
ileum 9, 12
ileus 20, 33(T)
illness and colic risk 88
inguinal hernia 43
internal parasites 77–85, **123–127**
  large strongyles 77–78, **142**
  small strongyles (cyathostomes) 78–81, **125–127**
  tapeworms 81–82, **124–125**
  roundworms 84–85, **143–144**
  deworming program 83, **123**
  recent deworming & colic 84
  climate and season 96
  fecal egg counts 123–124
intussusception **24**, 47, 82
ischemia (low blood flow) 22–25
jejunum 9, 11–12

K, L

large colon 9, 13–16
large colon displacement 15, 52–53, 61, **132–133**
large colon impaction 14, 28, 60, 72, **131**
large colon volvulus (twist) 42, **133–134**
large strongyles 77-78, **142**
larvicidal treatment 125
Lethal White Foal syndrome 56
lipoma, strangulating 24, **44**, 48

M, N

meconium impaction 43, 46, **143**
microbial fermentation 7, 15–16

Miniature Horses 41, 64, **135**
monitoring colic 163–164
mycotoxins 70
NSAIDs, or nonsteroidal anti-inflammatory drugs 91–92, **140**

O, P

pasture
  pasture access and colic risk 72, 74, 112, 114–115
  fresh grass 63, 110–111, 130
  calculating pasture intake 108
physical status (assessing) 153
  heart/pulse rate 154–156
  gum color 156–158
  capillary refill time 158
  hydration status 158–159
  extremities 159
  other changes 159
poisonous plants 96–98
  black locust 97
  castor bean 97
  nightshades 97
  oak/acorns 97–98
  oleander 98
  pokeweed 98
  tobacco 98
Potomac horse fever 26, 93, 94
proximal (anterior) enteritis
  duodenitis–proximal jejunitis 11
  and high-grain diets 61
  geographic distribution 94

R

recovery from colic 168–169
rectum 9, 17
recurrent colic 53–54
right dorsal colitis 91–92, **142**
rolling and displacements/twists 52–53

roughage
   colic risk   63–67
   fresh grass   63, 110–111, 130
   hay quality   64, **119**, 134–135
   coastal Bermuda grass hay
   65–66, **134–135**
   alfalfa hay   66–67
   daily requirements   108–109
roundworm (ascarid) impaction
   47, 84–85, **143–144**

S

Salmonella infection   26, 87
sand colic   26, 94, **136–137**
scrotal hernia   40, 41, 43
season/weather & colic risk   94–96
simple obstructions   21, 27, 28, 32–33(T)
small colon   9, 16–17
small intestine   9, 10–12
small strongyles (cyathostomes)   78–81, **125–127**
spasmodic colic   19, 28, 60, 63, **130–131**
spoiled feed   120–121
   also see feed contaminants
squamous-cell carcinoma   48, 69
stomach   8–10
stomach ulcers
   see gastric ulcers
strangulating lipoma   24, **44**, 48
strangulating obstruction   **23–25**, 27, 28
stress and colic risk   86–88
Strongid C®   84, 126–127
Strongylus vulgaris (redworm or bloodworm)   25, 77–78, **142**

T

tapeworms   81–82, **124–125**
teeth
   see dental care
thromboembolic colic   25, 78, 142
torsion   23
transport/shipping
   and colic risk   87–88
   for colicky horses   170–172

U, V, W

umbilical hernia   24, 46–47
unusual feeds   69, 120
use/activity and colic risk   49–51
vaccination and colic risk   92–93
verminous arteritis   25, 78, **142**
volvulus   23
water
   intake and colic risk   75–76
   requirements   75, 122
   heating water in winter   76
   transport and exercise   121–122
   importance of clean water   122
weather/season & colic risk   94–96

Georg Fohrer

Studien zur alttestamentlichen Theologie und Geschichte (1949—1966)

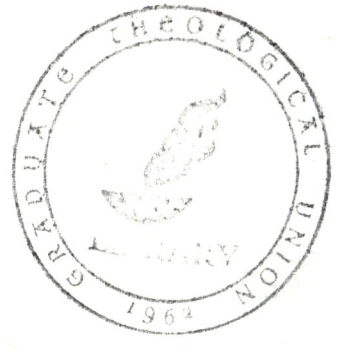

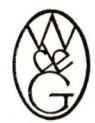

Walter de Gruyter & Co.
Berlin 1969

Beihefte zur Zeitschrift für die alttestamentliche Wissenschaft

Herausgegeben von Georg Fohrer

115

1969

by Walter de Gruyter & Co., Berlin 30, Genthiner Straße 13
Alle Rechte des Nachdrucks, der photomechanischen Wiedergabe,
der Übersetzung, der Herstellung von Mikrofilmen und Photokopien,
auch auszugsweise, vorbehalten.
Printed in Germany
Satz und Druck: Walter de Gruyter & Co., Berlin 30
Archiv-Nr. 3822694

Vorbemerkung

Die in diesem Sammelband erneut vorgelegten Studien behandeln vornehmlich religions- und theologiegeschichtliche, theologische und historische Fragen. Alle sind überarbeitet, manchmal gekürzt oder erweitert und, soweit erforderlich, geändert worden. Auch die seit der Erstveröffentlichung erschienene Literatur wurde berücksichtigt. Gelegentliche inhaltliche Wiederholungen sind belassen worden, damit jede Studie gesondert für sich gelesen werden kann. Nach der Bearbeitung ist die jetzige Fassung der Studien und nicht mehr diejenige der Erstveröffentlichung maßgeblich.

Für die Hilfen bei der Herstellung des Manuskripts und des Registers sowie bei der Korrektur des Buches schulde ich Frau Hildegard Hiersemann und Herrn Dr. Gunther Wanke meinen Dank, der auch an dieser Stelle ausgesprochen sei.

Erlangen, im Mai 1969   Georg Fohrer

Inhaltsverzeichnis

Vorbemerkung V
Abkürzungsverzeichnis IX

I. Religions- und Theologiegeschichte

Die wiederentdeckte kanaanäische Religion 3
Universale Vorstellungen in der kanaanäischen und der israelitischen Religion . . 13
Die zeitliche und überzeitliche Bedeutung des Alten Testaments 23
Die Judenfrage und der Zionismus 39
Tradition und Interpretation im Alten Testament 54
Altes Testament — »Amphiktyonie« und »Bund«? 84
Das sogenannte apodiktisch formulierte Recht und der Dekalog 120
»Priesterliches Königtum« (Ex 19 6) 149
4QOrNab, 11QTgJob und die Hioblegende 154

II. Theologie

II. Theologie 161
Das Gottesbild des Alten Testaments 163
Theologische Züge des Menschenbildes im Alten Testament 176
Zion-Jerusalem im Alten Testament 195
Die Weisheit im Alten Testament 242
σῴζω, σωτηρία, σωτήρ und σωτήριος im Alten Testament 275

III. Geschichte

Die Vorgeschichte Israels im Lichte neuer Quellen 297
Israels Staatsordnung im Rahmen des Alten Orients 309
Der Vertrag zwischen König und Volk in Israel 330
Eisenzeitliche Anlagen im Raume südlich von $nā'ūr$ und die Südwestgrenze von Ammon 352

Quellenverzeichnis 367

Register der Bibelstellen 368

Abkürzungsverzeichnis

ABR	Australian Biblical Review.
AcOr	Acta Orientalia.
AfO	Archiv für Orientforschung.
AJA	American Journal of Archaeology.
AJSL	American Journal of Semitic Languages and Literatures.
ALBO	Analecta Lovaniensia Biblica et Orientalia.
ANET	J. B. Pritchard (ed.), Ancient Near Eastern Texts relating to the Old Testament, 1955^2.
AnSt	Anatolian Studies.
AOT	H. Greßmann (hrsg.), Altorientalische Texte zum Alten Testament, 1926^2.
ArOr	Archiv Orientální.
ARW	Archiv für Religionswissenschaft.
ASTI	Annual of the Swedish Theological Institute in Jerusalem.
AThR	Anglican Theological Review.
BA	The Biblical Archaeologist.
BASOR	Bulletin of the American Schools of Oriental Research.
BEThL	Bibliotheca Ephemeridum Theologicarum Lovaniensium.
Bibl	Biblica.
BiOr	Bibliotheca Orientalis.
BJRL	Bulletin of the John Rylands Library.
BZ	Biblische Zeitschrift.
CBQ	The Catholic Biblical Quarterly.
ColG	Collationes Gandavenses.
ELKZ	Evangelisch-Lutherische Kirchenzeitung.
EThL	Ephemerides Theologicae Lovanienses.
EvTh	Evangelische Theologie.
Exp	The Expositor.
GCS	Die Griechischen Christlichen Schriftsteller der ersten drei Jahrhunderte, 1897 ff.
HdO	Handbuch der Orientalistik.
HUCA	Hebrew Union College Annual.
IEJ	Israel Exploration Journal.
JAOS	The Journal of the American Oriental Society.
Jb	Jahrbuch.
JBL	Journal of Biblical Literature.
JCS	Journal of Cuneiform Studies.
JJS	The Journal of Jewish Studies.
JNES	Journal of Near Eastern Studies.
JPOS	Journal of the Palestine Oriental Society.

JSOR	Journal of the Society of Oriental Research.
JSS	Journal of Semitic Studies.
JThSt	The Journal of Theological Studies.
KAT	E. Schrader, Die Keilinschriften und das Alte Testament, 1903³.
KuD	Kerygma und Dogma.
MGWJ	Monatsschrift für Geschichte und Wissenschaft des Judentums.
MIOr	Mitteilungen des Instituts für Orientforschung.
MPL	J. P. Migne (ed.), Patrologia, Series Latina, 1844—64.
NF	Neue Folge.
NkZ	Neue kirchliche Zeitschrift.
NS	New Series.
NThT	Nieuw Theologisch Tijdschrift.
NT	Novum Testamentum.
NTSt	New Testament Studies.
OLZ	Orientalistische Literaturzeitung.
OTSt	Oudtestamentische Studiën.
PEQ	Palestine Exploration Quarterly.
PJB	Palästinajahrbuch.
RB	Revue Biblique.
RE	Realencyklopädie für protestantische Theologie und Kirche, 1896—1913³.
RGG	Die Religion in Geschichte und Gegenwart.
RHPhR	Revue d'Histoire et de Philosophie Religieuses.
RHR	Revue de l'Histoire des Religions.
SEA	Svensk Exegetisk Årsbok.
ThBl	Theologische Blätter.
ThLZ	Theologische Literaturzeitung.
ThQ	Theologische Quartalschrift.
ThR	Theologische Rundschau.
ThSt	Theological Studies.
ThW	Theologisches Wörterbuch zum Neuen Testament.
ThZ	Theologische Zeitschrift.
VT	Vetus Testamentum.
VTSuppl	Supplements to Vetus Testamentum.
WZ	Wissenschaftliche Zeitschrift.
WZKM	Wiener Zeitschrift für die Kunde des Morgenlandes.
ZA	Zeitschrift für Assyriologie.
ZAW	Zeitschrift für die alttestamentliche Wissenschaft.
ZDMG	Zeitschrift der Deutschen Morgenländischen Gesellschaft.
ZDPV	Zeitschrift des Deutschen Palästina-Vereins.
ZEE	Zeitschrift für evangelische Ethik.
ZKTh	Zeitschrift für katholische Theologie.
ZThK	Zeitschrift für Theologie und Kirche.

I. Religions- und Theologiegeschichte

Die wiederentdeckte kanaanäische Religion

I.

Die Religion der Kanaanäer ist niemals völlig tot gewesen; manche ihrer bezeichnenden Vorstellungen und Gebräuche wirken in der modernen Kultur nach oder leben in ihr fort, wenn auch so umgestaltet und umgebildet, daß sie nicht leicht zu erkennen sind. Dies wird noch dadurch erschwert, daß bis vor kurzer Zeit nur wenig über die kanaanäische Religion bekannt war und dieses Wenige zudem aus zweiter Hand stammte: aus den meist polemischen Äußerungen des Alten Testaments über die Kanaanäer; aus ägyptischen und mesopotamischen Texten, den Amarna-Briefen und späten phönizischen Inschriften, die einige Anspielungen auf kanaanäische Gottheiten und kultische Bräuche enthalten; und aus einigen griechischen Schriftstellern, die gelegentlich einige Bruchstücke kanaanäischer Mythologie überliefern. Alles in allem war es äußerst wenig und mit fremden, nichtverstehenden oder gar übelwollenden Augen gesehen. Die Wissenschaft befand sich etwa in der gleichen Lage wie gegenüber den mesopotamischen Kulturen und Religionen, bevor die Keilschrifttexte aufgefunden und entziffert worden waren.

Diese Lage hat sich seit 1929 plötzlich grundlegend geändert. Es ist gewiß übertrieben zu sagen, daß wir nun von Angesicht zu Angesicht sehen und nicht mehr nur wie in einem Spiegel, aber immerhin sprechen die Kanaanäer einer bestimmten Zeit und Gegend nunmehr durch ihre Urkunden selber zu uns. Der Boden Syriens hat die ersten Überreste der kanaanäischen religiösen Literatur hergegeben, und immer noch fördern die Ausgrabungen, die im Auftrage der Pariser Académie des Inscriptions et Belles Lettres in Ras Schamra vorgenommen werden, Neues zutage. Ras Schamra ist die frühere phönizische Stadt Ugarit, ein kanaanäischer Stadtstaat und Hafen an der nordsyrischen Küste; seine Blütezeit fällt in die 2. Hälfte des 2. Jt. v. Chr., bis er um 1200 der Überflutung des westlichen Alten Orients durch die sog. Seevölker erlegen ist.

Die Funde in den Ruinen dieser Stadt gewähren zunächst neue Erkenntnisse in staatlichen, sozialen, wirtschaftlichen und künstlerischen Fragen sowie in sprach- und schriftgeschichtlicher Hinsicht; vor allem aber haben sie religionsgeschichtliche Bedeutung. Es handelt sich sowohl um Statuen und Reliefs von Gottheiten, Tempel und Altäre mit Kultgeräten, Grabanlagen mit Beigaben und Vorrichtungen für bestimmte Riten, als auch um zahlreiche Tontafeln mit Texten, die in einer bis dahin unbekannten Kceilshrift geschrieben waren[1]. Entgegen der in Mesopotamien gebräuchlichen war sie alphabetisch, und nach ihrer schnell gelungenen Entzifferung[2] erwies sich die Sprache als ein kanaanäischer Dialekt, der als solcher dem Hebräischen nahesteht. Die religiösen Texte sind kultisch-rituelle Formulare (z. B. Aufzählungen von Göttern mit ihren Heiligtümern, Listen von Opfern, rituelle Vorschriften) und mythologische Dichtungen, die teilweise recht umfangreich sind.

Freilich enthüllt sich sogleich eine mehrfache Problematik. Es handelt sich 1. um religiöse Texte und Denkmäler, die aus dem Ugarit des 14./13. Jh. v. Chr. stammen, zunächst also lediglich ein örtlich und zeitlich begrenztes Bild geben können. Inwieweit sind Rückschlüsse auf die kanaanäische Religion anderer Orte und Zeiten zulässig? Es handelt sich 2. vielfach um Dichtungen, die sich der herrschenden religiösen Vorstellungen und Bräuche als ihres Stoffes bedienen. Inwieweit sind sie als Dichtung trotz aller inneren Bindung frei und selbständig gegenüber der damaligen lebendigen Religion und inwieweit ihr unmittelbarer Niederschlag? Es handelt sich 3. um Texte aus einer Stadt mit einer stark gemischten Bevölkerung, zu der nicht zuletzt hurritische Elemente gehörten. Inwieweit sind Vorstellungen und Bräuche davon beeinflußt worden und inwieweit wirklich kanaanäisch?

II.

Bisher sind diese wiederentdeckten Reste der kanaanäischen Religion hauptsächlich von Orientalisten und Alttestamentlern bearbeitet worden, die sich durch ihr Fachinteresse daran gewiesen sahen. Doch dabei sollte es nicht bleiben. Zwar sind die philologischen Kenntnisse und das Einfühlungsvermögen in die Eigenart semitischen Vorstellens und Denkens außerordentlich wichtig und oft unerläßlich. Darüber hinaus aber geht es nunmehr, nachdem auf diesen Gebieten viel erreicht worden ist, um die Untersuchung der kanaanäischen Religion nach den allgemeinen religionswissenschaftlichen Methoden und um ihre Eingliederung in den bisher gewonnenen religionsgeschichtlichen Erfahrungskreis — gerade wegen der Problematik der ugaritischen Texte und Denkmäler und mancher ihrer religiösen Vorstellungen.

Diese Notwendigkeit eingehender religionswissenschaftlicher Erforschung zeigt sich 1. daran, daß es bisher keine ausreichende und um-

---

[1] Vgl. Cl. F.-A. Schaeffer (ed.), Le Palais Royal d'Ugarit, II—V 1955—1965; Ugaritica, I—IV 1939—1962.

[2] Vgl. H. Bauer, Entzifferung der Keilschrifttafeln von Ras Schamra, 1930; Das Alphabet von Ras Schamra, 1932. Gleichzeitig gelang E. Dhorme die Entzifferung.

fassende Gesamtdarstellung der kanaanäischen Religion gibt[3]; ausführlicher sind besonders einzelne Texte[4], einige sachliche Fragen[5] und die Beziehungen zum Alten Testament[6] untersucht worden. Es ist 2. bezeichnend, daß auch in neueren Darstellungen der Religionsgeschichte[7] zwar die sumerisch-akkadische, babylonisch-assyrische und ägyptische Religion, nicht aber die kanaanäische behandelt wird.

Die Voraussetzungen für die Mitarbeit der Religionswissenschaft sind weithin erfüllt. Die Texte sind in der Reihenfolge ihrer Entdeckung[8] oder gesammelt[9] herausgegeben worden, wobei ein Vergleich allerdings zeigt, daß die Ausgaben in der Deutung mancher Worte und Stellen mehr oder weniger voneinander abweichen. Es gibt auch Übersetzungen[10], jedoch weichen sie oft beträchtlich voneinander ab.

---

[3] Vgl. z. B. die kurzen Darstellungen von W. F. Albright, Archaeology and the Religion of Israel, 1946[2], 68—94; E. Dhorme — R. Dussaud, Les religions de Babylonie et d'Assyrie, les religions des Hittites et des Hourrites, des Phéniciens et des Syriens, 1949, 355—388; Th. H. Gaster, The Religion of the Canaanites, in: V. Ferm, Forgotten Religions, 1950, 111—143; O. Eißfeldt, Kanaanäisch-ugaritische Religion, in: HdO I 8, 1, 1964, 76—91.

[4] So z. B. H. L. Ginsberg, The Legend of King Keret, 1946; C. H. Gordon, The Loves and Wars of Anat, 1943; J. Obermann, How Danel was blessed with a Son, 1946; Ugaritic Mythology, 1948; K.-H. Bernhardt, Anmerkungen zur Interpretation des KRT-Textes von Ras Schamra-Ugarit, WZ Greifswald 5 (1954/55), 102—121; J. Gray, The Krt Text in the Literature of Ras Shamra, 1964[2]; W. Herrmann, Yariḫ und Nikkal und der Preis der Kuṯarāt-Göttinnen, 1968.

[5] So z. B. U. Cassuto, The Goddess Anath, Canaanite Epics of the Patriarchal Age, 1951; O. Eißfeldt, El im ugaritischen Pantheon, 1951; A. S. Kapelrud, Baal in the Ras Shamra Texts, 1952; M. H. Pope, El in the Ugaritic Texts, 1955.

[6] So z. B. R. Dussaud, Les découvertes de Ras Shamra et l'Ancien Testament, 1937; R. de Langhe, Les textes de Ras Shamra-Ugarit et leurs rapports avec le milieu biblique de l'Ancien Testament, 2 Bände 1945; E. Jacob, Ras Shamra-Ugarit et l'Ancien Testament, 1960; J. Gray, The Legacy of Canaan, 1965[2]. Ferner J. H. Patton, Canaanite Parallels in the Book of Psalms, 1944; O. Kaiser, Die mythische Bedeutung des Meeres in Ägypten, Ugarit und Israel, 1962[2]; M. J. Mulder, Kanaänitische goden in het Oude Testament, 1965; W. H. Schmidt, Königtum Gottes in Ugarit und Israel, 1966[2]; K.-H. Bernhardt, Aschera in Ugarit und im Alten Testament, MIOr 13 (1967), 163—174.

[7] F. König, Christus und die Religionen der Erde, 3 Bände 1951.

[8] Vor allem Ch. Virolleaud in Syria.

[9] H. Bauer, Die alphabetischen Keilschrifttexte von Ras Schamra, 1936; C. H. Gordon, Ugaritic Textbook, 1965 (mit Grammatik und Glossar); A. Herdner, Corpus des tablettes en cunéiformes alphabétiques découvertes à Ras Shamra-Ugarit de 1929 à 1939, 1963.

[10] C. H. Gordon, Ugaritic Literature, 1949; vgl. ferner die Auswahlen von H. L. Ginsberg, Ugaritic Myths, Epics, and Legends, in: ANET 129—155; Th. H. Gaster, Thespis-Ritual, Myth and Drama in the Near East, 1950, 115—313 (kommentiert);

Voraussetzung für die weitere Arbeit ist eine kritische Neuausgabe der Texte in Umschrift, die für den des Hebräischen Kundigen wichtig wäre, mit gleichzeitiger Übersetzung und Kommentierung.

III.

Warum ist nun die Wiederentdeckung der kanaanäischen Religion, die doch nur eine unter vielen ist, so bedeutsam? Warum ist bisher schon soviel im einzelnen über sie geschrieben worden[11], warum muß die Religionswissenschaft aufgefordert werden, sich eingehender als bisher mit ihr zu befassen? Es sind vor allem zwei Gründe: Die kanaanäische Religion besitzt innerhalb des Alten Orients in sich selbst eigene Prägung und besondere Werte, und sie hat weltweite Nachwirkungen gehabt.

IV.

Es ist unbestreitbar, daß die kanaanäische Kultur und Religion zäh und lebenskräftig gewesen ist. Sie hat nicht nur die verschiedenen Herrenschichten aufgesogen, die sich des öfteren in Syrien festsetzten (z. B. die vermutlich hurritischen Hyksos und die indogermanischen Philister), sondern auch die israelitischen Stämme von ihrer Landnahme bis tief in die Königszeit hinein nachhaltig beeinflußt. Vor allem aber hat sie sich trotz der Einwirkungen von seiten der übrigen altorientalischen Kulturländer, denen Syrien infolge seiner zentralen Lage ständig ausgesetzt war und die vor allem in der Zeit des ägyptischen Mittleren Reiches und der Hyksos zu beobachten sind, im wesentlichen rein und unverfälscht erhalten. Außer den Assyrern sind es nur die phönizischen Kanaanäer, die den hurritischen und hetitischen Bergvölkern bei ihrem Vordringen (seit etwa 1450) trotz zeitweiliger Überfremdung und politischer Überwältigung dauernden Widerstand geleistet haben. Auch der kyprische und mykenische Einfluß, der bis zum 13. Jh. v. Chr. erkennbar ist, hat die Eigenart der phönizischen Kunst nicht brechen können und nicht eigentlich schöpferisch gewirkt. Während die Befestigungsanlage von Ugarit mykenisch-troisch-hetitische und der neuerdings ausgegrabene Königspalast kretische Züge aufweist[12], ist bei den übrigen Gebäuden dergleichen wenig oder nicht festzustellen. Die Phönizier haben dem

---

A. Jirku, Kanaanäische Mythen und Epen aus Ras Schamra-Ugarit, 1962; J. Aistleitner, Die mythologischen und kultischen Texte aus Ras Schamra, 1964².
[11] Für die Literatur bis 1941 vgl. W. Baumgartner, Ras Schamra und das Alte Testament, ThR NF 12 (1940), 163—188; 13 (1941), 1—20. 85—102. 157—183.
[12] Vgl. den Bericht The Royal Palace of Ugarit in: The Manchester Guardian vom 5. Mai 1952.

allen ihr eigenes Volkstum und ihre eigene Kultur und Religion schließlich mit Erfolg entgegengestellt und ihre selbständige Prägung beibehalten.

So erschöpft sich das Wesen des Kanaanäertums nicht darin, als Mittler zwischen den großen Kulturländern des Alten Orients aufzutreten. Die kanaanäische Kultur und Religion besaß außerdem etwas Eigenes und bildete inmitten der internationalen Kultur des Alten Orients einen besonderen Kulturkreis. Er war denjenigen Ägyptens, Mesopotamiens und Kleinasiens benachbart und teilweise verwandt, stand aber selbständig und auf gleicher Höhe neben ihnen.

Die kanaanäische Religion ist Volksreligion mit all ihren Kennzeichen: Ein Kulturvolk ist ihr Träger und ihr Geltungsbereich; sie bezieht sich auf eine politisch konstituierte Gesamtheit in diesem Volk, den Stadtstaat, während persönliche Erfahrung und Heil des einzelnen als zweitrangig gelten; ein allgemeiner Heilszustand ist vorgegeben, der zugunsten des Ganzen erhalten und immer wieder erneuert werden muß. Inhaltlich läßt sie sich als Religion des sich erneuernden Lebens und der Fruchtbarkeit bezeichnen; wie alle ähnlich bestimmten Religionen ist sie sinnlich und orgiastisch. Daher gehört zum Ritus der heiligen Hochzeit im Kultus die sakrale Prostitution, die die Gottheit stärken und die großen Mächte des Lebens in Gang halten soll.

Um die kanaanäische Religion zu kennzeichnen sei auf einige wichtige Züge ihrer Göttergestalten hingewiesen.

1. Im kanaanäischen Pantheon dominieren die beiden Götter El und Baal, um die sich andere Gottheiten gruppieren. El nimmt in den mythologischen Dichtungen und rituellen Formularen eine bedeutsame Stellung ein. Als »Schöpfer der Schöpfung« und »Vater der Menschheit« gilt er als Schöpfer und Vater der Götter und Menschen. Die Bezeichnung »König« veranschaulicht seine Macht und Stärke, neben denen Weisheit und ewiges Leben stehen. Vielleicht muß man tatsächlich annehmen[13], daß er zumindest um 1400 v. Chr. für einen Teil der Bevölkerung von Ugarit nicht nur der höchste Gott, sondern die Gottheit schlechthin gewesen ist, so daß die anderen Götter ihre Bedeutung zu verlieren und als bloße Ausstrahlung seiner göttlichen Potenz betrachtet zu werden begannen.

Baal[14] ist vielleicht mit dem Regen- und Sturmgott Hadad zu identifizieren und der Sohn des Korngottes Dagan. Als Regen- und Sturmgott, dessen Stimme in Blitz und Donner erschallt, ist er der Spender aller Fruchtbarkeit und der Repräsentant der grünenden Vegetation. Wenn er abstirbt, siecht die Natur dahin, alles Wachstum hört auf. Baal ist außerdem ein mächtiger Kämpfer, Tempelbauer und

---

[13] Vgl. O. Eißfeldt a. a. O. 60—70.
[14] Vgl. A. S. Kapelrud a. a. O.

Kultstifter, als Gott der Gerechtigkeit der Schrecken der Übeltäter. Wie El gilt er auch als Herrscher über Götter und Menschen, dessen Königtum ewig dauert.

2. Bemerkenswert ist die Zusammenstellung von Götterdreiheiten. Neben Baal stehen Jam (»Fürst Meer und Regent Strom«) als Repräsentant der dem Kulturland gefährlichen Überschwemmungen[15], den Baal alljährlich an seinem Vorhaben, die Erde durch Überflutung in Besitz zu nehmen, in erbittertem Kampfe hindern muß, und Mot (»Tod«) als Repräsentant der Trockenheit und Leblosigkeit, dem Baal jährlich unterliegt. Dieser sich wiederholende Kampf um die Herrschaft über die Erde bildet ein zentrales Thema der ugaritischen Texte.

Eine zweite Dreiheit findet sich bei den Göttinnen: Aschera als Frau und Mutter, als gesetzte Hausherrin und weibliches Familienhaupt; Astarte als Geliebte und Mätresse, die verführerische und wollüstige Verkörperung sexueller Leidenschaft; und Anat als schönes, jungfräuliches Geschöpf, voll jugendlicher Süße und Kraft, dem Kampf und der Jagd hingegeben. Insgesamt stellen sie verschiedene Aspekte des Weiblichen dar.

3. Kennzeichnend für diese und andere Göttergestalten ist zunächst das sexuelle Moment, das für die Göttinnen bereits an amulettartigen goldenen Halsgehängen mit Darstellungen der nackten Göttin unter Hervorhebung ihrer Geschlechtsteile erkennbar wird. Von El erzählt man, wie er zwei Göttinnen verführt und auf der Weide die Aschera begattet wie Baal die Anat. Baal wird zudem als »Jungstier« bezeichnet und unter dem Bild des zeugungskräftigen Stiers dargestellt.

Die meisten Gottheiten haben ferner einen doppelten Aspekt und sind polare Wesen. In den Göttinnen vereinen sich oft Jungfrauschaft und Fruchtbarkeit, in den Göttern Entmannung und Zeugungskraft. El kastriert nicht nur seinen Vater, sondern nach anderer Darstellung auch sich selbst, obwohl er zugleich der Göttervater ist. Der Gott des Todes und der Zerstörung ist zugleich der des Lebens, der die Wunden heilt, die er geschlagen hat. Der machtvolle Regen- und Sturmgott ist zugleich der dahinwelkende und wiederauflebende Gott.

Diese Gestalt des dahinwelkenden und wiederauflebenden Gottes, selbst wieder eine polare Vorstellung, ist ebenfalls kennzeichnend. Baal ist der Gott der Vegetation; mit seinem Abscheiden hört alles Leben auf Erden auf und erlischt alle Fruchtbarkeit, um mit seiner Wiederkehr von neuem zu erblühen. Mot, ursprünglich der Todesgott,

---

[15] So Th. H. Gaster a. a. O.; doch ist vielleicht statt dessen die Inbeziehungsetzung zu den Sturmfluten an der syrisch-palästinischen Mittelmeerküste zu bevorzugen. Dagegen ist seine Deutung des Aschtar als des Gottes der künstlichen Bewässerung des Ackers durch Kanäle und als weiteren Gegenspielers Baals unwahrscheinlich.

scheint in diesen Vorstellungskreis hineingezogen worden zu sein. Wie das Korn wird er zerhauen (gedroschen), geworfelt, aufs Feld gesät, um wiederaufzuleben.

Allerdings ist in der kanaanäischen Religion noch vieles problematisch und ungeklärt. Ist das Nebeneinander von El und Baal so zu erklären, daß der letztere ein junger Gott ist, der El von seinem Platz im Pantheon verdrängt? Oder verkörpern sie zwei verschiedene Gottesvorstellungen: El das transzendente Numen, demgegenüber der Mensch der Empfangende ist, sich wie der Sklave zum Herrn verhält und ihm in Anbetung und Verehrung naht; Baal aber die Projektion dessen, wovon der Mensch selbst ein Teil ist, worin er lebt und handelt und sein Wesen hat, so daß Baal immanent vorzustellen und das Verhältnis des Menschen zu ihm das des Eintauchens in ihn und der Gemeinschaft mit ihm ist?

Darf man ferner die Möglichkeit, daß El für einen Teil der Einwohner von Ugarit der Gott schlechthin gewesen zu sein scheint, als Grund für einen El-Urmonotheismus der Westsemiten in Anspruch nehmen, oder darf man besser nur von einem Hauptgott El sprechen? Ist es möglich, auch die vormosaischen Israeliten, die wohl vornehmlich aramäischer Herkunft waren, dennoch als Verehrer dieses Gottes zu denken?

Wie verhalten sich nach den ugaritischen Funden Mythos und Ritus zueinander? Sind Mythen und Kultlieder zu einem erheblichen Teil aus Jahreszeitspielen herausgewachsen, bieten sie in abgeblaßter und umgestalteter Form deren wesentlichen Gehalt[16]? Oder sind die Versuche, ugaritische Texte als Textbücher kultdramatischer Spiele oder ihre Nachklänge zu erweisen, als mißlungen zu bezeichnen und handelt es sich vielmehr um freie literarische Schöpfungen? Begleitet also der Mythos den Ritus, oder müssen sie anders verstanden werden? Trifft die augenblicklich zu beobachtende Überbewertung des kultischen Elements für die kanaanäische Religion tatsächlich zu?

Dieselbe Frage gilt in Hinsicht auf die vielerörterte Stellung des Königs im Alten Orient und seine angebliche Beziehung zur Gottheit. Stehen beide wirklich in Wechselbeziehung, so daß der König ein Avatar des Gottes ist? Stellt das, was der König im Ritual vollzieht, nur eine Realisierung dessen dar, was die Gottheit auf der überirdischen Ebene vornimmt? Umgibt den kanaanäischen Stadtkönig wirklich eine Aura des Numinosen? Bedeutet es in diesem Zusammenhang etwas, daß die Urkunden aus der königlichen Kanzlei von Ugarit das dynastische Siegel tragen, d. h. das Siegel des Gründers der Dynastie und nicht dasjenige mit dem Namen des regierenden Königs[17]?

---

[16] Th. H. Gaster a. a. O.
[17] Cl. Schaeffer nach dem Bericht: The Royal Palace of Ugarit a. a. O.

Ist schließlich mit der Vorstellung des dahinwelkenden und wiederauflebenden Gottes bereits der Glaube an eine Auferstehung gegeben oder vorgeformt, muß sein Ursprung im Parsismus gesucht werden, oder ist er israelitischen Wurzeln entsproßt?

Über solchen Fragen, die sich ergeben, soll jedoch nicht vergessen werden, daß die kanaanäische Religion ihre eigenen Werte besitzt, die über ihrer Einkleidung in rohe und unfertige Formen leicht übersehen werden. Sie sucht einen tieferen Zugang zur Welt und ihrer Erscheinung und stellt eine Vertrautheit zwischen Mensch und Natur her, die ein technisches Zeitalter nur zu leicht zerstört. Sie sucht die menschliche Existenz dadurch zu heben und zu festigen, daß sie den Menschen in den fortwährenden Schöpfungsvorgang einbezieht und seine demütige Abhängigkeit von der Gottheit durch die Erhebung zu ihrem Helfer ausgleicht.

V.

Betrachten wir die Nachwirkungen der kanaanäischen Religion, soweit es nach den bisherigen Erkenntnissen möglich ist, so liegen offensichtliche Beziehungen zum Alten Testament und damit zum Judentum, Christentum und Islam wie auch zur griechisch-römischen Antike und damit zum humanistischen Element der modernen Kultur vor.

1. Die Bühne, auf der sich das geschichtliche Werden der israelitischen Kultur und Religion nach der Landnahme in Palästina in Übernahme und Ablehnung kanaanäischen Gutes und in schärferer Erfassung der eigenen Werte vollzogen hat, ist für uns nunmehr heller beleuchtet worden. Beschränken wir uns auf das Gebiet der israelitisch-jüdischen Religion, so sind die kanaanäischen Einwirkungen auf sie in fast all ihren Strömungen und Aspekten deutlich.

Die magische Daseinshaltung, von der das israelitische Volk wohl mehr hielt, als man gewöhnlich anzunehmen geneigt ist, scheint in erster Linie durch die kanaanäische Vegetations- und Fruchtbarkeitsreligion geformt worden zu sein, obwohl die Israeliten schon aus ihrer nomadischen Frühzeit entsprechende Vorstellungen und Bräuche mitgebracht haben und andere in der späten Königszeit infolge der Vasallität und Bündnispolitik von außen hinzukamen.

Die kultische Frömmigkeit verfolgte eine mittlere Linie, die weder die restlose Ablehnung der kanaanäischen Elemente noch die völlige Anpassung des eigenen Glaubens bezweckte, sondern die lebensfähigen, berechtigten und dem Jahweglauben nicht widersprechenden Elemente einzubeziehen suchte. Unvereinbar mit Jahwe waren die Gedanken der geschlechtlichen Aufspaltung und des Sterbens der Gottheit. Konnte aber El nicht als Gatte und Vater in Jahwe aufgehen, so doch als Gott des Himmels und der Weisheit. Ließ sich die Stiernatur Baals und sein rhythmisches Sterben und Wiederaufleben nicht auf Jahwe übertragen, so doch seine Herrschaft über das Kulturland und seine segensreiche Gewährung aller Fruchtbarkeit. Fast der gesamte israelitische Kultus ist durch die kanaanäische Religion geprägt worden. Es ist bezeichnend, daß der salomonische Tempel nach kanaanäischem Vorbild errichtet worden ist, wie die 1936 entdeckte Parallele von Tell Ta'jīnāt in Nordsyrien erweist[18]. Oft genug ist Israel dabei zu weit gegangen, so daß zwischen einem kanaanisierten Jahwekult und einem jahwistisch beeinflußten Baalkult nur schwer zu unterscheiden war. Von da aus werden die ständige Gefahr des Synkretismus und die mehrfachen Kultusreformen verständlich.

Ähnlich wie in der kultischen Frömmigkeit ist manches in der national-religiösen Haltung der vorexilischen Quellenschichten des Hexateuchs zu beurteilen. Neben der Ablehnung fremder Erzählungselemente stehen wieder ihre Übernahme und Aneignung. Nicht nur sind kanaanäische Mythen auf Jahwe übertragen worden, auch die sumerisch-babylonischen müssen vielleicht als durch die Kanaanäer vermittelt gelten.

Schließlich ist die Gesetzesfrömmigkeit allein auf dem Boden der apodiktischen Lebens- und Verhaltensregeln Israels gänzlich undenkbar. Ihre wichtigste Wurzel liegt in dem kasuistischen Recht der Kanaanäer, das seit der Richterzeit in Israel heimisch wurde.

Da die Weisheitslehre wegen ihrer fremden, ausländischen Herkunft außer Betracht bleiben muß, kann als israelitische Bewegung gegen den kanaanäischen Einfluß zunächst nur die besonders von Nasiräern und Rechabiten vertretene konservative Haltung genannt werden. Sie lehnte die gesamte kanaanäische Kultur und Religion zugunsten der nomadischen Lebensweise rundweg ab. Dadurch hat sie zweifellos dazu beigetragen, die Impulse des mosaischen Jahweglaubens lebendig zu erhalten, ihr Sieg jedoch hätte Volk und Glaube zur Unfruchtbarkeit verdammt.

Lediglich den Propheten ist es gelungen, in Auseinandersetzung mit all den erwähnten Strömungen einen neuen und vollendeten Glauben zu erreichen und in den Formen ihrer Zeit auszusprechen und anzuwenden. Gerade angesichts des neuen und schärferen Bildes der israelitisch-jüdischen Religion mit ihren so verschiedenen, fast konfessionsähnlichen Richtungen auf dem Hintergrund der kanaanäischen Einwirkung wird die epochale, weltweite und ewig gültige Bedeutung der Prophetie deutlicher als je zuvor. Sie stellt sich als eine einmalige Erscheinung dar, die weder aus Israel noch aus der kanaanäischen oder einer anderen altorientalischen Religion geschicht-

---

[18] Vgl. den Plan von C. W. McEwan in: AJA 41 (1937), 9 Abb. 4.

lich abgeleitet werden kann. Angesichts der Wiederentdeckung der kanaanäischen Religion ist es also nicht nur erforderlich, die israelitisch-jüdische Religionsgeschichte neu zu betrachten, sondern auch wesentlich theologische Folgerungen zu ziehen, die für den christlichen Glauben eine noch schwer übersehbare Bedeutung erlangen könnten[19].

2. Lassen wir in den Beziehungen der Kanaanäer zur griechisch-römischen Antike wieder allgemeine kulturelle Errungenschaften wie die alphabetische Schrift, nautische Erkenntnisse sowie die Wirkungen der zeitweiligen Seeherrschaft im Mittelmeer und der kolonisatorischen Tätigkeit unbeachtet, so bleibt allein schon der Einfluß der kanaanäischen Religion auf das frühe Griechentum beachtenswert. Es mag genügen, auf drei bereits beobachtete Einzelheiten hinzuweisen, die sich offenbar aus der beiderseitigen Neigung zu ästhetischem Empfinden und spekulativem Denken ergeben haben[20]: die Gemeinsamkeiten des kanaanäischen Pantheons mit dem homerischen Olymp, die teilweise Abhängigkeit der griechischen Theogonie und Kosmogonie von der kanaanäischen Mythologie und die anthropomorphisierende Götterdichtung Ugarits als Vorbereitung der griechischen Religionsphilosophie.

Auf diese Weise gestatten die ugaritischen Texte Einblicke in die Vorgeschichte der Geisteskultur der Antike, durch die wiederum unser Dasein mitbestimmt ist. Dadurch und durch die Beziehungen zu Israel erhalten sie eine nachhaltigere Bedeutung und ein größeres Gewicht als die Funde, die man seit vielen Jahrzehnten im übrigen Alten Orient gemacht hat.

---

[19] Vgl. G. Fohrer, Die zeitliche und überzeitliche Bedeutung des Alten Testaments, s. u. 23—38.

[20] O. Eißfeldt, Die religionsgeschichtliche Bedeutung der Funde von Ras Schamra, ZDMG 88 NF 13 (1934), 180—184; Phönikische und griechische Kosmogonie, in: Éléments orientaux dans la religion grecque ancienne, 1960, 1—16 (= Kleine Schriften, III 1966, 501—512).

Universale Vorstellungen in der kanaanäischen und der israelitischen Religion

I.

Der Kongreß findet statt als Abschluß des »Vivekananda Birth Centenary Celebration Year«. Zweifellos gehört Vivekananda zu den großen Männern Indiens, denen wir gern unseren Tribut zollen, wie auch jeder vernünftige Mensch den Grundgedanken dieses Kongresses[1] fördern wird, »to bring about and strengthen a spirit of understanding, tolerance and co-operation in matters of the spirit and of the world around us, and to help peace on earth and good will among men«. Als Vivekananda 1893 am Weltkongreß der Religionen in Chicago teilnahm, haben seine Reden großen Anklang gefunden, und auch in Europa hat er mit Erfolg die Vedanta-Lehre Ramakrishnas gepredigt. Was seine Ideen wichtig macht, sind die Toleranz gegenüber anderen Religionen und die Auffassung, daß der Geist des Vedanta einen Hindu zu einem besseren Hindu und einen Christen zu einem besseren Christen machen soll. Wer sollte nicht immer besser werden, als er ist?

Die christliche Religion ist in Europa oft der Gefahr ausgesetzt, von der materialistischen Zivilisation überwältigt zu werden, und wird durch einen kämpferischen Atheismus bedrängt. Ihre unvergänglichen Grundzüge aber sind die Liebe Gottes zum Menschen und die Liebe des Menschen zu Gott und zum Mitmenschen. Als Jesus von einem Mann gefragt wurde, was er tun müsse, um das ewige Leben zu erwerben, ließ er sich aufsagen, was das Gesetz darüber sagt: »Du sollst den Herrn, deinen Gott, lieben aus deinem ganzen Herzen und mit deiner ganzen Seele und mit deiner ganzen Kraft und mit deinem ganzen Denken« und »deinen Nächsten wie dich selbst«. Und Jesus sagte dazu: »Tue das, so wirst du leben!« (Luk 10 25ff.).

Immer wieder lesen wir in der Bibel, daß Gott Liebe ist (I Joh 4 16), daß sein Wort das wahre Licht ist, das jeden Menschen erleuchtet (Joh 1 9), daß er sich nicht unbezeugt gelassen hat (Act 14 17) und daß er will, daß alle Menschen gerettet werden und zur Erkenntnis der Wahrheit kommen (I Tim 2 4). Darin begegnen wir dem universalen Aspekt seiner Offenbarung. Gott ist nicht ein Gott allein der Juden oder der Christen. Die Anhänger der anderen Religionen sind von

---

[1] »Parliament of Religions« 29. 12. 1963 — 5. 1. 1964 in Calcutta als Abschluß des »Vivekananda Birth Centenary Celebration Year«.

seiner Liebe nicht ausgeschlossen. Das ist die Lehre der Bibel, die Gottes Wollen und Handeln nicht auf die wenigen Stämme Israels und die christlichen Kirchen beschränkt, sondern die alle Menschen und Völker von der Entstehung der Menschheit bis zum Ende unserer Welt von seiner Liebe umfaßt sieht.

Solche universale Auffassung hat es in der christlichen Theologie von den frühen Tagen an gegeben. Augustin erklärte um 400 n. Chr. daß das durch den christlichen Glauben gebrachte Heil niemals für einen seiner würdigen Menschen unerreichbar war[2]. Im 15. Jh. drang Nikolaus von Cues zu der Erkenntnis vor, daß Gott in den verschiedenen Religionen auf verschiedenen Wegen gesucht und unter verschiedenen Namen angerufen wird, daß er in den verschiedenen Zeitaltern verschiedene Propheten und Lehrer zu den verschiedenen Völkern gesandt[3]. Sicher hätte Nikolaus nicht gezögert, Vivekananda zu diesen Lehrern zu zählen.

Als gegen Ende des 18. und im 19. Jh. die Kenntnis der östlichen Religionen mehr und mehr im Westen verbreitet wurde, waren es viele der größten Geister der westlichen Welt, die sich für die östliche und besonders für die indische Weisheit begeisterten. Die vergleichende Religionswissenschaft enthüllte manche Parallelen zwischen dem Christentum und nichtchristlichen Religionen. Umgekehrt erwiesen sich andere Religionen, insbesondere diejenigen des Alten Orients, als die Quelle von biblisch-christlichen Vorstellungen und von gottesdienstlichen und organisatorischen Zügen des Christentums. Sogar das Neue Testament ist von seiner jüdischen und hellenistisch-orientalischen Umwelt stark beeinflußt worden. So wurde der biblisch-christliche Glaube wie jede andere Religion in einem langen geschichtlichen Vorgang innerhalb des großen Stromes der universalen Geschichte der Religion vorbereitet, geboren und weitergebildet. Dabei hat er von Anfang an eine Tendenz zu universalen Vorstellungen besessen und diese Vorstellungen gegen den Widerstand in den eigenen Reihen weiter entwickelt.

Wenn wir nunmehr solche universalen Vorstellungen im Alten Testament aufweisen wollen, müssen wir uns klarmachen, daß diese Vorstellungen nicht aus sich selbst heraus entstanden sind, sondern wenigstens teilweise ihre Quellen in der altkanaanäischen Religion haben, die die Israeliten in Palästina kennenlernten. Das ist ein gutes Beispiel sowohl für die Interdependenz von Religionen als auch für den Universalismus, der Verstehen, Toleranz und Zusammenarbeit wecken oder fördern kann.

---

[2] Augustin, Ep. CII, 5.
[3] Nikolaus von Cues, De pace seu concordantia fidei, 1453, ed. Faber Stapulensis, 1514, I fol. CXIVb.

II.

Seit der frühen Bronzezeit im 3. Jt. v. Chr. haben die Menschen semitischen Ursprungs die Masse der Bevölkerung in Syrien und Palästina gebildet. Im 19.—18. Jh. kam die neue semitische Schicht der Kanaanäer hinzu, sodann in den folgenden Jahrhunderten als weiteres Element der Bevölkerung eine Gruppe von Hurritern und eine Herrenschicht indo-europäischer Abstammung. Diese und andere Menschen bildeten eine bunte Mischung, in der allerdings das kanaanäische Element überwog. Das war auch in den phönizischen Hafenstädten der Fall. Von diesen Städten ist für uns eine besonders wichtig geworden, die seit 1929 ausgegraben wird: das alte Ugarit an der syrischen Küste gegenüber der Ostspitze von Cypern. Dort sind Texte in 8 Sprachen gefunden worden, die uns ein recht klares Bild von den Beziehungen zu anderen Ländern und Zivilisationen und von der kanaanäischen Religion geben.

Ugarit lebte in wechselnder politischer Abhängigkeit von Ägypten und vom Reich der Hetiter in Kleinasien; es weist ferner manche kulturellen Einflüsse Babyloniens und der Hurriter auf, von denen die ersteren allerdings nur widerwillig geduldet wurden. Desto bereitwilliger nahmen Ugarit und andere phönizische Hafenstädte die Beziehungen zur Welt des Mittelmeers auf. Damit haben die Ausgrabungen uns gelehrt: Der Alte Orient war kein in sich geschlossener, monolithischer Block, sondern nach dem Westen hin offen. Die kanaanäischen Phönizier waren die Mittler zwischen den Zivilisationen und Religionen in Ost und West. Daher dürfen wir nicht mehr scharf zwischen dem Alten Orient und der antiken Welt des Mittelmeers, zwischen Semiten und Indo-Europäern trennen. Vielmehr standen beide miteinander in Verbindung und gegenseitiger Durchdringung — einmal auf dem Wege über die Hetiter sowie ferner vor allem über die semitischen Phönizier.

Die universale Wirkung dieser Beziehungen bemerken wir zunächst an der ugaritischen Schrift. Sie ist eine Keilschrift nach der Art der babylonischen Schrift. Aber im Gegensatz zu dieser bedeutet jedes Zeichen nicht eine Silbe, sondern einen Buchstaben. Die Schrift ist also dem Alphabet angepaßt, das ebenfalls von den kanaanäischen Phöniziern erfunden worden ist. Das Alphabet und die alphabetische Schrift haben dann einerseits die Israeliten und andere orientalische Völker übernommen, andererseits um 900 v. Chr. die Griechen. Unser Alphabet und unsere Schrift sind letzten Endes ein Erbe der Phönizier. Doch die Leute von Ugarit haben nicht nur ihre Beziehung zum Osten, zu Babylonien, benutzt, indem sie die Zeichen der Keilschrift verwendeten, sondern haben es auch der griechischen Welt des Mittelmeers erleichtert, ihre Schrift zu lesen. Während nämlich das semitische

Alphabet gewöhnlich nur Konsonanten und keine Vokale enthält, gibt das ugaritische Alphabet die drei Vokale a, i und u an.

Die universale Wirkung der Phönizier bemerken wir ferner in den Vorstellungen über das Werden der Götter und das Werden der Welt bei den Griechen[4]. Wenn wir die Darstellung des Phöniziers Sanchunjaton, über die später Philo Byblios ein wenig berichtet hat, mit den Darstellungen der Griechen bei Hesiod, Anaximander und Demokrit vergleichen, dann ergeben sich viele Ähnlichkeiten, die sicherlich nicht zufällig sind. Die Priorität liegt bei Sanchunjaton, der schon im 2. Jt. v. Chr. gelebt hat; von ihm sind die später lebenden Griechen abhängig. Die Phönizier waren die Gebenden und die Griechen die Empfangenden.

Diese universalen Wirkungen der phönizischen Zivilisation sind dem weltweiten, universalen Geist der Phönizier entsprungen, und diesem Geist entsprechen universale Vorstellungen in der kanaanäischen Religion.

Obwohl es niemals einen monotheistischen Zug in der kanaanäischen Religion gegeben hat, hat in ihr der Gott El — der auch in Ugarit ursprünglich der wichtigste Gott war — eine grundlegende Rolle gespielt und universale Eigenarten besessen. Er leitet die Versammlung aller Götter als deren König; er heißt Vater der Götter und Vater der Erhabenen (der Götter), Vater der Menschheit und Schöpfer der Geschöpfe. Die anderen in der Götterversammlung zusammentretenden Götter heißen Kreis bzw. Familie Els und Kreis der Söhne Els. Daß El nicht nur als »Vater« der Götter und Menschen gilt, sondern daß seine Schöpferkraft in umfassender Weise wirkt, ergibt sich daraus, daß er in westsemitischen Inschriften als Schöpfer der Erde bezeichnet wird. Sein Wesen ist »the highest virtue the Arabs knew in a ruler, ḥilm. This means a mixture of goodness, friendliness and wisdom, which results in moderation and tolerance, but after all is based on self-reliance and belief in one's own power, so that one is able to let the forces have free scope while standing in the point of balance«[5].

In Ugarit hat El während des 15. Jh. in zunehmendem Maße an Gewicht und Bedeutung verloren, während Baal der junge und aufstrebende Gott war. In Palästina dagegen war El noch bei der Landnahme der Israeliten der Hauptgott und wurde erst später durch Baal verdrängt. Dieser Umstand ist von größter Bedeutung für die

---

[4] Vgl. O. Eißfeldt, Taautos und Saanchunjaton, 1952; Phönizische und griechische Kosmogonie, in: Éléments orientaux dans la religion grecque ancienne, 1960, 1—16 (= Kleine Schriften, III 1966, 501—512).

[5] F. Løkkegaard, A Plea for El, the Bull, and other Ugaritic Miscellanies, in: Pedersen-Festschrift, 1953, 233.

Israeliten geworden, die El noch als den kanaanäischen Hauptgott kennenlernten. Zeitweilig haben sie die El-Religion übernommen. Vor allem haben sie El und Jahwe miteinander identifiziert und die universalen Züge im Bilde Els auf Jahwe übertragen. Dies begründete dann das universale Gepräge des Gottes Israels. Er übernahm die Funktionen des Schöpfers der Welt und des Königs der Götter, wobei die letztere dahin umgebildet wurde, daß er der König aller Menschen wurde. Er war es, der nicht mehr bloß die Herrschaft über sein Volk Israel beanspruchte, sondern der im Geschick aller Völker und Menschen handelte. Das ergab den Anstoß zu einer Entwicklung, die die ihm ursprünglich eigenen Züge der gefährlichen Unheimlichkeit und eifernden Leidenschaftlichkeit durch die Züge der Besonnenheit und Weisheit, der Mäßigung und Geduld, der Nachsicht und Barmherzigkeit ergänzte[6].

Auch Baal besaß universale Züge, vor allem im Bereich der Natur, die Jahwe übernehmen konnte. So wurde er nicht nur derjenige, der im Geschick der Völker und Menschen handelte, sondern auch derjenige, der Regen und Fruchtbarkeit schenkte oder versagte und dessen Walten mit der leisen Windstille vergleichbar war.

Aber am wichtigsten waren die von El übernommenen universalen Züge. Wohl mit Recht hat man zusammenfassend gesagt: »El is the special contribution of Canaan to the world. He is fused with the stern God Yahve, and thus he has become the expression of all fatherliness, being mild and stern at the same time.«[7]

III.

Wie Israel in einem religiösen Austausch mit der kanaanäischen Religion stand, so geriet es in kulturelle und kommerzielle Beziehungen zu den phönizischen Städten (besonders zu Tyrus) und vielleicht durch sie, durch hetitische Herrengeschlechter in Palästina und durch die Philister, sogar in Berührung mit der Welt der Indo-Europäer. Daraus, vor allem aus dem Einfluß der kanaanäischen Religion, werden die universalen Züge in der israelitischen Religion leichter verständlich. Sie wirken dann weiter und werden verstärkt durch das Drängen zum Monotheismus, d. h. zu dem Glauben, daß nur ein Gott existiert, der der Gott der ganzen Welt und aller Menschen ist.

Die universale Auffassung ist aber nichts Selbstverständliches, sondern hat sich immer wieder gegen eine national-partikularistische Auffassung durchsetzen müssen. Die Behauptung, daß Gott nur Israel erwählt habe und nur zu ihm — und zu keinem anderen Volk — in

---

[6] O. Eißfeldt, El and Yahweh, JSS 1 (1956), 36f. (= Kleine Schriften, III 1966, 397).
[7] F. Løkkegaard a. a. O. 232.

einem einzigartigen Verhältnis stehe, ist ein nationaler Irrglaube. Der Prophet Amos lehnt ihn denn auch ab und kehrt ihn dahin um, daß er für seine Zuhörer daraus lediglich das Recht Gottes ableitet, das ungehorsame und glaubenslose Israel zu vernichten. Das Alte Testament stellt immer wieder fest, daß Gott im Geschick aller Völker und Menschen und nicht nur im Geschick Israels handelt; man kann höchstens sagen, daß Israel als erstes Volk erkannt hat, daß es sich so verhält.

Daher beginnen die frühen Erzähler damit, daß sie die Entstehung und Entfaltung der Menschheit schildern: die Entwicklung der Stadtkultur neben dem Zeltleben der Nomaden, das Auftreten der Musikanten und Techniker neben den Hirten und Bauern. Wenn sie dann außerdem eine Übersicht über die damals bekannten Völker der Erde geben, ist es deutlich, daß sie die Völkergeschichte als eine Einheit verstehen. Und Abraham erhält den Segensspruch: »In dir sollen alle Geschlechter der Erde gesegnet werden« (Gen 12 3). Damit allerdings verengt sich der Blick der Erzähler auf das, was das in einer besonders engen Beziehung zu Gott lebende Israel für die übrige Welt bedeutet, wenn es auch seine Geschichte zugunsten der ganzen Menschheit leben und wenn auch das letzte Ziel die Vereinigung der in viele Völker und Sprachen aufgespaltenen Menschheit sein soll. Solche Verflochtenheit von universalen und nationalen oder partikularistischen Ideen findet sich häufig.

Daneben dringt jedoch immer wieder die rein universale Auffassung durch, besonders bei den alttestamentlichen Propheten. Wenn die Israeliten sich auf die Rettung aus Ägypten als Beweis der göttlichen Gnade berufen, hält Amos dem entgegen:

> Seid ihr mir nicht wie die Kuschiten,
> ihr Israeliten? (sagt Jahwe).
> Habe ich nicht Israel heraufgeführt
> aus Ägypten,
> aber auch die Philister aus Kaphtor
> und die Aramäer aus Kir? (Am 9 7)

Daher zieht Gott nicht allein Israel für seine Vergehen zur Rechenschaft, sondern auch andere Völker — selbst dann, wenn sie sich gegeneinander verfehlt haben und nicht gegen Israel. Das betrifft z. B. Moab,

> weil es die Gebeine des Königs von Edom
> zu Kalk verbrannt hat. (Am 2 1)

Genauso handelt Gott durch verschiedene Völker, die er dazu beruft, aber auch wieder verwerfen kann, wenn sie ihm nicht dienen wollen. In dieser Weise betrachtet Jesaja die damalige Weltmacht Assyrien:

Universale Vorstellungen in der kanaanäischen und der israelitischen Religion

> Wehe Assur,
> der Waffe meines Zorns,
> dem Stock meiner Verwünschung!
> Ich sende es gegen eine gottentfremdete Nation
> und biete es gegen das Volk meiner Wut auf. (Jes 10 5)

Analog erklären andere Propheten, daß Gott die Weltherrschaft an den König Nebukadrezzar von Babylonien oder den König Cyrus von Persien verliehen hat (Jer 27 6 Jes 45 1).

In der späteren Zeit werden solche universalen Ideen ebenfalls ausgesprochen. Ein unbekannter Prophet verkündet, daß alle Völker zu Gott wallfahren werden,

> damit er uns seine Wege lehre
> und wir in seinen Pfaden wandeln.

Das wird das Ende aller Kriege sein:

> Er wird zwischen den Völkern richten
> und zwischen vielen Nationen entscheiden.
> Da schmieden sie ihre Schwerter zu Pflugscharen um
> und ihre Speere zu Winzermessern.
> Nicht mehr hebt Volk gegen Volk das Schwert,
> noch lernt man fernerhin das Kriegführen. (Jes 2 2-4)

Ein anderer Prophet erwartet, daß die alten Feinde Ägypten, Assyrien und Israel sich versöhnen und Gott gemeinsam anbeten werden. Dann wird Gott sagen:

> Gesegnet sei mein Volk Ägypten und das Werk meiner Hände Assur und mein Erbbesitz Israel! (Jes 19 25)

Die Erzählung vom Propheten Jona zieht daraus die praktischen Folgerungen. Sie schildert, wie der Prophet von Gott gezwungen wird, die assyrische Hauptstadt wegen ihrer Sünde zur Buße zu rufen, wie Gott ihr gnädig und liebevoll vergibt und ihr das gleiche Heil schenkt wie Israel. Diese Erzählung der Bibel war ein kräftiger Schlag gegen alle nationalen oder partikularistischen Ideen. Ja, ein Prophet sprengt alle Schranken für Gott:

> Vom Sonnenaufgang bis zum Sonnenuntergang
> ist mein Name bei den Völkern groß.
> An allen Orten
> wird mir reine Gabe dargebracht,
> denn mein Name ist bei den Völkern groß,
> sagt Jahwe Zebaot. (Mal 1 11)

Schließlich ist der »Knecht Jahwes« zu erwähnen, mit dem wohl Deuterojesaja gemeint ist und der — wie seine Anhänger glaubten —

die Schuld aller Menschen getragen und für die Sünder in Israel und in der Völkerwelt gestorben ist, damit sie leben blieben:

> Er trug unsere Krankheiten,
>   unsere Schmerzen lud er sich auf,
> während wir ihn für gezeichnet hielten,
>   von Gott geschlagen und erniedrigt.
> Er war durchbohrt ob unserer Auflehnung,
>   zerschlagen wegen unserer Vergehen.
> Er wurde zu unserem Heil gezüchtigt,
>   durch seine Wunde wurden wir geheilt.   (Jes 53 4 f.)

Auf diese Weise

> trug er die Sünde der Vielen
>   und trat für die Empörer ein.   (Jes 53 12)

Das sind die großen universalen Ideen des Alten Testaments: die Gemeinschaft und Verbundenheit Gottes mit allen Völkern und Menschen, deren Leben und Geschick er in Natur und Geschichte, in Vergangenheit, Gegenwart und Zukunft leitet; die Gemeinschaft und Verbundenheit der Menschen untereinander, die eine große Gemeinde bilden und keine Kriege mehr kennen sollen; und die Gemeinschaft und Verbundenheit eines gottbegnadeten Menschen mit den anderen, für die er sein Leben opfert und die er mit Gott versöhnt. Diese Ideen wirken bis heute weiter.

IV.

Nun sind allerdings auch theoretische Einwände und praktische Vorwürfe gegen das Christentum erhoben worden, in dessen Bibel sich jene universalen Ideen finden. Man hat manchmal gesagt, daß es voll Dogmatismus und Intoleranz sei und daß es im täglichen Leben versage. Und man hat vorgeschlagen, daß es seine mystischen Züge wieder entdecken und entwickeln solle, um eine Synthese mit anderen ähnlichen Auffassungen einzugehen und mit diesen eine universale mystische Religion für alle Menschen zu bilden. Aber wäre das mehr als eine gekünstelte Konstruktion, die nur wenige Menschen befriedigen könnte? Vor allem ist das mystische Element in der biblischen Tradition sehr gering, so daß schwer zu sagen ist, was denn eigentlich entwickelt werden soll.

Statt dessen können wir von stärkeren Zügen der biblischen Tradition ausgehen, insbesondere von ihren universalen Ideen. Danach verhält es sich doch so, daß Gott jedes Volk, jede Klasse, jedes Alter und jede Person umfaßt.

Außerdem weist der alttestamentliche Glaube weitere Züge auf, die die Christenheit stärker betonen müßte und die dann eine Brücke zu anderen schlagen könnten. Jener Glaube ist nämlich nicht statisch, starr und bewegungslos, sondern dynamisch, lebendig und wirksam. Er kennt kein Dogma. Er schafft eine persönliche Gemeinschaft mit Gott, die die ganze menschliche Existenz umfaßt. Und er ist nicht ein frommes Fühlen und Sehnen, sondern soll sich im täglichen Leben auswirken und bewähren.

Gerade der letzte Punkt ist wichtig. Denn an ihm entscheidet sich, ob wir bei der Probe bestehen können, die Jesus in der Bergpredigt als ein Kriterium lebendigen Glaubens genannt hat: »An ihren Früchten werdet ihr sie erkennen« (Matth 7 14). Dem entspricht, was der Mönch Salvian im 5. Jh. n. Chr. erklärte: »Wenn unser Glaube gut ist, dann ist es nicht unser Verdienst, aber wenn unser Leben schlecht ist, dann ist es unsere Schuld. Es ist ohne Nutzen für uns, wenn unser Glaube gut, unser Leben und Verhalten dagegen nicht gut ist.« Denn »für unser schlechtes Leben sind wir selbst verantwortlich«[8].

Ebenso wichtig wie der Glaube ist das richtige Leben auf der Grundlage der Religion. Von ihm können wieder universale Wirkungen ausgehen. Wie das Verhältnis des Westens zum Osten in früheren Jahrhunderten von Alexander dem Großen an mißverstanden wird, wenn man es einfach als den Versuch imperialistischer Beherrschung darstellt, und wie vielmehr eine gegenseitige Beeinflussung und Befruchtung stattgefunden hat, so wirkt sich dieses Verhältnis auch in der praktischen sozialen Tätigkeit aus, die mit Liebe und Barmherzigkeit im Hinduismus begonnen zu haben das große Verdienst der Ramakrishna Mission ist.

Unsere Zeit benötigt die Zusammenarbeit aller religiösen Menschen zur Bewältigung der großen ethischen und erzieherischen, sozialen und politischen Aufgaben der Menschheit. Die meisten Religionen proklamieren die Bruderschaft aller Menschen und fordern Gerechtigkeit und Liebe. Darin liegt die gemeinsame Grundlage, die solche Zusammenarbeit ermöglicht. Schon mehrfach ist sie versucht und begonnen worden, aber wir sollten sie von neuem versuchen und beginnen. Wie es eine ökumenische Vereinigung der meisten christlichen Kirchen gibt, so sollte es auch eine ökumenische Bewegung der Religionen oder besser: der religiösen Menschen geben. Ihr Ziel kann nicht Vereinigung oder Relativierung der Religionen sein, wohl aber die praktische Zusammenarbeit aller religiösen Menschen gegen die gemeinsamen Feinde der Menschheit: Krankheit und Armut, Tyrannei und Krieg. Es ist unsere Pflicht, daß wir uns auf einer breiten Grundlage darum bemühen, zur Lösung der schwierigen Probleme unserer Zeit beizutragen: dem Verlangen nach Frieden, Toleranz und Bruder-

---

[8] Salvian, De gubernatio Dei.

schaft an Stelle von politischem und ideologischem Haß; Gleichheit an Stelle der Verachtung anderer Rassen; Freiheit, Lebensunterhalt und Bildung für alle Menschen. Ein solches universales Bemühen scheint mir sowohl den Ideen der biblischen Religion als auch den Absichten Vivekanandas gerecht zu werden.

Die zeitliche und überzeitliche Bedeutung des Alten Testaments

I.

In den letzten Jahrzehnten sind Raum und Zeit des Alten Orients durch eine umfassende Ausgrabungstätigkeit neu erschlossen worden. Diese Ausgrabungen ließen eine ganze Welt wiedererstehen, von der man bis dahin nur unzureichende Kunde aus dem Alten Testament und den griechischen Historikern gehabt hatte. Mitten in dieser Welt des Alten Orients lag auch Kanaan, die Heimstätte Israels; und obwohl es nur einen kleinen Ausschnitt aus ihr darstellte, bildete es infolge seiner zentralen Lage doch den Schauplatz der Begegnung und des Ringens der verschiedenen Kulturen jenes Raumes.

Zeitlich konnte man das Werden des Alten Orients bis ins 4. Jt. zurückverfolgen. Gegenüber diesen Anfängen und den Höhepunkten im 3. Jt. erscheint die Zeit Moses und Josuas als Spätzeit. Zugleich rückte die Geschichte Israels in weite Zusammenhänge. Die Landnahme in Kanaan erfolgte im Zuge der Völkerbewegungen aus der Wüste ins Kulturland, die Gründung von Staat und Königtum in Schwächezeiten der Großstaaten, der Untergang Israels und Judas in Zusammenhang mit dem neuen Aufstieg Assyriens und Babyloniens.

Als bedeutsamste Funde haben sich mehr und mehr die aus dem nordsyrischen Ras Schamra, dem alten Ugarit, erwiesen. Seit 1929 fand man immer neue Texte, durch die wir ein plastisches Bild der dortigen Kultur und Religion im 14./13. Jh. v. Chr. erhalten und durch die die Kanaanäer für uns Wesen von Fleisch und Blut zu werden beginnen. Diese Texte entstammen dem eigenen Boden Kanaans und sind die ersten wirklichen Überreste der kanaanäischen Literatur. Sie zeigen uns das Bild einer Hochkultur, die auf gleicher Stufe wie die ägyptische und babylonische steht — nur daß sie mehr als diese ihren bäuerlichen Charakter bewahrt hat. Dasselbe gilt für die ugaritische Religion. Die Fruchtbarkeit des Bodens und der Ertrag der Ernte bilden den Hauptgegenstand ihrer Mythen und Kulte. Diese Religion entsprach den Naturnotwendigkeiten Kanaans und war — wie alle derartigen Religionen — grausam, sinnlich und orgiastisch[1]. Neben den unzähligen Dämonen und Lokalgöttern, denen ein gut organisierter Tempelkult galt, gab es eine Reihe von Hochgöttern, die ein Pantheon in der Art des babylonischen bildeten.

---

[1] W. Baumgartner, Ugaritische Probleme und ihre Tragweite für das Alte Testament, ThZ 3 (1947), 92.

Angesichts der Fülle der erkannten Übereinstimmungen mit Israel auf sprachlichem und lexikalischem, stilistischem und literarischem, kultur- und religionsgeschichtlichem Gebiet erhebt sich in verschärftem Maße die alte Frage nach dem Verständnis und der Geltung des Alten Testaments: Wieviel vom Alten Testament ist überhaupt noch israelitisch und nicht altorientalisches Erbgut? Und damit eine weitere Frage: Das Alte Testament hat eine andere Anschauung der Welt und andere Denkformen als wir. Mit innerer Wahrhaftigkeit können wir sie uns nicht zu eigen machen, sonst leben wir im Glauben in einer anderen Welt als im täglichen Leben. Das Eigentümliche des Glaubens aber ist es, gerade das ganze Leben und den ganzen Menschen zu umfassen. Es ergibt sich also die Frage: Ist in jener Welt des Alten Testaments, in ihren Vorstellungen und Begriffen noch etwas enthalten, das uns angeht? Ist das Alte Testament nur die Literatur eines Volkes mit einer orientalischen Mischkultur oder anderes und mehr als das, so daß es heute noch Geltung beanspruchen kann? Hat es lediglich zeitliche Bedeutung gehabt, so daß es heute nur noch den Historiker interessiert, oder besitzt es bleibende, überzeitliche Bedeutung, so daß es nach wie vor jeden Menschen angeht und Gegenstand theologischer Forschung sein kann?

Es ist keine Lösung dieser Frage, wenn man die Bezeugung der Offenbarung im Alten Testament ignoriert und es einfach beiseite schiebt oder in ihm nur den Ausdruck des typischen Daseinsverständnisses des Menschen vor der Offenbarung Gottes gegenüber dem besonderen des Neuen Testaments erblickt. Es ist aber ebensowenig eine Lösung, wenn man die Ergebnisse der kritischen Wissenschaft mißachtet, die geschichtliche Bedingtheit des Alten Testaments verkennt und es entweder als Einheit versteht, die aus sich heraus zu interpretieren wäre, oder es in mehr oder weniger handgreiflicher Form als Christuszeugnis deutet.

Deutlich wird daran nur die Schwere des Problems. Entweder sieht man im Alten Testament nur Überzeitliches, wenn auch vielleicht in zeitbedingter Einkleidung, oder nur Zeitliches mit dem unberechtigten Anspruch auf Überzeitlichkeit. Entweder nimmt man die Offenbarung buchstäblich, dann kann man die Ergebnisse der kritischen Wissenschaft nicht brauchen, oder man verzichtet auf die Annahme von Offenbarung, dann ist man allen kritischen Erkenntnissen offen, aber verfehlt das Eigentümliche des Alten Testaments.

Der richtige Weg muß der geschichtlich-menschlichen Seite und der Bezeugung der göttlichen Offenbarung im Alten Testament gleicherweise gerecht werden. Beides aber, damit zugleich seine überzeitliche und seine nur zeitliche Bedeutung und damit wiederum seine Beziehung zu uns, wird deutlich, sobald man das Daseinsverständnis des alttestamentlichen Menschen vor Gott ins Auge faßt. Im Daseinsverständnis ist jene Schicht gegeben, in der die Reaktion des Menschen auf die Offenbarung und damit zugleich der Einbruch dieser Offenbarung in das menschliche Dasein deutlich wird. Es kann wiederum nur mit den Mitteln der kritischen Wissenschaft erforscht und dargestellt werden, die also die unentbehrliche Voraussetzung für das Verständnis des Alten Testaments bildet. Je kritischer sie ist, desto genauer kann das Daseinsverständnis des alttestamentlichen Menschen mit seinen Voraussetzungen und Grundlagen erkannt werden.

Dieses Daseinsverständnis stellt sich im Alten Testament in einer bestimmten Geschichte dar, in deren Rahmen es in verschiedener Weise Wirklichkeit geworden ist. Es gilt, diese seine Ausprägung und mehrfache Umgestaltung im Ablauf dieser Geschichte zu erkennen. Ihr äußerer Verlauf ist längst bekannt, während der innere erst infolge der Erschließung des Alten Orients einsichtig wird. Diese innere Geschichte aber ist die Geschichte der Auseinandersetzung des alttestamentlichen Glaubens mit zwei ihm feindlichen Mächten, die in Anerkennung und Abwehr das typische menschliche Daseinsverhältnis bestimmt haben: mit der Magie und der Lebensweisheit. Es handelt sich um die Auseinandersetzung mit den beiden großen Versuchen des Menschen, seines Lebens Herr zu werden und sich seiner sicher zu fühlen, sein Dasein vor dem Einbruch jener mehr oder weniger bekannten überweltlichen, jenseitigen Macht zu sichern, die es erschüttert und in Frage stellt.

II.

Aus ihrer eigenen Vorzeit brachten die israelitischen Stämme zunächst den Glauben der mosaischen Zeit mit, der in vieler Hinsicht undeutlich ist. Der Gottesname Jahwe scheint fremden Ursprungs zu sein. Sicher ist, daß dieser Jahwe der einzige Gott der Israeliten sein sollte. Der Glaube Israels an den Einen wird stets auf Mose zurückgeführt, obwohl er die Existenz anderer Götter für andere Völker wohl noch nicht bestritten hat. Im Namen dieses Gottes hat Mose den um ihn versammelten Israeliten neue, das ganze Leben bestimmende Verhaltensregeln verkündet, die solch unauslöschlichen Eindruck gemacht haben, daß noch viele Jahrhunderte später neue Anordnungen mit der Autorität Moses begründet worden sind. Jahwe ist von Anfang an der Volksgott; er zieht mit seinem Volke mit. Und er ist mächtiger als alle anderen Götter, darum konnte er die Seinen aus Ägypten retten. Entsprechend dem Erlebnis am Sinai ist er gewaltig und erhaben, leidenschaftlich und grimmig. Ein Gott des Rechts und der Gerechtigkeit, ernst und fordernd, der Sitte und Sittlichkeit will. Ein kriegerischer Gott der die Seinen schützt und zornig auf die Feinde losfährt, dem man im Kriege dienen soll. Ein Gott heiligen Willens, der unbedingtes Vertrauen und rücksichtslosen Gehorsam fordert.

Daneben jedoch ist das Daseinsverständnis des alttestamentlichen Menschen weitgehend durch die Magie bestimmt. Außer dem Glauben der mosaischen Zeit brachten die israelitischen Stämme auch manche magischen Vorstellungen und Praktiken mit. Vermehrt wurden sie durch das Einströmen ägyptischer und babylonischer Kulte, die teilweise oder völlig von der Magie durchsetzt waren[2]. Am gefährlichsten aber war die kanaanäische Vegetations- und Fruchtbarkeitsreligion, die erst recht auf magischer Grundlage beruhte. In ihr diente alles dazu, die Gottheit zu stärken, die großen Mächte des Lebens in Gang zu halten und Fruchtbarkeit zu gewährleisten. Dieses magisch bestimmte sexuelle Moment zeigt sich in der israelitischen Volksreligion in der sakralen Prostitution, die lange Zeit sogar an den Jahweheiligtümern im Schwange war, in den wiederholten Versuchen, Jahwe ein Weib zu geben und es in den Tempel einzuführen, und in der Darstellung des Gottes durch das Bild des zeugungskräftigen Stiers.

Dem seßhaft gewordenen Israeliten erschien die Wüste von Dämonen bevölkert, deren einem, Asasel, man alljährlich ein Abwehropfer darbrachte. Die Fruchtbarkeit der Felder hing von anderen Dämonen ab. Ihretwegen dürfen die Bäume nicht ganz abgeerntet werden und muß eine letzte Getreideecke stehenbleiben. Sonst werden sie zornig und ziehen fort; dann verdorrt das Feld, und der Baum geht ein.

Die Bedeutung der Magie für das Volk und seinen Glauben kann schwerlich überschätzt werden. Eine erstaunlich große Zahl von Handlungen und Gebräuchen, deren magischer Charakter noch ganz deutlich ist, erfüllte das tägliche Leben des Israeliten. Er brauchte sie bei der Geburt und als Trauergebräuche beim Tode, bei der Arbeit und in der Liebe, bei der Ablegung des Eides und zur Ermittlung der Wahrheit; er führte sie im Tanz und in der Blutrache aus; er schützte sich vor fremder Macht durch Amulette und suchte durch all dies auf die göttlichen und dämonischen Mächte Einfluß zu gewinnen oder sie sich dienstbar zu machen. Was es also auch sein mag — stets sind die magischen Vorstellungen und Gebräuche Ausdruck eines bestimmten Daseinsverständnisses. Der Mensch, der in ihnen lebt, glaubt die großen Mächte des Lebens zu seinem Nutzen und zum Schaden des anderen beeinflussen und lenken zu können. Sie sollen dazu dienen, des eigenen Daseins Herr zu werden, es gegen alle Gefahren zu sichern und zu seinem Höhepunkt zu führen. Sicherung vor den Mächten des Schicksals und Dienstbarmachung dieser Mächte — das ist das typische Daseinsverständnis des magischen Menschen!

Demgegenüber steht die schroffe Ablehnung alles Kanaanäischen in den Kreisen der Jahweorden, als deren Exponent die Rechabiten

---

[2] Vgl. z. B. G. Contenau, La magie chez les Assyriens et les Babyloniens, 1947.

betrachtet werden dürfen. Sie haben die Gefahr klar erkannt, die mit der Übernahme der religiös verankerten kanaanäischen Kultur gegeben war. Daher lehnten sie Ackerbau und Stadtkultur ab und verboten den Genuß von Wein und das Wohnen in Häusern.

So bewundernswert das Festhalten am alten Glauben war, so gefährlich war dieses konservative Daseinsverständnis. Hätte es sein Ziel erreicht, so wären Volk und Glaube zur Unfruchtbarkeit verurteilt gewesen. Inmitten des Kulturlandes das Leben der Wüste zu führen, war nicht Gottes Wille, sondern sterile Reaktion. Es galt gerade, sich nicht in die Vergangenheit zu flüchten, sondern Gottes Willen in der lebendigen Gegenwart zu erkennen und im Dasein Gestalt gewinnen zu lassen.

Ein solcher Versuch liegt in dem durch Kultus und Gesetz bestimmten Glauben vor, der vom Priestertum immer neue Impulse erhielt und weitgehend als der offizielle Glaube Israels betrachtet werden darf. Dieser kultische Glaube hat sich in der Auseinandersetzung mit der Magie gebildet und ist eine der Ausgestaltungen des alttestamentlichen Glaubens.

Er ist gekennzeichnet durch ein Nebeneinander von Verbot und Kompromiß. Man wollte weder völlige Anpassung des Jahweglaubens noch völlige Ablehnung des Kanaanäischen, sondern ging einen mittleren Weg.

Verboten und scharf verfolgt wurde alles, was unmittelbar mit Magie und Zauberei in Zusammenhang stand, also ein wesentlicher Teil des Volksglaubens. Wenn man ein Böckchen nicht in der Milch seiner Mutter kochen soll, so ist dies das Verbot einer offenbar auf Milchzauber beruhenden Sitte, die in den ugaritischen Texten erwähnt wird: »Sie kochten ein Ziegenböckchen in Milch, ein Lamm (?) in Rahm!«[3]

Übernommen und assimiliert wurde, was mit dem eigenen Glauben vereinbar und in der neuen Lage erforderlich schien. An Els Statt wird Jahwe zum Gott des Himmels und der Weisheit, an Baals Statt zum Herrn des kanaanäischen Kulturlandes und Spender aller Fruchtbarkeit. Man überträgt die kanaanäischen Mythen vom Drachenkampf mit Leviatan und Tannin und von der Bändigung der aufrührerischen Urgewässer auf ihn. Der Tempel wird nach ausländischem Muster gebaut, der Kultus nimmt kanaanäische Züge an, zumindest ein Teil der Opfer ist kanaanäischen Ursprungs[4]. Die Priester erteilen Orakel, sprechen das Beschwörungsgebet, den Segen und den Fluch.

---

[3] Text 52, 14 (zitiert nach C. H. Gordon, Ugaritic Textbook, 1965).
[4] Schlachtopfer in ugaritischen Texten: 1, 17; 19, 13; 51, III passim. Dankopfer: 1, 8; 3, 17. 52 u. a. Schuldopfer: 27, 4. 9. Räucheropfer: 2 Aqht I, 28; 3 Aqht 26. 37.

Das Daseinsverständnis wird nun durch den Kultus geprägt. Durch ihn kann der Mensch an der göttlichen Sphäre Anteil erlangen und in gefühlsmäßigem Überschwang oder ekstatischer Erhebung in sie eindringen. Gewährt Gott dem Bauern seinen Segen, der die Ernte reifen und die Viehherden gedeihen läßt, so bringt dieser ihm dafür seine Opfer als Dank und Bitte dar. An den Heiligtümern sitzt er mit Gott zu Tisch und ist fröhlich in der Gewißheit, daß er auch im nächsten Jahre reichen Segen erlangen kann.

Darauf — von Gott etwas zu erlangen — ist der ganze Kultus abgestimmt. Während Bußgebet und Lobpreis in der älteren Literatur selten begegnen, ist das Bittgebet häufig. Man sucht dabei durch Weinen, Klagen und Trauergebräuche das Mitleid Gottes zu erwecken oder durch Versprechen von Opfern die Erhörung der Bitte zu sichern.

Auch das Gesetz, an dessen Überlieferung und Weiterbildung das Priestertums bereitwillig gearbeitet hat, dient der Gewinnung von Gottes Gunst und der Vergewisserung seiner Gnade. Zwar spielt es in der vorexilischen Zeit bei weitem nicht die entscheidende Rolle wie im späteren Judentum. Aber die Voraussetzungen sind geschaffen. Nicht umsonst wird demjenigen, der das Gesetz hält, Gottes Segen verheißen, demjenigen aber, der es nicht beachtet, sein Fluch angedroht. Man kann dem weder einen tiefen Ernst noch die Bereitschaft zum Gehorsam gegen den göttlichen Willen absprechen. Die innere Zustimmung zum Gesetz ist immer wieder spürbar, die über den Buchstaben hinausgehende Erfüllung fehlt durchaus nicht. Die einzelnen Gesetze können sogar dem grundlegenden Verhalten gegenüber dem Mitmenschen untergeordnet und dieses in umfassender Weise als Liebe zum Nächsten (Lev 19 18) bezeichnet werden.

Demgegenüber ist zu beachten, daß die kultischen Gebote dasselbe Schwergewicht wie die ethischen erhalten, wenn ihre Bedeutung nicht sogar überwogen hat. Neben der dadurch geförderten Sakralisierung und Ritualisierung des Lebens steht seine Einengung in die Grenzen des Rechts, seine Regulierung und Schematisierung. Nur das äußere Tun und Lassen kann als Maßstab dienen, da sich die innere Zustimmung und Hingabe der Beobachtung entziehen. Fromm und gerecht ist derjenige, der die im Gesetz niedergelegten Forderungen Gottes erfüllt. Der Mensch sucht durch sein Tun Gottes Herrschaft in seinem Volk in sichtbarer Gestalt zu verwirklichen und Gottes Gnade für sich selbst zu erlangen.

Das Große an dieser Umgestaltung des Glaubens ist zweifellos die Befreiung des Menschen von der Magie durch die restlose Beziehung des Kultus auf Jahwe und die Betonung der Einheit von Glaube und Sittlichkeit durch das Gesetz — mag es auch im zeitbedingten Gewande jenes Kultus und jenes Gesetzes geschehen. Letztlich aber sind magisches und kultisch-gesetzliches Daseinsverständnis nicht grundsätzlich, sondern nur gradweise unterschieden. Denn der Mensch sucht durch sein kultisches Handeln und das Befolgen des Gesetzes Gottes Segen für sein Volk und sich selbst zu erlangen. Er sucht — wie der magische Mensch — sein Dasein mit Hilfe Gottes zu sichern. Die Offenbarung, die dieses Dasein in Frage stellt, wird damit übersehen oder umgedeutet. So steht der entschlossenen Wendung gegen die Magie das Steckenbleiben in dem für den Menschen typischen Versuch gegenüber, sein Dasein mit Hilfe des durch Kultus und Gesetz erreichbaren Gottes zu sichern[5].

Genauso wie die Volksreligion mit ihrem magisch begründeten Daseinsverständnis forderte auch die volkstümliche Überlieferung der Erzählungen aus der Vorzeit des Volkes die Kritik heraus. Genauso wie in der Auseinandersetzung mit ihr werden von den großen Erzählern in den Quellenschichten des Hexateuchs die kanaanäischen und anderen fremden Einflüsse ausgeschaltet, wo es möglich ist. Genauso wird anderes übernommen und assimiliert. Daher überträgt man die Heiligtümer des Landes auf Jahwe, indem man sie mit den Ahnen des Volkes in Verbindung bringt. Sie haben sich dort aufgehalten, und Jahwe hat sich ihnen dort unter anderen Namen geoffenbart. Infolgedessen gehören jene Heiligtümer rechtmäßig ihm[6].

Entscheidend für diese neue Umgestaltung des Glaubens aber ist weniger dieses kultische[7] als das nationale Element. Angesichts der Trennung der beiden Reiche Israel und Juda verankert man den großisraelitischen Gedanken mittels der Vätertradition in der Vorzeit: eine Ahnenreihe — ein Glaube — ein Volk! Demselben nationalen

---

[5] E. Würthwein, Der Sinn des Gesetzes im Alten Testament, ZThK 55 (1958), 255—270, hat dagegen eingewendet, daß es sich bei den aus dem »Bund« Jahwes mit Israel erwachsenen apodiktischen Gesetzen anders verhalte: »Wer sie beachtet, tut das Selbstverständliche und Notwendige, nichts Verdienstliches« (266). Der Gehorsam werde als Antwort des Volkes erwartet. »Der Imperativ folgt aus dem Indikativ« (267). Demgegenüber ist zu sagen, daß diese Auffassung als eine theologische Theorie möglich wäre, ohne daß ihr jedoch die Praxis des Lebens entsprechen müßte oder entsprochen hätte. Es geht aber gerade um diese Praxis, nämlich um die gesetzliche Frömmigkeit. Zudem hat die genannte Theorie gar nicht bestanden, vielmehr war der Gedanke der Korrelation zwischen Gott und Mensch grundlegend; vgl. G. Fohrer, Action of God and Decision of Man in the Old Testament, in: Biblical Essays 1966, 1967, 31—39. Ferner geht Würthwein von der Singularität des als genuin israelitisch betrachteten »apodiktischen Rechts« aus. Doch diese Auffassung ist nicht länger haltbar. Weder sind die apodiktisch formulierten Sätze genuin israelitisch und singulär, noch stellen sie Rechtssätze dar (abgesehen von einigen Sätzen kasuistischen Rechts, die apodiktische Form erhalten haben); vgl. G. Fohrer, Das sogenannte apodiktisch formulierte Recht und der Dekalog, s. u. 120—148.

[6] Vgl. A. Alt, Der Gott der Väter, 1929 (= Kleine Schriften zur Geschichte des Volkes Israel, I 1953, 1—78).

[7] Vgl. auch E. Sellin — G. Fohrer, Einleitung in das Alte Testament, 1965[10], § 22—23.

Gedanken dient der Glaube an die Erwählung Israels durch Jahwe. Beim Jahwisten strebt die Erzählung von der düsteren Urgeschichte schnell zu Abraham und der Erwählung der Erzväter hin; der Elohist verzichtet völlig auf die Urgeschichte. Dann zieht sich der Gedanke an die Gefährdung der erwählten Sippe und an die Weisheit Jahwes, der seinen Plan der Erwählung zu einem glücklichen Ende führt, als Leitgedanke durch die verschiedenartigsten Geschichten hindurch.

Obwohl nicht übersehen werden darf, daß bei diesen Erzählern auch prophetische Einflüsse wirksam sind und das Wissen um das Handeln Gottes in Leben und Geschick von Menschen und Völkern anstatt im naturhaften Kreislauf des Jahres sich durchsetzt, ist es doch bedenklich, daß Volks- und Glaubensgrenzen zusammenfallen. Jahwe überschreitet wohl die Landes-, nicht aber die Volksgrenzen. Das Volk gar hofft auf den »Tag Jahwes«, an dem der Feind von der Katastrophe ereilt wird und Israel über alle Welt herrschen wird. So wird Gott nun auch noch in die Schranken der Nation eingeschlossen. Nicht nur durch die Ausübung des Kultus, sondern ebenso durch seine Zugehörigkeit zum auserwählten Volk glaubt der Mensch sich gesichert. Auch dieses auf den nationalen Glauben gegründete Daseinsverständnis ist demnach ein für den Menschen typisches, also ein bleibendes im zeitbedingten Gewande.

III.

Den Höhepunkt der Geschichte des alttestamentlichen Glaubens bildet das Auftreten der großen Einzelpropheten. Die Überlieferung weiß nur von wenigen solcher Männer, deren Worte ganz oder teilweise bewahrt worden sind. Von diesen sogenannten Schriftpropheten sind andere, die herkömmlich ebenfalls als Propheten bezeichnet werden, wohl zu unterscheiden. Es sind die Kultpropheten, die neben den Priestern an den Heiligtümern amtierten und im Rahmen des Kultus dem Volke oder einzelnen Menschen die Zukunft oder Jahwes Willen verkünden sollten (Nahum, Habakuk, manche Psalmen). Es sind ferner die Hofpropheten, die unter dem Einfluß des nationalen Machtwillens den König verherrlichen und seine und der Politiker Pläne aus dem Sumpf brutalen und selbstsüchtigen Machtstrebens in das reine Licht des göttlichen Geistes zu heben suchten (I Reg 22 Jer 27f.; mit kultischen Motiven verbunden in manchen Psalmen).

In den großen Einzelpropheten aber leben die Erfahrungen, Eindrücke und Impulse der mosaischen Zeit in geläuterter Form wieder auf. Sie erfahren von neuem Gottes wunderbares Wesen und seinen heiligen, Entscheidung fordernden Willen. Sie wissen sich von Gott gerufen, von ihm gedrängt und gezwungen. Der göttliche Geist ist über sie gefallen und hat sie bezwungen, die göttliche Kraft hat sie überwältigt und treibt sie zum Reden und Handeln. Darum verkünden sie das Wort, das ihnen unauslöschlich vor die Seele getreten ist und das sie in Stunden gehört und geschaut haben, in denen sie sich von Gott ergriffen wußten.

Hieraus ergibt sich das grundlegende theologische Merkmal der Offenbarung. Sie bestätigt nicht einfach das typische menschliche Daseinsverständnis, sondern erschüttert es und stellt es in Frage. Darüber hinaus läßt sie ein neues Daseinsverständnis erstehen, das von dem bisherigen nicht nur gradweise, sondern grundsätzlich verschieden ist. In ihm gibt der Prophet alle magischen, kultisch-gesetzlichen und nationalen Sicherungen preis, die sonst so eifrig gepflegt werden. Der Sinn der prophetischen Berufung ist eine solche Preisgabe des typischen Daseinsverständnisses und das Hineingestelltwerden in ein neues. Sie bildet weder das Ergebnis eines inneren Zusammenbruchs mit anschließender Bekehrung noch das einer befreienden Aufklärung, sondern ist die Beugung unter das Gericht Gottes, das der Prophet anzukündigen hat oder wie Jesaja an sich selbst erfährt (Jes 6). Der Prophet gibt jede Sicherung und sich selber auf; und indem er es tut, nimmt Gott ihn in all seiner Ungesichertheit auf und schenkt ihm ein neues Dasein. Dieses neue Dasein aber bedeutet beides: Überwindung und Erfüllung des typischen menschlichen Daseinsverständnisses.

Die Propheten haben die Magie überwunden und erfüllt, wie das Beispiel ihrer symbolischen Handlungen zeigt. Sie führen sie aus, um an und mit einem ausgewählten Symbol, das einen anderen Gegenstand darstellt, eine Handlung zu vollziehen, die symbolisch nachahmt, was sich in Wirklichkeit ereignen soll. Es gab nun viele magische symbolische Handlungen, die nach dem Willen dessen, der sie ausführt, ihre Wirksamkeit in sich selber tragen. Der Prophet dagegen erwartet nicht, daß die Gegenstände seiner Handlung kraftwirkend sind, daß auf den Vollzug seiner Handlung die Wirkung mechanisch erfolgen muß, sondern symbolisiert statt dessen den gewünschten Erfolg. Ihn Wirklichkeit werden zu lassen, bleibt Gott anheimgestellt.

Ist dadurch die Magie überwunden, so wird die symbolische Handlung doch in der Gewißheit ausgeführt, daß das symbolisierte Geschehen sich tatsächlich ereignen wird. Sie ist die wirksame Ankündigung eines Geschehens, das Gott nach seinem Willen heraufführen wird. Damit ist das berechtigte Moment erfüllt, das die magische Handlung enthält: das Bewußtsein, daß eine die Zukunft symbolisierende Handlung von Erfolg gekrönt sein muß — wenn sie aus der Gemeinschaft mit Gott geboren ist. Diese Voraussetzung, die der Magie fehlt, ist in der Prophetie gegeben. Daher wird in der prophetischen Handlung — neben der Überwindung der Magie — der tiefste

Wunsch des magischen Menschen erfüllt: Das Symbolisierte kann eintreffen[8]!

Die Propheten zerschlagen ebenso die kultisch-gesetzlichen Schranken, die zur Sicherung des Daseins errichtet worden sind. Sie haben die Wirklichkeit Gottes als die völlige Infragestellung ihres Daseins neu erfahren. Angesichts dieses Gottes muß der ganze Kultus zerbrechen und seinen Untergang finden. Priestertum und Tempel sind für die Vernichtung reif. All das, womit man Gott zu dienen und worin man ihn zu fassen geglaubt hat — Gottesbilder und Altäre, Opfer und Gebete, Gesänge und Reigen, Gelübde und Feiertage — all dies sind untaugliche Mittel, um sich Gottes Segen zu sichern. Darum verfluchen die Propheten den Kultus und verwenden die Namen der Heiligtümer zu höhnischen Wortspielen (Am 5 5). Der ganze kultische Betrieb dient letztlich nur der Sünde, ja ist im Grunde selber schon die Sünde! Er bewirkt nicht nur, daß man Gottes in ihm sicher zu sein glaubt, sondern verleitet auch dazu, daß das Volk sich auf die Erfüllung der kultischen Pflichten beschränkt und in ihrer Ableistung Gottes Willen erfüllt glaubt. Es befolgt seine angelernten Rituale und wähnt, damit vollen Gehorsam geleistet und im Leben des Alltags freie Hand zu haben. Es läßt Gott nicht die bestimmende Macht des Daseins sein und nimmt seine sittlichen Forderungen nicht mehr ernst. Darum sollten an Stelle des Kultus Recht und Gerechtigkeit gepflegt werden.

Damit soll nicht das Gesetz an die Stelle des Kultus treten. Auch seine einwandfreie Erfüllung besagt noch nichts. Denn durch sie beansprucht der Mensch nur wieder Rechte gegenüber Gott, anstatt seinen Willen anzuerkennen; durch sie will er sich Gottes Belohnung sichern, anstatt sich von ihm in Anspruch nehmen zu lassen. Vielmehr muß an die Stelle einer sachlichen Leistung und äußeren Befolgung die persönliche Hingabe treten. Man darf nicht beim Wortlaut des Gesetzes stehenbleiben, sondern muß das starre Gebot lebendig machen und seinem Geiste nach erfüllen.

Ist so das kultisch-gesetzliche Daseinsverständnis überwunden, so liegt in der Prophetie auch seine Erfüllung beschlossen. Die Propheten sprechen ethische Mahnungen aus, weil sich in ihrer Befolgung in erster Linie die Ergriffenheit des Menschen durch Gott und die gläubige Hingabe an seinen Willen ausdrückt. Es sind Forderungen Gottes, die der Mensch nur gehorsam erfüllen kann. Und das Anliegen des Kultus erfüllt sich im Gebet eines solchen Menschen. Das bezeichnendste Beispiel ist das Leben Jeremias, das erfüllt ist von innerem Ringen mit Gott im Gebet, von Fürbitten für sein irrendes Volk und

---

[8] Vgl. G. Fohrer, Die symbolischen Handlungen der alttestamentlichen Propheten, 1968².

von der Versenkung in Gott im Gebet, durch das ihm Gottes Weisung zuteil wird.

Die Propheten haben schließlich auch die nationalen Schranken gesprengt. Der Gott, der sie gesandt hat, läßt über sich nicht zugunsten eines Volkes oder Staates verfügen und ist nicht der Garant der nationalen Macht oder der völkischen Kultur. Vor der schrecklichen Offenbarung seines Willens verblassen Volk und Staat, Königtum und Erwählungsglauben, vorteilhafte Bündnisse und siegreiche Schlachten. Vor ihm muß die ganze israelitische Kultur zerbrechen und in einem schauerlichen Gericht ihren Untergang finden.

Die alleinige Bindung Gottes an Israel wird überwunden. Sein Walten ist im Schicksal aller Völker zu erkennen. Er hat Israel aus Ägypten geleitet, aber auch die Philister aus Kaphtor und die Aramäer aus Kir (Am 9 7). Wie für Jesaja Assyrien Jahwes Werkzeug war, so war es Babylonien für Jeremia und Ezechiel. Er führt Nebukadnezar auch gegen Tyrus und Ägypten.

Aus dem Nationalgott wird der Herr der Welt. Der Blick erhebt sich über die Grenzen des Volkes zu einer gläubigen Deutung des Weltgeschehens. Darin liegt zugleich wieder die Erfüllung des nationalen Glaubens, der Gottes Handeln nicht im Ablauf der Jahreszeiten und in der Fruchtbarkeit des Ackers, sondern in Ereignissen des Völker- und Menschenlebens sah. Allen Völkern aber gilt nun Gottes Wille; daher wenden die Propheten sich oft mit einem Jahwewort an sie. Alle Menschen wissen, was gut ist und was der Herr von ihnen fordert; daher wird ihnen das Gericht angedroht, wenn sie sich dagegen vergangen haben (vgl. bes. Am 2 1 ff.). Alle dienen letztlich dem einen Gott; daher kann es heißen:

> Vom Aufgang bis zum Untergang der Sonne
> mein Name groß unter den Völkern ist;
> und allerorten wird ihm Rauchopfer
> und reine Gabe dargebracht. (Mal 1 11)

Und alle Völker werden an der künftigen Heilszeit teilhaben, alle werden Gottes Wege kennenlernen und seine Pfade wandeln (Jes 2 2-4).

Insgesamt überwindet das prophetische Daseinsverhältnis also die typischen menschlichen Versuche der Lebenssicherung durch den Zwang der Magie, durch das Einfangen Gottes im Kultus, durch den Leistungsgedanken und die Werkgerechtigkeit des Gesetzes und durch die Bindung Gottes an das Volk im nationalen Glauben. An die Stelle dieser Sicherungen tritt die völlige Hingabe des glaubenden Menschen an Gott — als Merkmal dieses besonderen und überzeitlichen Daseinsverständnisses.

Das bedeutet freilich kein weltabgeschiedenes Leben, sondern gerade die entschlossene Hinwendung zur Welt und eine leidenschaftliche Wirksamkeit im Dienste Gottes und zur Anerkennung seines Willens auf allen Lebensgebieten. Es fordert zugleich einen Gehorsam, der nur Gehorsam, aber keine Leistung und Sicherung sein will; einen Glauben, der die Hingabe eigener Kraft und Sorge einschließt; ein Vertrauen, das die Hingabe eigenen Mühens und Planens voraussetzt.

Dieses prophetische Daseinsverständnis ist nichts Selbstverständliches, sondern letztlich nur als Geschenk zu begreifen. Freilich ist es auch vom Menschen nicht unabhängig. Denn die Propheten unterscheiden sich in manchen Dingen voneinander und stehen »dem« prophetischen Daseinsverständnis verschieden nahe. Sie wandelten auch nicht unangefochten auf lichten Höhen, sondern haben — wie besonders das Beispiel Jeremias zeigt — immer um ihren Glauben ringen müssen. Wenn sie also begnadet waren — und sie waren es —, dann nur so, daß sie immer wieder begnadet wurden. Das prophetische Daseinsverständnis ist nicht statischer, sondern dynamischer Art.

IV.

Im prophetischen Daseinsverständnis liegt schließlich die Überwindung der zweiten Macht beschlossen, die neben der Magie der orientalischen Kulte die Ausprägung und Umgestaltung des alttestamentlichen Glaubens bestimmt hat: die Überwindung der Weisheitslehre.

Diese Lehre von der Lebensweisheit hat ihren Ursprung vor allem in Ägypten. Ihr Daseinsverständnis ist klar zu erkennen. Da sucht der alte Weise seinem Sohne die Gesetze der Welt zu erläutern und ihn über sein Verhalten in allen Lebenslagen zu belehren: Wie hat er sich am Hofe zu benehmen, wie gegen den Bittsteller, wie im Hause des Vornehmen, wie gegen die Frau? Es ist eine ausgesprochen praktisch orientierte Lebensweisheit, der es darum geht, wie man am besten des Lebens Herr wird. Das ist die Frage, die den aufgeklärten Weisen beschäftigt, der eingesehen hat, daß es mit der Magie nun einmal nicht geht. Und die Antwort ist von dem zuversichtlichen Glauben getragen: Es ist möglich, die bösen Klippen des Lebens klug und vorsichtig zu meiden und allen Gefahren zu entkommen, wenn man nur auf die ehrwürdigen und bewährten Lebensregeln achtet. Nur der Tor geht zugrunde[9].

Das ist das optimistische Daseinsverständnis des orientalischen Weisen, das auch in Israel Anhänger fand, zunächst unter den könig-

---

[9] Nach W. Zimmerli, Die Weisheit des Predigers Salomo, 1936. Vgl. A. Erman, Die Literatur der Ägypter, 1923; M. Pieper, Die ägyptische Literatur, 1928.

lichen Beamten wohl seit der Zeit Salomos, später in weiten Kreisen des Volkes. Eins der wichtigsten Dogmen des Judentums, die Vergeltungslehre, ist hauptsächlich durch diese Lebensweisheit geprägt worden.

Ihre Überwindung ist bereits bei Jesaja gegeben[10]. Er wendet sich gegen die Weisen, die ihre politischen Pläne selbstsicher auf ihre Weisheit gründen, die sich auf die eigene Weisheit und die ihrer ägyptischen Bundesgenossen verlassen. Sie vergessen in ihrer Selbstsicherheit, daß Jahwe allein weise ist und die Klugheit aller irdischen Weisen zunichte macht. Es gilt nicht, klug und vorsichtig nach einem Ausweg zu suchen und behutsam nach rechts und links zu schauen, sondern aus dem Glauben heraus zu handeln. Nur wer glaubt, wird bleiben (Jes 7 9)! Nur aus Stillesein und Vertrauen kann man Kraft schöpfen (Jes 30 15)!

Hauptsächlich vollzieht sich die Auseinandersetzung mit der Weisheitslehre jedoch in nachexilischer Zeit. Aber obwohl sie auf dem Grunde ihrer prophetischen Überwindung erfolgte, vermochte man nur ganz selten einen dem prophetischen ähnlichen Höhepunkt zu erreichen.

Meist wird die Weisheitslehre in den eigenen Glauben eingebaut, vor allem im Buch Proverbia. Aus ihm ergibt sich die Normalgestalt des israelitischen Weisen: Klug und rechtschaffen, mit frommer Scheu vor Gott, aber in guter Zuversicht, daß er das Leben meistern wird, scharf und verachtungsvoll sich vom Toren abgrenzend, der seine Einsichten nicht hat[11]. Freilich macht sich auch der prophetische Einfluß bemerkbar. Gottesfurcht, Gerechtigkeit und Weisheit können einen untrennbaren Zusammenhang bilden, und die Lebensregeln werden auf den einen Gott begründet und bezogen. Letztlich triumphiert aber das Daseinsverständnis des sich weise gegen alle Gefahren sichernden Menschen.

Demgegenüber zeigt das Buch Kohelet den Typ des Weisen, der das theologische System der Weisheitslehre mit Skepsis betrachtet. Die selbstsichere Haltung der Schulweisheit erscheint falsch und unsinnig. Denn die Welt ist eine ungeheuere, eherne Gesetzmäßigkeit, die dem Menschen dennoch nicht einsichtig ist und daher als Willkür und Regellosigkeit erscheint. Gott ist verhüllt und unerkennbar. Der Glaube an seine Gerechtigkeit und Vergeltung, an einen erkennbaren Sinn des Lebens ist zerbrochen.

In dieser Lage ist der Prediger aber nicht etwa den Weg gegangen, unter ein Dasein, das für den Lebenswillen des Menschen nur ein Nein

---

[10] Vgl. J. Fichtner, Jesaja unter den Weisen, ThLZ 74 (1949), 75—80 (= Gottes Weisheit, 1965, 18—26), ohne daß man aber sagen müßte, daß Jesaja selbst aus solchen Kreisen stammt.

[11] W. Zimmerli a. a. O. 11.

kennt, den Schlußstrich zu setzen und es fortzuwerfen. Er hat sich beschieden: Ist dem Menschen die Erfüllung des Lebens und seine Sicherung verwehrt, so halte er sich an das, was ihm gegeben ist — und das, solange er kann. Er erkenne, was »sein Teil« ist, und genieße es, solange es ihm gewährt wird.

Das ist nicht der einzig mögliche Weg. Es gibt auch den auf der Höhe der prophetischen Überwindung, den die Dichter des Buches Hiob und des 73. Psalms gegangen sind. »Der Mensch erkennt seine ausweglose Situation — und anerkennt sie als seine Situation. Er erkennt hinter allem Geschehen den Herrn der Welt, der ihm immer wieder alle eigenen Sicherungen aus der Hand schlägt — und anerkennt ihn als seinen Herrn. Seine autonome Lebenshaltung, in der er fordernd der Welt und Gott entgegengetreten war, bricht zusammen. Er erkennt in ihr seine tiefste Schuld, verliert sein Leben vor Gottes Gericht.« Und er erlebt dann, daß Gott sich ihm gerade jetzt zuwendet: »Daß Gott dem Menschen da, wo er an dem Leben aus irdischer Möglichkeit verzweifelt, das Leben aus seiner Möglichkeit verspricht.« Er kann sie als Glaubender ergreifen[12].

Der Mensch erfährt die Nähe Gottes und erhält, wie der Dichter des 73. Psalms[13], in aller Not die Gewißheit restlosen Geborgen- und Geführtseins. Gott ist ihm immer nahe, auch in dunklen und undurchsichtigen Stunden. Bei ihm liegen Sinn und Ziel des Daseins, ja sie bestehen in der vorbehaltlosen Hingabe und völligen Gemeinschaft mit Gott. Demgegenüber gibt es nichts Höheres, nicht einmal gleich Begehrenswertes:

> Wen könnt ich neben dir im Himmel suchen?
>   Nichts außer dir begehr ich sonst auf Erden!
> Wenn sich auch Leib und Seel verzehren,
>   bleibt Gott doch allezeit mein Teil!
> Ja, die dich lassen, kommen um;
>   du tilgest jeden, der dir treulos wird.
> Für mich aber ist Gott das Glück,
>   beim Herrn hab Zuflucht ich gefunden! (Ps 73 25-28)

V.

Prüfen wir die verschiedenen Umgestaltungen des alttestamentlichen Glaubens, so erblicken wir in ihnen einerseits Ausprägungen des typischen menschlichen Daseinsverständnisses, das auf Sicherung bedacht ist. Es tritt uns entgegen im Bild des magischen, kultisch-gesetzlichen, nationalen und weisen Menschen. Wir finden andererseits das besondere Daseinsverständnis des prophetischen Menschen in

---

[12] W. Zimmerli a. a. O., 35f.
[13] Zum Buche Hiob vgl. G. Fohrer, Das Buch Hiob, 1963.

seiner gläubigen Hingabe an Gott. Der innere Zusammenhang dieser verschiedenen Glaubensrichtungen und damit die Einheit des Alten Testaments ist gegeben in der Auseinandersetzung um das menschliche Streben nach Sicherung — in der Welt und vor der Offenbarung — und in der Überwindung dieses Strebens durch die Preisgabe an den sich offenbarenden Gott und durch den hingebenden Gehorsam vor ihm.

Zeitlich bedingt und daher nur von zeitlicher Bedeutung ist die Art, in der das typische Daseinsverständnis des Menschen uns entgegentritt: im Gewand der antiken Magie, des israelitischen Kultus und Gesetzes, des Glaubens an die Erwählung Israels, des Verflochtenseins in die orientalische Weisheitslehre.

Überzeitlich ist das darin sich ausprägende Streben nach Sicherheit — Sicherheit in der gefahrbringenden Welt und Sicherheit angesichts der das Dasein in Frage stellenden Offenbarung. Denn dieses Streben nach Sicherheit liegt dem Denken und Wollen des Menschen in jedem Zeitalter zugrunde, nur in jeweils wechselndem Gewand, das durch seine Zeit und die in ihr herrschenden Vorstellungen bestimmt wird.

Von überzeitlicher Bedeutung sind aber auch die Bekämpfung der Magie im Kultus und die Befreiung von ihr durch die Weisheitslehre, die Einheit von Glaube und Ethos im Gesetz, das Wissen um das Handeln Gottes in Leben und Geschick von Menschen und Völkern (wenn man dabei auch zunächst nur an Israel denkt).

Überzeitlich ist vor allem das besondere Daseinsverständnis der Propheten. Denn es enthält das Letzte und Eigentliche, über das es kein Hinaus mehr geben kann — freilich auch teilweise in zeitbedingter und zeitgebundener Einkleidung. In seinem Kern aber, als Dasein in gläubiger Hingabe und gehorsamem Dienst aufgrund der völligen Gemeinschaft mit Gott, gilt es heute wie vor 2500 Jahren.

Kehren wir nun zum Judentum zurück, wenn wir dem prophetischen Daseinsverständnis bleibende Bedeutung und damit bleibenden Anspruch zuerkennen? Keineswegs! War es die Aufgabe Israels, sein Dasein nicht aus eigenem Willen und mit eigenen Zielen zu führen, sondern ein durch Gottes Willen geformtes Dasein vorzuleben — als einzige Möglichkeit, die nicht zum Scheitern verurteilt ist —, und das als Beispiel und Vorbild für eine aus sich heraus unfähige Welt, als Zeichen und Hinweis auf ein neues Dasein, so ist Israel und in seiner Nachfolge das Judentum an dieser seiner göttlichen Aufgabe schuldig geworden, insofern es immer wieder aus der ihm auferlegten Daseinsform herausgefallen ist und Gott nur als metaphysische Sicherung für sein eigenwilliges Leben hat benutzen wollen. Daher ist das Daseinsverständnis des Judentums nicht das prophetische, sondern im Anschluß an das kultisch-gesetzlich-nationale das typische menschliche, das durch die Prophetie gerade überwunden ist. Nicht um Rückkehr zum Judentum handelt es sich also, sondern auch um seine Überwindung — zugleich um die tiefste Erfüllung dessen, was es eigentlich hätte sein sollen.

Beides ist in der Botschaft Jesu noch einmal offensichtlich geworden. Denn sie ist ihrem Inhalt nach nichts anderes als die Fortsetzung der prophetischen Verkündigung — mit der Weiterführung des begonnenen Weges, indem der einzelne unmittelbar vor Gott gestellt und die Herrschaft Gottes als unmittelbar bevorstehendes Heil verstanden wird. Indem nun die Urgemeinde darüber hinaus Jesu Gekommensein selbst als die entscheidende Gottestat glaubt, erkennt sie dadurch das prophetische Daseinsverständnis als gottgewollt an. Und ihr Glaube, daß der eschatologische Richter und Retter Jesus Christus der gekreuzigte und auferstandene Jesus von Nazareth sei, besagt in diesem Zusammenhang nichts anderes, als daß für das Verhältnis Gottes zum Menschen bezeichnend ist, daß der glaubende Mensch die Worte und Forderungen des Jesus von Nazareth als für ihn geltende Worte und Forderungen Gottes versteht, d. h. daß er das auch von Jesus Christus verkündete prophetische Daseinsverständnis als für sich maßgebend anerkennt. Die Botschaft Jesu und der Glaube an ihn heben es also nicht auf, sondern bestätigen es als gottgewollt. Es wird ausgeführt, begründet und aktualisiert. Seine erste und grundsätzliche Ausprägung aber hat es bereits im Alten Testament gefunden. Hier ist ein Glaube bezeugt, der nicht mehr überboten werden kann und daher nach wie vor verpflichtende Kraft besitzt.

Die Judenfrage und der Zionismus

I.

Durch eine umfassende Ausgrabungstätigkeit ist während der letzten Jahrzehnte eine ganze Welt wiedererstanden, von der man bis dahin nur unzureichende Kunde gehabt hatte: die Welt des Alten Orients. Mitten in dieser Welt lag Palästina, infolge seiner Mittellage der Schauplatz der Begegnung und des Ringens der politischen, kulturellen und religiösen Mächte jener Welt. Die in das Land eindringenden israelitischen Stämme übernahmen Sprache und Kultur der kanaanäischen Einwohner und wurden fortan auch von ägyptischen und babylonisch-assyrischen Kulturelementen beeinflußt. Sie traten zudem erst in das Licht der Geschichte, als der Alte Orient seinen Höhepunkt bereits überschritten hatte. Schon Mose und Josua sind in einer Spätzeit geboren, und die spätere Geschichte Israels ist ein Geschehen am Rande umfassender Zusammenhänge: Die Landnahme in Palästina erfolgte als eine der zahlreichen Völkerbewegungen aus Steppe und Wüste ins Kulturland; Staat und Königtum entstanden und blühten in Zeiten politischer Schwäche der Großmächte; der Untergang der getrennten Staaten Israel und Juda war durch den neuen Aufstieg Assyriens und Babyloniens bedingt.

Und doch ist an diesem Volk, das im Raume einer altorientalischen Mischkultur in der Spätzeit gegenseitiger Beeinflussung und Abhängigkeit als ein für das Ganze unwichtiger Faktor gelebt hat, etwas Besonderes, das es so sehr unterschieden und hervorgehoben hat, daß aus ihm zwei Weltreligionen hervorgehen und eine dritte wichtige Impulse erhalten konnte.

Dieses Besondere beruht ursprünglich auf den Erfahrungen der Mosezeit. Obwohl die geschichtlichen Erinnerungen von Sagen und Märchen überwuchert sind, ist das Entscheidende noch erkennbar, weil von ihm alles Spätere abhängt. Nachdem eine größere Gruppe von Israeliten aus ägyptischer Fronherrschaft geflohen war — wie ihnen ihr Führer Mose immer wieder versicherte: weil der Gott Jahwe, der sie bei sich in der Wüste haben wollte, geholfen und sie aus der Knechtschaft gerettet hatte —, sammelte Mose am Sinai die eigenwillige, »murrende« Schar und einte sie untereinander und mit dem neuen Gott. Nach Aufgehen der Moseschar in den israelitischen Stämmen im mittleren Palästina bildete sich allmählich ein Volk, das sich sein Land eroberte und einen Staat schuf. Zugleich wurde der Glaube der Moseschar allmählich zum Glauben des ganzen Volkes, der auf sein Leben wie auf das Leben jedes einzelnen in ihm bestimmend einwirken wollte. Der Gott Jahwe sollte der einzige Gott Israels sein. Er ist gewaltig und erhaben, leidenschaftlich und grimmig; ein Gott des Rechts und der Gerechtigkeit, ernst und fordernd, der Sitte und Sittlichkeit will; ein Gott heiligen Willens, der unbedingtes Vertrauen und rücksichtslosen Gehorsam fordert. Ist er Israels Gott, so ist Israel sein Eigentum. Er hat es »erwählt«; das bedeutet nicht Bevorzugung und Bevorrechtung, sondern die Bestimmung und Zuweisung einer Aufgabe. Israel sollte ein Dasein besonderer Art führen, das der seines Gottes entsprach.

Die Propheten haben dieses Daseinsverständnis aktualisiert und für ihre Gegenwart wirksam gemacht. Sie traten in einer Zeit auf, die die Erkenntnis der besonderen Lage Israels zu verfälschen drohte. In der Auseinandersetzung mit den magischen Vorstellungen und Gebräuchen der fremden, vor allem der kanaanäischen Fruchtbarkeitsreligion, hatte sich ein durch den Kultus bestimmter Glaube gebildet, in dem auch das Gesetz eine Rolle spielte.

Der Gott Israels nahm in Palästina die Merkmale der Landesgötter an und wurde wie sie verehrt. Der starke ethische Wille trat zugunsten der geheimnisvollen Lebensmacht der Gottheit und ihres Wirkens im Raum der Natur zurück. Der Kultus schloß sich an den des eroberten Landes an; an seinen Heiligtümern, auf seinen Altären, mit seinen Riten wurde er ausgeübt, nur auf den Gott Israels als den alleinigen Herrn bezogen. Gewährt Gott dem Bauern seinen Segen, so bringt dieser ihm dafür seine Opfer als Dank und Bitte dar. Man sitzt mit Gott zu Tisch und ist fröhlich in der Gewißheit, daß man auch im nächsten Jahr wieder reichen Segen erlangen kann.

Ebenso diente das Gesetz der Gewinnung von Gottes Gunst und der Vergewisserung seiner Gnade. Seine Forderungen wurden zur Richtschnur menschlichen Handelns, ihre Erfüllung zur gültigen Lebensform. Demjenigen, der es hält, wird Gottes Segen verheißen, demjenigen aber, der es nicht beachtet, sein Fluch angedroht.

Daneben entstand ein durch das nationale Element bestimmter Glaube. Er suchte seine geschichtliche Berechtigung in dem Nachweis des mächtigen Handelns Gottes im Seßhaftwerden Israels im verheißenen Kulturland. In Auseinandersetzung mit Mythologie und Sage, gegenüber den kanaanäischen Vorstellungen von der Offenbarung des dahinwelkenden und wiederauflebenden Gottes im naturhaften Kreislauf des Jahres setzte sich in diesem Glauben das Wissen um das göttliche Handeln in Leben und Geschick von Menschen und Völkern durch — vor allem in Leben und Geschick des eigenen Volkes. Der Glaube an die Erwählung Israels begründet nun seine bevorrechtete Stellung, der großisraelitische Gedanke wird durch den Hinweis auf die Vorzeit gestützt: eine Ahnenreihe — ein Land — ein Volk!

Der Mensch sucht also durch sein kultisches Handeln und das Befolgen des Gesetzes Gottes Segen und Gnade zu erlangen. Er sucht ihn ferner in die Schranken der Nation einzuschließen und auf das erwählte Volk zu verpflichten. Er sucht sein Dasein mit Hilfe Gottes zu sichern; die göttliche Offenbarung, die es erschüttert und in Frage stellt, wird übersehen oder umgedeutet, über den sich offenbarenden Gott durch menschliches Handeln verfügt.

Demgegenüber erneuern die Propheten das echte Daseinsverständnis des glaubenden Menschen. Sie haben den gewaltigen und welterhabenen Gott, dessen Willen der Mensch in Eingriff und Erschütterung seines Daseins erlebt, von neuem als heilige Leidenschaft und lodernde Glut erfahren. Angesichts dieses Gottes muß der Kultus zerbrechen und seinen Untergang finden. Das Volk glaubt durch ihn Gottes Schutz erlangen zu können, so daß es seine sittlichen Forderungen nicht mehr ernst nimmt und seinen Willen nicht die bestimmende Macht des Lebens sein läßt. An die Stelle des Kultus sollten daher Recht und Gerechtigkeit treten. Und das Gebet des glaubenden Menschen ist besser als aller Gottesdienst.

Der Gott, von dem die Propheten ergriffen sind, ist auch anders, als die Anhänger des nationalen Glaubens ihn sich vorstellen. Er läßt über sich nicht zugunsten eines Volkes oder Staates verfügen und ist nicht der Garant der nationalen Macht oder völkischen Kultur. Vor der schrecklichen Offenbarung seines Willens muß die ganze israelitische Kultur, die ihn verharmlost, in einem schrecklichen Gericht vergehen. Die alleinige Bindung Gottes an Israel wird überwunden. Aus dem Nationalgott wird der Herr der Welt, aus dem Gott des Volkes beginnt der Gott zu werden, der den einzelnen fordert.

Scheint dem Menschen vor diesem Gott zunächst nur der demütige Verzicht auf alles eigene Handeln, die hingebende Beugung und völlige Unterwerfung unter seinen Willen offenzustehen, so sieht er sich doch vor die Entscheidung gestellt, ob er zu diesem Gott und seinem Willen Ja oder Nein sagen will. Das Ja aber bedeutet: Glaube als unbedingtes Vertrauen auf den unsichtbaren Gott, Liebe als gehorsame Hingabe des Menschen mit all seinen Kräften, Gotteserkenntnis als Gemeinschaft mit Gott und Bestimmtsein des eigenen Lebens durch sein Wesen.

So erwarten die Propheten von ihrem Volk ein Dasein in gläubiger Hingabe und gehorsamem Dienst aufgrund der völligen Gemeinschaft mit Gott. An die Stelle der Versuche der Lebenssicherung durch das Einfangen Gottes im Kultus, durch den Leistungsgedanken und die Werkgerechtigkeit des Gesetzes und durch die Bindung Gottes an das Volk im nationalen Glauben tritt die Hingabe des glaubenden Menschen an Gott.

Aber dieses prophetische Daseinsverständnis hat sich nicht durchsetzen können. Schon in vorexilischer Zeit hat die altorientalische Weisheitslehre in Israel Anhänger gefunden — als profaner, der Magie entgegengesetzter Versuch der Lebenssicherung. Der Weise hält es für möglich, klug und vorsichtig alle Anstöße zu vermeiden und allen Gefahren zu entkommen, wenn er auf die weisen Lebensregeln achtet, die sich bewährt haben. Mit ihrer Hilfe kann er sein Dasein zum Höhepunkt hinaufführen und es sichern.

Hatte Jesaja solcher klugen, vorsichtigen und weltgewandten Weisheit ein Leben aus dem Glauben gegenübergestellt, so verfolgt die spätere Zeit diese prophetische Linie nur selten (Hiob, Ps 73), baut vielmehr die Weisheit in den eigenen Glauben ein und schafft ein umfassendes theologisches System oder setzt ihr die Überzeugung von der doch nicht zu behebenden Unsicherheit des Daseins entgegen.

Aus der Geschichte Israels ergibt sich demnach ein Doppeltes. Es war die Aufgabe Israels, sein Dasein nicht aus eigenem Willen und mit eigenen Zielen zu führen, sondern ein durch Gottes Willen geformtes Dasein zu leben, wie es im prophetischen Daseinsverständnis vorliegt. Israel sollte es vorleben als Beispiel und Vorbild für eine aus sich heraus unfähige Welt, als einzige Möglichkeit, die nicht zum Scheitern verurteilt ist, als Zeichen und Hinweis auf ein neues Dasein.

Israel jedoch ist an dieser seiner göttlichen Aufgabe schuldig geworden, insofern es immer wieder aus der ihm auferlegten Daseinsform herausgefallen ist und Gott nur als metaphysische Sicherung für sein eigenwilliges Dasein hat benutzen wollen. Kultus, Gesetz, Nation und Weisheit sind die Elemente dieses sich Gott versagenden Daseins.

II.

In der Zeit nach dem babylonischen Exil beginnt sich das Judentum zu bilden. Unter der persischen und griechisch-ptolemäischen Herrschaft bleibt es ungestört; als es dann unter syrisch-seleukidischer Herrschaft hellenisiert werden soll, erkämpfen die Makkabäer einen selbständigen Staat, der bis zur römischen Herrschaft bestehen bleibt. Von dieser abhängig, regieren einige Jahrzehnte die Herodianer, bis das ganze Land unter römische Prokuratoren oder unmittelbare römische Verwaltung kommt. Die Aufstände von 66—70 und 132 n. Chr. enden mit der Vernichtung der bisherigen staatlichen Daseinsform.

Während der Tempelkultus allmählich zugunsten des kultlosen Gottesdienstes der Synagoge zurücktritt, wird das Judentum von einem immer stärkeren national-religiösen Erwählungsbewußtsein getragen, das seine Isolierung von andern Völkern und seinen Abschluß gegen die Forderungen der Gegenwart zur Folge hat. Je bedrückender die Lage, desto inbrünstiger die Hoffnung und desto fester die Überzeugung, daß Gott das geknechtete Volk befreien und zu der ihm gebührenden Herrlichkeit führen wird; entweder durch die Wiederherstellung des Davidreiches unter einem davidischen König (»Messias«) oder durch die Ablösung des jetzigen Zustandes von Leid und Not durch einen neuen Äon, in dem die Toten auferstehen — die Frommen zum ewigen Leben, die Gottlosen zu ewiger Schmach. Keine Enttäuschung vermag diese Hoffnung zu entmutigen, sondern steigert die Ungeduld und Erregung nur, bis schließlich aus der schwelenden Glut die hellen Flammen der Aufstände schlagen.

Gott vergilt dem Menschen nach seinen Taten. Da aber das, was zu tun ist, sich im Gesetz findet, gewinnt dieses eine ständig wachsende Bedeutung. Alles neue Werden ist jedoch ausgeschlossen. Das im Alten Testament kodifizierte Gesetz wird lediglich auf die verschiedenen sich neu ergebenden Fälle angewandt. Dabei wird nicht etwa eine richtige Auslegung vertieft oder eine falsche und veraltete überwunden, sondern lediglich eine neue daneben gestellt; zwischen ihnen hat man die Wahl.

Das ganze Leben wird durch dieses Gesetz geregelt. Es gilt eine Unmenge von Vorschriften zu beachten über Essen und Trinken, über Schlachten und Zubereiten der Speise, über die Gefäße, in denen man sie zubereitet, über Reinhalten des Leibes von Unreinigkeiten, über Waschungen, über Unreinheiten und vieles andere. Im 3. Jh. zählt jemand 365 Verbote und 248 Gebote, zusammen 613 Vorschriften.

Durch dieses Gesetz wird die Beziehung des Menschen zu Gott nicht mehr als gläubige Hingabe und vertrauende Gemeinschaft, sondern als juristisches Verhältnis bestimmt. Der Mensch erfüllt die göttlichen Forderungen und sichert sich dadurch seinen Lohn. Und da es sich nicht um völligen Gehorsam handelt, der den Geist des Gebotes erkennen und erfüllen will, sondern nur um äußere Befolgung, so bleibt Raum für eigenmächtige Entscheidungen oder besondere Leistungen, wenn einmal keine Vorschrift vorliegt.

Demgegenüber ist die Botschaft Jesu eine Aktualisierung und Konkretisierung des Daseinsverständnisses, wie es nach Mose die Propheten gelebt und verkündigt hatten. Wie jene sich gegen den kultisch-gesetzlich-national-weisen Glauben wandten, so Jesus gegen den nationalen Erwählungsglauben und die rituale Gesetzlichkeit des Judentums. Er stellt dem das Dasein des glaubenden Menschen gegenüber.

Zugleich führt Jesus den durch die Propheten beschrittenen Weg weiter. Es geht nun um das Verhältnis des einzelnen zu Gott. Vor ihm gibt es keine Sicherung — weder durch Leistung noch durch

Besitz. Denn Gott beansprucht den Menschen ganz und verlangt Gehorsam und Vertrauen im Bewußtsein der Abhängigkeit von ihm. Er fordert nicht nur äußeres Tun, sondern den Willen des Menschen. Der Mensch wird ganz mit Beschlag belegt und kann daher keine Ansprüche stellen, sondern gleicht dem Sklaven, der nur seine Schuldigkeit tun kann. Angesichts der jüdischen Gesetzlichkeit fordert Jesus daher Buße als Selbstbesinnung, Bekenntnis der Schuld vor Gott und Warten auf seine Gnade.

Gottes Wille gegenüber dem einzelnen aber ist Liebe — als Vertrauen auf Gott und Sorge für den Nächsten. Diese Liebesforderung ist allumfassend und unbegrenzt; weder kennt sie Grenze und Einschränkung, noch bedarf sie bestimmter Vorschriften.

Auch darin führt Jesus den von den Propheten begonnenen Weg weiter, daß er die Gottesherrschaft als unmittelbar bevorstehend verkündigt. Er verwirft das Bild des nationalen Glaubens von der Weltherrschaft und dem vollendeten Glück Israels und erwartet einen neuen Äon. Im Gegensatz zum gleichartigen jüdischen Gedanken aber betont er lediglich, daß Gott dann herrschen wird und daß jetzt, gerade jetzt die Zeit gekommen ist, in der diese Herrschaft hereinbricht. Und auf die Frage, woran das zu erkennen sei, verweist er auf sich selbst, sein Auftreten, seine Worte und Taten. Sein Auftreten wird damit zum Ruf zur Entscheidung für oder gegen Gottes Herrschaft. Alle müssen sich darüber klar werden, woran sie ihr Herz hängen wollen: an Gott oder die Güter dieser Weltzeit. Diese Entscheidung muß grundsätzlich gefällt und rücksichtslos verwirklicht werden.

Greift Jesus so die alte Aufgabe Israels auf und aktualisiert sie, so hat die christliche Gemeinde dies bejaht. Indem sie Jesu Gekommensein selbst als entscheidende Gottestat glaubt, erkennt sie die ursprünglich Israel gestellte Aufgabe eines Lebens der Gemeinschaft mit Gott als für sich bindend an, ohne daß sie allerdings dem Judentum damit abgenommen würde.

Damit wird es zugleich Sache der Kirche, das Judentum auf seine Aufgabe aufmerksam zu machen, vor der es bisher versagt hat, ohne es missionieren zu wollen; es die Propheten als vollgültige Verkünder seiner Aufgabe und Jesus als ihren Fortsetzer verstehen zu lehren, der den einzelnen Juden in die Entscheidung ruft; und es das aus ihren Worten sich ergebende Dasein des Menschen vor Gott und in der Welt erkennen und für die Gegenwart fruchtbar machen zu lassen.

In der Botschaft Jesu und ihrer Bestätigung durch die christliche Gemeinde ist also das gesetzlich-nationale Judentum überwunden und zugleich das erfüllt, was es eigentlich hätte erfüllen sollen und wozu die prophetische Verkündigung es aufgefordert hatte. Jesus hätte das Judentum von seinem falschen Wege und aus seiner Erstarrung herausreißen können. Seine Ablehnung bewirkte nur die Versteifung jener falschen Daseinshaltung; seine Verwerfung war die Weigerung des Judentums, seine göttliche Aufgabe zu erfüllen. Auch das Daseinsverständnis des Judentums ist also nicht das prophetische, sondern ein typisch menschliches, das auf Lebenssicherung bedacht ist; das gilt auch für die Form der pharisäischen Gesetzesfrömmigkeit, die sich als maßgeblich durchgesetzt hat. Israel und Judentum haben trotz Mose, den Propheten und Jesus gegenüber ihrer Aufgabe versagt. In diesem Nebeneinander von Aufgabe und Versagen aber liegt das Schicksal des Judentums beschlossen.

III.

Das Daseinsverständnis des Judentums hat sich nicht mehr geändert, sondern ist grundsätzlich gleich geblieben. Ein Grundzug ist der alte nationale Glaube, der die Messiaserwartung gestützt hat. In die Hunderte geht die Zahl der angeblichen Messiasse, deren Auftreten immer wieder Erregung, himmelstürmendes Hoffen und beschämende Enttäuschung hervorgerufen hat. Erst als Preis für die Gleichberechtigung der Juden wird die Aufgabe des Bewußtseins verlangt, eine Nation zu bilden. Jener Glaube äußert sich darin, daß für den ins Judentum aufgenommenen Heiden oder Christen seine frühere Verwandtschaft nicht mehr gilt, so daß er theoretisch diese seine allernächsten Verwandten heiraten könnte, ohne Blutschande zu begehen.

Daneben findet sich gelegentlich die im Alten Testament heftig bekämpfte Magie. So im Gebrauch des Tetragramms, der vier Buchstaben des Gottesnamens JHWH, deren Verwendung als wirksame Zauberformel Abraham Abulafia aus Saragossa lehrte. So vor allem die Zahlenzauberei, die die Kabbala außer einer mystischen Geheimlehre mit sich brachte, und der unerfreuliche Inhalt der 6.—10. Bücher Mose.

Der bezeichnendste Zug des Judentums ist seine Gesetzlichkeit geblieben. Das Heiligtum jeder Synagoge bilden die Schriftrollen mit der Tora, dem Pentateuch. Der Blick des eintretenden Juden wird auf die Wand hingelenkt, an der sich der Kasten befindet, in dem sie aufbewahrt werden. Er legt die Hand aufs Herz und verneigt sich dagegen. Der feierliche Augenblick des Gottesdienstes ist das Herausnehmen und Enthüllen der Rollen. Wenn sie umhergetragen werden, berührt man sie mit einem Finger und küßt diesen.

Zum Gesetz tritt die Tradition, in der möglichst viele der zum Gesetz geäußerten Meinungen aufbewahrt werden. Außer der Mischna und Tosephta sind vor allem der jerusalemische und babylonische Talmud zu nennen, ferner die Targume, umschreibende Übertragungen alttestamentlicher Bücher ins Aramäische, und die Midrasche, Kommentare zu solchen Büchern.

So besteht das Gesetz, das die Rolle des Mittlers zwischen Gott und Mensch einnimmt, aus ungezählten Einzelheiten, durch die das Tun und Lassen des ganzen Lebens geregelt werden soll. Wenn etwa ein Mann am Morgen aufsteht, muß er das Hemd liegend überziehen, über den linken Arm möglichst vor dem rechten. Dann zieht er den rechten Strumpf und Schuh an, darf ihn aber erst zubinden, nachdem er den linken angelegt hat. Das alles, damit der Körper bedeckt und man vor Gott nicht schamlos ist. Nur wenn es um Leben und Existenz geht, darf der Jude einzelne Gesetze übertreten oder sich über die meisten Vorschriften hinwegsetzen. Auch hier das Streben nach Sicherung des Daseins!

Als Protest gegen diese Gesetzlichkeit entstand freilich, parallel zum Pietismus der Reformationskirchen, in Osteuropa die jüdische Erweckungsbewegung des Chassidismus (»Frömmigkeit«). Sie will das Gesetz von innen her verstehen und geistlich halten lehren. Durch Gebet und Tanz sucht man sich für den Empfang des göttlichen Geistes als Gnadengabe zu öffnen. Ist so schon eine künstlich erzeugte Empfangsbereitschaft grundlegend, so teilt sich die Bewegung bald in eine mehr beschaulich-mystische und eine um Wunderrabbinen sich sammelnde Richtung.

*

Die Geschichte des Judentums ist mit Blut geschrieben. Sieht man von kleineren Gruppen ab — den Mograbim in Nordafrika, den Lawambu-Juden an der afrikanischen Loangoküste und den schwarzen Juden in Indien — so handelt es sich hauptsächlich um das Geschick der Ost- und Westjuden. Sie konnten in Mittel- und Westeuropa bis zu den Kreuzzügen (12. Jh.), in Spanien während der maurischen Herrschaft durchweg in glücklichen Verhältnissen leben. Von gelegentlichen Störungen abgesehen, lebten sie nach ihrer Ordnung und kamen zu Wohlstand und Ansehen. Dann aber änderte sich das Bild.

Mit dem Beginn der Kreuzzüge wich für die Ostjuden (Askenazim) der Friede dem Sturm. In ihm brach der Zorn über die Juden als Mörder des Gottessohnes und als finanzielle Gläubiger der Herren los. Als durch einen päpstlichen Erlaß den Kreuzfahrern die Zinsen ihrer jüdischen Gläubiger erlassen wurden, begann man sich ihrer durch brutale Gewalt ganz zu entledigen oder ließ sie die gesamten Unkosten der Kreuzfahrer tragen. Die grausigen Berichte aus jener Zeit bergen ein ungeheures Maß von Schuld und Leid. Um die Mitte des 14. Jh. wurden dann die Judengemeinden am Rhein vernichtet; manchmal hat man in Anfällen von Großmut schwangere Frauen und Kinder vor dem Tode bewahrt. Es folgte schließlich die Vertreibung der

Juden. Ihrer Ausweisung aus England (1290) folgte die Vertreibung aus den deutschen Gebieten im 15. Jh. Sie wanderten nach Osteuropa, wo sich auf diese Weise die Juden zusammenballten. Zur Zeit des ersten Weltkriegs schätzte man sie auf etwa 7 Millionen, von denen besonders die russischen qualvolle Jahrzehnte hinter sich hatten.

Die Westjuden (Sephardim) haben ihre Heimat in Spanien. Sie hatten, nachdem sie jahrzehntelang bedrückt, gequält und zwangsgetauft worden waren, die Araber als Befreier begrüßt; es folgte eine glänzende Zeit jüdisch-arabischer Kulturblüte. Nach Aufhören der arabischen Herrschaft brach 1391 der Sturm los; das Zeichen des Kampfes gab ein Pogrom, durch das die 30 000 Seelen große Gemeinde von Sevilla vernichtet wurde. Es darf freilich nicht übersehen werden, daß dies alles weitgehend durch den Mißbrauch der in jüdischer Hand liegenden Machtbefugnisse hervorgerufen wurde — ein Mißbrauch, der seine Ursache wiederum in dem alten Abfall von der Aufgabe Israels und dem typisch menschlichen Streben nach Lebensgenuß und -sicherung hatte. Viele Juden ließen sich taufen, da sie ja in Gefahr das Gesetz preisgeben durften. Diese Marranen wurden aber ebenso überwacht, wie man die ungetauften Juden auszurotten suchte. Die in den Händen der Dominikaner liegende Inquisition feierte Triumphe; allein 1482 wurden 2000 Ketzer, also vor allem Juden, verbrannt. Als alles nichts nutzte, wurden die Reste ausgewiesen; sie verstreuten sich von Portugal bis zur Türkei. Aber nach Verkäufen als Sklaven, Zwangsheiraten von Frauen und Mädchen mit Christen forderte Spanien von Portugal bei Heiratsverhandlungen wieder ihre Ausweisung. Sie erfolgte auch — mit Ausnahme der Vier- bis Zwanzigjährigen, die zwangsgetauft wurden. Die anderen wanderten weiter, vor allem nach Holland und Deutschland. Auch bei den Westjuden also eine Geschichte voll Blut und Tränen!

Da die Kirche zeitweilig offiziell das Zinsnehmen verboten hatte (etwa 1100—1500), fiel währenddessen das ganze Geldgeschäft an die Juden. Da man ihnen zugleich das bürgerliche Recht des Haus- und Landbesitzes nahm und sie aus den Zünften ausschloß, blieb ihnen tatsächlich auch nur das Geld- und Pfandgeschäft übrig. Und weltliche wie geistliche Herren brauchten sie dringend dazu! Sie lebten unter dem Schutz der Landesherren, die dafür aus ihnen herauszupressen suchten, was möglich war.

Aufgrund ihrer finanziellen Bedeutung erhielten die Juden häufig besondere Vorrechte, zu denen durchweg gemeindliche Selbstverwaltung und eigene Gerichtsbarkeit gehörten — Vorrechte, die sie ebenso häufig mißbrauchten. Demgegenüber aber standen noch mehr einschränkende Gesetze. Papst Innozenz III. ordnete an, daß die Juden eine besondere Kleidung tragen sollten, die deshalb entwürdigend war, weil sie außerhalb der normalen Standes- und Berufskleidung stand. Die Juden mußten ferner in den Quartieren (Ghetto) wohnen bleiben, in die sie sich früher zurückgezogen hatten, ohne Rücksicht auf ihre Vermehrung; sie mußten sich mit den ungeheuerlichen Verhältnissen begnügen, die sie vorfanden. Sie waren vom Handwerk, von freien Berufen und vom Studium ausgeschlossen und nur auf den Handel beschränkt; es ist verständlich, daß sie sich hierin zu Meistern entwickelten. Sie unterlagen Ehebeschränkungen, insofern die Familienzahl festgelegt war, so daß viele erst dann heiraten konnten, wenn ein Familienvater gestorben war. Sie mußten häufig auch für die christliche Obrigkeit beten, die ihnen das alles auferlegte, oder in der Passionszeit christliche Predigten anhören. Theodor Herzl hat den Nagel auf den Kopf getroffen: »Wir sind, wozu man uns in den Ghetti gemacht hat«.

*

Lang und schwer war daher der Kampf, der von verschiedenen Seiten um die Gleichberechtigung der Juden geführt wurde. Er begann im Jahrhundert der Aufklärung, die im Namen der Vernunft und Menschlichkeit für sie eintrat, und wurde seit der französischen Revolution unter dem Motto der Freiheit, Gleichheit und Brüderlichkeit auf dem Feld der Politik ausgetragen. Grundsätzlich wurden Freiheit und Gleichheit den Juden zuerst in den USA gewährt, während die praktische Durchführung allerdings nicht so einfach war. In Europa ging es nicht so schnell. In Preußen verweigerte noch Friedrich Wilhelm IV. den Juden die Zuerkennung der vollen politischen Rechte seiner christlichen Untertanen. Auch die Revolution von 1848 konnte keine grundlegende Änderung herbeiführen; bis 1918 waren ungetaufte Juden von hohen Beamtenstellen und der Offizierslaufbahn ausgeschlossen. Erst die Weimarer Verfassung brachte ihnen die volle Gleichberechtigung; kein Wunder, daß sie sie nun ausnutzten und dadurch ungewollt das Umsichgreifen des Antisemitismus begünstigten.

Der Gleichberechtigung entsprach innerhalb des Judentums die Emanzipation (Selbstbefreiung von gewissen Bindungen) und die Assimilation (Anpassung an die Umwelt). Hier bietet sich dem Beobachter ein buntes, aber letztlich uninteressantes Bild. Wesentlich ist nur die Entstehung des Reformjudentums, dessen Wurzeln in der Aufklärung liegen. Die Gleichberechtigung hatte als unerbittliche Forderung mit sich gebracht, daß das Judentum sich nicht mehr als Volk, sondern als Konfession verstehen mußte. Nun wurde — außer der Angleichung des Lebensstils an den der Umwelt — der Versuch gemacht, auch die Konfession zu reformieren. Der synagogale Gottesdienst wurde dem protestantischen nach Möglichkeit angeglichen; aus den Gebeten wurde entfernt, was mit der nationalen und messianischen Hoffnung zusammenhing; ein neues Gesangbuch wurde geschaffen, für das man christliche Lieder übertrug; die Praxis der Sabbatheiligung wurde gemildert und die Beschneidung als nicht mehr erforderlich betrachtet. Es war ein Abbau, ohne daß Neues an die Stelle des Beseitigten getreten wäre. Es war lediglich die Verneinung des eigentlich Jüdischen zugunsten der politisch-rechtlichen Sicherung und darum die Verneinung der Aufgabe des Judentums. Hatte es bisher die Aufgabe falsch verstanden und vor ihr versagt, so wurde sie nun überhaupt nicht mehr erkannt. Das Reformjudentum konnte daher die Judenfrage nicht lösen und mußte scheitern. Es trug sogar noch zum Wiederaufleben des Antisemitismus bei, da der Jude nun, wenn er aus seiner Konfession austrat, als rassisch unterschieden betrachtet wurde und im Sehnen nach Freiheit, Betätigungsmöglichkeit und Anerkennung im internationalen Kommunismus wirkte.

Die Frage des Antisemitismus ist schwierig und vielschichtig. Er findet sich schon in der Antike, in der er allerdings eher eine Abart des allgemeinen Fremdenhasses als eigentlicher Judenhaß zu sein scheint. Er hat, besonders im Mittelalter, häufig wirtschaftliche und politische Gründe gehabt, die in dem den Juden aufgezwungenen Geld- und Pfandgeschäft, aber auch in ihrer oft bedenkenlosen Machtausnutzung lagen. Es gab auch einen kirchlichen Antisemitismus, der sich schon im 4. Jh. voll entfaltete und von Hetzpredigten in der Anwesenheit von Juden und Geldbußen am Palmsonntag über Zwangsdisputationen und -taufen bis zur Inquisition führt. Eigentlich aber sollte Antisemitismus in jeder Form in der Kirche ausgeschlossen sein. Er zerstört ihre Grundlagen, weil er das Wort entleert, daß Gott sich aller Menschen erbarmt. Und der rassische Antisemitismus, der mit Dühring und H. St. Chamberlain beginnt, ist ein Unding. Er muß außer acht lassen, daß die Juden ebenso das Produkt einer Rassenmischung sind wie die Deutschen. Er muß sich ferner, wörtlich genommen, auch gegen die Araber richten. Berücksichtigt man dies aber, so bleibt nur eine brutale Gegnerschaft übrig, die sich mit einem pseudowissenschaftlichen Mäntelchen zu tarnen sucht.

Eins lehrt die Geschichte mit unerbittlicher Klarheit: Wie immer der Antisemitismus begründet wird, ob er gar vom Staat sanktioniert oder privilegiert wird — er wirkt sich stets als Aufforderung zum Raubmord aus. Diese Feststellung kann von aktueller Bedeutung sein. Man hat mehrfach die Notwendigkeit einer Gesetzgebung gegen den Antisemitismus erwogen. Sie erscheint jedoch überflüssig oder sogar irreführend, sobald erkannt und anerkannt ist, daß jede Form des Antisemitismus als Anstiftung zum Raubmord betrachtet werden muß.

*

Welches ist nun die tiefere Ursache für die entsetzlichen Leiden, die das Judentum immer wieder betroffen haben? Sie sind nicht einfach — wie die Christen vielfach glaubten — die Folge der Verwerfung Jesu oder gar Strafe dafür. Diese falsche Auffassung rief mehrfach Verfolgung oder gewaltsame Bekehrungsversuche an Juden hervor. Ihre Leiden ließen sich höchstens als Folge des die Verwerfung Jesu einschließenden Versagens vor der Aufgabe des Judentums oder der Verneinung dieser Aufgabe verstehen.

Die Leiden des Judentums sind auch nicht — wie die Juden vielfach glauben — die Folge der Erfüllung der göttlichen Aufgabe Israels, durch die es sich der Menschheit verhaßt gemacht hätte; denn das Judentum hat diese seine Aufgabe ja gerade nicht erfüllt.

Es leidet zwar wegen jener über ihm schwebenden Aufgabe, durch die es — ohne es zu wollen oder sogar zu wissen — gezeichnet ist, die es als Fremdkörper in einer Welt erscheinen läßt, für die es Beispiel und Vorbild, Zeichen und Hinweis auf ein in Gott gegründetes Dasein und — bei Erfüllung der Aufgabe — ein ständiger Ruf zur Entscheidung für Gott werden sollte. Es leidet aber auch, weil es vor dieser Aufgabe immer wieder versagt hat, indem es sie falsch verstand, sich der Erfüllung verweigerte oder die Aufgabe überhaupt verneinte und statt dessen auf seine Art Sicherheit in der Welt suchte.

IV.

Für das Judentum hat Jerusalem nie seine Bedeutung verloren. Es gab stets einen frommen Zionismus, ein Heimweh nach dem von Gott den Vätern geschenkten Lande. Immer sind fromme Juden im Alter nach Jerusalem ausgewandert, um dort unter kümmerlichen Verhältnissen ihr Leben in Gebeten an der Mauer des einstigen Tempels zu beenden. Sie starben in der Gewißheit ihrer künftigen Auferstehung, da ihr Grab in der Erde des heiligen Landes liegen würde.

Der politisch-nationale Zionismus ist das Werk Theodor Herzls (1860—1904), der seine Erkenntnisse in dem aufwühlenden Erlebnis des Dreyfus-Prozesses empfing. Im Gegensatz zur osteuropäischen Bewegung der »Freunde Zions« forderte er ein politisches Recht des Judentums auf eine Heimstätte in Palästina, danach erst die Besiedlung aufgrund dieses Rechtes. Angesichts des Scheiterns des Reformjudentums erblickte er in seinen freidenkerischen und politischen Plänen die Lösung der Judenfrage: »Ich halte die Judenfrage weder für eine soziale noch für eine religiöse Frage, wenn sie sich auch noch so und anders färbt. Sie ist eine nationale Frage, und um sie zu lösen, müssen wir sie vor allem zu einer politischen Weltfrage machen, die im Rate der Kulturvölker zu regeln sein wird. Wir sind ein Volk, ein Volk!«

Nach langen, teilweise heftigen Kämpfen innerhalb des Judentums begann in den Verhandlungen Weizmanns und Sokolows mit der englischen Regierung die Frucht zu reifen. Am 2. November 1917 schrieb der Außenminister Balfour an Rothschild: »Sr. Majestät Regierung betrachtet mit Wohlwollen die Errichtung einer nationalen Heimstätte für das jüdische Volk in Palästina und wird die größten Anstrengungen machen, um die Erreichung dieses Zieles zu erleichtern, wobei selbstverständlich nichts unternommen werden soll, was den bürgerlichen und religiösen Rechten bestehender nichtjüdischer Gemeinschaften in Palästina oder der staatsrechtlichen Rechtstellung der Juden in irgendeinem Lande Abbruch tun könnte«. Die Verwirklichung dieses Zieles konnte nach der Mandatserteilung über Palästina an England durch den Völkerbund (24. Juli 1922) beginnen.

Für England als Vormacht des Orients waren vor allem politische Gründe maßgebend gewesen. Es suchte Ölinteressen und Handelsmonopole im Orient und See- und Luftweg nach dem Osten durch das Mandat zu sichern und dazu im Mandatsgebiet eine verläßliche Bevölkerung anzusiedeln. Freilich geriet es dadurch in Konflikt mit den Arabern, die für die Unterstützung Englands im Kriege einen arabischen Großstaat erwartet hatten und sich nun »verraten« sahen. Die wirtschaftliche und kulturelle Überlegenheit der Juden, ihr politischer Einfluß bei den Großmächten und der umfangreiche Erwerb palästinischen Bodens riefen Angst und Haß hervor. Es kam zu immer stärkerem Widerstand der Araber gegen die jüdische Einwanderung, bis schließlich der Aufstand 1936/39 und der drohende Anschluß der Araber an die »Achse« England veranlaßten, die Einwanderung und den Bodenerwerb der Juden erheblich einzuschränken.

Dadurch aber wurden diese zu heftigen Gegnern Englands. Schon während des zweiten Weltkrieges begannen Geheimverbände den Kampf gegen es; und nach seiner Beendigung tobte zwei Jahre lang der Aufstand, der erbittert und mit großen Opfern geführt wurde. Schließlich legte England sein Mandat nieder, widersetzte sich aber auch dem Beschluß der UN, Palästina zu teilen und einen jüdischen Staat zu bilden, und suchte sich zuletzt wenigstens die militärischen Stützpunkte im Negeb und in Aqaba zu sichern.

Inzwischen hatte der zweite Weltkrieg angesichts der neuen ungeheuerlichen Verfolgung der Juden nicht nur eine beschleunigte Einwanderung, sondern auch eine Radikalisierung des jüdischen Nationalismus mit sich gebracht. Es ging nicht mehr um eine Heimstätte in Palästina, sondern um ganz Palästina als Heimstätte des Judentums. Die Folge war, daß nun doch »den bürgerlichen und religiösen Rechten bestehender nichtjüdischer Gemeinschaften in Palästina« Abbruch getan wurde. Durch Diplomatie, Kampf und Terror wurde der Staat Israel errichtet und das arabische Element in eine hoffnungslose Lage gedrängt.

Schon nach dem ersten Weltkrieg hatten die Juden in Palästina beachtliche Erfolge erzielt. Die Stadt Tel Aviv wuchs aus dem Nichts hervor, eine hebräische Universität machte von sich reden, weite Gebiete wurden landwirtschaftlich genutzt. Auch die Anstrengungen Englands zur Verteidigung Palästinas im zweiten Weltkrieg kamen dem Land zugute. Das inzwischen Erreichte ist bewundernswert — ob es sich um die Verschmelzung der verschiedenen Kulturen der Einwanderer zu einem gleichartigen jüdischen Volkstum handelt, um das Erziehungswesen vom Kindergarten bis zur Universität, um die Arbeiterbewegung mit ihren Gewerkschaften oder um die verschiedenen Arten der landwirtschaftlichen Besiedlung vom eigenen Hof über die Genossenschaften auf der Grundlage des Privatbesitzes bis zu den Gemeinschaftssiedlungen (private Besitzlosigkeit, aber gemeinschaftlicher Besitz ohne staatlichen Einfluß).

Die Entwicklung zur kulturellen und wirtschaftlichen Blüte ist jedoch noch nicht gesichert. Es fehlt immer noch an ausreichendem Kapital, vor allem für den Ausbau der Industrie, die Erschließung neuen Bodens für die Landwirtschaft und den Wohnungsbau. Die passive Handelsbilanz muß allmählich ausgeglichen werden. Die benötigten Geldmittel kann allein das amerikanische Judentum aufbringen. Wird es aber dazu willens sein?

Es fehlt ebenso an Menschen, die das Bestehen des Staates sichern könnten. Das erworbene Land nützt nichts, wenn es nicht besiedelt werden kann. Nachdem das Sammelbecken der verschleppten und dem Tode entronnenen Juden in Mittel- und Westeuropa nahezu ausgeschöpft ist, bleiben in erster Linie die noch in Osteuropa lebenden Juden, bei denen Wunsch und Wille zur Auswanderung nach Palästina stets lebendig waren. Aber werden die Volksdemokratien sie ziehen lassen, nachdem sich die Theorie durchgesetzt hat, daß es im Grunde keine Juden gebe, jeder vielmehr dort Aufbauarbeit leisten solle, wo er geboren ist?

Gegenüber dem Reformjudentum betont der Zionismus das eigentlich Jüdische, die nationale Haltung und die Nichtassimilation. Damit ist er bewußte Verweltlichung, die Säkularisierung der Hoffnung Israels und die letzte Folgerung aus der allmählich vollzogenen Preisgabe der ursprünglichen Aufgabe Israels. An die Stelle der Hingabe an Gott ist das Streben nach Sicherung getreten. Daß Herzl auch an Uganda und Argentinien als Heimstätten für sein Volk dachte, zeigt deutlich, daß er einfach eine sichere Zuflucht wollte.

Doch wie zur Zeit des Alten Testaments ist Israel wieder zum Pufferstaat zwischen den Großmächten geworden, das sich denjenigen Bundesgenossen auswählt, der ihm Vorteile und Sicherheit verspricht. Wieder hat sich ein nationaler Staat konstituiert, der seine Ansprüche gegenüber anderen mit allen verfügbaren Mitteln durchzusetzen sucht.

Wieder ist in bestimmten Kreisen der Wunsch lebendig, das Gesetz zur Richtschnur des ganzen Lebens zu erheben. Damit ist eine Lage wiederhergestellt, die derjenigen ähnelt, in der Israel einst versagt hat. Wird es dem Judentum besser ergehen?

An sich wäre es für die Erfüllung seiner alten Aufgabe nebensächlich, ob es zerstreut in der Welt oder als Volk in Palästina lebt. Jedoch bot die erstere Lage mehr Möglichkeiten; das Judentum hätte ein ständiger Stachel im Fleisch der Völker, ein ständiger Aufruf zu einem besonderen Dasein sein können. In Palästina ist es allen ferner gerückt. Zudem erfolgte die Gründung des Staates als letzte Stufe der Verweltlichung, die alle Kräfte für politische und wirtschaftliche Aufgaben beansprucht. Werden sie nicht von der eigentlichen Aufgabe noch mehr ablenken?

Auch der Zionismus ist nicht die Lösung der Judenfrage, es sei denn, daß er wider Erwarten und entgegen seiner ursprünglichen Idee dazu beiträgt, daß das Judentum die alte Aufgabe Israels wieder erkennt, bejaht und zu verwirklichen beginnt: die Herrschaft Gottes in der Welt zu wollen als seine Herrschaft in jedem einzelnen Menschen durch dessen gläubige Hingabe und liebenden Gehorsam in völliger Gemeinschaft mit diesem Gott.

Tradition und Interpretation im Alten Testament

I.

Das Bemühen um das genaue Erkennen und Bestimmen der Rede- und Literaturgattungen hat für das Verständnis des Alten Testaments viele wichtige Ergebnisse erbracht. Freilich sind die Gattungsforschung und die aus ihr folgende formgeschichtliche Untersuchung manchmal der Gefahr der Einseitigkeit ausgesetzt, die die Form zu hoch bewertet. Denn nicht die Gattung, sondern der Inhalt der Rede ist das Primäre; vom Inhalt aus bestimmt sich die gewählte äußere Form. Jedoch darf man nicht immer umgekehrt von der gewählten Form auf den Inhalt schließen wollen. Damit, daß der Inhalt das Primäre ist, hängt es vielmehr zusammen, daß die ursprüngliche Gattung in ihrer Verwendung innerhalb einer Rede oder eines Buches eine neue Funktion erhält, die vom ursprünglichen »Sitz im Leben« abweicht[1]. Daher ist stets die Doppelheit von Form und Funktion zu beachten.

Eine ähnliche Doppelheit zeigt sich in der Verwendung inhaltlicher Stoffe und Motive innerhalb alttestamentlicher Texte und in dem Verhältnis, in dem sie jeweils zu anderen und älteren Traditionen stehen. Daß überhaupt ältere Traditionen und Motive benutzt worden sind, ist nun zwar keine neue Einsicht der Forschung, sondern zumindest hinsichtlich der Verwendung und Deutung alttestamentlicher Traditionen im Neuen Testament immer schon bekannt gewesen. Für die neuere Zeit genügt es, auf die Bemerkung von H. Schmidt zu Jes 6 hinzuweisen[2]:

> »Die menschliche Phantasie erschafft im allgemeinen keine neuen Bilder. Sie vermag empfangene Eindrücke zu ordnen, zu gruppieren, zu steigern und dadurch das Wesentliche in ihnen hervorzuheben, oft mit so überraschender Klarheit und Kraft, daß wir bewundernd wie vor einer Neuschöpfung stehen, aber das Material selbst nimmt sie vom Empfangenen. Auch der größte Künstler schafft nicht aus dem Nichts, sondern schafft nach, was ihm durch Erfahrung oder Überlieferung begegnet.«

Aber der heftige Streit über »Babel und Bibel« und in den letzten Jahren die nicht weniger laute Auseinandersetzung über das Verhältnis des Alten Testaments zu einem angeblichen »cultic pattern« im

---

[1] Vgl. G. Fohrer, Form und Funktion in der Hiobdichtung, ZDMG 109 (1959), 31—49 (= Studien zum Buche Hiob, 1963, 68—86).
[2] H. Schmidt, Die großen Propheten, 1923², 28.

Alten Orient hatten eine Hauptursache darin, daß man sich über die Art und Weise der Verwendung anderer Traditionen nicht genügend klar war. Tatsächlich werden im Alten Testament die Traditionen nur selten übernommen, in aktualisierender Art von neuem verkündigt oder wieder in Erinnerung gerufen. Vielmehr werden sie gewöhnlich in einer bestimmten Interpretation verwendet. Wie es bei der äußeren Form und Gattung zugleich um die Funktion geht, der sie dienen soll, so bei der Tradition zugleich um ihre jeweilige Interpretation. Die Tradition wird bei ihrer Übernahme und Verwendung gewöhnlich gleichzeitig interpretiert; und sie wandelt sich meist in der Interpretation, so daß sie einen anderen und sogar den gegenteiligen Sinn erhalten kann. Darin handelt es sich zumeist um eine jeweils eigene Verarbeitung und Bewältigung der Tradition. Sie macht die alten Vorstellungen und Stoffe dann zu bloßen Hilfsmitteln, mittels deren der Bearbeiter seine Gedanken ausdrückt. Angesichts dessen besteht die Aufgabe der Exegese darin, nicht nur die verwendeten Traditionen eines alttestamentlichen Textes und die traditionsmäßige Heimat seines Verfassers zu bestimmen, sondern auch das Ineinander von Tradition und Interpretation zu beachten.

Gewiß gibt es andere Verhaltensweisen gegenüber der Tradition als ihre immer neue Interpretation. So können wir ein einfaches Nachwirken der nomadischen Tradition in Israel feststellen, wenn man Ahnenreihen für einzelne Menschen und Sippen oder für das ganze Volk zusammentrug[3] oder wenn ein Teil der »Richter« und der Könige als gottgerufene Führer auftrat[4]. Gelegentlich wird eine Tradition lediglich auf eine neue Situation angewendet, wie Nahum die geschichtliche Tradition von der Eroberung Thebens durch die Assyrer drohend auf deren Hauptstadt Ninive angewendet hat (Nah 3 8ff.). Oder eine fremde Tradition wird unverändert übernommen, wobei die Übernahme kanaanäischer religiöser Vorstellungen und Bräuche am deutlichsten zeigt, welche Gefahren damit verknüpft sind. Daher hat Israel solche Traditionen, die sich dem Jahweglauben nicht dienstbar machen ließen, häufiger abgelehnt und bekämpft als übernommen[5]. Stets aber handelt es sich wenigstens um eine — positive oder negative — Auseinandersetzung mit der Tradition. Das einfache starre Festhalten an ihr führt zur geistigen Erstarrung und beraubt sich der Möglichkeit, auf die zeitgeschichtliche Lage einzuwirken. Daß die Rechabiten mit dem Jahweglauben zugleich die kulturellen Traditionen der Wüstenzeit festhielten und die neuen Errungenschaften des Kulturlandes wie Haus- und Weinbau ablehnten, war gewiß

---

[3] Gen 10 11 10-26. 27 22 20-24 25 2-4. 13-16 29 31—30 24 49 Num 1 5-15 26 Dtn 33. Die Sechser- und Zwölfersysteme von Stämmen bilden wohl verkürzte volkstümliche Genealogien nach nomadischem Muster.

[4] Vgl. A. Alt, Das Königtum in den Reichen Israel und Juda, in: Kleine Schriften zur Geschichte des Volkes Israel, II 1953, 116—134.

[5] Vgl. J. Fichtner, Die Bewältigung heidnischer Vorstellungen und Praktiken in der Welt des Alten Testaments, in: Baumgärtel-Festschrift, 1959, 24—40 (= Gottes Weisheit, 1965, 115—129).

achtenswert, verurteilte sie aber zur Bedeutungslosigkeit. Indem sie im Kulturland ein nomadisches Leben führen wollten und führten, versagten sie davor, im Ringen mit den neuen Verhältnissen den rechten Weg zu finden. Überwiegend aber hat sich die Auseinandersetzung mit der eigenen und der fremden Tradition als ein Merkmal geistigen und religiösen Lebens im geschichtlichen Werden Israels weithin vollzogen, vor allem nun eben mittels der immer neuen Interpretation der Tradition.

Noch eine weitere Abgrenzung ist erforderlich. Neue Einsichten sind nicht nur mittels der Neuinterpretation der Tradition, sondern auch spontan und unabhängig von einer Tradition erlangt worden[6]. Dies gilt insbesondere für die Propheten, sofern sie das neue und unerwartete göttliche Handeln ankündigen und die Ereignisse und Geschicke der Völker- und Menschenwelt als Wirkungen des Eingreifens Gottes deuten. Durch die unmittelbare existentielle Erfahrung werden auf diese Weise neue Traditionen geschaffen, dann allerdings häufig mittels der Interpretation älterer Traditionen ausgedrückt und verständlich gemacht.

Im folgenden wollen wir uns weder den selteneren Verhaltensweisen gegenüber der Tradition noch der Gewinnung spontaner Einsichten unabhängig von der Tradition zuwenden. Vielmehr soll uns das Problem der Doppelheit von Tradition und Interpretation beschäftigen. Es handelt sich darin einmal um die wichtigste und häufigste Form der Auseinandersetzung mit der Tradition, die man in den sich wandelnden Verhältnissen und angesichts neuer Fragen zum Sprechen zu bringen sucht und durch deren Interpretation man zu neuen Einsichten gelangt. Und ferner gehen besonders die Propheten nicht selten den Weg, ihre anderweitig gewonnenen neuen Einsichten durch eine eigene Interpretation von Traditionen auszudrücken.

II.

Daß im Alten Testament nur eine begrenzte kleine Auswahl aus dem israelitischen Schrifttum vorliegt, hängt bereits mit dem Problem von Tradition und Interpretation zusammen. Hatten schon die deuteronomische und priesterschriftliche Theologie zu einer tiefgreifenden Bearbeitung der alten Traditionen geführt, so sind in den Kanon des Alten Testament nur mehr diejenigen Schriften aufgenommen worden, die dem auf dieser Grundlage sich bildenden spätantiken Judentum unanstößig waren, während alle Schriften ausgeschlossen worden sind, die seinen Lehrern anstößig erschienen. Infolgedessen ist vieles verlorengegangen, was unter anderen Gesichtspunkten als denjenigen des spätantiken Judentums durchaus hätte Wert und Bestand haben und mit nicht geringerem Recht die gleiche Autorität wie manche der erhaltenen Schriften beanspruchen können. Zugleich sind auf diese Weise viele der Schwierigkeiten geschaffen worden, die ein rich-

---

[6] Vgl. z. B. A. Alt, Die Deutung der Weltgeschichte im Alten Testament, ZThK 56 (1959), 129—137.

tiges Verständnis vieler alttestamentlicher Texte erschweren oder sogar verhindern; es fehlen eben so viele Texte, daß wir oft ärgerliche Lücken antreffen, wenn wir einer Einzelfrage genauer nachgehen. Dies alles beruht vorwiegend auf einem umfassenden Interpretationsvorgang, der sich über Jahrhunderte erstreckt hat. Dadurch sind gewiß viele Schriften dem gleichfalls möglichen Untergang entrissen worden; zugleich aber wird die Anerkennung einer Schrift als kanonisch davon abhängig, ob ihre unter den Gesichtspunkten des spätantiken Judentums erfolgte Anerkennung weiterhin als gültig betrachtet werden kann, und findet ihre Grenze darin.

Damit nicht genug, ist auch der Text des Alten Testaments nicht bloß tradiert, sondern gleichzeitig interpretiert worden. Allerdings ist es fraglich, ob zunächst durchgehend mit einer langen mündlichen Überlieferung und innerhalb dieser mit einer ständigen Umformung und Interpretation oder wenigstens mit der durch sie beeinflußten Umgestaltung der gleichzeitig schriftlichen Überlieferung zu rechnen ist. Während diese Annahme für die meisten prophetischen Worte, die sich auf eine bestimmte geschichtliche Situation beziehen, sehr unwahrscheinlich ist[7], trifft sie für andere alttestamentliche Bücher in etwas abgewandelter Art wohl zu. Am deutlichsten lassen vielleicht die Erzählungen der Genesis die Stadien des Umgestaltens und Interpretierens erkennen, die ihrer — wiederum verschiedenartigen — schriftlichen Fixierung in den einzelnen Quellenschichten vorangegangen sind. Wie sich dergleichen noch bei anderen Erzählungskomplexen beobachten läßt[8], so sind vielleicht manche Psalmen, die einen jungen Eindruck machen, durch einen vor der jetzigen schriftlichen Fixierung liegenden Umgestaltungsprozeß aus älteren Psalmen entstanden. So könnte der endgültigen Form des Ps 78 ein altes, aus der Zeit Davids oder Salomos stammendes Lied zugrunde liegen, das in den Erfolgsjahren Josias neu bearbeitet worden ist[9].

---

[7] Vgl. neuerdings die Auseinandersetzung mit dieser Frage bei C. Stuhlmueller, The Influence of Oral Tradition upon Exegesis and the Senses of Scripture, CBQ 20 (1958), 299—326; A. H. J. Gunneweg, Mündliche und schriftliche Tradition der vorexilischen Prophetenbücher als Problem der neueren Prophetenforschung, 1959; dazu E. Sellin—G. Fohrer, Einleitung in das Alte Testament, 1965^{10}, § 3.

[8] Vgl. z. B. G. S. Glanzman, The Origin and Date of the Book of Ruth, CBQ 21 (1959), 201—207; G. Fohrer, Überlieferung und Wandlung der Hioblegende, in: Baumgärtel-Festschrift, 1959, 41—62 (= Studien zum Buche Hiob, 1963, 44—67).

[9] O. Eißfeldt, Das Lied Moses Deuteronomium 32 1-43 und das Lehrgedicht Asaphs Psalm 78 samt einer Analyse der Umgebung des Mose-Liedes, 1958, möchte den Psalm aus der Zeit vor Salomos Tod herleiten. Doch daß dessen Geschichtsbetrachtung nur bis zu David bzw. Salomo führt, muß nicht mit seiner Abfassungszeit zusammenhängen, sondern kann genau so gut in seiner sachlichen Tendenz begründet sein. Auch andere Beobachtungen und Überlegungen führen für die gegenwärtige

Es fragt sich ferner, wie weit die sprachgeschichtliche Entwicklung des Hebräischen bis zu seiner masoretischen Form gleichzeitig Interpretationsvorgänge in sich schließt. Auf einer solchen Voraussetzung beruhen letztlich die zahlreichen Versuche, aufgrund anderer semitischer Sprachen im Alten Testament neue Vokabeln oder Wortbedeutungen zu entdecken, die in späterer Zeit nicht mehr bekannt waren oder mißverstanden wurden. Während dabei freilich vieles ungewiß oder fragwürdig bleibt, läßt sich das interpretierende Eingreifen in die Textüberlieferung in vielen anderen Fällen deutlich erkennen. Manchmal erfolgte es zurückhaltend und konservativ wie in der Anwendung des Ketib/Quere oder auch noch in den Fällen der Tiqqune und Itture Sopherim[10]. Außerdem sind aber vermutlich besonders in älterer Zeit allerlei Eingriffe in den Text ohne irgendeine Kennzeichnung erfolgt. Die interpretierende Absicht liegt schließlich zahlreichen Glossen zugrunde, die dem Text im Lauf der Zeit hinzugefügt worden sind. Gliedert man sie nach ihren verschiedenen Arten auf[11], so zeigt sich, daß sie in der Mehrzahl in irgendeiner Weise das Verständnis des überlieferten Textes fördern sollen, indem sie ihn interpretieren. Meist entsprechen sie den hermeneutischen Regeln der talmudischen Schriftauslegung, die zwar erst jüngeren Datums sind, jedoch nur die älteste erhaltene schriftliche Fassung von längst bekannten Methoden und den konkreten Ausdruck einer schon viel früher geübten Art der Textauffassung und -behandlung darstellen.

III.

Der Blick auf Text und Kanon läßt erkennen, daß bei der Entstehung des Alten Testaments selbst die Tradition in der verschiedensten Weise interpretiert worden ist. Gehen wir der Frage weiter nach, so zeigt sich, daß dies nicht allein für die Spätzeit zutrifft, sondern daß der ganze Verlauf der religiösen Geschichte Israels weithin dadurch bestimmt ist. In ihr findet eine ständige Auseinandersetzung mit den zeitgeschichtlichen Verhältnissen und mit den Einflüssen fremder Kulturen und Religionen statt. Dabei ist sowohl das entschiedene Be-

---

Form des Psalms eher in die Zeit Josias, vgl. G. Fohrer in: WZKM 55 (1959), 177; H. Junker, Die Entstehungszeit des Ps 78 und das Deuteronomium, Bibl 34 (1953), 493; H.-J. Kraus, Psalmen, 1960, 540f.

[10] Vgl. die Aufzählung und Charakteristik bei E. Würthwein, Der Text des Alten Testaments, 1963², 20f.

[11] Für ein einzelnes Buch vgl. G. Fohrer, Die Glossen im Buche Ezechiel, ZAW 63 (1951), 33—53 (= Studien zur alttestamentlichen Prophetie [1949—1965], 1967, 204—221); P. R. Ackroyd, Some Interpretative Glosses in the Book of Haggai, JJS 7 (1956), 163—167. Vgl. ferner G. R. Driver, Glosses in the Hebrew Text of the Old Testament, in: L'Ancien Testament et l'Orient, 1957, 123—161.

harren auf wesentlichen Grundsätzen der Traditionen des Jahweglaubens unter schroffer Ablehnung fremder Vorstellungen und Bräuche als auch die Abwandlung eigener und die Übernahme fremder Traditionen zu beobachten. Wir bemerken einerseits, wie die eigenen Traditionen des Jahweglaubens jeweils neu interpretiert, den verschiedenartigen zeitgeschichtlichen Verhältnissen angepaßt und dadurch in ihnen lebendig erhalten werden. Andererseits ist nicht zu verkennen, daß ursprünglich fremde, nichtisraelitische und nichtjahwistische Vorstellungen und Bräuche mit einer entsprechenden Interpretation übernommen werden, um den Jahweglauben zu erweitern und zu bereichern. Dessen Geschichte ist weithin die Geschichte der immer neuen Anpassung der jahwistischen Traditionen und der Aneignung fremden Gutes.

Dem dienen schon die vielfach als Wortspiel geformten etymologischen Ätiologien für Personen- und Ortsnamen, die sich überwiegend in den Erzählungstraditionen für die Zeit vor der Landnahme in Palästina finden[12]. Mit ihrer Hilfe, d. h. mit einer etymologisch-ätiologischen Interpretation, gliedert besonders der Jahwist die Personen und Orte in den Ablauf der Geschichte Israels und seiner Ahnen mit Jahwe ein. Gerade der wortspielartige Charakter der Ätiologien, der sie den ägyptischen Wortspielen annähert, weist darauf hin, daß sie wie diese die Funktion haben, alten Traditionen einen neuen Sinn zu verleihen[13].

Nicht weniger bezeichnend ist der Vorgang, den man als »interpretatio israelitica et jahwistica« einer Reihe von palästinischen Heiligtümern bezeichnen kann. Viele von ihnen wie Betel, Gilgal und Sichem sind, bevor sie israelitisch wurden, kanaanäische Heiligtümer gewesen und reichen bei der Zähigkeit, mit der solchen Stätten durch Jahrhunderte und Religionen hindurch ein heiliger Charakter zugeschrieben zu werden pflegt, zweifellos weit in die Vorzeit zurück. Die Israeliten haben sie mitsamt dem an ihnen geübten Kultus übernommen, indem sie die vorhandenen Kultlegenden in zweifacher Weise interpretierten: Sie bezogen die die Heiligkeit der Stätte und den Kultus begründende Offenbarung auf eine Gestalt ihrer eigenen Vergangenheit, vorzugsweise auf einen der Patriarchen, und ersetzten die bisherige Gottheit — meist eine lokale Form des Gottes El — durch Jahwe, wie etwa die Diskrepanz in Gen 16 13 28 16. 19 deutlich macht. In manchen Fällen mag sich der Interpretationsvorgang in zwei Stadien vollzogen haben, da nach der Landnahme einer israelitischen Gruppe das Heiligtum zunächst zu einem ihrer Ahnen und erst nach der späteren Annahme des von der Moseschar mitgebrachten Jahweglaubens auch zu Jahwe in Beziehung gesetzt wurde.

Gleiches gilt für viele Einzelheiten des Kultus und des Brauchtums. Das nomadische Passafest mit seinen Riten wird mittels der Deutung auf den Exodus legitimiert (Dtn 16 1); solche historisierende Interpretation und Aneignung wiederholt sich bis hin zum ursprünglich heidnischen Purimfest, dessen Übernahme durch die östliche Diaspora das Buch Esther zeigt. Die uralte Sitte der Beschneidung wird mit geschicht-

---

[12] Vgl. im einzelnen J. Fichtner, Die etymologische Ätiologie in den Namengebungen der geschichtlichen Bücher des Alten Testaments, VT 6 (1956), 372—396.
[13] Vgl. S. Morenz, Wortspiele in Ägypten, in: Akten des Vierundzwanzigsten Internationalen Orientalisten-Kongresses München, 1959, 91f.

lichen Gestalten oder Situationen in Verbindung gebracht (Gen 17 Ex 4 23-26 Jos 5 2 ff.), die eherne Schlange des Jerusalemer Tempels — an sich das Bild eines Heildämons — bis auf Hiskia mit Hilfe ihrer mosaischen Interpretation beibehalten (Num 21 4-9 II Reg 18 4) und die Mazzebe bis zum deuteronomischen Verbot (Dtn 16 22) als Denkstein interpretiert (Gen 28 18 31 45 35 20 usw.). Während das deuteronomische Gesetz die Mazzebe verbietet, interpretiert es selbst wiederum manches ursprünglich heidnische Brauchtum und ordnet es dadurch in den Jahweglauben ein — so die Freistellung vom Kriegsdienst (Dtn 20 5-8), das Abnehmen eines Gehenkten vor Anbruch der Nacht (Dtn 21 22 f.), die Quasten der Kleidung (Dtn 22 12, vgl. Num 15 38 ff.) und die Behandlung der Erntereste (Dtn 24 19-21). In I Sam 5 4 f. wird sogar der nicht übernommene (und Zeph 1 9 gerügte) Kultbrauch des Springens über die Schwelle in Asdod geschichtlich aus einer Wirkung der Lade Jahwes erklärt.

In alledem handelt es sich um Ausschnitte und Einzelerscheinungen aus einem umfassenden und langwierigen Interpretationsprozeß. Er hat sich auf religiösem Gebiet nach zwei Richtungen hin vollzogen: in der Auseinandersetzung des Jahweglaubens mit dem nomadischen Traditionsgut Israels und in derjenigen mit der fremden, vor allem der kanaanäischen Kultur und Religion.

Freilich stehen wir hinsichtlich der Frühzeit der Israeliten vor einer schwierigen religionsgeschichtlichen Frage: Haben sie die sog. Vätergötter mit bestimmten Eigenarten und verschiedenen Namen verehrt[14] oder der für die Semiten überhaupt charakteristischen Elreligion gehuldigt? Oder besteht zwischen diesen Auffassungen gar kein Gegensatz, sondern handelt es sich entweder um zwei aufeinander folgende Stadien mit der Ablösung der später als fragwürdig geltenden Vätergottkulte durch die Elreligion[15], oder sind die Vätergötter mit ihren verschiedenen Namen einzelne Variationen der Gottheit El, wie deren lokale Formen in Palästina durch verschiedene Zusätze zum Namen El gekennzeichnet waren[16]? Jedenfalls ist ein zweifacher Interpretationsvorgang anzunehmen: Die altisraelitischen Vätergötter oder Elformen sind zunächst mit den lokalen Formen des palästinischen El aus dem kanaanäischen Pantheon und dann nach der Annahme des Jahweglaubens mit Jahwe identifiziert worden. Die Gleichsetzung mit Jahwe als Interpretation der früheren Religionsgeschichte erfolgt durch den Elohisten, der zuvor den Jahwenamen vermieden hat, in Ex 3 13ff. und durch die Priesterschrift in Ex 6 3, nunmehr ausgeweitet und systematisiert zu einem Schema von vier Offenbarungsperioden mit teilweise unterschiedlichen Gottesnamen.

---

[14] A. Alt, Der Gott der Väter, 1929 (= Kleine Schriften zur Geschichte des Volkes Israel, 1953, 1—78), dazu die überlieferungsgeschichtliche Kritik von J. Hoftijzer, Die Verheißungen an die drei Erzväter, 1956.

[15] O. Eissfeldt, Religionshistorie und Religionspolemik im Alten Testament, VT Suppl III, 1955, 94—102 (= Kleine Schriften, III 1966, 359—366).

[16] Vgl. dazu B. Gemser, Vragen rondom de Patriarchenreligië, 1958.

Tiefergreifend und folgenreicher haben sich die Beziehungen zwischen der kanaanäischen Religion und dem Jahweglauben ausgewirkt. Auch wenn man die strittigen Fragen nach Herkunft und Bedeutung der Lade beiseite läßt[17], ist doch fast der gesamte israelitische Jahwekult in Palästina durch die interpretierende Übernahme kanaanäischer Riten geprägt, der salomonische Tempel nach kanaanäischem Vorbild gebaut und nicht zuletzt das Gottesbild mehrfach durch die Einbeziehung neuer Elemente erweitert worden. Konnte El nicht als Gatte und Vater in Jahwe aufgehen, so doch als Herrscher der Götter und als Gott des Himmels und der Weisheit. Ließen sich die Stiernatur Baals und sein rhythmisches Dahinwelken und Wiederaufleben nicht auf Jahwe übertragen, so doch seine Herrschaft über das Kulturland und sein segensreiches Gewähren aller Fruchtbarkeit. So ist das Bild Jahwes einerseits vom Gott El her neu interpretiert worden[18], indem er zunächst in Baalat zum Herrn der Zebaot erklärt (II Sam 6 2)[19], dann in Jerusalem im Zusammenhang mit dem Tempel Salomos mit dem — sich zugleich auch an das Königtum Baals anschließenden — Königstitel versehen[20] und später als Weltschöpfer verstanden wurde[21], andererseits vom Gott Baal her, indem ihm wie diesem die Verfügungsgewalt über den Regen und damit über Fruchtbarkeit und Gedeihen des Kulturlandes zugeschrieben wurde[22].

---

[17] Vgl. den gut unterrichtenden Überblick von E. Kutsch in: RGG³, IV 197—199, ferner J. Maier, Das altisraelitische Ladeheiligtum, 1965. Manches scheint mir für die Annahme zu sprechen, daß die Lade das außerpalästinische und vorjahwistisch-israelitische Wanderheiligtum der mittelpalästinischen Stämmegruppe oder der Ephraimiten und späteren Benjaminiten gewesen ist.

[18] Zum Verhältnis El-Jahwe vgl. besonders O. Eißfeldt, El and Yahweh, JSS 1 (1956), 25—37 (= Kleine Schriften, III 1966, 386—397).

[19] Vgl. aber auch O. Eißfeldt, Jahwe Zebaoth, Miscellanea Acad. Berol. II 2, 1950, 128—150 (= Kleine Schriften, III 1966, 103—123); V. Maag, Jahwäs Heerscharen, Schweiz. Theol. Umschau 20 (1950), Nr. 3/4, 27—52.

[20] Vgl. besonders O. Eißfeldt, Jahwe als König, ZAW 46 (1928), 81—105 (= Kleine Schriften, I 1962, 172—193); A. Alt, Gedanken über das Königtum Jahwes, in: Kleine Schriften zur Geschichte des Volkes Israel, I 1953, 345—357; H. Schmid, Jahwe und die Kulttraditionen von Jerusalem, ZAW 67 (1955), 168—197 (bes. 171—178); A. Caquot, Le Psaume 47 et la Royauté de Yahwé, RHPhR 39 (1959), 311—337; V. Maag, Malkût Jhwh, VTSuppl VII, 1960, 129—153; W. H. Schmidt, Königtum Gottes in Ugarit und Israel, 1966².

[21] H. Schmid a. a. O. bes. 181—183. Doch hat dieser Gedanke für die frühe Königszeit noch keine wesentliche Rolle gespielt. Abgesehen von der Schöpfungserzählung des Jahwisten, die auf andere Quellen als Jerusalemer Kulttraditionen zurückgeht, tritt der Schöpfungsgedanke erst später stärker hervor.

[22] Vgl. im einzelnen G. Fohrer, Elia, 1968². Anders C. A. Keller, ThZ 16 (1960), 298—313, der gegenüber allen Fragen nach der Eigenart Elias bei dem (von niemandem bestrittenen) Allgemeinplatz verharrt, daß die Tradition ihn als Diener Gottes,

Mit alledem haben sowohl die kultische Frömmigkeit als auch die national-religiöse Theologie der vorexilischen Erzähler der Hexateuchschichten eine mittlere Linie verfolgt. Sie lehnten weder die kanaanäischen Elemente grundsätzlich ab, noch paßten sie den eigenen Glauben völlig an die Kulturlandreligion an; vielmehr suchten sie deren lebensfähige, berechtigte und dem Jahweglauben nicht widerstrebende Elemente durch eine entsprechende Interpretation in diesen einzubeziehen[23].

Handelt es sich in dieser Auseinandersetzung mit der kanaanäischen Religion überwiegend um die Stellungnahme zu dem Versuch der Weltbewältigung und Lebensgestaltung mittels magischer Vorstellungen und Bräuche, so muß wenigstens kurz darauf hingewiesen werden, daß sich die israelitische Oberschicht während der Königszeit zugleich mit der anderen menschlichen Möglichkeit dessen auseinanderzusetzen hatte: mit der überwiegend rational bestimmten Weisheitslehre, die seit der Zeit Salomos zunächst die Bildung und Moral der regierenden Kreise beherrscht hat. Daß dieses auf praktische Erfolge gerichtete Klug- und Kundigsein offenbar gern übernommen und praktiziert worden ist, wird an den kritischen Worten Jesajas deutlich (vgl. Jes 5 20. 21 31 1-3)[24]. Doch ist nicht zu übersehen, daß die von der Umwelt übernommene Lebensweisheit in immer stärkerem Maße israelitisch-jahwistisch interpretiert worden ist; darauf wird noch zurückzukommen sein.

Aus solchen Interpretationen eigener und fremder Traditionen hat sich eine gewisse Normalform des offiziellen Jahweglaubens ergeben. Sie ist grundlegend dadurch bestimmt, daß sie Israel in einem vorgegebenen Heilszustand erblickt. Es kann diesen zwar durch einzelne Verfehlungen stören, durch entsprechende Sühnemaßnahmen aber jederzeit wiederherstellen. Demgemäß erwartet es den »Tag Jahwes«, an dem dieser in seinem wunderbaren Glanz unter den Begleiterscheinungen der Theophanie sichtbar wird, immer als etwas unbeschreiblich Herrliches und Glückseliges, da die Katastrophen die Feinde Israels treffen, ihm selbst aber die heilvollen Wirkungen der Gotteserscheinung zugute kommen werden.

---

nicht als Helden zeige. Die Behauptung allerdings, daß diese Tradition das geschichtliche Bild Elias wiedergebe und daß der Exeget und Historiker sie anzunehmen habe, wie sie ist, würde — nähme man sie ernst — das Ende der Wissenschaft vom Alten Testament zugunsten eines Rezitierens der Tradition bedeuten.

[23] Als Beispiel vgl. O. Kaiser, Die mythische Bedeutung des Meeres in Ägypten, Ugarit und Israel, 1962².

[24] Vgl. auch J. Fichtner, Jesaja unter den Weisen, ThLZ 74 (1949), 75—80 (= Gottes Weisheit, 1965, 18—26); R. T. Anderson, Was Isaiah a Scribe ?, JBL 79 (1960), 57f., obwohl schwerlich anzunehmen ist, daß Jesaja selbst aus dem Stand der »Weisen« hervorgegangen ist.

Die großen Einzelpropheten der vor- und frühexilischen Zeit haben diese Auffassung des herkömmlichen Jahweglaubens uminterpretiert. Sie sehen den Menschen nicht in einer vorgegebenen Heilssituation, sondern wegen seiner Sünde, die den Kern seines Wesens verderbt, in einer grundsätzlichen Unheilssituation. Nach ihrer Botschaft droht nicht mehr eine einzelne, vorübergehende Strafe, sondern wird das schuldverhaftete Dasein Israels oder anderer Völker und Menschen völlig zunichte. So wird auch die Vorstellung vom Tag Jahwes uminterpretiert. Amos sagt, daß dieser Tag für Israel nicht Heil (Licht), sondern Unheil (Finsternis) bedeutet (Am 5 18-20). Jesaja läßt zwar die leuchtenden Farben bestehen, sieht aber als Folge der glanzvollen Erscheinung gleichfalls Verderben statt Glück, Freude und Frieden für Juda, wenn Gewittersturm und Erdbeben alles Überragende und Hohe niederreißen und einstürzen lassen (Jes 2 12-17). Auch wenn die Gerichtszeit wie in Jer 25 11 ff. 29 10 auf 70 Jahre begrenzt wird, gilt dies nur als angemessene Strafzeit, nach deren Ablauf die sündige und verurteilte Generation ausgestorben ist; es handelt sich um die Verhängung einer lebenslänglichen Strafe über die Verbrecher, nicht aber um eine vorübergehende Unterbrechung eines Heilszustandes. Angesichts des drohenden Untergangs halten die großen Einzelpropheten allerdings eine Rettung noch für möglich. Sie setzt aber nicht eine Sühnemaßnahme, sondern die grundlegende innere und äußere Wandlung des schuldigen Volkes oder Menschen mittels der Umkehr zu Gott (Ez 18 30f.) oder der Erlösung durch ihn (Hos 14 2-9) voraus. Statt der Zuteilung des Heils an Israel und des Unheils an seine und Jahwes Feinde ist daher für die Propheten das Entweder-Oder der Vernichtung oder der Rettung grundlegend. Charakteristisch für dieses Entweder-Oder ist Jes 1 19f.:

> Wenn ihr willig seid und gehorcht,
> sollt ihr das Gut des Landes essen.
> Wenn ihr euch aber weigert und widerspenstig seid,
> müßt ihr das Schwert 'fressen'[25].

Vom Exil an hat die eschatologische Prophetie das Entweder-Oder in ein zeitliches Vorher-Nachher uminterpretiert. Ist dies schon aus dem in zeitlichen Kategorien sich vollziehenden Denken und Vorstellen des alttestamentlichen Menschen erklärlich, so wirkte außerdem die alte, nicht zuletzt in kultprophetischen Kreisen verbreitete Auffassung vom ständigen Heil Israels darauf ein. Wie man deswegen nach wie vor mit einer grundlegenden Heilssituation rechnen und einseitig den göttlichen Heilswillen betonen zu dürfen glaubte, so verstand man zugleich den Untergang Judas und das Exil als das von den

---

[25] Oder es ist zu lesen: »sollt ihr 'vom' Schwert gefressen werden«.

großen Einzelpropheten angedrohte Gericht. Und da es nicht mehr als ständig drohende Möglichkeit, sondern als einmaliges geschichtliches Ereignis galt, konnte nach seinem Ablauf nur mehr eine endgültige und ewige Heilszeit folgen. So unterscheidet die eschatologische Prophetie zwischen zwei Zeitaltern, an deren Grenze sie sich stehen glaubt, und malt den Übergang vom einen zum anderen und das Bild des künftigen Zeitalters in mannigfacher Weise aus[26]. Der Tag Jahwes wird wieder im alten, für das Israel der Endzeit heilvollen Sinn mit dem Endgericht über die Völker interpretiert (z. B. Joel 4 14 Jes 34 8).

> Die eschatologische Interpretation hat sich auch auf die äußere Gestaltung der Prophetenbücher ausgewirkt. Einige von ihnen sind dreigeteilt: Unheil für Israel — Unheil für andere Völker als Übergang zum Kommenden — Heil für Israel und vielleicht für andere Völker. So verhält es sich deutlich in den Büchern Ezechiel, Zephanja und der LXX-Fassung Jeremias, nicht ganz durchgeführt in Jes 1—35. Diese Gliederung entspricht dem eschatologisch-apokalyptischen Schema, das also für die Ordnung und Aneinanderreihung der schon vorliegenden Spruchsammlungen der vorexilischen Propheten entgegen ihrer eigenen Theologie angewendet worden ist. Hat diese Deutung der prophetischen Korpora als eschatologischer Bücher oder gar als Apokalypsen keine bleibende Wirkung ausgeübt, so desto mehr die ebenfalls der eschatologischen Auffassung entspringende Methode, auf eine Spruchsammlung mit scheltenden und drohenden Worten eine oder mehrere Verheißungen, durchweg eschatologischer Art, folgen zu lassen und auf diese Weise das Vorher-Nachher der Eschatologie äußerlich sichtbar zu machen. Während dazu im Hoseabuch ausnahmsweise ein Heilswort Hoseas selbst benutzt werden konnte (Hos 14 2-9), handelt es sich in Am 9 8 ff. um spätere Worte Unbekannter. Ebenso verhält es sich mit Jes 2 2-4 als Abschluß von Kap. 1[27]; 4 2-6 als Abschluß von 2 6—4 1; 9 1-6 als Abschluß von Kap. 6—8; 11 1-16 als Abschluß der in sich schon erweiterten Sammlung 9 7—10 34 (mitsamt dem abgesprengten Teil 5 25-29); Kap. 12 als Abschluß von Kap. 1—11. Im Michabuch ist dies zweimal zu beobachten; auf Kap. 1—3 folgen die Verheißungen in Kap. 4—5, auf 6 1—7 7 wieder 7 8-20. Diese interpretierende Methode bewirkt bis heute, daß manche dieser eschatologischen Heilsworte den vorexilischen Propheten selbst zugeschrieben werden.

Derartige Neuinterpretationen des Glaubens finden sich in der Folgezeit wieder — in der durch die Tätigkeit Esras inaugurierten Gesetzesfrömmigkeit und in der Apokalyptik als der jüngeren und sozusagen moderneren Form der Eschatologie, ja weit über die Zeit des Alten Testaments hinaus. All diese Interpretationen der Tradition suchen den Gegensatz zu vermeiden oder zu beheben, der sich für den in einer geprägten und festgelegten Form bestehenden Glauben inner-

---

[26] Vgl. im einzelnen G. Fohrer, Die Struktur der alttestamentlichen Eschatologie, ThLZ 85 (1960), 401—420 (= Studien zur alttestamentlichen Prophetie [1949—1965], 1967, 32—58).

[27] Die Überschrift 2 1 war für die Sammlung 2 6—4 1 bestimmt und ist sekundär vor 2 2 ff. gesetzt worden.

halb einer sich wandelnden Welt nur zu leicht gegenüber dem täglichen Leben und seiner Bewältigung ergibt. Die vorgegebenen Traditionen als solche sind stets der Gefahr ausgesetzt, in Denkweise, Geist und Sprache nicht mehr Grundlage, Vorbild oder Ausdruck des Glaubens und der Lebenswirklichkeit in einer Zeit und Welt zu sein, die sich seit dem Entstehen der Traditionen verändert hat. Die jeweils neue Interpretation kann sie dessen wieder fähig machen und ist daher grundsätzlich berechtigt und sogar notwendig. Freilich gelingt sie insofern nicht immer, als sie den Sinn und Gehalt der Tradition in Mitleidenschaft ziehen und verfälschen kann. Das ist bereits in der kultischen und national-religiösen Interpretation des vorexilischen Jahweglaubens bis zu einem gewissen Grad zu beobachten. Manchmal fragt es sich, ob noch ein mit Hilfe uminterpretierter kanaanäischer Vorstellungen und Bräuche den palästinischen Verhältnissen angepaßter Jahweglaube oder nicht vielmehr eine baalisierte Jahwereligion oder gar eine bloß jahwistisch getönte Baalreligion vorliegt. Und wie die Glaubensinterpretation der eschatologischen Prophetie letztlich eine epigonale Entartung der vorexilischen Prophetie darstellt, so haben das Vorgehen Esras und die Apokalyptik den alttestamentlichen Glauben in bedenkliche Bahnen gelenkt. Sie sind Beispiele dafür, daß eine Interpretation der Tradition nicht nur als Zeichen lebendigen Werdens und Wachsens gelten und nicht immer positiv beurteilt werden muß, sondern auch auf einen Irrweg führen kann.

Daraus ergibt sich zugleich, daß das Verhältnis von Tradition und Interpretation zueinander nicht so zu verstehen ist, daß eine ursprünglich »kompakte«, verdichtete Symbolik allmählich »differenziert«, in ihre einzelnen Bestandteile auseinandergelegt wird und daß jede spätere Auslegung eine bestimmte Einzelheit einer Tradition hervorhebt und in zutreffender Weise aus ihr folgert, weil alles schon im alten Symbol enthalten wäre[28]. Wenn man auf die Begriffe »Fortschritt« und »Entwicklung« im Sinne eines evolutionistischen Schemas verzichtet, ist es darum nicht nötig, die entgegengesetzte Annahme der Differenzierung einer gegebenen Tradition zu vertreten. Denn das jeweils Neue ist nicht schon von vornherein in der alten Vorstellung enthalten, so daß es aus ihr abgeleitet werden könnte, sondern wird gewöhnlich aus der schöpferischen Auseinandersetzung mit einer andersgearteten Situation oder aus einer unmittelbaren existentiellen Erfahrung gewonnen und mittels der Neuinterpretation der altehrwürdigen Tradition gleicherweise verständlich gemacht und legitimiert. Dabei treten die entscheidenden Gesichtspunkte in der neuen Interpretation und in ihrem Unterschied zur Tradition zutage.

---

[28] E. Voegelin, Order and History, I: Israel and Revelation, 1956, z. B. 410f.

IV.

In besonders starkem Maße sind die erzählenden Bücher des Alten Testaments dadurch gekennzeichnet, daß sie Traditionen verschiedenster Art in immer neuer und anderer Weise interpretieren. Allein ein Vergleich des chronistischen Geschichtswerks mit den älteren Darstellungen zeigt, welche Umwandlung der Überlieferung noch in nachexilischer Zeit möglich war. Nicht anders verhält es sich mit den älteren Darstellungen selbst.

Die Traditionen, die den erzählenden Büchern zugrunde liegen, sind mannigfacher Art. Allein für die Genesis ergibt sich eine bunte Reihe. In der sog. Urgeschichte, die beim Jahwisten besser als Vorgeschichte und in der Priesterschrift als Frühgeschichte zu bezeichnen wäre, sind vor allem mancherlei Mythen oder mythische Motive in geschichtlicher Interpretation verwendet worden, am besten erkennbar in den Erzählungen über Schöpfung und Fall, Engelehen und Sintflut.

Dabei hat sich neuerdings herausgestellt[29], daß der eigentliche Platz der mesopotamischen Sintfluterzählung nicht das Gilgamesch-Epos, sondern das Atrachasis-Epos ist: Enlil sendet die Flut, weil der Lärm der zahlreicher werdenden Menschheit ihn am Schlafen hindert, wie denn die mesopotamischen Götter auch sonst durch Lärm erheblich gestört scheinen. Demgegenüber wird die jahwistische Neuinterpretation am deutlichsten in der völlig anderen Begründung der Flut in Gen 6 5-7. Die Hauptbedeutung des Atrachasis-Epos, das die Schöpfung der Menschen, den Beginn der Kultur, die Königsliste und die Flut darbietet, liegt aber darin, daß es als ganzes eine Parallele zu Gen 1—10 darstellt. Nicht bloß in einzelnen Episoden der sog. Urgeschichte sind also ältere Traditionen verarbeitet, sondern der Aufbau und die Abfolge der gesamten Darstellung haben ihr Gegenstück im mesopotamischen Epos.

In den Erzählungen über die Patriarchen geht die Interpretation so weit, daß es kaum mehr möglich ist, die im Mittelpunkt stehenden Gestalten in ihrer wirklichen Geschichtlichkeit zu erfassen, obwohl sie sicherlich geschichtliche Einzelgestalten gewesen sind. Gerade die in den Quellenschichten des Hexateuchs erfolgte letzte Interpretation hat offenbar bezweckt, die Erzählungen so zu gestalten, daß die Patriarchen geradezu als verschiedene Typen des Menschen vor Gott und in der Welt erscheinen. So ist Abraham der Typ des glaubenden Menschen, Isaak der des duldend hinnehmenden, Jakob der des zuerst falsch und dann richtig hoffenden und harrenden und Joseph der des hochmütigen, der zur Demut geführt wird. Die dieser Auffassung zugrunde gelegten und schon vorher wiederholt uminterpretierten Traditionen sind mannigfachen Ursprungs.

Die Nuzi-Texte haben gelehrt, daß manche Genesis-Erzählungen mesopotamische Rechtsbräuche des 15./14. Jh. widerspiegeln — wie Gen 15 die Erbfrage,

---

[29] W. G. Lambert, New Light on the Babylonian Flood, JSS 5 (1960), 113—123; W G. Lambert—A. R. Millard, Atra-ḫasīs, 1969.

Gen 16 und 30 die stellvertretende Geburt durch die Sklavin und Gen 21 deren Rechte, Gen 29 29 ff. die Übertragung des Erstgeburtsrechts und Gen 31 den Nachweis der Erbberechtigung. Andere Erzählungen gehen auf kanaanäische Kultlegenden zurück — wie die Begründung der Heiligkeit der Stätte von Betel in Gen 28 10 ff., die Lokalsage von Peniel bzw. Penuel in Gen 32 25 ff. (dazu in v. 33 die Erklärung eines Opferbrauchs) und die Sage von der Ablösung des Menschenopfers zu Jeriel bzw. Jeruel in Gen 22 mit der späteren Umdeutung auf Jerusalem durch Einfügung des Namens Moria (vgl. II Chr 3 1). Hinzu treten zahlreiche lokale Erinnerungen und Erzählungen, die schon im vorjahwistischen Stadium im Zuge der Landnahme der Israeliten auf die gleichfalls nach Palästina versetzten Vätergestalten übertragen und in einem weiteren Stadium dem Jahweglauben angepaßt worden sind. Die neueste Untersuchung der Joseph-Novelle von der Ägyptologie her hat zu dem Schluß geführt, daß sie auf eine sehr alte Erzählung gegründet sei, die in die ramessidische Epoche Ägyptens zurückreiche[30]. Freilich ist diese genaue Zeitbestimmung ebensowenig gesichert, wie die aus der Untersuchung gefolgerte Abfassung durch Mose an Wahrscheinlichkeit gewinnt. Es ist nicht zu übersehen, daß die Begründung des Übertritts von Israeliten nach Ägypten und des Aufstiegs des Josephstammes sowie die Überflügelung Manasses durch Ephraim eng und unauflöslich in und mit der Joseph-Novelle verknüpft sind[31]. Muß man auf dieser Grundlage die vom Jahwisten und Elohisten als Vorlage benutzte ältere Joseph-Erzählung um 1100 v. Chr. ansetzen, so kann man angesichts des ägyptologischen Materials außerdem vielleicht annehmen, daß die Erzählung die israelitische Umarbeitung einer ägyptischen Geschichte darstellt. Noch in sehr später Zeit sind in Gen 14 einige Bruchstücke historischer Traditionen über einen nur mehr mit vielen Unsicherheiten und Vorbehalten zu bestimmenden Feldzug in Palästina und über einen priesterlich amtierenden Stadtkönig von Jerusalem mit der Gestalt Abrahams zu einer midraschartigen Erzählung verbunden worden, um das Bild des friedfertigen Patriarchen zu korrigieren und die Pflicht zur Demut gegenüber dem Hohenpriester in Jerusalem einzuschärfen. Die darin verborgene Beziehung auf die Gegenwart des Erzählers tritt gleicherweise in den zahlreichen ätiologischen Erklärungen hervor, die ja von auffälligen Tatbeständen ausgehen, die »bis auf diesen Tag« bestehen, und sie dem Zeitgenossen deuten wollen[32].

Daß die Interpretation einer Tradition sich auf zeitgeschichtliche Fragen der Erzähler bezieht, ist auch aus anderen Erzählungen ersichtlich. Es mag ausreichen, auf die Auseinandersetzungen um priesterliche Rechte hinzuweisen, die sich in Num 12 und 16 widerspiegeln.

In Num 12 benutzt der Elohist eine Erzählung vom Murren Mirjams und Arons gegen Mose wegen seiner »kuschitischen« Frau dazu, um die Bestreitung des Priesterrechts der Nachkommen Moses abzuwehren. Er tritt damit für diejenigen nordisraelitischen Priester ein, die sich von den Eliden in Silo als Nachkommen Moses herleiteten

---

[30] J. Vergote, Joseph en Égypte, 1959.
[31] So mit Recht O. Eißfeldt in: OLZ 55 (1960), 39—45.
[32] Zur Auseinandersetzung über Tradition und Ätiologie vgl. J. Bright, Early Israel in Recent History Writing, 1956, 91—100; M. Noth, Der Beitrag der Archäologie zur Geschichte Israels, VTSuppl VII, 1960, 262—282 (bes. 278ff.); S. Mowinckel, Tetrateuch—Pentateuch—Hexateuch, 1964, 78—86; E. Sellin—G. Fohrer a. a. O. 100f.

und denen die als Nachkommen Arons geltenden Zadokiden des Jerusalemer Tempels gegenüberstanden. In dem priesterschriftlichen Anteil an Num 16 bestreitet der Laie Korach das alleinige Priestertum Arons, für das die Priesterschrift sich einsetzt, während eine jüngere Bearbeitung, nach der der Levit Korach priesterliche Rechte für sich in Anspruch nimmt, sich gegen den Widerstand der nachexilischen Leviten wendet, die ihre Einstufung als niedere Tempeldiener wenigstens zeitweilig nicht hinzunehmen gewillt waren[33].

Daß schließlich sogar die Quellenschichten als ganze die Tradition im Blick auf ihre zeitgenössischen Verhältnisse interpretieren, lassen die jüngeren Darstellungen des Deuteronomiums und der Priesterschrift wohl am deutlichsten erkennen. Mit Recht ist darauf hingewiesen worden, daß das Deuteronomium ältere kultgesetzliche Materialien homiletisch interpretiert und paränetisch darbietet[34]. Auch wenn man bezweifelt, daß der Aufbau des Buches unter dem Zwang der kultischen Form eines postulierten Bundeserneuerungsfestes steht, ist nicht zu verkennen, daß z. B. das Gebot 14 22 in v. 23. 27 und v. 24-26 und das Gebot 15 19 in v. 20-23 von der neuen Forderung der Kultuszentralisation aus interpretiert werden. Es ist nicht zu verkennen, daß die politisch-militärischen Bestimmungen nach dem Versagen des Königtums ein neues Verständnis unter Verwertung der prophetischen Kritik anstreben, nach der Zerschlagung des Berufsheeres die frühere Einrichtung des milizartigen Heerbanns erneuern wollen und das am Jerusalemer Tempel eingesetzte oberste Gericht nach der Zersetzung der örtlichen Rechtsgemeinde die Verpflichtung gegenüber dem im göttlichen Willen gegründeten Recht in neuer Weise wahrnehmen soll. Gleicherweise sieht sich die Priesterschrift einem völlig anderen Israel als demjenigen der Frühzeit, aber auch des deuteronomischen Gesetzes gegenüber. Für dieses Israel entwirft sie programmatisch eine Lebensordnung unter Verwendung älterer Gesetze, Kultordnungen und Sammlungen priesterlichen Berufswissens[35], wobei gerade die gesetzlichen Abschnitte mehrfach bearbeitet und auf den neuesten Stand gebracht worden sind. Zugleich wird die Geschichte, aus der das Gesetz abgeleitet worden ist[36], durch einen abgestuften Übergang von der

---

[33] Dagegen betont die letzte Behandlung des Abschnitts durch G. Hort, The Death of Qorah, ABR 7 (1959), 2—26, sehr stark die historische Glaubwürdigkeit der Erzählung.

[34] F. Horst, Das Privilegrecht Jahwes, 1930 (= Gottes Recht, 1961, 17—154); G. von Rad, Deuteronomium-Studien, 1947.

[35] Vgl. R. Rendtorff, Die Gesetze in der Priesterschrift, 1954; K. Koch, Die Priesterschrift von Exodus 25 bis Leviticus 16, 1959.

[36] Die enge Verbindung von Geschichte und Gesetz in der Verknüpfung von Periodenschema und Sinaigesetzgebung spricht gegen die Annahme, daß P ein ursprünglich reines Erzählungswerk mit nachträglich eingeschalteten Gesetzen sei; so M. Noth,

Geschichte des Kosmos zu derjenigen Israels und durch die Gliederung in vier, der allmählichen Offenbarung Jahwes angepaßte Perioden (Schöpfung-Noah-Abraham-Mose) neu interpretiert.

Darüber hinaus ist auch die Entstehung der älteren Hexateuchschichten unter anderem ein Problem der ständig neuen Interpretation der Überlieferungen Israels. Man hat versucht, sie teils aus einem kultisch verwurzelten Bekenntnis (Dtn 26 5-9, vgl. 6 21-23 Jos 24) als Keimzelle und Leitfaden, teils — soweit es die darin nicht einbezogene Sinaitradition betrifft — aus der Feier eines Bundeserneuerungsfestes herzuleiten[37], oder zerlegt das Kernelement in mehrere große, voneinander zu trennende Themen[38]. Neuerdings ist auf Ex 19 3b-8 hingewiesen worden[39]. Aber es ist doch fraglich, ob die genannten Texte auf kultische Begehungen und bestimmte Feste schließen lassen und ob sie als Keimzelle für das Werden der Hexateuchüberlieferung betrachtet werden dürfen.

Es ist zwar beliebt, immer neue israelitische Feste zu postulieren, von denen die Überlieferung nichts weiß, oder wenigstens die erkennbaren Feste mit einer Fülle von Traditionen zu verbinden, deren während der Festtage schon aus zeitlichen Gründen gar nicht alle gedacht worden sein kann. Aber einem solchen Bemühen stehen, besonders wenn es zur Methode entartet, grundsätzliche Bedenken entgegen. Sobald man denn auch derartigen postulierten Festen genauer nachgeht, ergeben sich mannigfache Schwierigkeiten[40]. Sie zeigen, daß nicht jeder Text, der von einem Geschehen berichtet, damit ein ursprünglich kultisches Geschehen meint, und nicht jeder Text, der formularartigen Charakter hat, eine Festagende überliefert.

Ferner können Dtn 26 5-9 und verwandte Texte kaum als Keimzelle der Hexateuchüberlieferung betrachtet werden. Sie sind literarisch und überlieferungsgeschichtlich vielmehr so jung, daß in ihnen eher eine nachträgliche konzentrierende Zusammenfassung vorliegt, die in Dtn 26 5-9 mit dem Anfangs- und Endpunkt des früheren Heilshandelns Jahwes an Israel das Ganze umspannt. Wie darin die Brücke von der Rettung aus Ägypten zur Landnahme unter stillschweigendem Einschluß alles dessen, was dazwischen liegt, geschlagen wird, so in Ex 19 3-6 von der Rettung bis zur Verpflichtung am Gottesberg. Stets handelt es sich um eine konzentrierende Interpretation[41].

Überlieferungsgeschichtliche Studien I, 1957², 180—217; K. Elliger, Sinn und Ursprung der priesterlichen Geschichtserzählung, ZThK 49 (1952), 121—143 (= Kleine Schriften zum Alten Testament, 1966, 174—198).

[37] G. von Rad, Das formgeschichtliche Problem des Hexateuch, 1938 (= Gesammelte Studien zum Alten Testament, 1958, 9—86).

[38] M. Noth, Überlieferungsgeschichte des Pentateuch, 1948.

[39] H. Wildberger, Jahwes Eigentumsvolk, 1960.

[40] Vgl. E. Kutsch in RGG³, II 914—916.

[41] C. H. W. Brekelmans, Het »historische Credo« van Israël, Tijdschrift voor Theologie 3 (1963), 1—10; A. S. van der Woude, Uittocht en Sinaï, 1961; L. Rost, Das kleine geschichtliche Credo und andere Studien zum Alten Testament, 1965, 11—25; W. Richter, Beobachtungen zur theologischen Systembildung in der alttestament-

Demgegenüber läßt sich von der Doppelheit von Tradition und Interpretation aus die Hexateuchüberlieferung, wie sie in den älteren Quellenschichten gesammelt und bearbeitet worden ist, auf drei Traditionsreihen zurückführen, die ursprünglich selbständig und voneinander unabhängig waren. Die erste Reihe ging von den Väterüberlieferungen aus, die — wie die mesopotamischen Elemente aus verschiedenen Jahrhunderten zeigen — teilweise in vorpalästinischer Zeit entstanden und sekundär nach Palästina verpflanzt worden sind, um die Ansprüche der einzelnen israelitischen Gruppen nach ihrer Landnahme zu begründen und zu rechtfertigen. Ihr Kern sind die Verheißungen der Vermehrung und des Landbesitzes, deretwegen sie in Palästina benutzt werden konnten. Dort schildern sie die Patriarchen in verschiedenartigen Stadien im Verhältnis zum Kulturland — von der flüchtigen Berührung bis zur Seßhaftigkeit und im Jakob-Esau-Laban-Kreis mit dem Anspruch auf ostjordanisches Gebiet — und in Beziehungen zu den Heiligtümern, die die Israeliten übernommen hatten. Die zweite Reihe enthielt die Traditionen der Moseschar, d. h. der einmal nach Ägypten verschlagenen Israeliten, und ihres Weges von Ägypten über den Gottesberg und durch die Wüste bis zum Eintreffen an der Grenze des westjordanischen Kulturlandes. Die dritte Reihe bildeten die Erzählungen von der Landnahme der israelitischen Stämme im Westjordanland unter der Führung Josuas. Alle Reihen sind miteinander verknüpft worden — einerseits durch die Joseph-Novelle, die von Palästina nach Ägypten hinüberleitet, und andererseits durch die Einführung Josuas in den Pentateuch, wobei Josua aus einem Stammesführer in Palästina zum Nachfolger Moses wurde.

Ebenso ist in den folgenden erzählenden Büchern zu beobachten, daß die Tradition immer wieder interpretiert worden ist. Durch den deuteronomischen Rahmen des Richterbuchs erscheinen die Helden und Führer einzelner Stämme als die Retter des ganzen Volkes, so daß sich aus der künstlichen Aneinanderreihung der einzelnen Episoden der Anschein einer fortlaufenden Darstellung der Geschichte Israels ergibt. Die Erzählung in Jdc 19—21, die ursprünglich vom Sich-Lossagen Benjamins von Ephraim und von seiner Verselbständigung gehandelt hatte, ist ebenfalls gesamtisraelitisch interpretiert worden, während die Kultlegende des Heiligtums von Dan in Jdc 17—18 vom jerusalemischen Standpunkt aus so überarbeitet worden ist, daß sie die unrühmlichen Umstände der Entstehung des Heiligtums spöttisch darstellt und es verächtlich macht. Auffällig ist die verschiedenartige Wertung Davids, d. h. die Interpretation seiner ge-

---

lichen Literatur anhand des »kleinen geschichtlichen Credo«, in: Schmaus-Festschrift, 1967, 175—212.

schichtlichen Gestalt. Die Erzählungen von seinem Aufstieg in I Sam 16—II Sam 5* 8* schildern den trotz aller unverdienten Anfeindungen stets edlen und untadligen Helden. Dagegen spielt er in der Thronfolgegeschichte II Sam 9—20 I Reg 1—2 eher eine ungünstige, wenig beachtenswerte und nicht gerade rühmliche Rolle. In den deuteronomistischen Bemerkungen der Königsbücher erscheint er wiederum als das Idealbild des gottesfürchtigen und gehorsamen Herrschers (I Reg 11 33. 38), der als Maßstab zur Beurteilung der anderen Könige dienen kann (I Reg 9 4 II Reg 18 3 22 2). In dieser Behandlung der nachdavidischen Königsgeschichte unter deuteronomistischem Vorzeichen tritt der interpretierende Charakter der Darstellung ganz deutlich zutage: in den Maßstäben, nach denen der Verfasser in den Rahmenformeln die Könige bewertet, in der Auswahl, die er aus den zur Verfügung stehenden Quellen trifft[42], und in der Reflexion über den Untergang des Nordreichs (II Reg 17 7-23).

Im Anschluß daran mag gleich auf die Psalmen hingewiesen werden, die gegenüber den erzählenden Büchern keine wesentlich neuen Gesichtspunkte erbringen. Wir beobachten wie dort die interpretierende Übernahme fremder Traditionen (z. B. Ps 19 2-7 29 68 104) und ausgesprochen mythischer Motive (z. B. in Ps 46 48) und ebenso die deutende Geschichtsbetrachtung mit jeweils eigener Akzentsetzung (z. B. Ps 78 105 106 136). Vermutlich bestehen ferner gewisse Zusammenhänge mit der nachexilischen eschatologischen Prophetie. Wie die Zionslieder in Jes 2 2-4 17 12-14 und verwandten Prophetenworten aufgenommen und interpretierend weitergebildet werden, um die Schau des endzeitlichen Heils ausmalen zu helfen, so sind die Jahwes königliche Herrschaft preisenden Psalmen am ehesten als kultische Interpretationen des deuterojesajanischen Monotheismus zu verstehen. Am wichtigsten aber ist die Möglichkeit, aus den in den Psalmen interpretierten Traditionen, soweit sie sich erfassen und mit einiger Sicherheit datieren lassen, Rückschlüsse auf die Entstehungszeit dieser Psalmen zu ziehen. Die Doppelheit von Tradition und Interpretation gibt dazu ein bisher wenig genutztes Mittel an die Hand.

Von den gemachten Beobachtungen aus fällt einiges Licht auf die heutige Auseinandersetzung über den Wert und Sinn der alttestamentlichen Geschichtsbetrachtung, in der entweder die Gültigkeit der historischen Fakten oder das der Darstellung zu entnehmende Kerygma betont wird. Für die alttestamentlichen Erzähler bestand dieser Gegensatz nicht, sondern bildeten Faktum und Deutung eine Einheit, so daß sie nach ihrer Absicht nicht gegeneinander ausgespielt werden dürften. Sie haben Traditionen benutzt, die nach ihrer Meinung

---

[42] Zur Vor-, Überlieferungs- und Bearbeitungsgeschichte eines Erzählungskomplexes vgl. G. Fohrer, Elia, 1968².

»geschichtlich« waren, und sie nach ihrem jeweiligen Verständnis interpretiert. Allerdings galten die Traditionen nicht in solchem Maße als »historisch« fixiert, daß sie nicht auf verschiedene Personen und Umstände anwendbar gewesen wären. Und sie waren nicht so vergangenheitlich bestimmt, daß die Erzähler sie nicht zur Erläuterung von Fragen ihrer eigenen Gegenwart hätten heranziehen können. »Geschichtliche« Überlieferungen erzählen von etwas, das als typisch betrachtet und daher immer wieder neu verwertet werden kann, wenn es wünschenswert scheint. Dies hängt mit dem Denken und Vorstellen des Israeliten zusammen, der die Geschichte unter dem Gesichtspunkt der Wiederholbarkeit versteht und an Stelle einer theoretischen oder allgemeingültigen Darlegung zum Mittel konkreter und als zeitliches Geschehen sich abspielender Erzählungen greifen muß. Daher bleibt im Einzelfall zu untersuchen, ob und wie weit die dazu verwendete Tradition sich an historische Tatsachen anschließt oder historische Erinnerungen enthält. So gewiß dies in vielen Fällen offensichtlich ist, ist auch manche Tradition für unseren Geschichtsbegriff ungeschichtlich; dann bleibt ihre Interpretation als wesentlich und für das Wollen des Erzählers maßgeblich übrig. Man darf aber keinen dieser Gesichtspunkte verallgemeinern, will man nicht Gegebenheiten übersehen, die für den anderen Standpunkt sprechen.

V.

In den zur Weisheitsliteratur im weiteren Sinn gehörigen Büchern läßt sich die Doppelheit von Tradition und Interpretation in einer für diese Literatur charakteristischen Eigenart erkennen. Der Weisheitslehre[43] liegt ein zunächst gemeinorientalisches Ideal der Bildung und Formung des ganzen Menschen zugrunde. Wie in Ägypten das angestrebte Ideal der »Schweigende« oder der »rechte Schweiger«, sein Gegenbild aber der »Heiße«, der seinen Begierden unterlegene, unbeherrschte Mensch ist[44], so in Israel der »Kaltblütige« (Prov 17 27) im Gegensatz zum »Hitzkopf« (Prov 15 18 usw.), der »Langmütige« im Gegensatz zum »Jähzornigen« (Prov 14 29), der Mensch mit »gelassenem Sinn«, der der verzehrenden Leidenschaft nicht nachgibt, sondern seine Affekte und Triebe beherrscht (Prov 14 30). Von da aus ist es nicht verwunderlich, daß die israelitische Weisheitslehre von den Traditionen der altorientalischen Weisheit zunächst stark beeinflußt,

---

[43] Vgl. A. Alt, Die Weisheit Salomos, ThLZ 76 (1951), 139—144 (= Kleine Schriften zur Geschichte des Volkes Israel, II 1953, 90—99); K. Galling, Die Krise der Aufklärung in Israel, 1952, 5—10; M. Noth, Die Bewährung von Salomos »Göttlicher Weisheit«, VTSuppl III, 1955, 225—237.

[44] Vgl. besonders H. Brunner, Die Weisheitsliteratur, in: HdO I 2, 1952, 93—96; H. Gese, Lehre und Wirklichkeit in der alten Weisheit, 1958, 11—21.

wenn nicht abhängig war. Die Übernahme solcher Traditionen reicht bis in die alttestamentlichen Texte hinein.

Wie Prov 22 17—23 11 Exzerpte aus der ägyptischen Lehre des Amen-em-ope darstellen[45] und 23 14 f. aus der Lehre des Achiqar entlehnt ist, so müssen wohl auch die »Worte Agurs, des Sohnes Jakes, 'des Massaiten'[46]« in Prov 30 1-14 und die »Worte Lemuels, des Königs von Massa« in Prov 31 1-9 von Angehörigen eines nichtisraelitischen Stammes hergeleitet werden[47].

Bald aber hat die israelitisch-jahwistische Interpretation der Weisheitslehre eingesetzt und diese schließlich völlig durchdrungen. Einmal wurde die Weisheit nationalisiert und in das israelitische Volkstum eingefügt. Das bedeutete einerseits, daß sich die Bindung an einen einzelnen Stand — das Beamtentum — lockerte und löste und die Lehre sich an das allgemein Menschliche jenseits der sozialen und soziologischen Grenzen wandte; ein Zeichen dafür ist die Aufnahme zahlreicher volkstümlicher Sprichwörter in die Proverbia-Sammlungen. Andererseits wurde die Weisheit bis in die Einzelheiten der Lage in Palästina angepaßt; so folgt das der Gottesrede im Hiobbuch vermutlich zugrunde liegende Onomastikon nicht dem ägyptischen Schema, sondern ist von Weltbild, landschaftlichen, klimatischen und zoologischen Besonderheiten Palästinas bestimmt.

Ferner wurde die interreligiöse Weisheitslehre dem Jahweglauben angepaßt und zugeordnet. Daraus erklärt sich die große Rolle, die gegenüber der bloßen Weltklugheit die ethische Weisung sowie das ethische oder fromme Verhalten — und zwar in sehr starkem Maße den Forderungen des Jahweglaubens entsprechend — einnehmen. Häufig ist der Jahwename statt der allgemeinen Bezeichnung »Gott, Gottheit« eingeführt und so der Schöpfer- und Weltengott mit Jahwe gleichgesetzt oder die »Jahwefurcht« geradezu als Anfang der Weisheit (Prov 9 10) oder als ihr Ausgangspunkt (Prov 1 7 Ps 111 10) bezeichnet worden.

Schließlich ist in einem letzten großen Interpretationsvorgang der Weisheitsbegriff theologisch durchdacht und ein systematisch-

---

[45] Mehrfach ist umgekehrt die Abhängigkeit Amen-em-ope's von Prov behauptet worden, besonders von W. O. E. Oesterley, The »Teaching of Amen-em-ope« and the Old Testament, ZAW 45 (1927), 9—24; R. O. Kevin, The Wisdom of Amen em-apt and its Possible Dependence upon the Hebrew Book of Proverbs, JSOR 14 (1930), 115—157; E. Drioton, Sur la Sagesse d'Aménémopé, in: Mélanges bibliques A. Robert, 1957, 254—280; Le livre des Proverbes et la Sagesse d'Aménémopé, in: Sacra Pagina, I 1959, 229—241. Doch ist diese Annahme unwahrscheinlich, vgl. zuletzt P. Montet, L'Égypte et la Bible, 1959, 111—128; B. Couroyer, L'origine égyptienne de la Sagesse d'Amenemopé, RB 70 (1963), 208—224.

[46] Es ist הַמַּשָּׂא statt »der Ausspruch« zu lesen.

[47] S. u. Die Weisheit im Alten Testament, Anm. 45.

theologisches Lehrganzes hergestellt worden, in dem das Wort *ḥåkmā* die Bedeutung »schulmäßige Lehrweisheit« annimmt (so in der Kritik daran in Koh 2 12f. 14. 16. 21 8 17 usw.)[48]. Außer in Prov 1—9 und Hi 28 findet sich dies teilweise in der inspirierten Weisheit Elihus, der sich durch offenbarende Erleuchtung in ihrem dauernden Besitz weiß[49], aber auch in der Gottesrede des Hiobbuchs, in der die Naturwelt als Schöpfung wenigstens andeutungsweise zu der an den Menschen ergehenden Offenbarung in Beziehung gesetzt wird.

Zweifellos stellt diese Interpretation der Weisheitstraditionen eine bedeutende theologische Leistung dar. Sie erfaßt durch die Einbeziehung von Schöpfung und Offenbarung in das Weisheitsdenken diejenigen Gebiete, die das Klug- und Kundigsein der früheren Bildungs- und Lebensweisheit beiseite gelassen hatte, und schafft ein umfassendes theologisches System[50]. Doch eben dieses System mußte wegen seiner unvermeidlichen Einseitigkeiten und Unzulänglichkeiten fast notwendig die Kritik wachrufen. Sie äußert sich in den Büchern Hiob und Kohelet und ist mit neuen, vom System abweichenden Interpretationen der Tradition verbunden[51].

Obwohl Kohelet der Schulweisheit einen gewissen relativen Wert einräumt (Koh 2 3. 14. 16 4 13 10 12), wendet er sich gegen die Selbstsicherheit, mit der das System das Ganze der Welt und des Lebens zu umgreifen sucht, und weist auf die Grenzen hin, die jede Lebenssicherung ausschließen (Koh 2 15f. 7 26) und es dem Menschen verwehren, mit menschlichen Mitteln zu seiner Eigentlichkeit zu gelangen. Es bleibt nur übrig, den Anteil am Leben, der dem Menschen gewährt wird, auszukosten — und zwar in einer tätigen Existenz (Koh 9 7-10). Der erste Teil dieses Rates Kohelets entspricht genau demjenigen der Götterschenkin im Gilgamesch-Epos, der auch die negative Abgrenzung enthält[52]:

> Gilgamesch, wohin läufst du?
> Das Leben, das du suchst, wirst du nicht finden!
> Als die Götter die Menschheit erschufen,
> teilten den Tod sie der Menschheit zu,

---

[48] G. von Rad, Theologie des Alten Testaments, I 1957, 439.

[49] Vgl. G. Fohrer, Die Weisheit des Elihu (Hi 32—37), AfO 19 (1960), 83—94 (= Studien zum Buche Hiob, 1963, 87—107).

[50] G. von Rad a. a. O. 449.

[51] Wie aus den beiden Büchern hinreichend deutlich wird, entsteht die Kritik nicht dadurch, daß im System der Kontakt mit dem Wirken Jahwes in der Geschichte verlorenzugehen drohte (so G. von Rad a. a. O. 451), sondern entzündet sich an dessen grundlegenden Behauptungen und letztlich am Vorhandensein eines Systems überhaupt.

[52] Tafel X: iii 1—13, zitiert nach der Übersetzung von A. Schott, Das Gilgamesch-Epos, durchges. und ergänzt von W. v. Soden, 1958, 77f.

nahmen das Leben für sich in die Hand.
Du, Gilgamesch — dein Bauch sei voll,
ergötzen magst du dich Tag und Nacht!
Feiere täglich ein Freudenfest!
Tanz und spiel bei Tag und Nacht!
Deine Kleidung sei rein, gewaschen dein Haupt,
mit Wasser sollst du gebadet sein!
Schau den Kleinen an deiner Hand,
die Gattin freu' sich auf deinem Schoß!

Der zweite Teil des Rates Kohelets entspricht dem Trost, den Gilgamesch in seinem großen, dauerhaften Werk findet: der Stadtmauer von Uruk, die er gebaut hat[53] — nur mit dem Unterschied, daß Gilgamesch in der Erkenntnis, daß das Werk bleibt und mehr als der todgeweihte Mensch ist, das Werk als Ergebnis des Tätigseins meint, Kohelet das Tätigsein selbst als tätige Existenz.

So hat Kohelet eine uralte Tradition aufgegriffen und dem System der Schulweisheit entgegengesetzt. Denn dies ist dem Streben Gilgameschs nach Erlangen der Unsterblichkeit gleich, weil es das Einmalige, Bleibende und Endgültige verschaffen soll. Indem Kohelet demgegenüber die beschränkten Möglichkeiten des Menschen aufweist, ist er nicht skeptisch und resigniert an sich, sondern nur im Hinblick auf die Möglichkeiten eines theologischen Systems, das als Allheilmittel betrachtet wird. Tatsächlich bleibt nur die Möglichkeit des Gilgamesch-Epos — aber nun neu interpretiert als von Gott gegebene Möglichkeit, die der Fromme als ihm beschieden aus seiner Hand entgegennimmt (Koh 2 14 f. 3 13 5 17 f.).

Kritik und eigene Lösung des Hiobbuchs unterscheiden sich von Kohelet. Das Buch richtet sich vor allem gegen den Vergeltungsglauben als eine der tragenden Säulen des weisheitlich-theologischen Systems und stellt der (von den Freunden Hiobs) geforderten Unterwerfung unter die theologische Tradition die eigene Erfahrung in der persönlichen Begegnung mit Gott entgegen, die zum Eigentlichen der menschlichen Existenz jenseits des bloßen Lebensvollzugs führt. Diese den großen Einzelpropheten verwandte Grundhaltung findet wie bei diesen ihren Ausdruck in der Neuinterpretation älterer Traditionen. Der Hiobdichter hat nicht nur die alte Hioblegende unter möglichst geringen Änderungen als Rahmenerzählung verwendet[54], sondern ist auch in seiner Dichtung zutiefst und in erster Linie in den Überlieferungen des alttestamentlichen Glaubens und den üblichen Stoffen und Motiven des Alten Testaments verwurzelt, so daß es im ganzen

---

[53] Vgl. Tafel XI, 302—307.
[54] Vgl. G. Fohrer, Zur Vorgeschichte und Komposition des Buches Hiob, VT 6 (1956), 249—267 (= Studien zum Buche Hiob, 1963, 26—43).

Buch nur wenige Verse gibt, in denen die Bezugnahme darauf fehlt. Das ist um so beachtenswerter, als man häufig gerade auf die altorientalischen Parallelen oder auf die neuen, gegen die Tradition gerichteten Gedanken des Dichters hingewiesen hat. Natürlich haben allerlei einzelne Redewendungen, Bilder und Motive ihre altorientalischen Parallelen; aber sie sind nicht zahlreicher als im übrigen Alten Testament[55]. Und natürlich richten sich die letzten Gedanken des Dichters gegen die Tradition des Weisheitssystems; aber er spricht dies mittels uminterpretierter traditioneller Vorstellungen aus, die vornehmlich aus den Bereichen der Weisheitslehre, der Psalmen und des Rechtslebens stammen[56] und daneben der Wissenschaft und Bildung der Zeit und Umgebung des Dichters entnommen sind. Wie er also in Berührung mit der altorientalischen Dichtung stand, den Plan für das eigene Werk aber ohne Vorbilder entwerfen mußte, so war er zwar mit den herkömmlichen alttestamentlichen Traditionen verbunden, mußte aber in der Erschütterung des systemgebundenen Glaubens seiner Zeit einen eigenen Weg zu tragfähigeren Grundlagen suchen, und benutzte zwar das ihm bekannte rationale Wissen und Bildungsgut, benötigte es aber zum Ausdruck von Zusammenhängen, in denen es um den Einbruch des Irrationalen und um Lebensstatt um Denkfragen geht. So dient ihm das Ineinander von Tradition

---

[55] Dagegen ist an ein altorientalisches Vorbild für das Ganze der Rahmenerzählung oder der Dichtung schwerlich zu denken. Zwar haben die von H. Gese a. a. O. 51—69 als Beleg dafür angeführten Texte — *Ludlul bēl nēmeqi*, AO 4462, STVC 1 + 2 (mit Ergänzungen), zu denen noch PBS I² 135 hinzuzurechnen ist — einiges miteinander und mit der Hiobdichtung gemeinsam. Doch sind ihre Unterschiede untereinander zu beträchtlich, als daß man sie einer Gattung des »Klageerhörungsparadigmas« zuweisen könnte. Sieht man von dem fragmentarischen 4. Text ab, so sind der 1. und 3. Text Monologe und Dankgebete mit ausführlicher Schilderung der einstigen Not, der 2. Text dagegen ist ein Dialog und eine Klage mit zusagendem Gottesspruch. Demgemäß sind alle Texte formgeschichtlich mit den Psalmen, nicht aber mit dem Hiobbuch vergleichbar. Auch inhaltlich berühren sie sich mit diesem nicht sonderlich eng, jedenfalls nicht enger als wiederum mit denjenigen Psalmen, die das Geschick des unschuldig Leidenden behandeln. Entgegen dem Hiobbuch enthält der 3. Text gerade ein Sündenbekenntnis des Beters, und zumindest der 2. und 3. Text schreiben ihm das Verhalten zu, das die Freunde Hiobs aufgrund ihres theologischen Systems im ersten Redegang empfehlen und das Hiob (und in seiner Gestalt der Hiobdichter) gerade ablehnt. Vorbereitet fand der Hiobdichter nur die Dialogform mit Rahmenerzählung und die Behandlung des Problems des ungerechten Menschenschicksals oder der ungerechten Weltordnung.

[56] Neuerdings hat auf die Psalmentraditionen C. Westermann, Der Aufbau des Buches Hiob, 1956, und auf die Rechtstraditionen H. Richter, Studien zu Hiob, 1959, hingewiesen. Die Grenze dieser Untersuchungen, die manche wertvollen Ergebnisse erbracht haben, liegt darin, daß sie jeweils nur einen der drei hauptsächlichen Traditionsbereiche berücksichtigen.

und Interpretation zur Erhellung der letzten Fragen menschlicher Existenz[57].

VI.

Anders als in den erzählenden Büchern sind in den Prophetenbüchern die verwendeten Traditionen nicht unter mehrfachen Interpretationen verborgen, sondern meist so gut erkennbar und bekannt, daß man von ihnen ausgehen und ihre prophetische Neuinterpretation beobachten kann. Um so erstaunlicher ist es, daß die ältere Forschung dies wenig berücksichtigt und die Eigenart der prophetischen Botschaft im ethischen Monotheismus erblickt hat. Damit hat sie zwar erkannt, daß sich eine grundlegende Änderung vollzogen hat, sie aber auf einem falschen Gebiet gesucht. Dagegen gliedern heute zwei andere Auffassungen die Prophetie in bestimmte Traditionen ein. Unterscheiden sie sich darin von der älteren Forschung, so gehen sie wiederum in der Bestimmung der für die Prophetie maßgeblichen Traditionen auseinander. Die eine Auffassung bezieht alle Propheten des Alten Testaments im Rahmen des »cultic pattern« in die altorientalische Kultprophetie ein, die andere versteht sie völlig als Träger altisraelitischer Traditionen, deren Institutionen und Rechtssätze aktualisiert und radikalisiert werden. Von beiden Auffassungen wird jedoch übersehen, daß Traditionen nicht nur aufgenommen, sondern gleichzeitig auch neu interpretiert werden, und daß sogar neue Einsichten, die unabhängig von der oder gegen die Tradition gewonnen worden sind, mittels uminterpretierter traditioneller Vorstellungen ausgedrückt werden. Beachtet man nicht, daß außer der verwendeten Tradition auch die Art ihrer Interpretation berücksichtigt werden muß, so läuft man Gefahr, die Eigenart der prophetischen Verkündigung zu verkennen.

Zweifellos haben — ganz abgesehen von den ohnehin im Bereich der Kultfrömmigkeit lebenden Kultpropheten — die großen Einzelpropheten mancherlei altorientalische und vor allem israelitisch-alttestamentliche Traditionen übernommen, wie sie sich auch der Formen der herkömmlichen prophetischen Verkündigung bedient haben. Mittels welcher Formen und Redemotive hätten sie sich sonst ausdrücken sollen? Selbst wenn der Prophet etwas Neues und Anderes als die bisherige Tradition zu sagen hat, ist er doch nicht dem chassidischen Rabbi Abraham »dem Engel«, dem Sohn des großen Maggid, vergleichbar, der dem Vatererbe entsagte[58]:

---

[57] Wie Koh 12 12-14 die Kritik und den eigenen Rat Kohelets kritisieren, so die Elihureden das Werk des Hiobdichters. Ihr Verfasser wendet sich sowohl gegen den häretischen Hiob und die Freunde, die der Dichter das Lehrsystem nicht zureichend vertreten läßt, als auch in feinerer Form gegen die Gottesrede.

[58] M. Buber, Die Erzählungen der Chassidim, 1949, 215.

»Nach dem Tod erschien der Maggid seinem Sohn und befahl ihm unter dem Gebot der Elternehrung, von seinem Weg der reinen Abgeschiedenheit zu lassen; denn wer ihn gehe, sei in Gefahr. Abraham antwortete: »Ich kenne keinen Vater nach dem Fleisch, nur den einen erbarmenden Vater alles Lebendigen.« »Daß du mein Erbe annahmst«, sprach der Maggid, »damit hast du mich auch nach meinem Abscheiden als Vater anerkannt«. »Ich entsage dem Vatererbe«, rief der Engel. Im gleichen Augenblick brach im Hause ein Brand aus, der die geringe Hinterlassenschaft des Maggids an seinen Sohn, und sie allein, verzehrte.«

Die Propheten haben dem Vatererbe zwar nicht entsagt, sondern es einerseits übernommen und verwendet. So ist denn mit Recht, obschon manchmal zu einseitig und mißverständlich, von verschiedenen Seiten her allerlei Material über die Traditionsbestimmtheit der Propheten zusammengetragen und in all seiner Vielfalt ausgebreitet worden[59]. Es ist so umfassend, daß in diesem Zusammenhang nicht einmal ein Auszug daraus wiedergegeben werden kann. Aber andererseits haben die Propheten diese übernommenen Traditionen nicht etwa nur rezitiert, aktualisiert, radikalisiert oder wie immer man eine Verwendung ohne gleichzeitige Umwandlung nennen mag, sondern haben sie gleichzeitig um- und neuinterpretiert, um ihre dem Vatererbe durchaus nicht immer entsprechenden Gedanken auf diese Weise auszudrücken. Ich möchte das Problem an Jes 1 16 b-17 erläutern:

> Hört auf, Böses zu tun,
>   lernt, Gutes zu tun!
> Trachtet nach Recht,
>   leitet 'den Unterdrückten',
> schafft der Waise Recht,
>   führt den Rechtsstreit der Witwe!

---

[59] Vgl. u. a. P. Humbert, Problèmes du livre d'Habacuc, 1944; H. A. Brongers, De scheppingstradities bij de profeten, 1945; A. Haldar, Studies in the Book of Nahum, 1947; A. Peter, Das Echo von Paradieserzählung und Paradiesmythen im Alten Testament unter besonderer Berücksichtigung der prophetischen Endzeitschilderungen, Diss. Würzburg 1947; G. von Rad, Die Stadt auf dem Berge, EvTh 8 (1948/9), 439—447 (= Gesammelte Studien zum Alten Testament, 1958, 214—224); H. F. D. Sparks, The Witness of the Prophets to Hebrew Tradition, ThSt 50 (1949), 129—141; A. Bentzen, The ritual Background of Amos I, 2—II, 16, in: OTSt VIII, 1950, 85—99; G. H. Davies, The Yahwistic Tradition in the Eight-Century Prophets, in: Studies in Old Testament Prophecy, 1950, 37—51; E. Würthwein, Amos-Studien, ZAW 62 (1950), 10—52; R. Bach, Die Erwählung Israels in der Wüste, Diss. Bonn 1952; K. Koch, Zur Geschichte der Erwählungsvorstellung in Israel, ZAW 67 (1955), 205—226; B. J. van der Merwe, Pentateuchtradisies in die prediking van Deuterojesaja, 1955; H. Schmid, Jahwe und die Kulttraditionen von Jerusalem, ZAW 67 (1955), 168—197; E. Rohland, Die Bedeutung der Erwählungstraditionen Israels für die Eschatologie der alttestamentlichen Propheten, Diss. Heidelberg 1956; H. W. Wolff, Hoseas geistige Heimat, ThLZ 81 (1956), 83—94; H.-J. Kraus, Die

Es ist nicht zu bestreiten, daß nicht erst die Propheten solche Rechtshilfe für die Witwen, Waisen und Unterdrückten gefordert haben. Sie wird sowohl im Epilog von Hammurabis Gesetz[60] als auch in ugaritischen Texten als Aufgabe des Königs angeführt[61]. So sind die entsprechenden einzelnen Weisungen Jesajas und anderer Propheten religionsgeschichtlich und soziologisch nichts Neues. Neu und einzigartig aber ist ihre Interpretation der altorientalischen Sozialtradition: Sie beziehen sie nicht nur auf den König, sondern auf jeden einzelnen Israeliten und Menschen überhaupt und rücken sie eindringlich und nachdrücklich in den Mittelpunkt der Einzelforderungen, um auf diese Weise die liebende Grundhaltung des Menschen zu beschreiben. Diese Grundhaltung gilt allein und ausschließlich als das dem Willen Gottes und seinem Verhältnis zu Israel entsprechende Verhalten, neben dem der Kultus zurücktreten muß.

Wie gegenüber der altorientalischen Tradition ist die prophetische Eigenart gegenüber der israelitischen Tradition zu erkennen, die das Gebot der Rechtshilfe für die Schwachen gleichfalls kennt (vgl. Ex 22 20-23 Dtn 10 18 24 17 27 19 u. ö. Ps 68 6 72 2. 4. 12-14 82 3 f. 146 9). Dafür ist zu beachten, daß Jesaja an die Spitze die Grundforderung stellt: Gutes tun, statt Böses tun. Die dann folgenden Einzelanweisungen erläutern dies und bilden nichts anderes als beispielhafte, konkrete Anwendungen der zusammenfassenden Grundforderung. Damit erfolgt ein wichtiger Schritt: An die Spitze und geradezu an die Stelle der Vielfalt der alten Rechtssätze, die zu bloßen Einzelbeispielen werden, tritt als ihre prophetische Interpretation die Konzentration des Gotteswillens in der einen grundlegenden Forderung »Gutes tun«, die damit zugleich dem Bereich des Rechts und des Gesetzes entnommen wird[62].

Die Neuinterpretation des herkömmlichen Glaubens, der sich der Prophet selber unterziehen muß, wird am Berufungsbericht Jesajas deutlich. Als er seinen Auftrag erhalten hat, fragt er: »Wie lange,

---

prophetische Verkündigung des Rechts in Israel, 1957; W. Beyerlin, Die Kulttraditionen Israels in der Verkündigung des Propheten Micha, 1959; M. Sekine, Davidsbund und Sinaibund bei Jeremia, VT 9 (1959), 47—57; R. Vuilleumier, La tradition cultuelle d'Israël dans la prophétie d'Amos et d'Osée, 1960.

[60] Rev. xxiv 60f.
[61] I Aqht i 23—25; II Aqht v 7f.; 127 (II K vi), 33f. 45—47.
[62] Die Auffassung von R. Hentschke, Gesetz und Eschatologie in der Verkündigung der Propheten, ZEE 1960, 46—56, daß die Propheten den Heilscharakter des Gesetzes weder bestritten noch angezweifelt, vielmehr den Glauben der Kultfrömmigkeit an seine lebenbewahrende Wirkung geteilt hätten, läßt sich aus diesen und anderen Stellen nicht belegen; die Auffassung, daß man bei ihnen vergeblich nach einer ähnlichen Überbietung oder Radikalisierung der alten Gebote wie in der Verkündigung Jesu suche, erweist sich an Jes 1 16b-17 als irrig.

Herr?« (6 11). Denn wie jeder Mensch ist er bestrebt, das neue Erleben in sein bisheriges Glauben und Denken einzuordnen. Dieses aber ist für den Israeliten durch die feste Erwartung bestimmt, daß Jahwe letztlich das Heil und nicht den Untergang Israels will. Daher ist es für Jesaja unvorstellbar, daß Verhärtung und Gericht den ganzen und ständigen Inhalt seines Auftrags bilden könnten. Jedoch die göttliche Antwort enthält ein entschiedenes Nein zu seiner Erwartung und verhängt die völlige Vernichtung. Sie stürzt die herkömmlichen Glaubenserwartungen Jesajas um, so daß er sie aufgeben und Neuland betreten muß[63].

Die auf solche Weise eingeleitete Wandlung zeigt sich an der Neuinterpretation vieler Ausdrücke und Begriffe in der prophetischen Verkündigung[64]. Auf die veränderte Auffassung des Tages Jahwes bei Amos und Jesaja wurde bereits hingewiesen. Amos wandelt ferner den Erwählungsglauben ironisch ab: Er kann sich nicht auf die Rettung aus Ägypten gründen, weil Jahwe auch die »Erbfeinde« Israels — Philister und Aramäer — geführt hat (Am 9 7). Daß Jahwe Israel »erkannt« hat, begründet höchstens, daß er seine Sünden an ihm heimsucht, nicht aber eine bevorzugte Behandlung (Am 3 1f.). Genauso wird der Glaubenssatz, daß die Israeliten Jahwes Söhne seien, neu interpretiert. Während sie sich selber als nach freier Wahl angenommene, adoptierte Kinder Gottes betrachtet hatten, wandelt Hosea dies dahin ab, daß das Kind Israel sich als undankbar erwiesen und gegen seinen Vater vergangen hat (Hos 9 10 11 1ff.). Jesaja verschärft das sogar: Söhne des himmlischen Vaters? Ja, aber schlechter als das Vieh des Vaters, weil sie sich gegen ihn aufgelehnt haben (Jes 1 2f.). Ebenso kehrt Hosea den Ehrentitel Israels »mein (Jahwes) Volk« in der Benennung seines Sohnes in »Nicht-mein-Volk« um (Hos 1 8) und spricht Jesaja nur noch verächtlich von »diesem Volk da«. Während Hos 10 1 und Jes 3 14 unbefangen das Bild des Weinstocks und Weinbergs als Symbol des bäuerlichen Palästina auf Israel anwenden, deutet Jeremia es wieder um: Die Edelrebe hat sich in eine entartete, wilde Rebe verwandelt (Jer 2 21). Und indem Ezechiel von der Frucht des Weinstocks absieht, fällt er über ihn das vernichtende Urteil, daß er nur als Brennholz taugt (Ez 15). In seinem Weinberglied hat Jesaja das Bild des Weinbergs aus der Liebesdichtung genommen, in der es die Braut oder Frau bezeichnet und dem Bild der Ehe ähnlich ist; aber dieser »Weinberg« Israel in seinem Verhältnis zu Gott ist ganz verdorben und muß zerstört werden (Jes 5 1-7). Das Bild der Ehe

---

[63] Vgl. im einzelnen G. Fohrer, Das Buch Jesaja, I 1966², 102; etwas anders E. Jenni, Jesajas Berufung in der neueren Forschung, ThZ 15 (1959), 321—339.
[64] Vgl. auch G. A. F. Knight, A Christian Theology of the Old Testament, 1959, 167—193: »Some Interpretations of Israel by Israel«.

selbst hat seine etwas bedenklichen Ursprünge letztlich in den kanaanäischen Fruchtbarkeitskulten. Wie man dort in der heiligen Hochzeit die Vermählung der Gottheit mit der Erde feierte, so nennt Hos 1 2 als älteste bekannte israelitische Anwendung noch das Land und nicht das Volk als Ehefrau Jahwes. Immerhin interpretieren Hos 1—3 Jes 1 21 Jer 2 2 3 1. 6-25 das Bild der Ehe zwischen Jahwe und Israel nur so, daß sie an ihm den Gegensatz zwischen der unschuldigen Frühzeit und der verderbten Gegenwart des Volkes illustrieren. Dagegen ändert Ezechiel die Deutung im Hinblick auf Jerusalem durch die weitere Tradition vom ausgesetzten und geretteten Kind (Ez 16). Er rechnet Jerusalem zur Welt des Heidentums, so daß die Sünde es von Anfang an bestimmt hat. Alles, was es war und ist, beruht allein auf Jahwes unbegreiflicher Liebe, so daß seine Sünde nicht nur im Abfall, sondern auch im schlimmsten Undank besteht.

Überhaupt ist die prophetische Interpretation der israelitischen Geschichtstraditionen sehr bezeichnend. Hosea versteht den gefeierten Ahnherrn Jakob als das hinterlistige, tückische Urbild des Israel seiner Zeit (Hos 12 3-7) und sieht die Sünde mit der Landnahme in Palästina in vollem Maße beginnen, als der Jahweglaube in eine Baalreligion verfälscht wurde (Hos 9 10 10 1f. 11 1-7 13 5-8). Jesaja gibt in 9 7-20 5 25-29 eine Interpretation verschiedener Stadien der Geschichte des Nordreichs Israel: der Nöte der Philister- und Aramäerkriege, der Ausrottung der Dynastie Omri und der noch schlimmeren Zeit der Dynastie Jehu, des Bürger- und Bruderkriegs während der folgenden revolutionären Unruhen und des schweren Erdbebens, nach dem man wahrscheinlich das Auftreten des Amos datiert hat. Im Gegensatz zur frommen Tradition ist sie keine Heilsgeschichte, sondern Entscheidungsgeschichte für das schuldige Volk. Und da es sich gewöhnlich falsch entscheidet, wird sie nur zu leicht zu einer Geschichte voller Unheil, das die widerspenstigen Sünder zunächst zur Umkehr bewegen soll, schließlich aber vernichtet. Auch Ezechiel interpretiert in 20 4-31a die Geschichte neu, indem er bestimmte Motive auswählt, beiseite läßt oder zusätzlich zur alttestamentlichen Geschichtsbetrachtung einführt. Er will zeigen, daß Israel von Anfang an sündig gewesen ist und schon in Ägypten Götzendienst getrieben hat und daß es trotz der immer härteren Drohungen und Maßnahmen Jahwes bis in die Gegenwart ungehorsam und aufrührerisch geblieben ist. Abgesehen von der fast gleichzeitigen deuteronomischen Beurteilung der Königszeit unterscheidet sich diese Auffassung stark von der älteren Interpretation der Geschichtstraditionen[65].

---

[65] Vgl. im einzelnen G. Fohrer, Prophetie und Geschichte, ThLZ 89 (1964), 481—500 (= Studien zur alttestamentlichen Prophetie [1949—1965], 1967, 265—293). Noch die spätere eschatologische Prophetie hat traditionelle Begriffe und Vorstellungen neu

Wozu dienen der großen Prophetie diese Interpretationen der Tradition? Sie sollen die neue Einsicht des prophetischen Glaubens ausdrücken, der sich in der Beurteilung der Situation des Menschen vor Gott von der außerprophetischen Auffassung wesentlich unterscheidet. Daher gibt es für die Propheten keine Rückkehr zur Tradition, sondern in weiterführender Interpretation der Traditionen des alten Jahweglaubens den Weg in ein neues Verhältnis zu Gott. Die Sünden erlauben es den Israeliten nicht, einfach zu Jahwe zurückzukommen (Hos 5 4); sie können ihre Art ebensowenig ändern wie ein Kuschit seine Hautfarbe oder ein Leopard die Zeichnung seines Fells (Jer 13 23). Wenn sie nicht im Gericht untergehen wollen, besteht die einzige Möglichkeit der Rettung darin, daß sie durch die Traditionen hindurch und über die Traditionen hinweg, die ihre Sünde nicht verhindert oder sie — wie die kultischen Traditionen — sogar herbeigeführt haben, den Weg in ein neues Dasein gehen. Der Umwandlung der Traditionen entspricht die völlige innere und äußere Wandlung des sündigen Menschen, die sich entweder durch eine radikale Umkehr oder durch die von Gott gewirkte Erlösung vollzieht. Und ebenso drückt die prophetische Interpretation der Tradition die theologische Wandlung aus, die sich in der prophetischen Verkündigung ereignet.

VII.

Die Erkenntnis der Doppelheit von Tradition und Interpretation könnte dazu beitragen, manche Spannungen in der heutigen alttestamentlichen Wissenschaft zu mildern. Sie läßt gegensätzliche Auffassungen, deren eine scheinbar die andere ausschließt, als zwei Aspekte eines einzigen Sachverhalts erkennen. Das gilt ebenso für den Streit um Wert und Sinn der alttestamentlichen Geschichtsbetrachtung (Fakten oder Kerygma) wie für die Frage des Verhältnisses zu den altorientalischen Traditionen und für diejenige der Eingliederung der Propheten in altorientalische oder israelitische Institutionen und Überlieferungen.

---

interpretiert, so diejenigen vom »Rest« und vom »Feind aus dem Norden«; vgl. dazu besonders B. S. Childs, The Enemy from the North and the Chaos Tradition, JBL 78 (1959), 187—198; doch wird man aus der richtig beobachteten Verwendung von ursprünglich mythischen Motiven schwerlich den Schluß ziehen dürfen, daß geschichtliche Traditionen »mythologisiert« würden. Die eschatologische Prophetie hat außer der erhofften Zukunft auch die Vergangenheit mittels der häufigen Entsprechungsmotive interpretiert, aufgrund deren man gern, aber nicht ganz zutreffend die »Endzeit« der »Urzeit« gleichsetzt; vgl. dazu im einzelnen G. Fohrer, Die Struktur der alttestamentlichen Eschatologie, ThLZ 85 (1960), 415—418 (= Studien zur alttestamentlichen Prophetie [1949—1965], 1967, 32—58).

Im weiteren Sinn rechtfertigt jene Doppelheit die Arbeit des Exegeten und Theologen — einmal in der sachgemäßen historisch-kritischen Interpretation der alttestamentlichen Texte mit dem Ziel, möglichst genau das zu erfassen, was sie meinen. Und ferner in der theologischen Interpretation alles dessen im Zusammenhang unseres heutigen Wahrheitsbewußtseins und Wirklichkeitsverständnisses, da wir vor einer Aufgabe des Übersetzens und Interpretierens stehen, die nichts einfach als selbstverständlich und eines neuen Nachdenkens nicht bedürftig hinnimmt. Die Interpretation der Tradition im Alten Testament, insbesondere bei den großen Propheten, kann uns dafür Wegweiser und Lehrmeister sein.

Altes Testament — »Amphiktyonie« und »Bund«?

Wir sind dessen gewiß, daß wir entgegen anderslautenden Ansichten Gott in der Bibel nicht nur suchen, sondern auch finden. Und daß wir ihn nur dort finden, nicht aber in Natur und Geschichte oder in einer kirchlichen, wissenschaftlichen oder sonstigen Tradition. Darum müssen wir gegenüber derartigen Traditionen, wie hoch oder niedrig wir sie einschätzen, auf die Bibel zurückgreifen. Dieser Grundsatz gilt gleicherweise für wissenschaftliche Hypothesen, die die Aussagen oder Geschichtsdarstellungen der Bibel in einen umfassenden Rahmen zu stellen suchen und ihr Gesamtbild zu bestimmen geeignet scheinen. Dazu gehören die fast schon zur Tradition gewordenen Hypothesen, daß die Israeliten bald nach ihrer Landnahme in Palästina einen sakralen Bund von zwölf Stämmen gebildet haben und daß das Verhältnis Gott-Israel grundlegend und stets durch einen »Bund« geformt worden sei.

Wenn ich »auf die Bibel zurückgreifen« sage, dann ist damit natürlich kein biblizistisches, sondern ein kritisches Verstehen der Bibel, in diesem Falle des Alten Testaments, gemeint. Denn die historisch-kritische, form- und überlieferungsgeschichtliche Untersuchung, wie sie seit Jahrzehnten im Gange ist, schließt eine naive biblizistische Betrachtung ein für allemal aus. Auch die genannten Hypothesen sind ja aus einem kritischen Verstehen erwachsen oder in es einbezogen worden. Daher handelt es sich im folgenden um die kritische Prüfung von Hypothesen aus dem Bereich der kritischen Erforschung des Alten Testaments mitsamt der Geschichte des alten Israel, wie ich anderwärts bereits einen Ausschnitt der Hypothesen über die Moseüberlieferung und die Hypothese vom apodiktisch formulierten Recht überprüft habe[1].

I.

Auf den ersten Blick scheint die Amphiktyonie-Hypothese klar und eindeutig formuliert und überall, wo man sich ihrer bedient, in ziemlich gleichmäßiger Form vertreten zu sein. Bei genauerem Zusehen ist freilich festzustellen, daß wir es in Wirklichkeit mit einer Mehrzahl von Hypothesenformen zu tun haben. Auch wenn wir nicht jede Spielart und jedes Abweichen von einer Grundform berücksichtigen, sind doch wenigstens fünf Formen zu erkennen:

---

[1] G. Fohrer, Überlieferung und Geschichte des Exodus, 1964; Das sogenannte apodiktisch formulierte Recht und der Dekalog (s. u. 120—148).

a) die Annahme einer Amphiktyonie der zwölf Stämme Israels in deren Frühzeit, der sog. Patriarchenzeit, vor Mose und der Annahme des Jahweglaubens, wie sie von H. Ewald vertreten und noch von H. Gunkel akzeptiert wurde: »Gewiß sehr plausibel. Also doch ein Zentralheiligtum in Israels Urzeit!«[2];

b) die Annahme einer »israelitischen Eidgenossenschaft« von wechselndem Umfang nach der Landnahme in Palästina während der sog. Richterzeit durch M. Weber, der sie als einen Kriegsbund unter und mit Jahwe als dem Kriegsgott des Bundes, Garant seiner sozialen Ordnungen und Schöpfer des materiellen Gedeihens der Eidgenossen, insbesondere des dafür nötigen Regens, verstand[3];

c) die vor allem von M. Noth begründete Annahme eines sakralen Stämmebundes, der ebenfalls in der Richterzeit entstanden ist, dessen Umfang jedoch grundsätzlich durch die Zwölfzahl von Mitgliedern analog den griechischen und italischen Amphiktyonien bestimmt war, dessen Kern nicht die Kriegsführung, sondern der Kultus am Zentralheiligtum, das den Kultus und die gegenseitigen Beziehungen der Mitglieder regelnde kodifizierte Amphiktyonenrecht und nichtkodifizierte Gewohnheitsrecht bildeten und der nur in Ausnahmefällen, nämlich bei Vergehen gegen eine Bestimmung des Amphiktyonenrechts, gegen ein Mitglied den Amphiktyonenkrieg führte[4]; abgewandelt in die Annahme eines lediglich zehn Stämme umfassenden sakralen Bundes in der Richterzeit durch S. Mowinckel, der das Zwölfstämmesystem als nachdavidisch beurteilte, durch A. Weiser u. a.[5] — obwohl mit der

---

[2] H. Ewald, Einleitung in die Geschichte des Volkes Israel, I 1864³, 519ff.; H. Gunkel, Genesis, 1910³ (1964⁶), 332.

[3] M. Weber, Gesammelte Aufsätze zur Religionssoziologie, III 1923², 90ff. Die Bezeichnung Israels als »kriegerische Eidgenossenschaft« stammt anscheinend von J. Wellhausen, Israelitische und jüdische Geschichte, 1914⁷, 23.

[4] M. Noth, Das System der zwölf Stämme Israels, 1930. A. Alt, mit dem M. Noth nach dem Vorwort seines Buches die meisten Fragen durchsprechen konnte und der in: Der Gott der Väter, 1929, 59 (= Kleine Schriften zur Geschichte des Volkes Israel, I 1953, 55), nur von einer Amphiktyonie von Mamre sprach und 63f. (59) auf das Kultwesen der griechischen Amphiktyonie für den Unterschied zwischen gemeinsamer Volksreligion und abweichenden Stammesreligionen verwies, hat die Annahme sogleich übernommen, zunächst sogar noch weiter ausholend durch die Vermutung, daß der Zwölferbund wenigstens in seinen Anfängen noch in Israels vorpalästinische Zeit und zu einem Heiligtum außerhalb des Kulturlandes gehöre, vgl. RGG², III 439; sodann: Die Staatenbildung der Israeliten in Palästina, 1930, 9ff. 26f. (= Kleine Schriften zur Geschichte des Volkes Israel, II 1953, 7f. 21f.).

[5] S. Mowinckel, Zur Frage nach dokumentarischen Quellen in Josua 13—19,1 946, 20ff.; »Rahelstämme« und »Leastämme«, in: Von Ugarit nach Qumran, Eißfeldt-Festschrift, 1958, 129ff. Für eine Zehnamphiktyonie auch A. Weiser, Das Deboralied, ZAW 71 (1959), 96; K.-D. Schunck, Benjamin, 1963, 48ff.

Annahme eines Zehnstämmebundes die für die Amphiktyonie-Hypothese wesentliche Analogie mit den griechischen und italischen Institutionen hinfällig wird;

d) die meist vorgenommene Vermischung der unter b) und c) genannten Annahmen, wozu eigentlich schon die soeben erwähnte Reduzierung der Mitglieder der Amphiktyonie auf die Zehnzahl gehört, unter Einbeziehung des sog. heiligen Krieges[6] und bis hin zur Ausweitung in eine politische Organisation der Stämme mit einem Anführer und einem Ältestenkollegium[7];

e) die Annahmen einer Reihe weiterer kleiner israelitischer Amphiktyonien vor oder neben dem Zwölfstämmebund — von der Frage nach nichtisraelitischen Amphiktyonien aufgrund der sechs oder zwölf Namen umfassenden Listen anderer Völker in der Genesis einmal ganz abgesehen —, so in Hebron durch A. H. Sayce[8] bzw. in Mamre durch A. Alt und M. Noth[9] oder in Kadesch und Hebron durch S. Mowinckel[10], in Gilgal durch K. Möhlenbrink[11], in Betel durch A. Jepsen[12] und in Sichem durch M. Noth und Th. J. Meek[13]; diese Auswahl mag genügen, da eine größere oder geringere Vollständigkeit nichts zur Sache beiträgt.

Da die Annahme einer patriarchenzeitlichen Zwölfstämme-Amphiktyonie durch die inzwischen gewonnene genauere Einsicht in das Werden der israelitischen Stämme, die teilweise erst auf dem Boden Palästinas entstanden sind, hinfällig geworden ist und da die Annahmen kleiner Amphiktyonien meist im Zusammenhang mit der Frage nach der Vorgeschichte der Zwölfstämme-Amphiktyonie erfolgt sind und mit dem Urteil über diese stehen und fallen, brauchen wir uns im folgenden nur mit der Annahme einer solchen israelitischen Zwölfstämme-Amphiktyonie zu befassen, wie sie in verschiedener Form unter b)—d) erwähnt worden ist. Sie ist denn auch gewöhnlich gemeint, wenn von der Existenz einer Amphiktyonie, eines sakralen

---

[6] G. von Rad, Der Heilige Krieg im alten Israel, 1951 (1965⁴).

[7] J. Dus, Die »Ältesten Israels«, Communio viatorum 3 (1960), 232—242; Die »Sufeten Israels«, ArOr 31 (1963), 444—469.

[8] A. H. Sayce, The Cuneiform Tablets of Tel El-Amarna, now preserved in the Boulaq Museum, Proceedings of the Society of Biblical Archaeology 11 (1888/89), 347.

[9] A. Alt, Der Gott der Väter, 1929, 58f. (= Kleine Schriften zur Geschichte des Volkes Israel, I 1953, 55); M. Noth a. a. O. 107f.

[10] S. Mowinckel, Kadesj, Sinai og Jahve, Norsk Geografisk Tidskrift 9 (1942), 13f.: Kadesch als älteres Zentrum der Hebron-Gruppe.

[11] K. Möhlenbrink, Die Landnahmesagen des Buches Josua, ZAW 56 (1938), 246ff.

[12] A. Jepsen, Zur Überlieferungsgeschichte der Vätergestalten, in: Alt-Festschrift, 1953/54, 273. 276.

[13] M. Noth a. a. O. 75ff.; Th. J. Meek, Hebrew Origins, 1936, 25. 139.

Stämmebundes, im alten Israel die Rede ist. Aus ihr leitet man zahlreiche andere Erscheinungen her oder bringt sie mit ihr in Verbindung. Auch dafür müssen einige Beispiele genügen, zumal es nahezu unmöglich ist, alle derartigen Hypothesen zu erfassen. Nehmen wir alles in allem, so bleibt in einer fast tausendjährigen Geschichte Israels kaum etwas übrig, was nicht als eine ursprüngliche Einrichtung oder als eine Folgeerscheinung der Amphiktyonie erschiene. Sie müßte, wichtiger als der Jahweglaube selber, die eigentliche Keimzelle Israels, des alttestamentlichen Glaubens und des Alten Testaments gewesen sein — und dies in der anscheinend allein schöpferischen Periode der Richterzeit. So versteht man die sog. kleinen Richter als Vertreter eines zentralen Richteramtes[14] oder gar als politische Führer[15], die $n^e\acute{s}i'im$ als die offiziellen Vertreter der Stämme bei den Bundesversammlungen am Zentralheiligtum[16], den unter Davids und Salomos Hofbeamten aufgeführten Mazkir als amphiktyonischen Amtsträger im Zusammenhang mit einem deklaratorischen Gesamturteil kultischen Gepräges[17] und sogar die Nabis als Träger eines mosaischen und dann amphiktyonischen Amtes der Rechtsverkündigung und -überlieferung[18]. Man erblickt das Amphiktyonenrecht in dem angeblich genuin israelitischen und mit dem Gottesrecht zu identifizierenden sog. apodiktischen Recht, dessen älteste Teile im Bundesbuch Ex 22—23 vorliegen und das in anderen Rechtsbüchern bis zum deuteronomischen Gesetz Dtn 12—26 und zum Heiligkeitsgesetz Lev 17—26 weitergebildet worden ist[19], findet den »Sitz im Leben« des Urbestandes der Stammessprüche Gen 49 Dtn 33 und Jdc 5 in der Theophaniebegehung der Amphiktyonie[20] und denjenigen der Sprüche Jdc 21 3 I Sam 2 27b-30 II Sam 7 5b-7 in einer amphiktyonischen Poesie[21]. Man schreibt der Amphiktyonie, wie bereits erwähnt wurde, sogar die Führung heiliger Kriege und die Rolle einer demokratischen politischen Organisation zu. Ja, letzten Endes soll der von der Person Moses los-

---

[14] M. Noth, Das Amt des »Richters Israels«, in: Bertholet-Festschrift, 1950, 404—417; Geschichte Israels, 1950, 88 f.; H.-W. Hertzberg, Die Kleinen Richter, ThLZ 79 (1954), 285—290 (= Beiträge zur Traditionsgeschichte und Theologie des Alten Testaments, 1962, 118—125).

[15] J. Dus, Die »Sufeten Israels«.

[16] M. Noth a. a. O. (Anm. 4) 151—162.

[17] H. Graf Reventlow, Das Amt des Mazkir, ThZ 15 (1959), 161—175.

[18] H.-J. Kraus, Die prophetische Verkündigung des Rechts in Israel, 1957.

[19] A. Alt, Die Ursprünge des israelitischen Rechts, 1934 (= Kleine Schriften zur Geschichte des Volkes Israel, I 1953, 278—332); M. Noth, Die Gesetze im Pentateuch, 1940 (= Gesammelte Studien zum Alten Testament, 1957, 9—141).

[20] A. H. J. Gunneweg, Über den Sitz im Leben der sog. Stammessprüche, ZAW 76 (1964), 245—255, im Anschluß an A. Weiser.

[21] J. Dus, Die altisraelitische amphiktyonische Poesie, ZAW 75 (1963), 45—54.

gelöste Glaube Israels auf dem Boden der Amphiktyonie aus den Ballungen der Väter-, Auszugs- und Sinaitraditionen und aus der religionsgeschichtlichen und historischen Konstellation erwachsen sein[22].

Die Amphiktyonie-Hypothese ist weithin mehr oder weniger unbesehen übernommen worden. Daher mag es wieder genügen, an Stelle der vielen Anhänger einige Stimmen derjenigen anzuführen, die sie einschränken oder ablehnen, wobei freilich zu beachten ist, daß sich bei weitem nicht alle zu Wort gemeldet haben, die eine solche Stellungnahme vertreten. So spricht M. A. Beek zwar von einer neuen Bekräftigung des Sinaibundes durch Josua in Sichem (Jos 24), vermag dem Text des Alten Testaments aber keine Mitteilung über ein Zentralheiligtum zu entnehmen, zu dem die israelitischen Stämme hätten pilgern können; das scheint ihm »ein deutlicher Beweis, wie locker das Band zwischen den Stämmen geworden ist, die sich über den Norden, die Mitte und den Süden verteilt hatten, ohne daß sie sogar einen gemeinschaftlichen religiösen Mittelpunkt besaßen«[23]. In anderer Hinsicht einschränkend äußerte sich S. Herrmann: »Die Amphiktyonie-These bleibt fruchtbar, solange sie den lockeren Zusammenschluß einzelner Stämme um ein gemeinsames Heiligtum als eine mögliche geschichtliche Erscheinungsform auch im Raume Israels zu erklären und zu rechtfertigen versucht. Sie wird problematisch, wo mit diesem äußeren organisatorischen Zusammenschluß auch eine weitgehende geistig-religiöse Vereinheitlichung des Bewußtseins verbunden wird, die sich zudem noch in der relativ kurzen Zeitspanne der Richterzeit ausgebildet und bewährt haben soll«, während sich die Entwicklung langsam und allmählich vollzogen und bis in die späte Königszeit fortgesetzt hat[24]. In wieder anderer Weise stellte R. Smend die angebliche Beziehung zwischen Amphiktyonie und »Jahwekrieg« in Frage. In Wirklichkeit hatte die Amphiktyonie mit solchen Kriegen nichts zu tun, da in den Kriegen der Richterzeit weder Gesamtisrael noch die amphiktyonische Institution, sondern jeweils ein kleinerer israelitischer Verband in Erscheinung trat. Vielmehr bestand ein Dualismus zwischen Amphiktyonie und Jahwekrieg, der darauf beruhte, daß die Rahelstämme das Element des Jahwekrieges und die Leastämme das amphiktyonische Element vertraten, und der erst spät und unvollkommen ausgeglichen wurde[25].

Völlig ablehnend hat sich schon vor Jahren Y. Kaufmann geäußert, in dessen Rekonstruktionen der frühen Geschichte Israels, der

---

[22] K. Koch, Der Tod des Religionsstifters, KuD 8 (1962), 100—123.
[23] M. A. Beek, Auf den Wegen und Spuren des Alten Testaments, 1961, 90f. 113.
[24] S. Herrmann, Das Werden Israels, ThLZ 87 (1962), 561—574.
[25] R. Smend, Jahwekrieg und Stämmebund, 1963, übrigens auch mit der Trennung von Lade und Zentralheiligtum.

freilich wenige zu folgen geneigt sein werden, die Institution einer Amphiktyonie keinen Raum findet: In der Richterzeit »authority was vested in two institutions. There was, first, the secular, ‚primitive democracy' of the elders. This authority, unlike that of the Greek amphictyony, was not religious in any way; it was not connected with temple and had no sacral functions . . . Above this primitive democracy there arose from time to time the ‚judges', men of ‚spirit', messengers of God« als eine »unparalleled political institution«[26]. Ausführlicher hat H. M. Orlinsky die Verhältnisse der Richterzeit mit folgendem Ergebnis analysiert: »Israel in the period of the Judges consisted of tribes and city-states that shared much in religious belief and practice and that spoke the same language; but their economic and geographical conditions, their disposition to commerce rather than to agriculture, the extent to which they were exposed to invasion and even conquest of varying might and duration — these were the factors that determined the actions of the tribes. The tribes and city-states came, or neglected to come, to each other's assistance insofar as they were, or were not, threatened seriously by the invading force. The concept and structure of amphictyony existed in Israel no more than it did in Transjordan or anywhere else in Western Asia at the time.«[27] Auch O. Eißfeldt hat zu der Amphiktyonie-Hypothese erklärt, daß »this theory, although it has had great attraction, rests mainly upon two passages, Joshua xxiv and Judges xix—xxi, which are too weak to support it«, da gewichtige Gründe für eine nachträgliche nationale Ausweitung dieser ursprünglich auf einzelne Stämme bezogenen Erzählungen bestehen und da die Annahme, daß überall dort, wo Zwölfergruppen erwähnt werden, »these represent regular amphictyonies with twelve members must seem artificial«[28]. Ja, B. D. Rathjen möchte vielmehr den philistäischen Fünfstädte-Bund im Gegensatz zu der Vereinigung der israelitischen Stämme als Amphiktyonie bezeichnen: »It . . . appears that the relationship of the Hebrew confederation during the period of the judges to the amphictyonies of Europe is

---

[26] So nach der Zusammenfassung und Übersetzung von Y. Kaufmann, The Religion of Israel, 1960, 256, durch M. Greenberg.
[27] H. M. Orlinsky, The Tribal System of Israel and Related Groups in the Period of the Judges, Oriens Antiquus 1 (1962), 11—20.
[28] O. Eißfeldt, The Hebrew Kingdom, The Cambridge Ancient History, Vol. II Ch. XXXIV, 1965, 16f. M. H. Woudstra, The Ark of the Covenant from Conquest to Kingship, 1965, erklärt ebenfalls, freilich von einem konservativen Standpunkt aus, daß kein alttestamentlicher Text die Amphiktyonie bezeuge, und betrachtet die Hypothese als »a desperate attempt to deny the very picture which the Bible itself presents« (125). Für die ebenfalls ablehnende Stellungnahme von C. H. J. de Geus, De richteren van Israël, NThT 20 (1965/66), 81—100, vgl. das Referat von A. S. van der Woude in ZAW 78 (1966), 245.

more or less superficial and coincidental. The Philistine league . . . fits the classical pattern of the ‚amphictyony' much better than does the Hebrew organization. For this reason it might be well to reexamine the use of the term amphictyony to refer to the Hebrew confederation.«[29] Fragen wir nach der Art der israelitischen »confederation«, insbesondere im Zusammenhang mit der Lade und dem Heiligtum in Silo, das gern als zeitweiliges Zentralheiligtum der Amphiktyonie betrachtet wird, so können wir mit der jüngsten Untersuchung des Ladeheiligtums durch J. Maier annehmen, daß im Gegensatz zu der Amphiktyonie-Hypothese in Silo der Mittelpunkt eines unter dem Druck der Philisternot entstandenen zeitweiligen militärischen Stämmebündnisses mit der Lade als dem dort angefertigten Behälter für das Bündnisdokument oder als Bundessymbol zu erblicken ist[30].

Die Gegenstimmen sind verhältnismäßig ausführlich zitiert worden, weil sie eine Sammlung erheblicher Gründe bilden, die gegen die Amphiktyonie-Hypothese sprechen, bisher jedoch kurzerhand übergangen worden sind: Sie erwähnen die Fragwürdigkeit der Analogie europäischer Institutionen, der Bewertung der Zwölfzahl, des Postulats eines (wechselnden) Zentralheiligtums und der Funktion der Lade, der Deutung einiger alttestamentlicher Texte und der Einschätzung der Verhältnisse während der Richterzeit. So stellt sich doch unüberhörbar die Frage, ob die Israeliten tatsächlich einen sakralen Stämmebund, vielleicht sogar mit einem oder mehreren kleinen Vorläufern gebildet haben und ob das gleiche für die anderen Stämme oder Völker gilt, die in der Genesis in Sechser- oder Zwölfergruppen aufgezählt werden. Mir scheint, daß die nunmehr vorzulegenden Gegengründe schwerer wiegen und die Annahme von Amphiktyonien ausschließen.

II.

1. Es ist sogleich auffällig und ungewöhnlich, daß es keinen hebräischen Ausdruck gibt, der die Amphiktyonie bezeichnet — auffällig und ungewöhnlich, weil es Ausdrücke für alle möglichen Einrichtungen und Lebensbereiche gegeben hat, während ein solcher für eine derart grundlegende Institution fehlen sollte. Obwohl für Sippe und Stamm sowie für ihre Lebensbereiche einerseits und für Heiligtum und Kultus sowie für diesen gesamten Bereich andererseits mannigfache Begriffe und Bezeichnungen geprägt worden sind, sollte dies für einen sakralen Stämmebund nicht geschehen sein? Schon diese begriffliche Lücke läßt Zweifel an der Existenz einer Amphiktyonie entstehen, zumal die Griechen, die diese Institution tatsächlich kann-

---

[29] B. D. Rahtjen, Philistine and Hebrew Amphictyonies, JNES 24 (1965), 100—104.
[30] J. Maier, Das altisraelitische Ladeheiligtum, 1965, 20 ff. 57 ff.

ten, dafür eben jenen Begriff gebildet haben — wie übrigens auch weitere Begriffe für Bünde anderer Art (»Symmachie«).

Der Name »Israel« kann nicht als Ersatz für den fehlenden Begriff angeführt werden. Es soll sich ja um eine auf den Jahweglauben gegründete Amphiktyonie gehandelt haben, die durch eine ausdrückliche Verpflichtung auf Jahwe geschaffen worden sein soll (Jos 24). Demgemäß wäre ein mit dem theophoren Zusatz »Jahwe« gebildeter Name für die Stämmegemeinschaft zu erwarten. »Israel« dagegen ist, wie immer man den ersten Bestandteil des Namens deutet, mit »El« gebildet. Daß man angesichts der sich anbahnenden Auseinandersetzung mit der kanaanäischen Religion ausgerechnet den mit der Bezeichnung eines der großen kanaanäischen Gegengötter versehenen Namen »Israel« für eine ausgesprochene Jahwe-Amphiktyonie gewählt hätte, muß als höchst unwahrscheinlich gelten. So bleibt die begriffliche Lücke bestehen.

2. Als Analogie zur angeblichen israelitischen Amphiktyonie oder gar als Modell für sie wird seit langem auf Erscheinungen hingewiesen, die zwar in räumlich ferner liegenden Landschaften begegnen, dort aber teilweise in so greifbarer Form, daß von ihnen aus das erwünschte Licht auf die Verhältnisse im alten Israel und in seiner Umgebung zu fallen scheint. Es handelt sich einmal um Stammesverbände der alten griechischen Geschichte, die nach der Sechs- und Zwölfzahl zusammengestellt sind und deren Mittelpunkt ein als Stätte des gemeinsamen Kultus dienendes Heiligtum bildete. Die bedeutendste Amphiktyonie war die pyläisch-delphische um die Heiligtümer der Demeter in den Thermopylen und des Apollon in Delphi, die zwölf Stämme umfaßt haben soll. Ferner erwähnt für den italischen Raum Livius I 8, 3 einen Verband von *duodecim populi*, dessen Mittelpunkt das Heiligtum der Göttin Voltumna im Gebiet der Stadt Volsinii war, und weiß die Tradition von weiteren Verbänden der Etrusker in der Poebene und in Kampanien sowie der Bruttier in Kalabrien, der nördlich anschließenden verwandten Lukaner und der illyrischen Japyger in Apulien. Die tatsächliche Bedeutung und Rolle solcher Amphiktyonien ist freilich kaum ersichtlich und darf jedenfalls nicht überschätzt werden[31].

Außerdem ist dazu sogleich zu bemerken, daß der Gang der griechischen Geschichte gerade nicht wie in Israel zur Entstehung größerer Staatsgebilde geführt hat, die an die Stelle der alten Stammesverbände getreten wären und ihnen ein Ende bereitet hätten. Es entstanden lediglich eine Fülle größerer oder kleinerer Stadtstaaten, so daß einerseits die alten Amphiktyonien bis in die späte Zeit hinein eine gewisse Bedeutung als Vereinigungen größerer Gruppen von

---

[31] Zum Ganzen vgl. I. Calabi, Ricerche sui rapporti tra le poleis, 1953.

Griechen behielten und andererseits sich nach ihrem Vorbild entsprechende Vereinigungen von Stadtstaaten bildeten, die ebenfalls Amphiktyonien hießen (so diejenigen von Delos zur Blütezeit Athens, von Kalaureia und Onchestos und ähnliche Verbände im kleinasiatischen Kolonialgebiet). Insofern hat B. D. Rahtjen wohl recht, wenn er nicht in Israel, sondern in der lockeren Vereinigung der philistäischen Stadtstaaten eine Amphiktyonie erblickt, zumal die philistäische Herrenschicht aus dem Umkreis des griechischen Mittelmeerraums nach Palästina gekommen ist. Der unterschiedliche Verlauf der staatlichen Geschichte in Griechenland und in Israel läßt jedenfalls wieder an der Existenz einer israelitischen Amphiktyonie zweifeln.

Vor allem sind zwei grundlegende Unterschiede zu beachten. Einmal ist die griechisch-italische Amphiktyonie offensichtlich eine Institution indogermanischer Völkerschaften, die man bei semitischen Gruppen nicht ohne weiteres in gleicher oder ähnlicher Weise annehmen kann — weder als Eigenschöpfung noch als übernommene Größe. Dazu sind die Gegensätze zwischen beiden Gruppen zu schwerwiegend. Tatsächlich sind im Alten Orient abgesehen von den fraglichen alttestamentlichen Texten zwar alle möglichen sakralen und staatlichen Institutionen und Formen belegt, nicht aber die Amphiktyonie. Gewiß könnte man auf die neuerdings stark betonten Beziehungen zwischen den Völkern des östlichen Mittelmeerraums und den phönizischen Stadtstaaten verweisen, wie sie sich insbesondere aus der Ausgrabung des alten Ugarit (Ras Schamra) bis zu dessen Untergang um 1200 v. Chr. erschließen lassen, um die Möglichkeit der Übernahme oder Bekanntschaft mit der Institution der griechischen Amphiktyonie auf diesem Wege nahezulegen. Doch gerade das phönizische Gebiet weist keine Spur einer solchen Einrichtung auf, auch nicht in der Form einer lockeren Vereinigung von Stadtstaaten wie bei den Philistern. Und auch von diesen kann Israel nicht beeinflußt worden sein, da sein Schema von zwölf Stämmen älter als jene Vereinigung ist. Wie eine semitische Analogiebildung scheidet eine Bekanntschaft mit dem griechischen System offenbar aus. Tatsächlich sind im Alten Orient außerhalb der fraglichen alttestamentlichen Texte zwar alle möglichen sakralen und staatlichen Institutionen und Formen belegt, nicht aber die Amphiktyonie[31a].

[31a] Eine solche meint W. W. Hallo, A Sumerian Amphictyony, JCSt 14 (1960), 88—114, für das sumerische Gebiet am Ende des 2. Jt., doch noch aus älterer Zeit stammend, entdeckt zu haben, weil bestimmte Städte zu monatlichen Lieferungen für den Kultus der großen nationalen Tempel in Nippur verpflichtet waren. Jedoch steht gar nicht eindeutig fest, daß die Lieferungen für die Tempel bestimmt waren. Vor allem scheint von Jahr zu Jahr eine wechselnde Gruppe die monatlichen Lieferungen übernommen zu haben und in einer unterschiedlichen Ordnung. Mit einer Amphiktyonie hat dies

Ferner ist zu bedenken: Was immer die griechisch-italischen Stämme in soziologischer Hinsicht gewesen sein mögen, bevor sie nach Griechenland und Italien kamen und nachdem sie dort seßhaft geworden waren — sie waren jedenfalls nicht Nomaden oder Halbnomaden nach Art der semitischen Gruppen, bei denen man Amphiktyonien vermutet. Zwischen beiden Völkergruppen bestehen grundlegende soziologische Unterschiede mit tiefgreifenden Folgen für die gesamte Lebenshaltung, die nicht übergangen werden dürfen[32]. Im Bereich des Alten Testaments handelt es sich ja nicht nur um die israelitischen Stämme, die zu Zwölfergruppen zusammengestellt sind, sondern auch um Nachbarvölker Israels, die in noch größerer Entfernung vom griechisch-italischen Raum lebten als Israel und bei denen eine Bekanntschaft mit dem dortigen System ganz unwahrscheinlich ist:

Gen 22 20-24 (Jahwist): zwölf Söhne Nahors als Ahnherren von Aramäerstämmen,

Gen 25 13-16 (Priesterschrift): zwölf Söhne Ismaels als Ahnherren von Ismaeliterstämmen.

Gen 36 10-14 (Jahwist): die Ahnherren der von drei Frauen Esaus hergeleiteten Edomiterstämme,

Gen 25 2 (Jahwist): sechs Söhne Abrahams und der Ketura als Ahnherren arabischer Stämme,

vielleicht außerdem

Gen 36 20-28 (Jahwist): die Ahnherren choritischer Stämme vom Gebirge Seïr, während die Königsliste 36 31-39 schwerlich heranzuziehen ist[33].

Es ist kaum anzunehmen, daß im Gegensatz zu den Amphiktyonien im Kulturland Griechenlands und Italiens im Vorderen Orient gerade die außerhalb des alten Kulturlandes oder an seinem Rand lebenden Stämme derartige Organisationen geschaffen hätten. Wie sollten diese denn funktionieren? Der regelmäßige Weidewechsel solcher Stämme in das Kulturland und wieder zurück in die Steppe schließt die regel-

---

nichts zu tun. Eher entspricht die Regelung den monatlichen Lieferungen der von Salomo eingerichteten Gaue Israels für den höfischen und staatlichen Bedarf.

[32] Vgl. z. B. B. S. Nyström, Beduinentum und Jahwismus, 1946; R. de Vaux, Das Alte Testament und seine Lebensordnungen, I 1964², 17—41. Die neueste Bestreitung dessen durch G. E. Mendenhall, The Hebrew Conquest of Palestine, BA 25 (1962), 66—87, der an Stelle einer Einwanderung von halbnomadischen Stämmen eine Revolte der Bauern gegen die Stadtstaaten unter dem Einfluß der religiösen Bewegung einer kleinen Gruppe von 70 Familien nach ihrer Flucht aus Ägypten postuliert, ist eher eine aus der Mischung von biblizistischem Fundamentalismus und Orientalistik hervorgegangene als geschichtlich haltbare Konstruktion. Vgl. dazu auch M. Weippert, Die Landnahme der israelitischen Stämme, 1967.

[33] Gegen J. R. Bartlett, The Edomite King-list of Genesis xxxvi. 31-39 and I Chron. i. 43-50, JThSt NS 16 (1965), 301—314.

mäßige, monatlich wechselnde Versorgung eines gemeinsamen Zentralheiligtums von vornherein aus. Hinzu kommt, daß es im Alten Testament zwar viele Beispiele für den lebendigen Zusammenhalt der Familie und Sippe, jedoch nahezu keine für eine gleiche gemeinschaftsbildende Kraft bei den israelitischen Stämmen gibt. Hinweise auf ein Solidaritätsgefühl zwischen den Stämmen liegen nur aus der Frühzeit vor wie im Deboralied Jdc 5[34]. Hat es also keine wesentliche gemeinschaftsbildende Kraft innerhalb des Stammes und ein bloß spärliches Solidaritätsgefühl zwischen den Stämmen gegeben, hat sich außerdem die Stammesorganisation bald nach der Landnahme infolge der veränderten Lebensbedingungen zersetzt, so ist erst recht nicht mit einem solchen Gemeinschaftsbewußtsein zu rechnen, wie eine Amphiktyonie es verlangt hätte. Auch der Verweis auf gemeinsame kriegerische Unternehmen in Amphiktyonenkriegen geht fehl, weil eine Amphiktyonie primär nicht eine politisch-militärische, sondern eine kultische Institution ist. Amphiktyonie und heiliger oder Jahwekrieg müßten verschiedenen Bereichen, dem kultisch-sakralen und dem politisch-militärischen angehören, wie S. Herrmann und R. Smend gezeigt haben[35]. Darüber hinaus ist es fraglich, ob überhaupt mit einem »heiligen Krieg« als sakraler Unternehmung zu rechnen ist und ob es sich nicht zunächst einfach um vor und nach dem Kampf vorzunehmende Kulthandlungen handelt, die erst wesentlich später zu einer Theorie vom heiligen Krieg systematisiert worden sind; Theorie und Wirklichkeit des »Bannes« lassen das letztere vermuten. Aus alledem folgt: Sechser- oder Zwölferlisten von Stämmen, die im nomadischen oder halbnomadischen Stadium leben oder im Seßhaftwerden begriffen sind, können grundsätzlich keine Amphiktyonien widerspiegeln oder auf deren Existenz hinweisen.

3. Eine Amphiktyonie besitzt ein gemeinsames Zentralheiligtum, das von den Mitgliedern abwechselnd versorgt wird. Hat es vor der deuteronomischen Kultuszentralisation in Jerusalem, genauer in der Richterzeit, in Israel ein derartiges Zentralheiligtum gegeben? Man behauptet, daß dies der Fall gewesen sei, daß die Lade Jahwes das Symbol der Amphiktyonie gebildet und daß mit ihr das Zentralheiligtum mehrfach gewechselt habe[36]. Es soll sich zumindest in Sichem, Betel und Silo befunden haben, bevor die Lade in die Gewalt der

---

[34] L. Wächter, Gemeinschaft und Einzelner im Judentum, 1961. Was R. de Vaux a. a. O. 31 ff. anführt, belegt gerade die Solidarität der Sippe und nicht des Stammes.
[35] Vgl. Anm. 24 und 25.
[36] Die Annahme von J. Dus, Ein richterzeitliches Stierbildheiligtum zu Bethel?, ZAW 77 (1965), 268—286, daß vor der allgemeinen Anerkennung der Lade ein Stierbild in Bethel das gesamtisraelitische Heiligtum dargestellt habe, ist unwahrscheinlich und beruht auf einer willkürlichen Interpretation von Ex 32.

Philister geriet und schließlich von David nach Jerusalem geholt wurde. Allerdings macht dieser mehrfache Wechsel stutzig, zumal er im Verlauf einer verhältnismäßig kurzen Zeit erfolgt sein soll; er widerspricht der konservativen Haltung in kultischen Fragen, die der ganzen Antike — und nicht nur ihr — eigen ist.

Nun wird die Lade in Verbindung mit Sichem überhaupt nicht erwähnt. Daß eine Mitteilung darüber verlorengegangen sein sollte, wäre verwunderlich, wenn sich in Sichem tatsächlich das Zentralheiligtum einer so grundlegenden Institution wie einer Amphiktyonie befunden hätte, ja, wenn diese dort gegründet worden wäre. Denn das ist der eigentliche Grund, aus dem man ein zeitweiliges Zentralheiligtum in Sichem annimmt: die Formierung des Zwölfstämmebundes unter maßgeblicher Mitwirkung Josuas nach Jos 24. Jedoch die gesamtisraelitische Perspektive dieser Erzählung vom sog. Landtag in Sichem beruht auf der fast allgemein zugestandenen Bearbeitung eines alten Sagenkerns, die bereits in der elohistischen Fassung erkennbar ist, erst recht in der deuteronomistischen Bearbeitung, die hier wie bei anderen Traditionen erfolgt ist. Jos 24 in der elohistischen und deuteronomistischen Fassung begründet nicht eine Einheit Israels, sondern setzt sie als schon bestehend voraus[37]. Die Zeit Josuas, in der die Landnahme seines Stammes noch nicht abgeschlossen und auch die anderen Stämme weithin in Bewegung waren, wäre für die Gründung eines Stämmebundes und die Herstellung eines einigen Israel so ungünstig wie nur möglich gewesen. Seine Siege bei Gibeon-Ajjalon (Jos 10 1-15) und am Wasser von Meron (Jos 11 1-9) waren zudem reine Stammesangelegenheiten und nicht dazu geeignet, ihm solches Ansehen zu verschaffen, daß ihm der Zusammenschluß aller Stämme hätte gelingen können. Wie sein Leben sich ganz im Rahmen seines eigenen Stammes abgespielt hat, so ist der alte Sagenkern, der Jos 24 zugrunde liegt, eine Stammeserzählung über einen geschichtlichen Vorgang, an dem Josua beteiligt war: die einmalige Verpflichtung des eigenen Stammes auf Jahwe durch Josua, nachdem er seine Erfolge im Namen Jahwes errungen hatte. Ob sich das tatsächlich in Sichem ereignet oder ob der Elohist, zu dessen Quellenschicht die Erzählung gehört hat, sie an diese Stätte, die er auch sonst bevorzugt, verlegt hat, läßt sich nicht mehr feststellen. Es ist immerhin wahrscheinlich, daß Sichem zur Zeit Josuas eine rein kanaanäische Stadt war, so daß der Vorgang von Jos 24 höchstens in der Umgebung, etwa auf den Bergen Garizim oder Ebal (vgl. Jos 8 30 Dtn 27 4), stattgefunden haben könnte. Außerdem bestehen viele auffällige Parallelen zwischen der Jakob- und der Josuatradition (vgl. Gen 34 35 1ff. 48 22), so daß H. H. Rowley es sogar für wahrscheinlich hält, »that the story

---

[37] So häufig, zuletzt G. Schmitt, Der Landtag von Sichem, 1964.

of Josh. xxiv represents the transfer to Joshua of an older tradition of a covenant between Israelites and Canaanites, but in an appropriately altered form«[38]. Wie sich das auch verhalten möge — eins ergibt die Analyse von Jos 24 deutlich: Von der Gründung einer Amphiktyonie und einem zeitweiligen Zentralheiligtum in Sichem kann keine Rede sein.

Ebensowenig hat sich das Zentralheiligtum zeitweilig in Betel befunden. Die Notiz über den dortigen Aufenthalt der Lade in Jdc 20 27 f. ist ein später Einschub in den Text[39], der in ungeschickter Weise die Einleitung der an Jahwe zu richtenden Frage auseinanderreißt: »Dann befragten die Israeliten Jahwe . . . (Ladenotiz) . . . folgendermaßen: . . .«. Der Einschub sollte in einer jungen Zeit begründen, warum sich die Israeliten — um welche es sich handelt, wird in Abschnitt 4. zu klären sein — ausgerechnet in Betel, das inzwischen als Staatsheiligtum des Nordreichs Israel verhaßt geworden war, zur Einholung eines Jahweorakels eingefunden hatten. Auch die elohistische Erzählung von der Wanderung Jakobs von Sichem nach Betel (Gen 35 1-5), die mit gewissen kultischen Handlungen und der »Entfernung der fremden Götter« verknüpft ist und in der man einen regelmäßigen Brauch vermutet hat[40], kann nicht für die Annahme verwertet werden, daß ein Zentralheiligtum von Sichem nach Betel verlegt worden sei. Abgesehen von der bezweifelten Voraussetzung, daß es sich einmal in Sichem befunden habe, wird die Wanderung der Jakobsippe zugeschrieben und vom Elohisten damit vielleicht als Brauch der vorjahwistischen Zeit gekennzeichnet. Doch auch wenn man ihn für die Zeit Josuas annehmen will, besagt die Erzählung im Zusammenhang mit Jos 24 nichts anderes, als daß Josuas Stamm im Anschluß an die Verpflichtung auf Jahwe nach Betel gepilgert ist, um nach der »Entfernung der fremden Götter« dort dem neuen Gott zu huldigen. Dann ergibt sich, daß sich damals im Unterschied von Sichem in Betel bereits ein Jahwe geweihtes Heiligtum befunden hat, das ein frischbekehrter Stamm aufsuchen konnte — nicht mehr.

---

[38] H. H. Rowley, From Joseph to Joshua, 1950, 128. Noch schärfer E. Auerbach. Die große Überarbeitung der biblischen Bücher, VTSuppl I, 1953, 3, der Jos 24 für eine deuteronomische Konstruktion exilischer Herkunft ohne jeden geschichtlichen Wert hält.

[39] Vgl. u. a. G. F. Moore, Judges, 1895 (1949[6]), 433f.; W. Nowack, Richter, Ruth und Bücher Samuelis, 1902, 170; H. Greßmann, Die älteste Geschichtsschreibung und Prophetie Israels, 1921[2], 266; G. Hölscher, Geschichtsschreibung in Israel, 1952, 363.

[40] Vgl. A. Alt, Die Wallfahrt von Sichem nach Bethel, in: Bulmerincq-Gedenkschrift, 1938, 218—230 (= Kleine Schriften zur Geschichte des Volkes Israel, I 1953, 79—88).

Dagegen ist Silo — und Silo allein! — der dauernde Standort der Lade vor ihrem Verlust an die Philister. Ist Silo darum das amphiktyonische Zentralheiligtum gewesen? Das hängt, abgesehen von den grundsätzlichen Fragen, davon ab, wie man Herkunft und Rolle der Lade beurteilt: mosaischer, palästinisch-kanaanäischer oder palästinisch-israelitischer Herkunft — Gottesthron oder Behälter[41]? Die erste Frage ist wegen des fast völligen Fehlens alter Bezeugungen kaum je mit einiger Wahrscheinlichkeit zu beantworten. Die Ansicht, daß die Lade das Wanderheiligtum der Moseschar gewesen sei, ist angesichts der Gegengründe in der sorgfältigen Untersuchung von J. Maier[42], die ebenso zwingende Gründe gegen palästinisch-kanaanäische Herkunft einschließt, kaum noch haltbar. Maiers eigener Auffassung, daß die Lade erst in Silo hergestellt und also palästinisch-israelitischer Herkunft sei, vermag ich mich freilich nicht anzuschließen. Denn in den Erzählungen Jos 3—4 und 6 ist ihre Erwähnung in den drei alten Quellenschichten JNE, die ich auch für das Josuabuch meine nachweisen zu können[43], fest verankert und durch scharfsinnige Aufteilung des Textes auf mehrere Bearbeitungsschichten nicht zu eliminieren. Dann lassen diese Vorkommen den Schluß zu, daß die Lade außerpalästinisch-israelitischer und vorjahwistischer Herkunft und von einer nach Palästina einwandernden Gruppe mitgebracht worden ist — am ehesten von der Gruppe, die die Traditionen über die Einwanderung durch den Jordangraben bewahrt hat und mit der der Name Josuas verbunden ist: das sog. Haus Joseph oder die Ephraimiten und die mit ihnen gemeinsam vorgehenden späteren Benjaminiten[44]. Dies erklärt sowohl die Erwähnung der Lade in den Erzählungen des Josuabuches als auch ihren Standort im ephraimitischen Silo[45]. Dort ist sie, darin stimme ich J. Maier wieder zu,

---

[41] Dies sind nicht die einzigen, wohl aber die wichtigsten Ansichten. Andere Auffassungen wie die als aus Ägypten mitgebrachter Josephsarg durch R. Hartmann, Zelt und Lade, ZAW 37 (1917/18), 209—244, oder als Miniaturtempel durch H. G. May, The Ark — a Miniature Temple, AJSL 52 (1935/36), 215—234, brauchen in diesem Zusammenhang nicht erörtert zu werden.

[42] Vgl. Anm. 30. Anders ursprünglich G. Fohrer, Tradition und Interpretation im Alten Testament, ZAW 73 (1961), 8 Anm. 17.

[43] E. Sellin—G. Fohrer, Einleitung in das Alte Testament, 1965^{10}, 29f.

[44] Zur Entstehung des Stammes Benjamin und zum Verhältnis zu Ephraim vgl. K.-D. Schunck a. a. O.

[45] Vgl. auch F. Horst in ThBl 12 (1933), 106f. Anders z. B. E. Nielsen, Some Reflections on the History of the Ark, VTSuppl VII, 1960, 63: ».. . there was once a special connection between the Benjaminites and the Ark«; A. S. Kapelrud, The Role of the Cult in Old Israel, in: The Bible in Modern Scholarship, 1965, 47: Die Lade ist von Gruppen mitgebracht worden, die von Süden her nach Palästina kamen. Die Verbindung der Lade mit Joseph bzw. Ephraim-Benjamin läßt zugleich die Möglich-

zum Symbol eines kurzzeitigen militärischen Stämmebündnisses geworden, das sich angesichts der Bedrängnis durch die Philister gebildet hat, oder hat gleichzeitig als Behälter für das Bündnisdokument oder -symbol — jedenfalls nicht als Gottesthron — gedient. So schließt die Bestimmung der Rollen Silos und der Lade die Annahme eines Zentralheiligtums auch in Silo aus. Daß die Lade nicht als Symbol einer Amphiktyonie gelten kann und die Existenz eines Zentralheiligtums nicht beweisbar ist, hat W. H. Irwin unter der Voraussetzung mosaischer Herkunft der Lade dargelegt[46]. Seine Gründe sind in jedem Falle stichhaltig.

Demnach ist es unwahrscheinlich, daß es in der Richterzeit ein gemeinsames israelitisches Zentralheiligtum gegeben hat. Darin liegt ein gewichtiger Grund gegen die Amphiktyonie-Hypothese vor. Natürlich schließt dies nicht aus, daß palästinische Jahweheiligtümer im Grenzgebiet mehrerer Stämme von diesen allen benutzt worden sind — so Gilgal von Benjamin, Ephraim und Manasse, der Tabor von Isaschar, Sebulon und vielleicht Naphtali, die »Steinkreise am Jordan« (Gelilot) von Ruben und Gad. Doch gleichzeitige Benutzung ist von einem sakralen Stämmebund wohl zu unterscheiden.

4. Eine weitere Frage, die unter Verweis auf andere Untersuchungen kurz beantwortet werden kann, stellt sich: Gibt es alttestamentliche Texte, die einen sakralen Stämmebund erwähnen oder von dessen möglichen Aktionen berichten? Bekanntlich fehlt jede unmittelbare Erwähnung, so daß man zwei Texte heranzieht, die anscheinend mittelbar eine Amphiktyonie bezeugen: das Deboralied Jdc 5 und die Erzählung vom Feldzug gegen die Benjaminiten Jdc 19—21.

Allerdings hat M. Noth seinerzeit Jdc 5 mit gutem Grunde aus seinen Erwägungen ausgeschlossen, während S. Mowinckel und A. Weiser den amphiktyonischen Charakter des Deboraliedes hervorheben[47] — jedoch zu Unrecht. Zunächst besteht eine erhebliche Differenz zwischen der alten Erzählung von der Prophetin Debora und von Barak in Jdc 4 4a. 5*. 6-10. 12-16, die als israelitische Teilnehmer an der Schlacht lediglich die Stämme Naphtali und Sebulon erwähnt, und dem ebenso alten Lied in Jdc 5, das sechs teilnehmende Stämme — Ephraim, Benjamin, Machir, Sebulon, Isaschar und Naphtali —

---

keit zu, daß die Lade vor Silo kurze Zeit in Gilgal gestanden hat. Ein langer Aufenthalt in Gilgal und die von H.-J. Kraus, Gilgal, VT 1 (1951), 181—199, vertretene Annahme, daß sich dort nach Sichem und kurz vor der Staatsbildung das Zentralheiligtum befunden habe, läßt sich mit Jos 3—4 nicht begründen, ebensowenig mit Jdc 2 1, wo man hinter dem Engel schwerlich die Lade vermuten darf.

[46] W. H. Irwin, Le sanctuaire central israélite avant l'établissement de la monarchie, RB 72 (1965), 161—184.

[47] M. Noth a. a. O. (Anm. 4) 5f. 36, ferner die Angaben in Anm. 5.

und vier abwesende Stämme — Ruben, Gilead, Dan und Asser — aufzählt. Auch wenn man von den Angaben des Liedes ausgeht und die Zehnzahl von für den Kampf in Frage kommenden Stämmen für zutreffend hält, muß man mit R. Smend — auf dessen Ausführungen über Jdc 5 der Kürze wegen verwiesen werden muß — sagen: »Läßt man die Zwölfzahl fallen, dann geht das sicherste und wesentlichste tertium comparationis verloren, das wir für den Vergleich zwischen dem israelitischen Stämmebund und den sakralen Bünden des alten Griechenland besitzen. Deutlicher gesagt: dann ist dieser Vergleich sinnlos und verboten; es ist dann nicht mehr erlaubt, das Israel vor der Staatenbildung mit dem von Hause aus den griechischen Zwölfer- (oder Sechser)bünden zukommenden Begriff einer Amphiktyonie zu bezeichnen.«[48] Schließlich wird, wie M. Noth mit Recht dargelegt hat, ein Amphiktyonenkrieg nur gegen ein Mitglied der Amphiktyonie geführt. Die Deboraschlacht jedoch wurde gegen die Kanaanäer geschlagen und kann schon aus diesem Grunde kein amphiktyonischer Krieg gewesen sein. An ihr war nur ein kurzzeitiges Stämmebündnis beteiligt, dem zweifellos Naphtali und Sebulon angehört haben und dem andere Stämme kleine Heerbannkontingente zu Hilfe geschickt haben mögen. Es hat sich wohl um ein ähnliches Bündnis wie das antiphilistäische von Silo gehandelt.

Dagegen könnte es sich bei dem in Jdc 19—21 geschilderten Ereignis um einen Amphiktyonenkrieg handeln: um ein Strafgericht, das der israelitische Stämmebund über sein Mitglied Benjamin verhängt und durchgeführt hätte. Doch dieser Interpretation hat O. Eißfeldt längst mit überzeugenden Gründen widersprochen[49]. Es ist ja höchst auffällig, daß lediglich in Jdc 19—21 anscheinend ein wirklich geschlossenes Israel zu einheitlich-planvollem Handeln auftritt, während sonst aus der Richterzeit immer nur von Aktionen einzelner Stämme oder kurzzeitiger Stämmebündnisse berichtet wird. Demgegenüber hat O. Eißfeldt gezeigt, daß an den Geschehnissen ursprünglich nur Beleidigter und Beleidiger, Ephraim und Benjamin, beteiligt waren, daß das wirkliche Vergehen Benjamins auf politischem Gebiet lag und daß es sich darin um die Auflehnung Benjamins oder einiger Städte des südephraimitischen Gebietes gegen das ephraimitische Kernland und um die Loslösung Benjamins von Ephraim, mit dem es gemeinsam eingewandert war, gehandelt hat. Daher läßt sich Jdc 19—21 nicht für die Amphiktyonie-Hypothese in Anspruch nehmen.

So gibt es kein alttestamentliches Zeugnis für die Existenz einer israelitischen Amphiktyonie, und das entspricht völlig den Verhältnis-

---
[48] R. Smend a. a. O. 12.
[49] O. Eißfeldt, Der geschichtliche Hintergrund der Erzählung von Gibeas Schandtat, in: Beer-Festschrift, 1935, 19—40 (= Kleine Schriften, II 1963, 64—80).

sen, in denen die Stämme während der Richterzeit lebten; für die Einzelheiten kann auf die Skizze verwiesen werden, die H. M. Orlinsky gerade im Blick auf die Amphiktyonie-Hypothese vorgelegt hat[50].

5. Welchen Sinn hat nun das Schema der Zwölfzahl, in das man die israelitischen Stämme gebracht hat? Um der Frage nachgehen zu können, ist es erforderlich, zunächst einen Überblick über die Formen, in denen das Schema im Alten Testament begegnet, zu gewinnen. Als Quellen kommen in Frage: die Erzählung von der Geburt der Kinder Jakobs Gen 29 31 ff., der Jakobsegen Gen 49, die Liste israelitischer Stammeshäupter Num 1, die Geschlechterliste Num 26 und der Mosesegen Dtn 33, während der priesterschriftliche Landnahmebericht Jos 13—19 wegen seines geringeren Quellenwertes außer acht bleiben kann. Aus diesen Quellen ergeben sich drei Formen des Zwölferschemas, nicht nur zwei, wie M. Noth annimmt. Die 1. Form ist in der Weise gegliedert, daß die zwölf Stämme in vier Gruppen nach den Frauen Jakobs und deren Sklavinnen angeführt werden; in der 2. und 3. Form werden einzelne Namen weggelassen und neue hinzugefügt, so daß die Zwölfzahl erhalten bleibt:

		1. Form	2. Form	3. Form
a) Lea:		1. Ruben	1. Ruben	1. Ruben
		2. Simeon	2. Simeon	2. Simeon
		3. Levi	3. Levi	
		4. Juda	4. Juda	3. Juda
		5. Isaschar	5. Isaschar	4. Isaschar
		6. Sebulon	6. Sebulon	5. Sebulon
		7. Dina		
b) Bilha:		8. Dan	7. Dan	6. Dan
		9. Naphtali	8. Naphtali	7. Naphtali
c) Silpa:		10. Gad	9. Gad	8. Gad
		11. Asser	10. Asser	9. Asser
d) Rahel:		12. Joseph	11. Joseph	10. Ephraim
				11. Manasse
			12. Benjamin	12. Benjamin

Danach läßt die 2. Form (Gen 49) gegenüber der 1. Form Dina weg und fügt statt dessen Benjamin hinter Joseph ein. Die 3. Form (Num 1 26) unterscheidet sich von der 2. Form dadurch, daß sie zusätzlich Levi wegläßt und dafür Joseph in Ephraim und Manasse zerlegt. Das zeigt, daß die Formen aus verschiedenen Situationen und Zeiten stammen und daß sie jeweils an inzwischen veränderte Verhältnisse angepaßt worden sind. Die älteste Form ist sicherlich die an erster Stelle angeführte, weil sie die Existenz des Stammes Benjamin noch nicht voraussetzt oder berücksichtigt und einen sonst un-

---

[50] Vgl. Anm. 27.

bekannten Stamm Dina nennt. Dagegen ist die zeitliche Aufeinanderfolge der 2. und 3. Form schwer zu bestimmen. Sie hängt davon ab, ob es einmal einen Volksstamm Levi gegeben hat oder die unter diesem Namen zusammengefaßten priesterlichen Leviten zur Erreichung der Zwölfzahl eingesetzt worden sind, und ob ein ursprünglicher Stamm Joseph später in die Stämme Ephraim und Manasse (und den nicht mehr in das Schema aufgenommenen Machir) geteilt oder umgekehrt diese nachträglich und künstlich in der höheren Einheit Joseph zusammengefaßt worden sind (was dann freilich auch in der 1. Form geschehen wäre). Zur absoluten Datierung genügen die Feststellungen, daß der Jakobsegen (2. Form) in seiner jetzigen Zusammenstellung wahrscheinlich aus der Zeit Davids oder Salomos stammt, die Einzelsprüche und die Zwölfzahl der Stämme jedoch einen älteren Zustand widerspiegeln, der nach M. Noth in der frühesten Periode der Richterzeit bestanden hat, daß M. Noth ferner Num 26 (3. Form) aus der zweiten Hälfte der Richterzeit, Num 1 (3. Form) aus einer etwas früheren Zeit herleitet[51] und daß das Deboralied Benjamin, Ephraim und Machir als selbständige Stämme nennt. Ist damit, wenn man von der Erwähnung Machirs an Stelle von Manasse absieht, die 3. Form praktisch für die Entstehungszeit des Deboraliedes, d. h. für das 12. Jh. v. Chr., belegt, so muß die 1. Form älter sein und der ausgehenden Landnahmezeit oder beginnenden Richterzeit angehören.

Es läßt sich also nicht bestreiten, daß man das Schema der zwölf Stämme in der Richterzeit aufgestellt und in drei Formen abgewandelt hat. Sicherlich handelt es sich darin nicht um eine bloße Theorie und fiktive Konstruktion, obschon die genannten Stämme weder gemeinsam Palästina erobert und sich dort angesiedelt noch nach dem in Wirklichkeit ganz anders verlaufenen Vorgang der Landnahme mehr oder weniger zufällig eine Zwölfzahl gebildet hätten. Zweifellos hat M. Noth darin Recht, daß das Schema weder eine historische Situation genau wiedergibt noch reine Theorie ist[52]. Eher läßt sich sagen: Es ist eine Theorie in Anpassung an die historische Situation. Primär ist die Grundidee der Zwölfzahl, an die die tatsächlichen Verhältnisse mehrfach angeglichen und angepaßt worden sind; daraus erklären sich in der Tat die verschiedenen Formen des Schemas.

Welchen Sinn hat die vorgegebene Zwölfzahl? Sie weist jedenfalls nicht gleich auf eine Amphiktyonie hin, sondern ist auch für andere Zusammenhänge typisch, z. B. für die Zwölfgöttersysteme Ägyptens, Griechenlands und Italiens oder für das römische Zwölftafelgesetz. Sie hat überhaupt für das antike Denken eine wichtige Rolle gespielt; sie ist eine kosmische Zahl, die Zahl des Tierkreises und der Monate

---

[51] M. Noth a. a. O. (Anm. 4) 14. 17f. 30.
[52] M. Noth a. a. O. (Anm. 4) 39ff.

des Jahres, die Grundzahl des Sexagesimalsystems, letztlich die runde Zahl einer Gesamtheit[53]. Aus der Zwölfzahl der israelitischen Stämme in den wechselnden Formen läßt sich nichts anderes ersehen, als daß die angeführten Stämme jeweils die Gesamtheit Israels darstellen sollten.

Wenigstens die 1. Form des Schemas kann aus einem weiteren Grunde nicht die Liste einer Jahwe-Amphiktyonie gewesen sein. Folgen wir M. Noth in der Datierung der 2. Form in die früheste Richterzeit und der 3. Form in deren zweite Hälfte, so gehört die 1. Form in die Periode unmittelbar nach der Einwanderung der letzten in ihr erwähnten israelitischen Stämme. In dieser Zeit befand sich die Moseschar, die nicht mit dem »Haus Joseph« identisch ist, erst auf dem Wege nach Palästina. Da sie den Jahweglauben mitgebracht hat, der dann allmählich von den israelitischen Stämmen angenommen wurde, wie es Jos 24 für den Stamm Ephraim zeigt, war vorher — also zur Zeit der 1. Form des Schemas — die Bildung einer israelitischen Amphiktyonie auf dem Boden des Jahweglaubens unmöglich. Dem entspricht es, daß die Gesamtheit der Stämme mit dem Namen Israel bezeichnet worden ist, d. h. mit einem nicht-jahwe-haltigen Namen.

Endlich stellen wir fest, daß das Schema noch in der Richterzeit erstarrt ist. Das Verschwinden von Ruben und Simeon und das Entstehen von Machir wird nicht mehr berücksichtigt. Sollte eine Amphiktyonenliste schon so früh gänzlich eingefroren sein? Daß man das Schema nicht weitergeführt hat, hängt doch wohl eher mit dem Abschluß des Seßhaftwerdens und der endgültigen Ansiedlung zusammen, woraufhin die frühere Rolle der Stämme von den inzwischen festgelegten Territorien ihrer Landgebiete übernommen wurde. Demgemäß entspricht das Schema in erster Linie den Verhältnissen der vorseßhaften Stammesgliederung der nomadischen oder halbnomadischen Zeit der Israeliten, wie denn auch die übrigen Sechser- und Zwölferlisten des Alten Testaments zunächst nicht seßhafte Nomadenstämme betreffen.

Wenden wir uns diesem Bereich zu, so wird sogleich deutlich, was das Schema der Zwölfzahl von Stämmen bedeutet: Es ist genau das, was es nach dem Willen des Alten Testaments sein soll — eine genealogische Liste zur Feststellung der Abstammungs- und Verwandtschaftsverhältnisse. Der Stamm besteht ja aus einer Reihe von Familien und Sippen, die sich von einem gemeinsamen Ahnherrn herleiten, dem Stamm dessen Namen geben, sich als sein »Haus« oder seine »Söhne« und gegenseitig als »Brüder« im weiteren Sinn verstehen.

---

[53] Vgl. vor allem F. Heiler, Erscheinungsformen und Wesen der Religion, 1961, 171f., mit weiterer Lit. 161f.

Das gilt sogar, wenn sich nicht miteinander verwandte Sippen zusammenschließen oder wenn fremde Sippen in einen Stamm aufgenommen werden. Diese Eingliederung läßt sich beispielsweise im Falle der in Juda aufgegangenen Sippe Kaleb vom ursprünglichen Bewußtsein ihrer Fremdheit bis zur Herstellung einer genealogischen Verbindung mit Juda deutlich verfolgen[54]. Wie für die einzelnen Stämme gilt das Verwandtschaftsschema für ihr Verhältnis zueinander. Auch die Beziehungen zwischen verschiedenen Stämmen werden in verwandtschaftlichen Kategorien ausgedrückt, so daß zwei Stämme ihre Gemeinsamkeit in der Weise umschreiben, daß sie sich auf zwei Ahnen zurückführen, die wirkliche Brüder gewesen sein sollen. Wie also die jeweils lebende Generation eines Stammes sich mit ihrem angeblichen Ahnen verwandt weiß und darum gemeinsam lebt, so weiß sie sich mit anderen Stämmen verwandt, deren Ahnen als Brüder des eigenen erscheinen. Dadurch ermöglichen sich das Zusammenleben mehrerer Stämme, die gemeinsame Benutzung eines Heiligtums und ein gelegentliches militärisches Bündnis.

Von da aus erklärt sich ungezwungen das Schema der zwölf israelitischen Stämme, das die Gesamtheit Israels in einer genealogischen Liste erfaßt. Anders als in den gelehrten und umfassenden Genealogien der Priesterschrift, der Chronik und des Islam[55] lebt in ihm die ältere und volkstümliche Tradition weiter. Es stellt eine kurze volkstümliche Genealogie dar und konstituiert die durch Bande der Blutsverwandtschaft zusammengehaltene Gemeinschaft Israel als vom Stammvater her verwandt, wie der gewöhnlich mit »Volk« übersetzte hebräische Ausdruck 'ăm besagt. Jener Ahn ist der mit Jakob gleichgesetzte Israel (vgl. Gen 32 29)[56]; ja, nach der genealogischen Aneinanderreihung der Patriarchen ist der 'ăm Israel eigentlich schon in der Familie Abrahams vorhanden. Natürlich hat nach der Annahme des Jahweglaubens auch dieser als einigendes Band gewirkt.

III.

Aus den angeführten Gründen scheint es mir ratsam, die Amphiktyonie-Hypothese durch die Annahme zu ersetzen, daß das Schema der zwölf Stämme Israels eine kurze volkstümliche Genealogie darstellt, die während der Frühzeit in wechselnden Formen entsprechend

---

[54] Vgl. R. de Vaux a. a. O. 22f.
[55] F. Wüstenfeld, Genealogische Tabellen der arabischen Stämme und Familien, 1852.
[56] Vgl. H. Seebaß, Der Stammvater Israel, 1966. Das Israel der Stele des Pharao Merneptah um 1220 kann die alte Israelsippe gewesen sein, die nach ihrer weitgehenden Vernichtung durch die Ägypter in einer anderen israelitischen Gruppe aufging, was die Gleichsetzung Israel-Jakob ermöglichte.

dem jeweiligen Bestand an Stämmen und unter Anpassung der Wirklichkeit an die vorgegebene Zwölfzahl die Gemeinschaft Israel konstituiert. Doch damit ist die gesamte Problematik noch nicht behandelt. Denn in Verbindung mit der Amphiktyonie-Hypothese, aber auch unabhängig von ihr, wird vielfach die Ansicht vertreten, daß das Verhältnis zwischen Jahwe und Israel grundlegend und stets durch einen »Bund« (b^{e}rît) geformt worden sei. Insbesondere scheint der amphiktyonische Bund der Stämme untereinander dem »Bund« zwischen Jahwe und dem amphiktyonisch organisierten Israel zu entsprechen. Ist aber die Amphiktyonie-Hypothese unwahrscheinlich, so legt sich die Frage nahe, wie es um die Vorstellung vom »Bund« zwischen Jahwe und Israel bestellt sein mag. Daher ist es nötig, dieser Frage in der gebotenen Kürze nachzugehen. Es handelt sich im folgenden weder um eine umfassende Untersuchung des Inhalts oder der wechselnden Inhalte der b^{e}rît-Vorstellung noch um eine Untersuchung der Bedeutung des Begriffs b^{e}rît; sie ließe sich auf wenigen Seiten keinesfalls vornehmen, wenn sich auch aus den Erwägungen in IV. ergeben wird, daß die Übersetzung mit »Bund« nicht sachgemäß ist und daher im folgenden vermieden wird. Außerdem muß zuvor die Frage geklärt sein, die hier in erster Linie behandelt werden soll: die Frage nach dem geschichtlichen Vorkommen der b^{e}rît-Vorstellung. Wie bei derjenigen nach der möglichen geschichtlichen Existenz einer israelitischen Amphiktyonie geht es bei dieser Frage darum, Auftreten und Rolle der b^{e}rît-Vorstellung festzustellen. Wann, wo, mit welchem Gewicht und welchem Einfluß auf den Gehalt des Jahweglaubens hat sie bestanden?

Seit alters hat es nahegelegen, die b^{e}rît-Vorstellung als grundlegend zu betrachten. Das bezeugen schon die Bezeichnungen Altes und Neues »Testament«, d. h. alter und neuer »Bund« im Blick auf den von Jahwe durch Mose mit Israel geschlossen alten und den in Jesus Christus gegebenen neuen »Bund« und im Blick auf die heiligen Schriften, die davon handeln und also die Bücher des alten und des neuen »Bundes« sind. Doch der weiteren Entwicklung kann und soll an dieser Stelle nicht nachgegangen werden. Wir stellen nur fest, daß sie immer wieder in Bewegung geraten und bis in die Gegenwart hinein zu wechselnden Auffassungen und neuen Hypothesen geführt hat. Über die jüngste Phase hat D. J. MacCarthy zusammenfassend und abwägend berichtet[57].

Dem steht gegenüber, daß sich mehr als eine Stimme gegen die Überschätzung der b^{e}rît-Vorstellung erhoben hat. Für sie alle mag das Ergebnis der umfangreichen Untersuchung von J. J. P. Valeton jr.

---

[57] D. J. McCarthy, Covenant in the Old Testament: the Present State of Inquiry, CBQ 27 (1965), 217—240; Der Gottesbund im Alten Testament, 1966.

stehen: »1⁰. Vor der deuteronomisch-jeremianischen Zeit kommt das Wort *Berith* in religiöser Anwendung nur vereinzelt vor. Von den pentateuchischen Quellen gebraucht es nur J, von den Propheten nur Hosea; außerdem steht es 1 Kön. XIX 14. — 2⁰. Der eigentliche Gebrauch des Wortes in religiöser Beziehung stammt aus der deuteronomisch-jeremianischen Zeit. Erwähnt wird da eine *Berith* mit den Vätern (eidliche Zusage des Landes Kanaan); — eine bei dem Auszug aus Ägypten, am Horeb und auf den Feldern Moabs geschlossene *Berith*, deren Urkunde das Hilkianische (deuteronomische) Gesetzbuch ist; eine *Berith* mit Levi und den Priestern (Deut. XXXIII 29, Maleachi, Neh. XIII 29, in einer dem Jeremia unterschobenen Stelle Jer. XXXIII 20 f. und in PC Num. XXV 12 f.); — eine *Berith* mit David, welche sich in der Zukunft bewähren wird (außer 2 Sam. XXIII 5, und in der obengenannten Jeremia unterschobenen Stelle, nur in der Chronik und im Psalter). — 3⁰. Im Großen und Ganzen ist *Berith* die stehende Benennung für ein freundliches, der göttlichen חסד entsprossenes Verhältnis zwischen Gott und dem betreffenden Menschen (Israel). Die Frage nach dem geschichtlichen Ursprung desselben tritt dabei in den Hintergrund. In einigen Stellen des B. Daniel wird die ganze jüdische Religion ihrem Wesen nach mit diesem Namen bezeichnet. — 4⁰. Die *Berith* offenbart sich einerseits in Verheißungen und Zusagen Gottes, andererseits in gewissen den Menschen vorgeschriebenen Verpflichtungen ... — 5⁰. In PC ist das Wort *Berith* ein theologischer Kunstausdruck ...«[58] Doch nicht nur Valeton, dessen Beurteilung erneuter Überprüfung bedarf[59], hat die $b^e rît$-Vorstellung kritisch eingeschätzt. Auch W. Eichrodt, der sie als Grundlage seiner alttestamentlichen Theologie gewählt hat, weist auf die Schwierigkeit hin, daß die »Bundes«-Vorstellung in der klassischen Prophetie bis zu Jeremia durchaus in den Hintergrund rückt. Er löst sie durch die Annahme, daß bei der kritischen Gesamteinstellung der Propheten zu dem geistigen Besitz ihres Volkes ihnen der »Bundes«-Gedanke im Kampf gegen alles *opus operatum* nicht helfen konnte und daß sie nur durch den Hinweis auf die Rettung aus Ägypten, nicht aber auf den Sinai-»Bund«, die zuvorkommende Gnade Jahwes in deutlicheres Licht

---

[58] J. J. P. Valeton jr., Bedeutung und Stellung des Wortes ברית im Priestercodex, ZAW 12 (1892), 1—22; Das Wort ברית in den jehovistischen und deuteronomischen Stücken des Hexateuchs, sowie in den verwandten historischen Büchern, ebd. 224—260; Das Wort ברית bei den Propheten und in den Ketubim, Resultat, ebd. 13 (1893), 245—279. Noch schärfer und entschiedener R. Kraetzschmar, Die Bundesvorstellung im Alten Testament in ihrer geschichtlichen Entwicklung, 1896.

[59] So ist z. B. die Frage des Vorkommens beim Elohisten neu zu prüfen, Hosea erwähnt den religiösen »Bund« nicht, weil 6 7 sich auf den Vertrag zwischen König und Volk bezieht und 8 1-3 ein späteres Wort ist.

setzen und die falsche Verkehrung seines Handelns in eine pflichtgemäße Leistung des »Bundes«-Gottes abwehren konnten[60]. Ganz so einfach, wie man vielfach vorausgesetzt hat, scheint der Sachverhalt sowohl bei den vordeuteronomischen Geschichtserzählern als auch bei den vorexilischen großen Einzelpropheten nicht zu sein.

So ist es verständlich, daß A. Jepsen eine andere Ansicht geäußert hat: Während sich für die vorexilische Zeit nur wenige Belege für eine göttliche $b^e rît$ finden, wird im deuteronomistischen und priesterschriftlichen Geschichtswerk, bei den Propheten des 6. Jh. und in meist späten Psalmen häufig davon gesprochen. »Das bedeutet doch wohl, daß *Berith* ein Theologumenon geworden ist, mit dessen Hilfe die Geschichte der Vergangenheit und Zukunft gedeutet wird« und das eine »feierliche Zusage Gottes« bedeutet[61]. Erst recht findet C. F. Whitley keine Grundlage für die Annahme, daß eine Sinai-$b^e rît$ die Einheit zwischen den Stämmen Israels hergestellt oder daß die $b^e rît$-Vorstellung von den Kanaanäern übernommen worden sei, zumal die vorexilischen Propheten die Beziehung Israels zu Jahwe nicht mittels der $b^e rît$, sondern durch die Bande natürlicher Verwandtschaft hergestellt sehen. Darum muß man bezweifeln, ob es in vordeuteronomischer Zeit eine »Bundes«-Vorstellung gegeben hat. Auch der Dekalog ist erst deuteronomischer Herkunft und vom priesterlichen Redaktor in die Sinaitradition aufgenommen worden[62]. Ebenso findet R. Smend die formelhafte Aussage, daß Jahwe der Gott Israels und Israel das Volk Jahwes sei, in ihrer vollen Form erst beim »Bundes«-Schluß Josias in der deuteronomischen Zeit vor. Weder in der vorstaatlichen noch in der frühen Königszeit hat es die zweiseitige Formel gegeben; sie setzt den entscheidenden Anstoß der prophetischen Krise voraus, wie sich denn auch bei Hosea der Übergang von Einzelwendungen zur Vorbereitung der vollen Formel vollzieht[63]. Schließlich hat E. Kutsch gezeigt, daß der Ausdruck $b^e rît$, den man meist mit »Bund« übersetzt, in Wirklichkeit als Selbstverpflichtung und als Verpflichtung eines anderen, daneben als gegenseitige Verpflichtung zu verstehen ist. Wo Jahwe Subjekt der $b^e rît$ ist, erscheint diese als seine Selbstverpflichtung in Form seiner gnädigen Zusage oder als die Verpflichtung, die er dem Menschen auferlegt. Doch während der Ausdruck im profanen Bereich geläufig war, begegnet er in Beziehung auf Gott und Mensch während

---

[60] W. Eichrodt, Theologie des Alten Testaments, I 1959[6], 19f.

[61] A. Jepsen, Berith, ein Beitrag zur Theologie der Exilszeit, in: Rudolph-Festschrift, 1961, 161—179.

[62] C. F. Whitley, Covenant and Commandment in Israel, JNES 22 (1963), 37—48. Die Annahme bezüglich des Dekalogs stellt die sogleich zu erwähnende Bundesformular-Hypothese in Frage.

[63] R. Smend, Die Bundesformel, 1963.

der vordeuteronomischen Zeit sehr selten. Daher wird die Ansicht, daß Israel seit seiner Frühzeit die Vorstellung von einem Jahwe-»Bund« als grundlegend erachtet habe, aufgrund der tatsächlichen Bedeutung von $b^e r\hat{\imath}t$ und der seltenen Verwendung des Ausdrucks in Beziehung auf Gott und Mensch während der vordeuteronomischen Zeit hinfällig[64].

Neuerdings schien sich eine Möglichkeit anzubieten, um alle Schwierigkeiten zu überbrücken und die Annahme einer fortdauernden »Bundes«-Vorstellung zu sichern. Man hat die altorientalischen, insbesondere die hetitischen Suzeränitäts- oder Vasallenverträge herangezogen[65], in denen weder zwei gleichwertige Partner einen Vertrag schließen noch ein Mächtiger gegenüber einem Schwächeren eine Selbstverpflichtung eingeht, vielmehr die Verpflichtungen dem schwächeren Empfänger, dem Vasallen, auferlegt werden, während der Mächtige sich auf allgemeine Treueversprechen beschränkt. Darin erblickt man vielfach das Vorbild und Muster für die alttestamentliche »Bundes«-Vorstellung und weist auf die Parallelität zwischen dem Formular der Vasallenverträge und der postulierten alttestamentlichen Gattung der »Bundes«-Urkunde, dem sog. »Bundes«-Formular, hin, vor allem in den Dekalogen Ex 20 und 34, ferner Dtn 4 29f. und Jos 24. In beiden sollen aufeinanderfolgen: Eröffnungsformel, Einzelbedingungen, Liste der Vertragszeugen, Segen und Fluch[66]. Danach erscheint die Form des »Bundes« von der alten bis in die junge Zeit als gleichbleibend. Diese Auffassung hat weitere Hypothesen nach sich gezogen, so über das Passa als »Bundes«-Schluß[67], über die prophetische Gerichtsrede als Ultimatum des Oberherrn an den Vasallen[68] und über die Flüche als Sanktionen im Alten Testament

---

[64] E. Kutsch, Gesetz und Gnade, ZAW 79 (1967), 18—35; Der Begriff בְּרִית in vordeuteronomischer Zeit, in: Rost-Festschrift, 1967, 133—143.

[65] Vgl. vor allem, V. Korošec, Hethische Staatsverträge, 1931; R. Borger, Zu den Asarhaddon-Verträgen aus Nimrud, ZA 54 (1961), 173—196; weitere Lit. für den ganzen Alten Orient bei F. Nötscher (Anm. 71).

[66] Nach ersten Andeutungen von E. Bikerman in: Archives d'Histoire du Droit Oriental 5 (1950/51), 153f., entwickelt von G. E. Mendenhall, Recht und Bund in Israel und im Alten Vordern Orient, 1960 (englisch 1954 und 1955); danach u. a. J. Muilenburg, The Form and Structure of the Covenantal Formulations, VT 9 (1959), 347—365; K. Baltzer, Das Bundesformular, 1966²; W. Beyerlin, Herkunft und Geschichte der ältesten Sinaitraditionen, 1961; J. L'Hour, L'alliance de Sichem, RB 69 (1962), 5—36. 161—184. 350—368; N. Lohfink, Das Hauptgebot, 1963; D. J. McCarthy, Treaty and Covenant, 1963.

[67] G. E. Mendenhall, Puppy and Lettuce in Northwest-Semitic Covenant-Making, BASOR 133 (1954), 26—30.

[68] J. Harvey, Le »Rîb—Pattern«, réquisitoire prophétique sur la rupture de l'alliance, Bibl 43 (1962), 172—196.

und vor allem in den prophetischen Drohworten[69]. Diese Beispiele mögen genügen, um die erkennbare Tendenz zu verdeutlichen.

Während demgegenüber E. Gerstenberger einen Zusammenhang solcher sozialen Gebote wie derjenigen des Dekalogs in Ex 20 mit den Bedingungen der Vasallenverträge für den Vertragspartner bestreitet und ihren Ursprung (wie auch denjenigen der Weisheitslehre) in der urtümlichen Ordnung des Vaters, des Weisen oder des Stammeshauptes sieht[70], hat F. Nötscher das Verhältnis zwischen den Verträgen und dem Alten Testament erstmals gründlich überprüft. Einerseits stellt er dabei wesentliche formale und inhaltliche Unterschiede zwischen den Vertragstexten und den Ausdrucksformen der Jahwe-$b^e r\hat{\imath}t$ fest und weist andererseits auf die heterogenetische Erklärungsmöglichkeit für Ausdrucksformen gleicher oder ähnlicher Erscheinungen hin. Das zwingt zur Zurückhaltung gegenüber der vorschnellen Annahme geschichtlicher oder gar literarischer Abhängigkeit[71]. Wegen ihrer grundlegenden Bedeutung sei auf diese Ausführungen nachdrücklich hingewiesen.

In der Tat sind die angeblichen Parallelen zwischen Vertrags- und alttestamentlichen Texten vielfach fragwürdig, wie das Beispiel Ex 20 2 zeigen mag: Die Selbsteinführung »Ich bin Jahwe« ist gattungsmäßig dem »So (spricht) die Sonne Murschilisch« nicht gleich; dessen Parallele läge eher in dem »So spricht Jahwe« vor. Die Erwähnung der Herausführung aus Ägypten, das grundlegende Bekenntnis Israels, ist nicht mit der Vorgeschichte des Vertragsschlusses gleichzusetzen (z. B. »obwohl du krank warst, habe ich, die Sonne, dich doch in die Stellung deines Vaters eingesetzt«), wie auch das Verhältnis Israels zu Jahwe — achtet man auf die alten Ansätze zu der ein ganz anderes Verhältnis umschreibenden sog. »Bundes-Formel«[72] — keineswegs der Bindung des Vasallen an seinen Oberherrn entspricht. Zudem gehört Ex 20 2 überhaupt nicht zum alten Bestand des Dekalogs, sondern ist eine deuteronomistische Erweiterung, so daß das angenommene »Bundes«-Formular zerfällt. Daß die Behauptung der Abhängigkeit alttestamentlicher Texte vom Vertragsschema ebensowenig zutrifft, zeigt das Beispiel der prophetischen Drohworte. Sie knüpfen an eine Tradition magischer Verwünschungen an, wie sie vor allem in Sammlungen

---

[69] F. Ch. Fensham, Malediction and Benediction in Ancient Near Eastern Vassal-Treaties and the Old Testament, ZAW 74 (1962), 1—9; Common Trends in Curses of the Near Eastern Treaties and *kudurru*-Inscriptions compared with Maledictions of Amos an Isaiah, ebd. 75 (1963), 155—175; auch VT 13 (1963), 133—143; D. R. Hillers, Treaty-Curses and the Old Testament Prophets, 1964.
[70] E. Gerstenberger, Covenant and Commandment, JBL 84 (1965), 38—51.
[71] F. Nötscher, Bundesformular und »Amtsschimmel«, BZ NF 9 (1965), 181—214.
[72] Vgl. Anm. 63.

von Beschwörungsritualen und -texten wie den babylonischen Serien Maqlû und Schurpu vorliegen. Die Vasallenverträge sind von diesen in gleicher Weise abhängig[73].

Wohin man fassen mag — die Vasallenvertrag-Hypothese erweist sich als brüchig und fragwürdig. Das gilt schließlich auch für die Frage nach der geschichtlichen Möglichkeit einer Übernahme des altorientalischen, insbesondere des hetitischen Formulars. Wie hätte denn die Sinai-b^{e}rît im Wüstengebiet Nordarabiens nach dem Muster hetitischer Verträge zwischen den kleinasiatischen Oberherren und ihren nordsyrischen und anderen angrenzenden Vasallen gestaltet werden können? Will man im Ernst annehmen, daß das Schema solcher Verträge den nomadischen Arabern oder Israeliten am Sinai genau bekannt gewesen wäre — ihnen, die vermutlich nicht einmal von der Existenz der Vertragspartner, geschweige denn der Abmachungen zwischen diesen wußten? Zudem gehörten die Verträge in den Bereich der großen Politik und besaßen für das tägliche Leben nomadischer Stämme nicht die geringste Bedeutung, so daß auf deren Seite kein Interesse an ihnen bestanden hat, aufgrund dessen sie sich um Einblick in die Verträge hätten bemühen können.

Es liegt wohl in der Ironie der Forschungsgeschichte, daß ein Vertreter der Vasallenvertrag-Hypothese selber das Vertrauen in diese erschüttert. N. Lohfink sucht eine »innerdeuteronomische Kritik am Bundesformular und an der damit verbundenen Institution des Gottesbundes Israels« nachzuweisen und führt als Grund für diese Kritik die rechtliche Herkunft und Bestimmtheit von »Bund« und »Bundes«-Formular an: »Der Bund Israels zeigt sich gerade in seinem formgeschichtlich erschließbaren Ansatz als eine theologisch durchaus nicht in jeder Hinsicht positiv zu bewertende Institution und Denkform.« Demnach rief sogar die »Bundes«-Vorstellung überhaupt, erst recht natürlich ihre vom Vasallenvertrag bestimmte Form, Schwierigkeiten hervor und brachte Gefahren mit sich[74]. Warum aber hätte man dann mit der Übernahme von »Bundes«-Vorstellung und -Formular einen solch verhängnisvollen Mißgriff tun und jahrhundertelang nicht beheben sollen — und dies trotz der Abneigung gegen fremde Einflüsse auf Glaube und Kultus bei den für die Übernahme und Beibehaltung verantwortlichen Vertretern des Jahweglaubens, ja, schon bei Mose selbst? Es ist nicht wahrscheinlich, daß ein im Ansatz gefährlicher Gedanke von Anfang an maßgeblich gewesen und nur unter einem Formzwang bis zur deuteronomischen Kritik beibehalten worden ist.

---

[73] G. Fohrer, Prophetie und Magie, ZAW 78 (1966), 38—40 (= Studien zur alttestamentlichen Prophetie [1949—1965], 1967, 242—264).

[74] N. Lohfink, Die Wandlung des Bundesbegriffes im Buche Deuteronomium, in: Rahner-Festschrift, I 1964, 423—444.

Daher kann die überbrückende Vasallenvertrag-Hypothese außer acht bleiben, so daß wir erneut vor der Frage nach dem geschichtlichen Vorkommen der b^{e}rît-Vorstellung stehen.

IV.

1. Überblicken wir den Bereich der drei älteren Quellenschichten des Hexateuchs[75] nach Erwähnungen einer göttlichen b^{e}rît — denn nur solche kommen für die Bewertung ernsthaft in Frage —, so müssen einige von ihnen, die man zunächst zu berücksichtigen geneigt sein könnte, aus zwingenden Gründen ausscheiden:

a) Ex 19 5 in dem erst aus dem Ende der judäischen Königszeit stammenden Abschnitt Ex 19 3b-8[76];

b) Ex 23 32 in der elohistischen Quellenschicht, das ein Abkommen mit den Kanaanäern und ihren Göttern, durch das sie von der Vertreibung verschont blieben, untersagt;

c) Num 10 33 14 44 Jos 3 3. 6 u. ö. mit Erwähnungen der Lade des »Bundes«, die sämtlich deuteronomistisch oder nachexilisch sind[77]; Num 25 12 f. als zur Priesterschrift oder späterer Bearbeitung gehörig[78];

d) Jos 24 25 in dem zuletzt deuteronomistisch bearbeiteten Abschnitt Jos 24 (s. o. II, 3), zumal die Verbindung »Satzung und Recht« noch in junger Zeit begegnet (Dtn 4 8 I Reg 9 4);

e) Jdc 2 1 b in dem späten Zusatz Jdc 2 1 b-5 a, zumal es sich lediglich um einen Rückverweis auf die Sinai-b^{e}rît handelt.

Von den verbleibenden Erwähnungen einer göttlichen b^{e}rît ist sogleich über Jos 7 11. 15 zu sagen, daß der Ausdruck dort die Sonderbedeutung »Gebot, Anordnung« besitzt: Achan hat mit seinem Diebstahl das Gebot Jahwes übertreten, sich nichts vom Banngut anzueignen, so daß der Zorn Jahwes entbrannte und die Israeliten im Kampf um Ai eine Niederlage erleiden ließ. Nun haben nach dem archäologischen Befund die Israeliten um die längst zerstörte und unbesiedelte Stätte von Ai überhaupt nicht kämpfen können, sind die Anschauungen der Erzähler über den Bann von recht theoretischer Natur[79] und ist das Banngebot zumindest für das Verständnis der älteren Zeit nicht mit einer b^{e}rît verknüpft und bei deren Setzung

---

[75] Vgl. dazu E. Sellin—G. Fohrer a. a. O. § 22—24. 30.
[76] E. Sellin—G. Fohrer a. a. O. 205 f.; G. Fohrer, »Königliches Priestertum« (Ex 19 6), ThZ 19 (1963), S. 359—362 (s. u. 149—153).
[77] Vgl. die Übersicht bei J. Maier a. a. O. 84 f.
[78] Vgl. die Nachweise bei O. Eißfeldt, Hexateuch-Synopse, 1922, 278*.
[79] Vgl. C. H. W. Brekelmans, De Ḥerem in het Oude Testament, 1959.

gegeben worden. So läßt sich aus Jos 7 jedenfalls für die b^{e}rît-Vorstellung nichts entnehmen.

Anders verhält es sich mit Gen 15 18, das mit 15 1 b β-2. 7-12. 17-19 zur Quellenschicht des Jahwisten gehört, während der übrige Teil des Abschnitts dem Elohisten zuzuweisen ist[80]. Der Jahwist erzählt, wie Abraham nach seiner Klage über seine Kinderlosigkeit auf Geheiß Jahwes aus getöteten und teilweise zerteilten Tieren eine Gasse bildet, durch die nach Einbruch der Dunkelheit ein rauchender Ofen und eine Feuerfackel hindurchfährt: »An jenem Tage schnitt Jahwe eine b^{e}rît mit Abram und sprach: Deinen Nachkommen will ich dieses Land geben, vom Strome Ägyptens bis zum großen Strome, dem Euphratstrome.« Will man nicht mit A. Caquot annehmen, daß Gen 15 einen Midrasch nach Art von Gen 14 bildet, eine patriarchalische Pseudotradition, die unter Benutzung einer Abraham-Tradition in Wirklichkeit David und seine Dynastie unter Rückprojizierung des die nationale Unabhängigkeit garantierenden Erbkönigtums in die Patriarchenzeit verherrlichen will[81], wofür wenig spricht, so bleiben die wahrscheinlichen Annahmen von A. Alt und A. Jepsen, daß der Erzählung des Jahwisten eine alte b^{e}rît-Tradition des »Gottes Abrahams«, eine Erinnerung an die Offenbarung des »Gottes Abrahams«, durch die dem Abraham Nachkommen und Landbesitz verheißen wurde, zugrunde liegt[82]. Nach unseren freilich geringen Kenntnissen des Vätergottglaubens bildet es in der Tat einen wesentlichen Teil dieser Sippen- oder Stammesreligionen, daß die Gottheit dem Sippenahnen, dem sie sich geoffenbart hat und von dem sie verehrt wird, eine verheißende Zusage macht und zu deren Verwirklichung eine dauernde Verpflichtung eingeht oder von sich aus auf sich nimmt. Die b^{e}rît ist also eigentlich die eidliche Zusicherung im Zusammenhang des gesamten Verhältnisses zwischen der Gottheit und dem Sippenahnen. Der dabei angewendete Ritus ist eine bedingte Selbstverfluchung oder -verurteilung, wie Jer 34 17 ff. und der Vertrag der Könige Bar-ga'jā von KTK und Matī'-'el von Arpad auf der Stele von Sfire I, A 39f. aus der Mitte des 8. Jh. v. Chr. zeigen[83]: Wenn derjenige, der sich verpflichtet

---

[80] Eine andere Aufteilung neuerdings wieder bei R. E. Clements, Abraham and David, 1967; O. Kaiser, Traditionsgeschichtliche Untersuchung von Genesis 15, ZAW 70 (1958), 107—126; N. Lohfink, Die Landverheißung als Eid, 1967; H. Seebaß, Zu Genesis 15, Wort und Dienst NF 7 (1963), 132—149.

[81] A. Caquot, L'alliance avec Abram (Genèse 15), Semitica 12 (1962), 51—66.

[82] A. Alt a. a. O. (Anm. 9); A. Jepsen a. a. O.

[83] Vgl. die Übersetzung in H. Donner—W. Röllig, Kanaanäische und aramäische Inschriften, II 1964, 240. Dagegen spielt der von J. Henninger, Was bedeutet die rituelle Teilung eines Tieres in zwei Hälften?, Bibl 34 (1953), 344—353, betonte Gedanke der mystisch-sakramentalen Vereinigung schwerlich eine Rolle.

hat, die getroffene Vereinbarung nicht einhält oder erfüllt, dann möge er wie die Tiere zerschnitten werden! Wie auch diese in bezug auf die Gottheit anthropomorphe Vorstellung nahelegt, meint die Erzählung des Jahwisten in Gen 15 ursprünglich wohl einen Teil des gesamten Vorgangs, in dem eine dauernde Beziehung zwischen Vätergott und Sippenahne hergestellt wurde. Ihm hat gewiß ein Gelöbnis des Menschen, z. B. das der kultischen Verehrung der Gottheit, entsprochen (wie Ex 34 27f.); auch ein Mahl, wie die Quellenschicht N es in Ex 24 9-11 für die Sinai-*berît* erwähnt (ohne den Ausdruck *berît* zu verwenden), kann der Herstellung der Gemeinschaft gedient haben.

Werden wir mit Gen 15 in die nomadische oder halbnomadische Frühzeit der Israeliten vor ihrer Bekanntschaft mit dem Jahweglauben zurückgeführt, so handelt es sich in einer derartigen *berît* um die Konstituierung einer nomadischen Religion. In ihr gilt die Gottheit mit der sie verehrenden Sippe als verwandt, als »Vater« oder »Bruder« des Menschen, wie noch die alten Personennamen zeigen[84]. Nicht anders ist die *berît* zwischen Jahwe und der Moseschar am Gottesberge Sinai oder Horeb zu verstehen, auf die die Quellenschicht N mit dem erwähnten Mahl anspielt und die der Jahwist im Zusammenhang mit dem sog. kultischen Dekalog in Ex 34 10. 27f. und der Elohist im Zusammenhang mit der Verpflichtung des Volkes, die sich ursprünglich auf den elohistischen Dekalog in Ex 20 bezogen hat, in Ex 24 7f. ausdrücklich nennen. Die Erinnerung an sie ist in den drei alten Quellenschichten fest verankert, so daß an einem entsprechenden Akt der Moseschar wohl nicht zu zweifeln ist. Offensichtlich handelt es sich wie in den Vätergottreligionen um ein einmaliges geschichtliches Ereignis, das die ständige Beziehung zwischen Jahwe und der Moseschar im Sinne einer fortdauernden Lebensgemeinschaft nach nomadischer Art begründen sollte. So ist denn das Verhältnis zwischen beiden ähnlich dem Verhältnis zwischen den Vatergöttern und den Patriarchensippen vorzustellen: als Verwandtschaftsverhältnis, in dem die Moseschar als *'ăm* Jahwes gilt. Demgemäß spricht nach R. Smend nichts dagegen, eher einiges dafür, daß die aus Ägypten gekommenen Israeliten außer der Verehrung des Gottes Jahwe auch den Ausdruck »Volk Jahwes« nach Palästina mitgebracht haben[85]; es ist ja auch auffällig, daß sich Suffixformen des Wortes *'ăm*, in denen das Suffix Jahwe bezeichnet, gerade in der Exodusüberlieferung gehäuft finden (vgl. Ex 3 7. 10 5 1. 23 7 16 8 16 ff. 9 1. 13 10 3).

---

[84] M. Noth, Die israelitischen Personennamen im Rahmen der gemeinsemitischen Namengebung, 1928.

[85] R. Smend a. a. O. 16. Nach seiner Statistik begegnet der Ausdruck etwa zehnmal; dazu kommen weniger als 300 Suffixformen, in denen das Suffix Jahwe bezeichnet (z. B. »mein Volk«).

Für die vor- und frühjahwistische Zeit ist also die Vorstellung einer b^{e}rît zwischen einem Vätergott und einer menschlichen Gruppe zur Begründung einer dauernden Lebensgemeinschaft im nomadischen Sinn, die durch das Verwandtschaftsverhältnis ausgedrückt wird, als sicher anzunehmen.

2. Von der Richterzeit an ändert sich das Bild völlig. Man weiß gewiß von der Sinai-b^{e}rît (und teilweise von einer Abraham-b^{e}rît wie der Jahwist), doch nicht sie, sondern die Rettung aus Ägypten wird zum grundlegenden Bekenntnis Israels. Die Sinai-b^{e}rît ist ein geschichtlicher Vorgang, der einmal der Konstituierung des »Volkes Jahwes« gedient hat. Damit hat sie ihre Schuldigkeit getan und tritt zurück. Das »Volk Jahwes«, von dem das Deboralied in Jdc 5 13 und erst recht die Zeit nach der Staatsbildung[86] in Gleichsetzung mit Israel reden, gibt die Überlieferung von der Sinai-b^{e}rît zwar weiter und weist ihr in den Quellenschichten des Hexateuchs einen entsprechenden Platz in den Gesamtüberlieferungen seiner Frühzeit zu, lebt aber nicht mehr aus ihr, nachdem es die nomadischen Lebensverhältnisse aufgegeben hat, sondern pflegt seine Existenz als »Volk Jahwes« vor allem durch den Kultus im Kulturlande. Aus der veränderten Situation wird das gänzliche Zurücktreten der b^{e}rît-Vorstellung erklärlich.

Die seltenen Erwähnungen der b^{e}rît in den die Richter- und Königszeit schildernden Büchern des Alten Testaments wie Jdc 2 20 I Reg 19 10. 14 stammen sämtlich aus jüngerer Zeit. Das gilt ebenso für die »ewige b^{e}rît« mit David, wie II Sam 23 5 die sog. Natanweissagung II Sam 7 interpretiert. In Wirklichkeit hat diese Erzählung ursprünglich lediglich von der Verhinderung des von David geplanten Tempelbaus berichtet (7 1-7. 17). Sie ist, wie die Einleitungsformel in 7 8 deutlich macht, später erweitert worden (7 8-16. 18-29 einschließlich zusätzlicher Erweiterungen und Umbildungen), wobei nicht mehr die Lade oder der Tempel, sondern David und seine Dynastie im Mittelpunkt stehen[87]. Den Ansatz dafür lieferte die ägyptische Königsnovelle[88], mittels deren Nachahmung die Legitimation Salomos als König erfolgt war (I Reg 3 4-15). II Sam 7 8-16 bildet eine nach dem Vorbild der Königsnovelle gestaltete und um ein Gebet in 7 18-29 bereicherte Sachparallele zur Legitimation Salomos, die jedoch jünger als diese ist. Denn nach einer Legitimation der ganzen Dynastie, wie sie in II Sam 7 8 ff. erfolgt, wäre eine eigene Begründung des König-

---

[86] Vgl. die Belege bei R. Smend a. a. O. 19.
[87] Die Einfügung wurde durch das mehrdeutige Wort *bájit* ermöglicht, dessen Bedeutung sich von »Haus« als Wohnung für Jahwe zu »Haus« als Dynastie wandelt.
[88] Vgl. S. Herrmann, Die Königsnovelle in Ägypten und in Israel, WZ Leipzig 3 (1953/54), 51—62; zum Gesamtzusammenhang G. Fohrer, Der Vertrag zwischen König und Volk in Israel, ZAW 71 (1959), 1—22 (s. u. 330—351).

tums Salomos nicht mehr erforderlich gewesen; dergleichen findet sich in der Folgezeit auch nicht. Was also in I Reg 3 4ff. die Person Salomos allein betraf, wurde in II Sam 7 8ff. auf die ganze Dynastie ausgedehnt und in späterer Zeit als *b^{e}rît* nach dem noch zu erwähnenden deuteronomischen Verständnis interpretiert (II Sam 23 5).

Offensichtlich spielt die nomadische *b^{e}rît*-Vorstellung von der Richterzeit an keine tragende Rolle mehr. Wie alles nomadische Erbe mehr oder weniger schnell und gründlich in den Hintergrund getreten ist, so auch sie. Es klafft infolgedessen eine jahrhundertelange Lücke — in gleicher Weise wie beim nomadischen Passa, das ebenso wie die *b^{e}rît*-Vorstellung erst vom Deuteronomium wieder erneuert worden ist[89]. Außerdem war die das Verhältnis zwischen Jahwe und Israel konstituierende Sinai-*b^{e}rît* als einmaliger geschichtlicher Akt nicht mehr wichtig. Er war lediglich das einmal angewendete Mittel zu einem bestimmten Ziel und Zweck gewesen. Nachdem Ziel und Zweck erreicht waren, galt es, das Ergebnis zu erhalten und zu pflegen: die dauernde Gemeinschaft zwischen Jahwe und Israel. Dem aber dienten primär der Kultus und sodann die Beibehaltung der verwandtschaftlichen Kategorien, nach denen der durch die Genealogien konstituierte *'ăm* Israel als ganzer den *'ăm* Jahwes bildete. Das bedeutet: Die Genealogien mit den zwölf Stammvätern Israels und die Sinai-*b^{e}rît* haben die gleiche Funktion als konstituierende Elemente — nicht weniger, aber auch nicht mehr.

Ausschließlich verwandtschaftliche Kategorien verwenden denn auch die vorexilischen großen Einzelpropheten bis in die Zeit Jeremias hinein. Da ich dies bereits dargelegt habe[90], kann ich darauf verweisen und brauche die jetzige Darstellung nicht mit den Belegstellen zu belasten. Entscheidend ist die Beobachtung, daß nach der Sinai-*b^{e}rît* jahrhundertelang von keiner weiteren *b^{e}rît* die Rede ist und daß jene während dieser Periode eine ganz untergeordnete, dienende Rolle spielte.

3. Noch einmal ändert sich das Bild grundlegend in der Zeit der prophetischen Tätigkeit Jeremias. Während in seiner Verkündigung vor der deuteronomischen Reform die *b^{e}rît*-Vorstellung nicht begegnet, vielmehr die von den anderen Propheten verwendeten verwandtschaftlichen Kategorien, verhält es sich in seiner Verkündigung nach der Reform umgekehrt — bis hin zum Wort von der »neuen *b^{e}rît*« (Jer 31 31-34). Damit wird der Einschnitt deutlich markiert: Die deuteronomische Theologie hat die *b^{e}rît*-Vorstellung aufgegriffen und zu einem grundlegend wichtigen Theologumenon gemacht. Erst damit beginnt

---

[89] Vgl. dazu G. Fohrer, Überlieferung und Geschichte des Exodus, 1964, 89ff.
[90] G. Fohrer, Prophetie und Geschichte, ThLZ 89 (1964), 481—500 (= Studien zur alttestamentlichen Prophetie [1949—1965], 1967, 265—293).

eine eigentliche »Bundes«-Theologie. Dazu trägt eine zweifache Bedeutungswandlung bei: Einmal gilt die $b^e r\hat{\imath}t$ nicht bloß als Konstituierung eines Lebensverhältnisses, das allein entscheidend wäre, sondern erhält den Sinn einer dauernd bestehenden Verpflichtung für Jahwe und Israel, so daß aller Nachdruck nunmehr auf die $b^e r\hat{\imath}t$ fällt. Ferner erzielt sie nicht mehr eine Lebensgemeinschaft aufgrund einer fiktiven Verwandtschaft, sondern zieht ein Verhältnis im Sinne des rechtlich gültigen und wirksamen Vertrages nach sich, bewegt sich also in rechtlichen Kategorien.

Es ist nicht ausgeschlossen, daß der zweite Zug auf dem Einfluß oder Vorbild zeitgenössischer — nicht längst vergangener — Staatsverträge beruht, wie R. Frankena eine Abhängigkeit von Dtn 28 20-57 von den Verträgen vermutet, die der assyrische König Asarhaddon im Jahre 672 mit mindestens neun Vasallen geschlossen hat[91]. Doch bedarf die Frage einer Einwirkung außenpolitischer Verträge noch sorgfältiger und nüchterner Untersuchung. Wahrscheinlicher ist der Einfluß innenpolitischer Verträge: derjenigen zwischen König und Volk — wie gerade auch Josia im Zuge der Annahme des deuteronomischen Gesetzes einen derartigen Vertrag geschlossen hat (II Reg 23 1-3). Jedenfalls ist der »Gedanke der Theokratie: Jahwe ist König ... dem des Gottesbundes nahe verwandt, so daß man den mit Gott geschlossenen Bund als einen Königsbund deuten darf«[92]. Einige weitere Hinweise habe ich an anderer Stelle gegeben: Dtn 26 16-19 Jer 14 21 und Ps 44 18 gehen geradezu vom Königsvertrag aus, Analogien zu Schwur, Vertragsurkunde und deren Aufbewahrung liegen vor, die Erwartungen einer künftigen $b^e r\hat{\imath}t$ bei Jeremia und Ezechiel knüpfen an den Königsvertrag an[93]. Doch da in diesem Zusammenhang das geschichtliche Vorkommen der $b^e r\hat{\imath}t$-Vorstellung wichtig ist, mögen die inhaltlichen Fragen auf sich beruhen[94].

Erwähnt das Deuteronomium außer der Sinai-$b^e r\hat{\imath}t$ eine nach deren Bruch (Ex 32) geschlossene Moab-$b^e r\hat{\imath}t$, so hat die nachexilische Priesterschrift die $b^e r\hat{\imath}t$-Vorstellung zu einem die ganze Geschichte umfassenden System ausgebaut: Das erste Stadium beginnt mit der Weltschöpfung, bei der Gott in einer unausgesprochenen $b^e r\hat{\imath}t$ den Menschen die vegetarische Nahrung als Ordnung der $b^e r\hat{\imath}t$ gebietet und den Sabbat als ihr Zeichen einsetzt. Als zweite folgt die Noah-$b^e r\hat{\imath}t$ mit den noachiti-

---

[91] R. Frankena, The Vassal-Treaties of Esarhaddon and the Dating of Deuteronomy, OTSt 14 (1965), 122—154.
[92] G. Quell in ThW II 123.
[93] G. Fohrer a. a. O.
[94] Beachtenswert ist noch, daß das Deuteronomium selber nicht nach einem Vertragsformular, sondern nach dem Muster altorientalischer Gesetzbücher angelegt ist; vgl. E. Sellin—G. Fohrer a. a. O. § 25.

schen Geboten als Ordnung mit dem Regenbogen als Zeichen, als dritte die Abraham-b^{e}rît mit der Ordnung und dem Zeichen der Beschneidung, als vierte und letzte die Mose-b^{e}rît am Sinai mit dem gesamten Kultprogramm.

Aus alledem ergibt sich, daß eine wirkliche »Bundes«-Theologie erst mit dem Deuteronomium beginnt und daß die b^{e}rît-Vorstellung nur einer von mehreren Vorstellungskreisen für das Verhältnis zwischen Jahwe und Israel ist, wobei in der Verwendung während der nomadischen Zeit der Gedanke der Gemeinschaft, während der Spätzeit der Gedanke der Herrschaft Gottes überwiegt.

V.

Hat es eine israelitische Amphiktyonie weder als sakrale noch als politisch-militärische Organisation gegeben und hat die b^{e}rît-Vorstellung in der Richterzeit (und in der vordeuteronomischen Königszeit) keine wesentliche Rolle gespielt, so stellen sich die Fragen nach dem geschichtlichen und religionsgeschichtlichen Verlauf dieser Periode und nach Vorstufen der Staatsbildung von neuem. Wenigstens einige Hinweise dürften erforderlich sein, um zu zeigen, daß ein Wegfall der Amphiktyonie-Hypothese und ein Zurückstellen der b^{e}rît-Vorstellung keine unschließbaren Lücken reißen.

1. Wie die israelitischen Stämme nicht gleichzeitig und unter einheitlicher Führung in Palästina eindrangen und es eroberten, sondern in einem längeren Zeitraum nacheinandern in einzelnen Gruppen von den Patriarchensippen bis zur Moseschar in das Land einwanderten, so blieb es in der Richterzeit beim Nebeneinander der Stämme ohne gemeinsame Führung, ohne umfassende Organisation und gewöhnlich auch bei militärischen Aktionen einzelner Stämme oder Sippen — nur mit dem genealogisch verankerten Bewußtsein der gemeinsamen Abstammung und der Verwandtschaft miteinander. Nachdem die Moseschar eingewandert und in die mittelpalästinischen Stämme eingegliedert worden war, erfolgte die allmähliche Übernahme des Jahweglaubens durch alle israelitischen Stämme, so daß der durch die Genealogien konstituierte 'ăm Israel insgesamt zum 'ăm Jahwes, also infolge der Übernahme des Jahweglaubens in die Lebensgemeinschaft mit Jahwe einbezogen wurde. Wie einerseits die Moseschar in den 'ăm Israel aufgenommen wurde, so andererseits Israel in den 'ăm Jahwes. Von da aus wird verständlich, warum Israel die Patriarchenüberlieferungen bewahrt und die Vätergötter mit Jahwe identifiziert hat. Es diente dazu, um die Kontinuität herzustellen, so daß der von Jakob-Israel hergeleitete 'ăm Israel wirklich von Anfang an als 'ăm Jahwes erscheinen konnte. Es ermöglichte ferner die dauernde Anwendung der Verwandtschaftskategorien auf das Verhältnis zwischen

Jahwe und Israel, wie sie sowohl der Väterreligion als auch dem Selbstverständnis Israels entsprach.

2. Die Richterzeit ist weithin die Zeit der kriegerischen Helden der sog. großen Richter, der Heerbannführer von Stämmen und Stammeshelden, von denen das Richterbuch in erster Linie erzählt. Nur im Falle der Deboraschlacht gegen die Kanaanäer und beim Vorgehen der Koalition von Silo gegen die Philister, also gegen weit überlegene Gegner, kam es zum gemeinsamen Handeln von Stämmegruppen, das naturgemäß das Gemeinbewußtsein stärkte. Es sind »Schlachten wie eben die im Deboraliede verherrlichte, die den eigentlichen Fortschritt der nationalen Idee bezeichnen«[95]. Und — so ist zu ergänzen — es sind Niederlagen wie diejenige der Koalition von Silo, die die Notwendigkeit des gemeinsamen Heerbanns aller Stämme und des israelischen Staates erwiesen. Auch die gemeinsame Benutzung von Heiligtümern durch mehrere Stämme und die einigende Kraft des Jahweglaubens sind nochmals zu nennen.

3. Ferner ist die Umbildung der nomadischen Organisation anzuführen. Diese war nach der Ansiedlung überholt und wurde durch den Orts- oder Gauverband ersetzt, so daß Stammesterritorien entstanden — ein Schritt auf dem Wege zum Territorialstaat. In solche Verbände wurden stammesfremde Israeliten und Kanaanäer aufgenommen, so daß nicht mehr die personelle Zugehörigkeit zu einem Stamm, sondern die Niederlassung in einer Ortschaft oder einem Gau maßgeblich wurde. Von großen Ortschaften aus werden neue Siedlungen gegründet, so daß man von der »Stadt A und ihren Tochterstädten« sprechen konnte. Darin liegt der Ansatz zur Bildung von Stadtstaaten, an denen Palästina seit der Hyksoszeit reich gewesen ist. Natürlich konnten die Schritte zu Territorien und Stadtstaaten zur völligen Zersplitterung führen, doch war die Zeit von der Landnahme bis zur Staatsbildung zu kurz und zu unruhig, als daß solche Gebilde sich hätten verfestigen können. So haben sie sich eher im Sinne von Vorstufen eines Gesamtstaates ausgewirkt.

4. Daß es tatsächlich zur Entstehung kleiner Herrschaften gekommen ist, wird man nach der beachtenswerten Untersuchung von W. Richter aus den Angaben über die sog. kleinen Richter folgern müssen[96]. Zu diesen gehören vor allem:

a) Tola in Samir auf dem Gebirge Ephraim (Jdc 10 1-2),

b) Jaïr in Gilead, wohl im Ort seiner Bestattung Kamon (Jdc 10 3-5),

---

[95] A. Bertholet, Kulturgeschichte Israels, 1919, 104.
[96] W. Richter, Zu den »Richtern Israels«, ZAW 77 (1965), 40—72. Vgl. ferner C. H. J. de Geus a. a. O.

c) Ibzan aus und in Betlehem (Jdc 12 8-10),
d) Elon in Ajjalon, wo er bestattet wurde (Jdc 12 11-12),
e) Abdon aus und in Piraton (Jdc 12 13-15).

Außerdem finden sich ähnliche Einzelangaben wie über diese »Richter« auch über Gideon (Jdc 6—8) und Jephta (Jdc 10 6—12 7). Wesentlich ist, daß das Schema der Notizen über sie den Notizen über Saul und die späteren Könige nachgebildet ist, und zwar der älteren Form I Sam 13 1 und der Form der Königsbücher I Reg 11 41f. usw., so daß sie als Herrscher hingestellt werden. Ihre Funktion war zwar nicht nur kriegerisch wie diejenige der Stammesführer und -helden des Richterbuches, hat aber ebensowenig allein die Gerichtspraxis umfaßt. Diese ist vielmehr als Teil eines herrscherlichen Waltens zu verstehen, wie ja das Verb *špṭ* »Recht schaffen« und »herrschen« bedeutet. Die fünf kleinen Richter im engeren Sinn stehen zudem nicht mit Stämmen, sondern mit Ortschaften in Verbindung. Ihre Sukzession ist sekundär, so daß sie gleichzeitig nebeneinander oder zu verschiedenen Zeiten in den Ortschaften, vielleicht sogar in einer ganzen Landschaft (Jaïr in Gilead) geherrscht haben können. Sie sind den kanaanäischen Stadtfürsten ähnlich und bilden also den Übergang von der Stammes- zur Stadtstaatverfassung[97]. Von da aus erscheint die Notiz Jdc 8 22f., daß dem Gideon die Königswürde angeboten worden sei, durchaus nicht abwegig, sofern man das Angebot von den Männern des Stammes Manasse und nicht von ganz Israel ausgehen läßt. Hätte Gideon es nicht abgelehnt, so wäre es wohl zu einem Stammes- oder Territorialkönigtum gekommen.

5. Daß dieser Weg möglich war und zugleich weiterführen konnte, ist aus den Erzählungen über die Erhebung Sauls zum König zu erschließen, wenn man der Interpretation von G. Wallis folgt[98]. Die Erhebung geschieht nach den überlieferten Erzählungen anscheinend mehrfach und an verschiedenen Orten. Da es schwer vorstellbar ist, wie ein einziger Akt an mehreren Orten in unterschiedlicher Weise als jeweils dort erfolgt dargestellt worden sein kann, legt sich eine andere einfache und einleuchtende Erklärung nahe: Saul ist nicht mit einem Male König über Gesamtisrael geworden, sondern von einzelnen Stämmen oder Territorien nacheinander in eigener Entscheidung dazu erhoben worden — so durch Akklamation in Gilgal über Benjamin (I Sam 11), durch Salbung zum *nagîd* in Ephraim (I Sam 9 1—10 16)

---

[97] Abimelech (Jdc 9) nennt man in diesem Zusammenhang besser nicht, weil er wohl ein Kanaanäer war, dessen Vater Jerubbaal später mit Gideon gleichgesetzt worden ist.

[98] G. Wallis, Die Anfänge des Königtums in Israel, WZ Halle-Wittenberg 12 (1963), 239—247.

und kraft der Bestimmung durch das Losorakel in Mizpa über Gilead (I Sam 8 10 17-27*). Andere Stämme haben sich dem angeschlossen. Noch David ist in ähnlicher Weise, nur in größerem Rahmen, nacheinander König über Juda und über Israel geworden, nachdem das von Saul beherrschte Gebiet zuerst auf Ischbaal übergegangen war.

6. Schließlich ist für den letzten Schritt zu Königtum und Staatsbildung wohl das Beispiel der Nachbarvölker von Einfluß gewesen, vielleicht weniger das der philistäischen Stadtstaaten als das der ostjordanischen Ammoniter, Moabiter und Edomiter; sie hatten Territorialstaaten mit Königen gebildet, die mehr als Stammesfürsten waren. Von dort kam in der Zeit der Philisternot infolge des ammonitischen Angriffs auf das ostjordanische israelitische Gebiet dann auch der letzte Anstoß, der Saul zum Eingreifen und die Stämme zur Königserhebung veranlaßte.

Insgesamt ergibt sich für die Richter- und den Übergang zur Königszeit ohne Verwendung der Amphiktyonie-Hypothese und der $b^e r\hat{\imath}t$-Vorstellung als tragender Ideen ein ebenso klares Bild wie mit ihnen.

Das sogenannte apodiktisch formulierte Recht und der Dekalog

I.

In einer vielbeachteten Untersuchung hatte A. Alt im Jahre 1934 einen neuen Weg zum Verständnis der alttestamentlichen Rechtskorpora eingeschlagen, indem er zwischen dem kasuistisch und dem apodiktisch formulierten Recht unterschied[1]. Während er das erstere, das durch die genaue Beschreibung von Rechtsfall und -folge gekennzeichnet ist, dem Betätigungsbereich der normalen Gerichtsbarkeit der Rechtsgemeinde zuwies und es infolge seines Zusammenhangs mit der übrigen altorientalischen Rechtskultur von den Israeliten nach ihrer Landnahme in Palästina aus den kanaanäischen Ordnungen übernommen glaubte, beurteilte er die apodiktisch formulierten Rechtssätze, die häufig in kürzeren oder längeren Reihen von gleichartig aufgebauten Sätzen überliefert sind, völlig anders: »Alles in ihnen ist vielmehr volksgebunden israelitisch und gottgebunden jahwistisch, auch wo das in dem knappen Wortlaut keinen unmittelbaren Ausdruck findet.«[2] Sie unterscheiden sich vom kasuistisch formulierten Recht durch ihre Unbedingtheit. Sah Alt diese in der Form der Sätze durch das Du der Anrede und das Ich des gebietenden Jahwe gegeben, so im Inhalt durch die unmittelbare Bezogenheit auf den strengen Willen des Volksgottes. Ja, er nahm als feststehenden Ritus, der die Grundlage für das Aufkommen und Leben der apodiktischen Rechtsgattung bildete, den Rechtsvortrag vor der versammelten Volksgemeinde am Laubhüttenfest zu Beginn des jeweils 7. Jahres an, auf den seiner Ansicht nach Dtn 27 hinwies.

Allerdings ging Alt der Frage nach dem Ursprung des apodiktisch formulierten Rechts nicht bis zur letzten Konsequenz nach. Es erschien ihm als sicher, »daß die Voraussetzungen für das Aufkommen dieser Gattung sofort gegeben waren, als die Bindung an Jahwe und in ihrer Folge die Institution der Bundesschließung und Bundeserneuerung zwischen ihm und Israel ins Leben trat«. Dagegen schloß er die weitere Frage aus, »ob die israelitischen Stämme etwa schon vor ihrer Volk-

---

[1] A. Alt, Die Ursprünge des israelitischen Rechts, 1934 (zitiert nach: Kleine Schriften zur Geschichte des Volkes Israel, I 1953, 278—332).
[2] Alt a. a. O. 323.

werdung, d. h. vor ihren Zusammenschluß in der Bindung an Jahwe, ähnliche Rechtsformulierungen kannten oder besaßen«[3].

Während die These vom Unterschied zwischen dem kasuistisch und dem apodiktisch formulierten Recht und von der religiös-kultischen Verhaftung des letzteren weithin angenommen worden ist[4], dabei allerdings vielfach übereifrig aus dem historischen in den theologischen Bereich übertragen wurde, so daß das apodiktisch formulierte Recht als geoffenbartes »Gottesrecht« erschien, forderte die offengebliebene Frage zu weiterer Untersuchung auf. Gewiß fragt es sich ebenso, ob man aus der einleitenden Erzählung von Dtn 27 einen feststehenden Ritus herauslesen darf, zumal es bei den landschaftlichen Gegebenheiten schwer vorstellbar ist, daß die auf dem Berge Ebal ausgesprochenen Flüche auf dem Berge Garizim vernehmbar wären[5]. Es fragt sich ferner, welchen Sinn eine Feier der »Bundeserneuerung« in regelmäßigen Abständen haben sollte, zumal sie bestenfalls nach einem Bundesbruch angebracht sein könnte und außerdem — wie so manches andere postulierte Fest — im Alten Testament nirgends erwähnt wird[6]. Aber dergleichen tritt hinter den grundlegenden Fragen zurück, durch deren Beantwortung auch darauf Licht fallen mag: Wo liegt der eigentliche Ursprung der apodiktisch formulierten Satzreihen? Handelt es sich in ihnen um genuin israelitisches und Jahwerecht?

Im Versuch einer Antwort darauf hat G. Heinemann auf Bestimmungen der hetitischen Vasallenverträge hingewiesen, die im apodiktischen Stil gehalten sind, und also einen außerisraelitischen Ursprung angenommen — allerdings in einer indirekten Abhängigkeit, wobei

---

[3] Alt a. a. O. 330.
[4] Allerdings sind auch Gegenstimmen laut geworden, vgl. B. Landsberger, Die babylonischen Termini für Gesetz und Recht, in: Symbolae P. Koschaker, 1939, 223; Th. J. Meek in ANET 183 Anm. 24; H. Gese, Beobachtungen zum Stil alttestamentlicher Rechtssätze, ThLZ 85 (1960), 147—150; F. Ch. Fensham, The Possibility of the Presence of Casuistic Legal Material at the Making of the Covenant at Sinai, PEQ 93 (1961), 143—146; St. Gevirtz, West-Semitic Curses and the Problem of the Origins of Hebrew Law, VT 11 (1961), 137—158; R. Kilian, Apodiktisches und kasuistisches Recht im Licht ägyptischer Analogien, BZ NF 7 (1963), 185—202.
[5] Außerdem ist die Erzählung nicht einheitlich. Nach Dtn 27 13 sollen sechs Stämme den anderen sechs Stämmen, nach 27 14 die Leviten allen Israeliten die Flüche zurufen.
[6] Auch die Aufforderung »Moses« in Dtn 31 10f., »dieses Gesetz« alle sieben Jahre beim Laubhüttenfest vorzulesen, begründet kein altes Bundeserneuerungsfest, sondern läßt sich beim besten Willen nur als fingierte mosaische Anweisung verstehen, die das abermalige Vergessen des zur Zeit des Königs Josia gefundenen deuteronomischen Gesetzbuchs verhindern sollte, zumal der Ausdruck »dieses Gesetz« eben jenes Gesetzbuch, nicht aber den Dekalog meint.

das beim Garizim und Ebal gelegene Sichem als Kultort des »Bundesbaal« das Bindeglied gewesen sein könne[7]. Wie es seit der Behauptung von G. E. Mendenhall[8] mit wechselnden Ansichten in Einzelheiten mehrfach dargelegt worden ist[9], soll Israel die Form der hetitischen Vasallenverträge als sachgemäße Ausdrucksform für sein Bundesverhältnis zu Gott betrachtet und im Zusammenhang damit auch den apodiktischen Stil für das mit dem Bund gegebene Jahwerecht übernommen haben.

Doch dem steht die völlig andere These von E. Gerstenberger gegenüber, der sich freilich auf die reinen Verbote im apodiktischen Stil beschränkt und die Partizipialkonstruktionen und Fluchformulierungen als weithin zum kasuistischen Recht gehörig beiseite läßt[10]. Danach bilden die Verbote zwar ebenfalls kein ursprüngliches Jahwerecht, weil ihre Stilisierung als Jahwerede sich durchweg als sekundär nachweisen läßt. Die in den Verboten sprechende Autorität ist aber auch keine ursprünglich staatliche, sondern eine patriarchalische Institution: Die apodiktischen Sätze stammen aus dem semitischen Sippenverband und bilden autoritative Verbote des Sippen- oder Familienältesten, der seine Würde aus der von ihm vertretenen geheiligten Ordnung erhält. Von da aus wird das Vorkommen solcher Verbote im Alten Orient außerhalb Israels, nicht zuletzt in der Weisheitsliteratur, verständlich.

Sind die apodiktisch formulierten Sätze — oder genauer: die Satzreihen — nun israelitischen, außerisraelitischen (hetitischen) oder überisraelitischen (semitischen) Ursprungs? Statt dessen ist eher anzunehmen, daß die Reihen apodiktisch formulierter Sätze nach den bisherigen Kenntnissen bei den noch nicht seßhaft gewordenen Nomaden oder Halbnomaden gebräuchlich waren und daß der Ursprung der alttestamentlichen Reihen dort zu suchen ist:

1. Man muß zwischen dem apodiktischen Stil, nach dem sowohl einzelne Sätze als auch Satzreihen geformt sein können, und den apodiktischen Satzreihen, die aus mehreren, jeweils gleichartig aufgebauten Sätzen bestehen, grundsätzlich unterscheiden.

2. Der apodiktische Stil — »tu dies!« oder »tu jenes nicht!« — ist so alt wie das erste von Menschen formulierte Gebot oder Verbot und gehört zu den Urformen menschlicher Redeweise, so daß es sinn-

---

[7] G. Heinemann, Untersuchungen zum apodiktischen Recht, Diss. Hamburg 1958.

[8] G. E. Mendenhall, Recht und Bund in Israel und dem Alten Vordern Orient, 1960 (englisch 1954 und 1955).

[9] So K. Baltzer, Das Bundesformular, 1966²; W. Beyerlin, Herkunft und Geschichte der ältesten Sinaitraditionen, 1961.

[10] E. Gerstenberger, Wesen und Herkunft des »apodiktischen Rechts«, 1965. Zu den Partizipialformen vgl. auch Kilian a. a. O. 188—194.

los ist, nach einem gemeinsamen geschichtlichen Ursprungsort für die Vorkommen apodiktischer Einzelsätze in den verschiedenen altorientalischen Literaturen zu suchen.

3. Die Bildung von Reihen gleichartiger Gebots- oder Verbotssätze in apodiktischer Formulierung läßt sich im Alten Orient bisher für den (halb)nomadischen Lebensbereich wahrscheinlich machen, für dessen Analphabetentum eine derartige Bildung von Reihen mit etwa 10 oder 12 Gliedern ein brauchbares Hilfsmittel zum Erlernen bot[11] — ganz abgesehen davon, daß solche Zahlen symbolische oder gar magische Bedeutung besaßen[12].

4. Es gibt nicht eine einzige Gattung, sondern mehrere Gattungen in apodiktischer Stilform. Allein die Formen von Gebot und Verbot sind als zwei verschiedene Gattungen zu bezeichnen, zu denen im Lauf der Zeit weitere hinzugetreten sind.

5. Die Reihen apodiktisch formulierter Sätze enthalten durchaus nicht immer »Recht«; dies ist nur in bestimmten Ausnahmen der Fall (s. u. V, 3). Sonst aber können sie weder als grundlegende Bewertungsnorm, als norma normans, gelten, weil sie nicht auf gesetzliche Einzelregelungen hin angelegt sind, vielmehr Gesetze, die sich mit solchen Handlungen, die in apodiktisch formulierten Geboten oder Verboten angeordnet oder untersagt sind, strafrechtlich befassen, unabhängig von diesen entstanden sind, und weil sie schlicht und einfach dem Einzelmenschen ein bestimmtes Tun und Lassen befehlen oder empfehlen. Noch können sie als Bestimmungsnorm, als in der Gerichtsverhandlung verwendbare Gesetze, gelten, weil sie keine rechtlichen Sanktionen vorsehen und keine begangene Tat voraussetzen, die zu ahnden sie herangezogen werden könnten, sondern auf den Einzel-

---

[11] Daher wird die Zehnzahl als von der Summe der Finger genommene runde Zahl gern zur Bezeichnung von »vielmals« verwendet: Gen 31 7 Lev 26 26 Num 14 22 Hi 19 3. Aus dem (halb)nomadischen Lebensbereich ist die Reihenform in den Gebrauch im Kulturland übergegangen. Wie sich dies für Israel an dem sogleich zu erläuternden Beispiel Lev 18 nachweisen läßt, so läge es für die Verwendung in der ägyptischen Weisheitslehre nahe, aus der das bisher einzige außerisraelitische Beispiel stammt, falls eine wirkliche Reihe anzunehmen ist: A. H. Gardiner, A New Moralizing Text, WZKM 54 (1957), 44f. (auch zitiert von Kilian a. a. O. 196f.). Es handelt sich um jetzt 16, im ursprünglichen, unbeschädigten Text vielleicht um 18 moralische Anordnungen, die einander formal insofern ähnlich sind, als sie durch ein »Tue nicht« eingeleitet werden und in einem zweiten Satz die Folge der verbotenen Handlung nennen oder sie durch einen Vergleich erläutern. Ob es sich um eine primäre oder angesichts der merkwürdigen Zahl der Anordnungen um eine sekundär zusammengestellte Reihe von ähnlich aufgebauten Sätzen handelt, muß offenbleiben.

[12] Vgl. z. B. F. Heiler, Erscheinungsformen und Wesen der Religion, 1961, 161—176 mit weiteren Literaturangaben.

menschen einwirken wollen, damit er sein Leben in einer Weise gestaltet, die den Pflichten gegenüber der Gemeinschaft oder — im Bereich des Jahweglaubens — dem göttlichen Willen entspricht. Die apodiktisch formulierten Sätze sollen das Begehen einer strafwürdigen Tat oder Unterlassung gerade von vornherein verhindern und gehen sachlich dem Recht voraus. So ist z. B. der Dekalog in Ex 20 1-17 aus all diesen Gründen als solcher keineswegs »Recht«. Zu den meisten seiner Forderungen finden sich erst im anschließenden sogenannten Bundesbuch entsprechende rechtlich-gesetzliche Bestimmungen oder Prozeßvorschriften in der Form kasuistischer Sätze mit Angabe des Tatbestandes und der rechtlichen Sanktion. Diese Sätze sind völlig unabhängig vom Dekalog entstanden und insbesondere aus dem kanaanäischen oder sonstigen altorientalischen Recht übernommen. Darin drückt sich doch wohl aus, daß der Dekalog gerade nicht als »Recht« betrachtet worden ist und daß der Unterschied zwischen apodiktischer und kasuistischer Formulierung nicht auf der Linie des Unterschiedes zwischen israelitisch-jahwistischem und kanaanäisch-übernommenem Recht verläuft.

II.

Ein wesentlicher Beleg für diese Auffassung ergibt sich aus der Reihe apodiktisch formulierter Sätze in Lev 18 7-17 a. Sie ist in mehreren Stadien der Überlieferung bearbeitet worden und hat dabei außer dem sie zur Jahweordnung erhebenden v. 6 sowohl einen Anhang in v. 17 b-23 als auch einen paränetischen Rahmen in v. 2 b-5 und 24-30 erhalten. Es handelt sich um — sekundär durch Erläuterungen, Näherbestimmungen und Begründungen erweiterte — Verbote, die den Geschlechtsverkehr mit bestimmten weiblichen Personen, überwiegend Verwandten und Verschwägerten, ausschließen sollen und die in allen Fällen noch erkennbare Urform besessen haben:

Die Blöße der (Bezeichnuug der Person) decke nicht auf!

In einer eingehenden Analyse, deren Ergebnisse zwingend sind, hat K. Elliger dargelegt[13], daß die Verbotsreihe drei Stadien durchlaufen hat: Ursprünglich hat ein Dekalog vorgelegen, zu dem die Bestimmungen in v. 7-12. 14-16 gehört haben und von dem nach dem jetzigen v. 9 ein Satz (über die Tochter) ausgefallen ist. Berücksichtigt man die genannten Personen, so wird man für den Ursprung dieses Dekalogs eindeutig auf die Lebensverhältnisse der Großfamilie verwiesen, wie sie in der (halb)nomadischen Zeit Israels bestanden hat.

---

[13] K. Elliger, Das Gesetz Leviticus 18, ZAW 67 (1955), 1—25; vgl. jetzt: Leviticus, 1966, 229—242. Dem schließt sich M. Noth, Das dritte Buch Moses, Leviticus, 1962, 115—117, wenigstens grundsätzlich an.

Ihr Zusammenleben sollte geschützt und umhegt werden, indem man Sittenregeln festlegte, die sich offenbar nicht auf die Ehe, sondern auf die geschlechtliche Betätigung überhaupt bezogen. Im zweiten Stadium erfolgte durch v. 13 und 17 a eine Erweiterung zum Dodekalog, der durch die Überschrift v. 6 als Jahweordnung proklamiert und zum Verbot bestimmter Verwandtschaftsgrade für die dauernde Verbindung der Ehe uminterpretiert wurde, während das dritte Stadium die nur mehr 11 Sätze in ein allgemeines Gesetz gegen die Unzucht eingliederte, um den Heiligkeitscharakter und die Kultfähigkeit der Gemeinde (nicht mehr der Familie) zu sichern. So entspricht der zweimaligen Neuinterpretation eine sich steigernde Jahwisierung der ursprünglichen Sippenregeln.

Was ergibt sich aus Lev 18 7 ff. für die Fragen um die apodiktischen Satzreihen, wenn man die von Elliger begonnenen Linien auszieht?

1. In dem aus v. 7-12. 14-16 zu erschließenden ursprünglichen Dekalog mit seinen apodiktischen Formulierungen in der oben angegebenen Art liegt eine echte Reihe vor, die von vornherein als solche angelegt war und nicht erst sekundär aus Einzelsätzen zusammengestellt worden ist. Das ergibt sich sowohl aus den aufgezählten Personen, die — nach Ergänzung der Tochter — den gesamten in Frage kommenden Kreis der Großfamilie umfassen, als auch aus dem Satzbau, da die Objekte abweichend von der gewöhnlichen Syntax dem Verb vorangestellt sind, um sie voneinander zu unterscheiden, so daß von vornherein ihre Mehrheit vorausgesetzt ist.

2. Die konkreten Lebensverhältnisse, denen diese Mehrheit von Personen entspricht, sind diejenigen der (halb)nomadischen Großfamilie, so daß der ursprüngliche Dekalog von Lev 18 aus der (halb)nomadischen Zeit Israels herzuleiten ist. Auch Elliger kommt zu dem Schluß: »Die Begründungen könnten ihrem Gehalt nach ebenso wie die Verbote selbst noch aus der Nomadenzeit Israels stammen, ja sogar aus vorjahwistischer Zeit.« Offensichtlich ist es das Gewicht der Thesen Alts, das ihn danach jedoch einschränkend fortfahren läßt: »Nur die apodiktische Form läßt es geraten erscheinen, mit der jetzigen Formulierung der Verbote in die Zeit hinunterzugehen, wo das unter Jahwes Willen sich beugende Israel bereits in Palästina saß, oder doch auf dem Wege dahin sich befand.«[14] Das ist nun einfach ein Fehlschluß, der die Dinge einer Hypothese zuliebe auf den Kopf stellt. Es muß gerade umgekehrt heißen, daß die Zurückführung der Verbote in die nomadische und damit für fast alle israelitischen Stämme vorjahwistische Zeit zeigt, daß zwar nicht die uralte apodiktische Satzform, wohl

---

[14] Elliger a. a. O. 12.

aber die Reihenbildung apodiktischer Sätze nicht erst eine Eigenart des sich unter Jahwes Willen beugenden Israel, sondern bereits diejenige des (halb)nomadischen vorpalästinischen Lebensbereichs ist. Es ist doch bezeichnend, daß noch die Regeln der an der nomadischen Lebensart festhaltenden Rechabiten in Jer 35 6 in apodiktischer Form gehalten sind und als vom Gründer der Gruppe erlassen gelten[15].

3. Der ursprüngliche Dekalog von Lev 18 enthält keine Rechtsbestimmungen, zumal eine Strafandrohung fehlt, sondern verbietende Anweisungen, die das Zusammenleben schützen sollen. Es sind (halb)nomadische Sittenregeln für die Großfamilie[16], die man »Sippenethos«[17] nennen kann. In einem umfassenderen Sinn lassen sie sich als Lebens- und Verhaltensregeln bezeichnen, die das tägliche Leben normativ bestimmen sollen. Dem entspricht es, daß mahnende und warnende Sprüche der Lebensweisheit, die ja Verhaltensregeln erteilen will, nicht nur formal, sondern auch inhaltlich mit apodiktisch formulierten Sätzen übereinstimmen.

4. Der ursprüngliche Dekalog von Lev 18 war erst recht kein Jahwe- oder Gottesrecht, weil er zunächst gar nicht auf Jahwe bezogen war. Dies ist erst durch die nachträglich vorangestellte Überschrift v. 6 geschehen. Will man für die alte Form überhaupt eine sprechende Autorität annehmen — was an sich nicht erforderlich ist, weil es eigentlich nur um die Befolgung durch das angeredete Du geht —, so kann man analog Jer 35 6 an den Sippengründer oder, da die Verbote doch wohl für mehrere Sippen gelten sollten, an die geheiligte Sippenordnung selbst denken.

5. Erst im zweiten Stadium der Bearbeitung und Überlieferung ist die Satzreihe im Zusammenhang mit ihrer Umgestaltung und Neuinterpretation in die Jahwerede und damit in den Jahweglauben einbezogen worden. Mittels solcher Neuinterpretation wurden die Verbote auf Jahwe beziehbar und bezogen und von da an in steigendem Maße zu Rechtssätzen, zu »Satzungen« und »Rechtsentscheidungen« erklärt (v. 4f. 26, vgl. v. 30).

Im Gegensatz zur Behauptung von Alt ergibt sich demnach am Beispiel von Lev 18, daß die apodiktische Satzreihe nicht genuin israelitisch und jahwistisch, sondern vorpalästinisch-nomadisch und vorjahwistisch ist und daß die Beziehung auf Jahwe und die Proklamation als »Recht« nicht am Anfang, sondern am Ende der Entwicklung stehen.

---

[15] Vgl. auch Gerstenberger a. a. O. 110f.
[16] Elliger a. a. O. 8.
[17] Noth a. a. O. 116.

III.

Von den dargelegten Erkenntnissen aus fällt neues Licht auf die im engeren Sinn als »Dekalog« bezeichnete Sammlung von Geboten und Verboten in Ex 20 1-17, die außerdem mit einer Reihe geringfügiger und mit wenigen schwerwiegenden Textabweichungen in Dtn 5 6-22 überliefert ist. Da ihre zahlreichen Probleme trotz der immerwährenden Bemühungen darum[18] in vielen Fällen noch keine klaren und eindeutigen Lösungen gefunden haben (und vielleicht niemals finden werden), muß man jede zu ihrer Erhellung sich bietende Möglichkeit ergreifen.

1. Schon die Frage, ob der Dekalog im Rahmen einer alten *Quellenschicht* des Pentateuchs überliefert oder ein in späterer Zeit in die Erzählung eingeschaltetes Textstück ist, wird verschieden beantwortet. Die letztere Ansicht findet sich — wiederum sehr differenziert — z. B. bei G. Beer, nach dessen Ansicht er wegen seines deuteronomistischen Sprachgewandes aus einem verlorenen deuteronomistischen Zusammenhang stammt, in dem er während des babylonischen Exils entstanden war[19], und bei M. Noth, nach dessen Meinung er eine geschlossene, selbständige Einheit und in der Sinaierzählung ein literarisch sekundäres Stück darstellt, in seinem Grundbestand allerdings aus der Zeit vor der klassischen Prophetie herrührt[20].

Jedoch ist der deuteronomistische Sprachgebrauch durchweg nur in den noch zu erwähnenden Erweiterungen der ursprünglichen Dekalogsätze zu beobachten, die ohnehin aus einer späteren Zeit als die Sätze selber stammen; von den Erweiterungen läßt sich kein solch weitgehender Schluß auf Herkunft und Alter der Dekalogsätze ziehen, wie Beer ihn unternimmt. Dagegen trifft es gewiß zu, daß die Dekalogsätze nicht von der Prophetie beeinflußt sind, weil ihnen das für diese so wichtige Element der im engeren Sinn ethisch-sozialen Forderungen fehlt. Freilich läßt dies keinen sicheren Schluß auf ihr Alter zu, weil auch in und nach der Zeit der Propheten eine nichtprophetische Auffassung des Gotteswillens vertreten werden konnte und vertreten worden ist[21].

Die eigentliche Begründung Noths für seine Auffassung aber, daß nämlich der Dekalog nur lose in die Erzählung eingefügt sei, trifft

---

[18] Vgl. die zusammenfassende Darstellung von J. J. Stamm, Der Dekalog im Lichte der neueren Forschung, 1962², der auch die Textunterschiede zwischen beiden Versionen des Dekalogs behandelt; dazu ferner J. J. Stamm — M. E. Andrew, The Ten Commandments in Recent Research, 1967.

[19] G. Beer, Exodus, 1939, 103.

[20] M. Noth, Das zweite Buch Mose, Exodus, 1959, 124. 134.

[21] Die Frage, ob die Propheten (vor allem Hos 4 2) den Dekalog voraussetzen, muß in einem späteren Zusammenhang behandelt werden (s. u. III, 3).

keineswegs zu. Der Anstoß, daß die auf den Dekalog folgenden Verse 20 18-21, die überwiegend der Quellenschicht des Elohisten (E) angehören (vgl. »Elohim« in v. 19-20), nicht an den Dekalog, sondern an die Theophanieschilderung in 19 16 b. 17. 19 b anknüpfen, erledigt sich durch die alte Beobachtung, daß 20 18-21 sich ursprünglich an 19 16 b. 17. 19 b anschlossen und daß der Dekalog also auf 20 18-21 folgte[22]. Tatsächlich ergibt sich auf diese Weise ein glatter Zusammenhang: Das unter dem Eindruck der Theophanie erschrockene Volk wünscht, daß nicht Gott, sondern Mose zu ihm redet; nachdem dieser es beruhigt hat, naht er sich dem Dunkel, in dem Gott weilt und dann »diese Worte« (20 1) spricht. Daß 20 18-21 an den jetzigen Platz hinter den Dekalog umgestellt worden sind, hängt wohl mit der späteren Einschaltung des sogenannten Bundesbuchs in 20 22 ff. zusammen. Danach verkündet Gott sogleich bei der Theophanie den Dekalog, das Volk erschrickt über sein Erscheinen und Reden und wünscht nur mehr Mose sprechen zu hören; Gott geht darauf ein, spricht die als Ausführungsbestimmungen zum Dekalog gedachten Gesetze des Bundesbuchs zu Mose und beauftragt ihn, sie den Israeliten weiterzusagen (20 22).

Die sich daraus nahelegende und vielfach vertretene, ja geradezu herkömmliche Annahme, daß der Dekalog der Quellenschicht des Elohisten zuzurechnen ist, wird durch seinen einleitenden Satz in 20 1 bestätigt. Denn er weist — wie allgemein sein Inhalt[23] auch sein mag — ebenfalls die Gottesbezeichnung »Elohim« auf, die E nach der Offenbarung des Jahwenamens an Mose (Ex 3 14 f.) weiterhin mehrfach verwendet. Da er dies allerdings nicht ausschließlich tut, braucht das Vorkommen des Jahwenamens in 20 7 keinen Anstoß zu erregen, ganz abgesehen davon, daß es sich ja um ein von E unverändert übernommenes Verbot handeln kann.

So ist es am wahrscheinlichsten, daß der Dekalog zunächst im Zusammenhang der Quellenschicht E überliefert und von dort für eine erneute Verwendung in den Einleitungsreden des Deuteronomiums herangezogen worden ist. Sein Gegenstück in der Quellenschicht des Jahwisten (J) bildet der sogenannte kultische Dekalog in Ex 34 14-26 (28).

2. Unabhängig von dieser Frage stellt sich diejenige nach der ursprünglichen Textform des Dekalogs. Auch wer ihn nicht einer Quellenschicht des Pentateuchs zuweisen, sondern als selbständiges, literarisch sekundäres Stück betrachten will, stellt doch *Unebenheiten und Erweiterungen* fest, die auf eine mehrfache spätere Bearbeitung des Textes schließen lassen[24]. Dabei kann das Vorkommen zweier positiv gehaltener Gebote (v. 8. 12) neben den zahlreicheren negativ

---

[22] O. Eißfeldt, Hexateuch-Synopse, 1922, 148*.
[23] Noth a. a. O. 124 führt dies als Einwand gegen die Zugehörigkeit zu E an.
[24] Vgl. z. B. Noth a. a. O. 129.

gehaltenen Verboten außer acht bleiben, weil es gattungsmäßig und formgeschichtlich zu erklären ist. Auffällig ist aber:

a) der Unterschied zwischen den extrem kurzen Verboten in v. 13-15 bzw. den ebenfalls recht knappen Verboten in v. 3. 16-17 a und und den übrigen, durch Aufzählungen, Anweisungen und Begründungen überladenen Dekalogsätzen;

b) der sowohl in den Dekalogsätzen als auch in den Erweiterungen festzustellende Unterschied zwischen dem redenden »Ich« Gottes (v. 3. 5-6) und seiner Erwähnung in der 3. Person (v. 7. 10-12);

c) der Unterschied in den Begründungen des Sabbatgebots in Ex 20 und Dtn 5, die offensichtlich zu verschiedenen Zeiten sekundär hinzugefügt worden sind. Dies alles macht deutlich, daß der ursprüngliche Text des Dekalogs in den kurzen Verbots- bzw. Gebotssätzen vorliegt und daß ein Teil von diesen im Verlauf der Überlieferung allmählich erweitert worden ist.

Für die Bewertung dieses Erweiterungsvorgangs ist es freilich nicht unwichtig, ob man die Zugehörigkeit des Dekalogs zur Quellenschicht E als gegeben annimmt. Auch wenn es nicht der Fall ist, *kann* man gewiß die Erweiterung eines lange Zeit selbständig bestehenden Dekalogs als einen Vorgang der mündlichen Überlieferung oder sogar als einen literarischen Prozeß verstehen, ebenso aber an den stück- und schichtweisen Zuwachs im Rahmen einer kultisch-rituellen Verwendung denken[25]. Diese letztere Möglichkeit scheidet dagegen praktisch aus, wenn man darauf beharren muß, daß der Dekalog der Quellenschicht E angehört. In ihr muß er in der ursprünglichen Textform ohne die Erweiterungen der Dekalogsätze vorgelegen haben; denn für die Konzeption des E war neben dem redenden »Ich« Gottes dessen Erwähnung in der 3. Person in v. 7 b. 10-12 ausgeschlossen; zudem tragen die Erweiterungen, wie noch zu zeigen ist, ein völlig anderes Sprachgewand, als es dem E eigentümlich ist. Ist der Dekalog aber in der ursprünglichen Form kurzer Rechtssätze in der Quellenschicht E überliefert worden, so kann deren Erweiterung auf den jetzigen Textbestand ausschließlich als ein sekundärer literarischer Vorgang verstanden werden. Die Erweiterungen müssen dem schriftlich vorliegenden Dekalog in der Zeit nach der Entstehung der elohistischen Quellenschicht hinzugefügt worden sein.

Tatsächlich ist längst erkannt worden, daß ein großer Teil der Erweiterungen dem Stil und der Sprache des Deuteronomiums und der deuteronomistischen Literatur entspricht[26]. Denn der dort zu

---

[25] So am ausgeprägtesten H. Graf Reventlow, Gebot und Predigt im Dekalog, 1962.
[26] Vgl. die Zusammenstellung bei H. Schmidt, Mose und der Dekalog, in: Gunkel-Festschrift, I 1923, 85.

Wort kommende theologische Kreis hat sich genauso wie später die priesterschriftliche Quellenschicht des Pentateuchs eine ihm eigentümliche Ausdrucksweise geschaffen, die unverwechselbar ist. Man kann den daraus für die Erweiterungen des Dekalogs sich ergebenden Folgerungen nicht durch die Behauptung entgehen, daß keine Abhängigkeit vom deuteronomistischen Kreis vorliege, weil der Dekalog vielmehr von dem auch im Deuteronomium fließenden Strom einer das Gesetz auslegenden und also beiden vorangehenden »Predigt« ergriffen worden sei[27]. Diese Behauptung ist durch nichts zu begründen. Die stilistisch-sprachlichen Kriterien sind eindeutig. Es handelt sich nicht um eine das Gesetz auslegende Predigt schlechthin, sondern — wenn man schon den nicht unbedingt angemessenen Begriff »Predigt« beibehalten will — um die sachlich und zeitlich genau festzulegende *deuteronomistische* Predigt.

Zu den deuteronomistischen Erweiterungen, die in den Dekalogtext im 7./6. Jh. v. Chr. eingefügt worden sind, gehört zunächst der offenbar als Vordersatz und Begründung des folgenden 1. Verbots gedachte Vers 20 2:

Ich, Jahwe, bin dein Gott, der ich dich aus dem Lande Ägypten, aus dem Sklavenhaus, herausgeführt habe.

Der Satz, der fast ausschließlich aus deuteronomistischen Redewendungen besteht[28], bildet schwerlich einen Vorspruch zum ganzen Dekalog, den er nur unzureichend begründen könnte; besonders für die letzten Verbote — z. B. des Tötens, des Ehebrechens und des Stehlens — besagt der Hinweis auf die Rettung aus Ägypten überhaupt nichts. Wohl aber wird damit das Verbot, andere Götter an Stelle des Rettergotts zu verehren und seinen durch die Rettung erworbenen Anspruch auf Israel zu verletzen, ausgezeichnet begründet. Demgemäß muß der Anfang des Satzes in der obigen Weise übersetzt werden[29] und die andere mögliche Übersetzung »Ich bin Jahwe, dein Gott« ausscheiden, obwohl sie neuerdings häufiger vertreten wird[30].

---

[27] Reventlow a. a. O. 94.
[28] Deuteronomistisch sind: »Jahwe, dein Gott« (mehr als 200mal im Dtn), »herausführen aus dem Lande Ägypten« (15mal im Dtn) und »aus dem Sklavenhaus« (5mal im Dtn). P. Humbert, Dieu fait sortir, ThZ 18 (1962), 357—361 (Ergänzung 433—436), hat die Verwendung des Verbs »herausführen« im einzelnen untersucht. Da v. 2 sekundär ist, fällt die mit diesem Vers begründete Auffassung von G. von Rad, Theologie des Alten Testaments, I 1957, 193, daß sich mit der Ausrufung des Dekalogs die Erwählung Israels verwirkliche, dahin.
[29] So auch Alt a. a. O. 329 Anm. 2; M. Buber, Moses, 1952², 160; E. Auerbach, Moses, 1953, 199.
[30] So besonders W. Zimmerli, »Ich bin Jahwe«, in: Alt-Festschrift, 1953, 204f.; Noth a. a. O. 130 (anders in: Gesammelte Studien zum Alten Testament, 1957, 58). Vgl. auch K. Elliger, »Ich bin der Herr — euer Gott«, in: Heim-Festschrift, 1954, 9—34.

Daran ändert auch der Hinweis auf Ps 50 7 nichts, wo im sogenannten »elohistischen Psalter« der jetzige Text »Elohim, dein Gott, bin ich« ursprünglich gelautet haben muß: »Jahwe, dein Gott, bin ich«. Denn infolge des im Unterschied von Ex 20 2 nachgestellten »ich« ist die Redewendung keineswegs eindeutig und kann durchaus in dem Sinn des »Ich, Jahwe, bin dein Gott« verstanden werden. Für diese Fassung spricht in Ex 20 2 auch die verwendete volle Form des Wortes »ich«, die den Nachdruck darauf legt, daß der »Ich« und kein anderer der Gott Israels ist.

Erst von da aus erklärt es sich ferner, daß die deuteronomistischen Bearbeiter in den Wortlaut des 1. Verbots — und nur dieses Verbots! — eingegriffen haben. Der Ausdruck »andere Götter« ist deuteronomistisch und hat eine ältere Form ersetzt, die nach der Parallele in Ex 34 14 »einen anderen Gott« gelautet haben mag. Das anschließende »neben mir« oder »gegen mich« ist wahrscheinlich eine spätere, an sich überflüssige Erweiterung, wie sich bei der Frage nach der Urform der Dekalogsätze bestätigen wird.

Eine umfangreiche Erweiterung findet sich im Anschluß an das 2. Verbot in 20 4aβ-6. Zwar erscheint ihre atomisierende Aufsplitterung und Zuweisung an sieben Verkündiger oder Prediger in vielen Generationen durch H. Graf Reventlow recht gekünstelt[31], aber einheitlich ist sie nicht. Eine erste Zufügung ist »und keinerlei Abbild« (häufig in Dtn 4), die wohl das als zu eng empfundene Wort »Gottesbild« ergänzen sollte[32]. Dem folgte eine etwas jüngere, typisch deuteronomistische Erweiterung, die die Bereiche aufzählt, denen das Bild nicht entnommen werden darf, und seine Verehrung verbietet; sie setzt die beiden Ausdrücke für das »Bild« voraus (Rest von v. 4 und v. 5 a)[33]. Die anschließenden Sätze in v. 5 b-6 stammen aus anderen Zusammenhängen.

Sicher deuteronomistisch ist schließlich die Erweiterung des Elterngebots in 20 12 b, vielleicht auch der erste Teil der Bemerkungen über den Sabbat in 20 9-10, während sich die Begründung in 20 7 b nicht eindeutig klassifizieren läßt und die Aufzählung in 20 17 b angesichts der Umgestaltung, die das Verbot bzw. die Verbote des

---

[31] Vgl. Reventlow a. a. O. 29—40.
[32] Der Ausdruck »Abbild« ist eindeutig dadurch festgelegt, daß er nur von Gott (Num 12 8 Dtn 4 12. 15 Ps 17 15 Hi 4 16) oder von Götterbildern als Nachahmung der Erscheinung (Dtn 4 16. 23. 25) gebraucht wird. Zu Hi 4 16 vgl. G. Fohrer, Das Buch Hiob, 1963, z. St.
[33] Die pluralischen Suffixe, die W. Zimmerli, Das zweite Gebot, in: Bertholet-Festschrift, 1950, mit bewogen haben, die Erweiterung auf das erste Gebot zurückzubeziehen, betreffen dann in Wirklichkeit die beiden Substantive »Gottesbild« und »Abbild«.

»Begehrens« in Dtn 5 erfahren haben, eher vordeuteronomistisch sein mag.

Außer den deuteronomistischen Erweiterungen liegt in 20 5 b-6 eine andersartige Zufügung vor, die vom vergeltenden Handeln des eifernden Gottes redet. W. Zimmerli hat darin zwei alte Bekenntnisformeln erblickt[34]. Zweifellos entspricht das sich in den Sätzen aussprechende Denken nicht der deuteronomistischen Theologie, die beim menschlichen Richten eine Haftung der Kinder für ihre Väter (und umgekehrt) gerade ausschließt (Dtn 24 16) und auch die göttliche Vergeltung im Leben jedes einzelnen wirksam sieht (Dtn 7 10). Jedoch geht es nicht um die Frage nach dem letzten Ursprung der Vorstellungen oder Formeln der Erweiterung, sondern um diejenige, woher 20 5 b-6 stammen. Und da verhält es sich doch wohl so, daß die Formulierung aus Ex 34 7 (Num 14 18) herrührt: »Jahwe ahndet Väterschuld an den Söhnen und Enkeln, an der dritten und vierten Generation«[35], aber »bewahrt den Tausenden Verbundenheit«. Dies ist in Ex 20 5 b-6 eingetragen und dabei vor allem um die Worte »bei denen, die mich hassen« und »bei denen, die mich lieben« ergänzt worden. Zweifelhaft bleibt, ob diese Worte sich auf die Väter oder die Söhne beziehen. Wird die Schuld nur solcher Väter, die Jahwe hassen, oder das Verdienst solcher, die ihn lieben, an den Nachkommen vergolten? Oder wird Väterschuld und -verdienst nur an solchen Nachkommen vergolten, die ihrerseits Jahwe hassen oder lieben? Das Targum Onkelos versteht es im letzteren Sinn: »sofern die Söhne zusätzlich nach ihren Vätern sündigen«[36]. Da es weitere Beispiele für diese Art der Konstruktion gibt[37], legt sich die Deutung des Targums als wahrscheinlich nahe. Dann hat der Bearbeiter in Ex 20 5 b-6 die Bemerkung aus Ex 34 7 Num 14 18 (jüngere Zusätze zu J) aufgegriffen, sie jedoch in dem personalen Sinn der Beziehung auf die jeweils eigene Schuld nach den Vorbildern der deuteronomistischen Theologie, von Ez 18 1-20 usw. interpretiert. Das bedeutet, daß diese Erweiterung frühestens aus der Exilzeit stammen kann.

Übrig bleibt die Begründung des Sabbatgebots in 20 11. Während diejenige in Dtn 5 vom Geist der deuteronomistischen Theologie geprägt ist, verhält es sich in Ex 20 anders. Es ist längst erkannt und anerkannt, daß ein Zusammenhang mit der priesterlichen Schöpfungs-

---

[34] Zimmerli a. a. O. 555.
[35] Mit L. Rost, Die Schuld der Väter, in: R. Hermann-Festschrift, 1957, 229—233, wird man diese Ausdehnung auf vier Generationen daraus herleiten müssen, daß es sich um die in einer Familie zusammenlebenden Generationen handelt, an denen die Rechtsgemeinde den Bann vollstreckte.
[36] Vgl. A. Sperber, The Bible in Aramaic, I 1959, 122.
[37] C. Brockelmann, Hebräische Syntax, 1956, § 107 i α.

erzählung besteht, die die Sabbatruhe aus dem Ruhen Gottes nach der Schöpfung erklärt (Gen 1 1—2 4a). Obschon auch nach ihrer schriftlichen Fixierung eine wörtliche Übereinstimmung mit ihr für Ex 20 11 nicht erwartet und verlangt werden muß, ist es nicht ausgeschlossen, daß der Satz bereits vorher aus der mündlichen Überlieferung hinzugefügt worden sein kann. Auch in diesem Fall dürfte man angesichts der späten endgültigen mündlichen oder schriftlichen Fixierung der Priesterschrift zeitlich kaum vor die frühnachexilische Zeit zurückgehen.

So zeigen die Erweiterungen insgesamt, daß an der in der Quellenschicht E überlieferten Textform wenigstens vom ausgehenden 7. Jh. bis in die frühnachexilische Zeit gearbeitet worden ist. Im wesentlichen handelt es sich um Erweiterungen; nur das 1. Verbot ist in der Ausdrucksweise ein wenig geändert worden.

3. Nachdem die Erweiterungen entfernt sind, liegt klar zutage, daß die 10 Dekalogsätze apodiktisch formuliert sind. Der Dekalog des E bestand aus 8 verschieden langen Verboten und 2 Geboten in apodiktischer Form:

I Du sollst keinen 'anderen Gott' haben.
II Du sollst dir kein Gottesbild machen.
III Du sollst den Namen Jahwes nicht zu Nichtigem aussprechen.
IV Gedenke an den Sabbattag (ihn zu heiligen)[38].
  (Du sollst kein Werk tun 'am Sabbat'[39].)
V Ehre deinen Vater und deine Mutter.
VI Du sollst nicht töten.
VII Du sollst nicht ehebrechen.
VIII Du sollt nicht stehlen.
IX Du sollst nicht als Lügenzeuge gegen deinen Nächsten aussagen.
X Du sollst nicht nach dem Haus deines Nächsten trachten.

Angesichts der aus 10 (oder 12) Gliedern bestehenden Reihenform, in der apodiktische Sätze anderwärts auftreten, und der in solchen Fällen zu beobachtenden Gleichförmigkeit der Sätze hat sich nun ferner die Frage gestellt, ob es sich beim Dekalog in Ex 20 einmal genauso verhalten und ob es also einen *Urdekalog* von 10 gleichmäßig gebauten Sätzen in apodiktischer Formulierung gegeben habe. Muß man dergleichen nicht geradezu fordern, weil es sich zweifellos um eine Satzreihe handelt? Wegen der beiden verschieden langen Formen der vorkommenden apodiktischen Verbote bieten sich anscheinend sogar zwei Möglichkeiten an, die Frage zu beantworten und die Sätze eines Urdekalogs wiederherzustellen.

---

[38] Es kann sehr wohl sein, daß »ihn zu heiligen« eine Erweiterung darstellt, vgl. Anm. 51.
[39] Auch dieser aus v. 10 b stammende und zu ergänzende Satz ist in Erwägung gezogen worden.

So könnte man die kurze Fassung der aus zwei Wörtern bestehenden Verbote VI—VIII als Urform und Vorbild betrachten und die übrigen Sätze ihnen anzugleichen suchen. Jedoch stößt ein derartiger Versuch in den meisten Fällen auf solch große Schwierigkeiten, daß er praktisch gänzlich aussichtslos ist[40]. Wie sollte man beispielsweise die Verbote der Verehrung anderer Götter, der Herstellung von Gottesbildern oder der mißbräuchlichen Verwendung des Jahwenamens bloß durch eine verneinte Verbform ausdrücken?

Einen Schritt in Richtung auf die zweite Möglichkeit haben E. Sellin und A. Alt getan[41], indem sie annehmen, daß die positiv formulierten Gebote über den Sabbat und die Eltern ursprünglich ebenfalls Verbote waren und erst im Laufe der Zeit ihre jetzige Fassung erhalten haben. Dabei kann man für das erste aus v. 10b die Worte »Du sollst keine Arbeit tun« heranziehen und sie durch »am Sabbat« ergänzen. Für das zweite muß man freilich, der negativen Fassung zuliebe, ein anderes Verb benutzen, das man in Ex 21 17 findet, so daß sich ergibt: »Du sollst deinem Vater und deiner Mutter nicht fluchen.«

K. Rabast ist diesen Weg seines Lehrers Alt konsequent weitergegangen und hat für alle Sätze des Dekalogs eine gleichmäßige Form in metrischer Fassung mit je vier betonten Hebungen herzustellen gesucht[42]. Daß er außerdem einen Dodekalog anstrebt, kann als von vornherein mißglücktes Unternehmen beiseite bleiben. Denn der Satz in v. 2a »Ich, Jahwe, bin dein Gott« kann ebensowenig als erstes Gebot des angeblichen Dodekalogs gelten wie der Anfang von v. 5a »Du sollst sie nicht anbeten« als ein neues viertes; beide entsprechen den eigenen Maßstäben Rabasts nicht, weil sie nur je drei Hebungen aufweisen, v. 2a überhaupt nicht apodiktisch formuliert ist und in v. 5a das beziehungslose »sie« unzureichend ist.

---

[40] Die von Stamm a. a. O. S. 11f. als Beispiel für diesen Versuch angegebene Rekonstruktion von R. Kittel, Geschichte des Volkes Israel, I 1932⁶, 383f., hat lediglich die Erweiterungen entfernt, bemüht sich aber nicht um eine Reduzierung der Sätze auf je zwei Wörter. Dagegen erklärt B. Couroyer, L'Exode, 1968⁵, 96: »Chaque clause de l'Alliance était peut-être, à l'origine, exprimée sous une forme aussi brève que celle, par exemple, des cinquième, sixième, septième et huitième commandements. Les développements seraient alors dûs à des rédacteurs postérieurs soit deutéronomiques soit sacerdotaux.«

[41] E. Sellin, Geschichte des israelitisch-jüdischen Volkes, I 1935², 83f.; Alt a. a. O. 317f. Dagegen lehnt A. Jepsen, Beiträge zur Auslegung und Geschichte des Dekalogs, ZAW 79 (1967), 277—304, die Annahme einer Satzreihe überhaupt ab und versteht den ersten Teil des Dekalogs als Gottesrede, den zweiten Teil als Prophetenrede.

[42] K. Rabast, Das apodiktische Recht im Deuteronomium und im Heiligkeitsgesetz, o. J. (1949), 35—39.

Im einzelnen übernimmt Rabast die Gebote IV und V in der verbietenden Fassung von Sellin und Alt. Im Verbot III ändert er »den Namen Jahwes« in »meinen Namen«, so daß sich vier Hebungen ergeben. Die Kurzform der Verbote VI—VIII hat er mit je zwei weiteren Wörtern aufgefüllt[43]. So lauten nach diesem Vorschlag die Verbote III—VIII:

    III Du sollst 'meinen' Namen nicht zu Nichtigem aussprechen.
    IV Du sollst keine Arbeit 'am Sabbat' tun.
    V 'Du sollst' deinem Vater und deiner Mutter 'nicht fluchen'.
    VI Du sollst nicht töten 'einen Menschen an seiner Seele'.
    VII Du sollst nicht ehebrechen 'mit der Frau deines Nächsten'.
    VIII Du sollst nicht stehlen 'einen Mann oder eine Frau'.

Doch so glatt diese Lösung zu sein scheint und so gleichförmig sich der gewonnene »Urdekalog« darbietet, so groß sind die Bedenken gegen derartige Textmanipulationen. Schon die Änderung des »den Namen Jahwes« in »meinen Namen« im Verbot III ist völlig unbegründet, zumal es angesichts der den Dekalog als Jahwewort hinstellenden Einleitung in v. 1 unerklärlich bleibt, warum das zutreffende »meinen Namen« im Verlauf der Überlieferung geändert worden sein sollte. Da man ferner nicht damit rechnen kann, daß der verstümmelte Wortlaut des Verbots IV ausgerechnet mitten in der umfangreichen Erweiterung zum Sabbatgebot (v. 9-11) erhalten geblieben sein sollte, muß Rabast nicht weniger als fünf Dekalogsätze — genau die Hälfte! — in recht tiefgreifender Weise ändern oder ergänzen. Wenig ist ungerechtfertigter als ein solches Verfahren!

Es gibt keine Möglichkeit, die 10 Sätze des Dekalogs in eine gleichförmige Fassung zu bringen. Jeder Versuch der Änderung, Kürzung oder Erweiterung eines jeweils großen Teils von ihnen ist zum Scheitern verurteilt, weil er ganz und gar willkürlich ist. Da aber der Dekalog offensichtlich eine Reihe von apodiktischen Sätzen und nicht bloß eine zufällige Aneinanderreihung sein soll, bleibt die Annahme übrig, daß er nicht eine ursprüngliche Reihe gleichmäßig gebauter Sätze in apodiktischer Formulierung wie Lev 18 7-16, sondern eine sekundär hergestellte Reihe ist. Die Beobachtungen am parallelen Dekalog des J in Ex 34 werden dies bestätigen.

Ist dies erst einmal erkannt, so erklärt sich das Nebeneinander von drei verschiedenen apodiktischen Satzformen in Ex 20 3-17. Und obwohl sich kein zwingender Beweis führen läßt, ist es am wahrscheinlichsten, daß die Dekalogsätze dementsprechend drei verschiedenen apodiktischen Reihen entnommen sind:

---

[43] A. Alt, Das Verbot des Diebstahls im Dekalog, in: Kleine Schriften zur Geschichte des Volkes Israel, I 1953, 333—340, hat sich der Umwandlung in zehn vierhebige Verbote angeschlossen.

a) 5 Verbote können gemeinsam aus einer apodiktischen Reihe von Sätzen mit je 4 Hebungen stammen, die die Pflichten gegenüber Jahwe und dem Nächsten behandelte:

    I Du sollst keinen 'anderen Gott' haben[44].
    II Du sollst dir kein Gottesbild machen[45].
    III Du sollst den Jahwenamen nicht zu Nichtigem aussprechen.
    IX Du sollst nicht als Lügenzeuge gegen deinen Nächsten aussagen[46].
    X Du sollst nicht nach dem Haus deines Nächsten trachten[47].

Auch der Dekalog des J in Ex 34 14 ff. beginnt mit den gleichen Verboten I und II, wenn auch in etwas anderem Wortlaut. Dies läßt doch wohl darauf schließen, daß beide Dekaloge diese Sätze aus einer ursprünglich gemeinisraelitischen apodiktischen Reihe geschöpft haben, die sich im Nord- und Südreich zu verschiedener Ausdrucksweise weiterentwickelt hat — wie ja auch sonst die von J und E verwendeten Traditionen sich hinsichtlich der Ausdrucksweise und der Namengebung voneinander unterscheiden[48].

b) 3 Verbote stammen aus einer apodiktischen Reihe von Sätzen mit je 2 Hebungen:

    VI Du sollst nicht töten[49].
    VII Du sollst nicht ehebrechen.
    VIII Du sollst nicht stehlen.

---

[44] Aufgrund dieser formalen Erwägungen ist das jetzt den Satz schließende »neben mir« bzw. »gegen mich« als Erweiterung zu beurteilen. Die Auffassung von Reventlow a. a. O. 26, daß Ex 20 3 nicht ein Verbot, sondern eine Aussage darstelle (»Du hast keine anderen Götter neben mir«), ist eine spielerisch zu erwägende Möglichkeit und nicht mehr. Dagegen sprechen die zutreffende philologische Erklärung durch Alt (Die Ursprünge des israelitischen Rechts, 318), die Wiedergabe in den alten Übersetzungen, die formgeschichtlich und exegetisch notwendige Erklärung analog den folgenden Verbotssätzen und die ständige synkretistische Neigung Israels, der gegenüber die einfache Proklamation des Sieges Jahwes über die anderen Götter in den Wind gesprochen wäre.

[45] Daß damit bildliche Darstellungen Jahwes, nicht aber heidnischer Gottheiten gemeint sind, hat Stamm a. a. O. 43—45 erneut dargelegt.

[46] Das Verbot beschränkt sich auf die Zeugenaussage vor Gericht, wie die verwendeten Ausdrücke der Rechtssprache zeigen; vgl. im einzelnen Stamm a. a. O. 60f.

[47] Daß das Verb nicht einfach »begehren« als eine Willensregung meint, sondern die Machenschaften zum Erlangen des Begehrten einschließt, hat J. Herrmann, Das zehnte Gebot, in: Sellin-Festschrift, 1927, 69—82, gezeigt. Zur Illustration vgl. Mi 2 1 f.

[48] Daraus erklären sich auch die verschiedenen Ausdrücke für das Gottesbild in Ex 20 4 und 34 17.

[49] Der Sinn des Verbs ist noch nicht eindeutig bestimmt. Stamm a. a. O. 53f. denkt an das ungesetzliche, gemeinschaftswidrige Töten (durch Reventlow a. a. O. 71—75 dahin modifiziert, daß das in den Bereich der Blutrache fallende Töten gemeint sei).

Einen gewissen Beweis hinsichtlich dieser drei Verbote kann man aus Hos 4 2 Jer 7 9 entnehmen. Gewöhnlich führt man diese Stellen als Beleg dafür an, daß der Dekalog den Propheten bekannt gewesen und daher älter als sie sei[50]. Aber Hosea und Jeremia beziehen sich nur auf die Verbote VI—VIII des Dekalogs, während man die übrigen Glieder ihrer Sündenkataloge nur recht mühsam aus ihm herleiten kann. Sie stellen nebeneinander:

Hos 4 2:	*fluchen,*		
	lügen,		
	töten,	Jer 7 9:	*stehlen,*
	stehlen,		*töten,*
	ehebrechen,		*ehebrechen,*
	einbrechen.		*betrügerisch schwören,*
			dem Baal räuchern,
			anderen Göttern nachlaufen.

Daß drei Glieder der Aufzählung Hoseas — wenn wir den von ihm in mancher Hinsicht und vielleicht auch im Sündenkatalog beeinflußten Jeremia sowie die beiden anderen Aufzählungen einmal beiseite lassen — ausgerechnet mit den drei zweihebigen Verboten des Dekalogs übereinstimmen, ist auffällig. Da bei Hosea die drei weiteren Glieder ähnlich gelagerte Vergehen anprangern, kann man vermuten, daß er alle einer apodiktischen Reihe entnommen hat, aus der drei Sätze auch in den Dekalog geflossen sind. Dies kann um so mehr der Fall sein, als sowohl der den Dekalog überliefernde E als auch Hosea im Nordreich Israel beheimatet waren. Dann bezeugt Hos 4 2 noch für die zweite Hälfte des 8. Jh. die Existenz einer nordisraelitischen Reihe apodiktischer Verbotssätze, aus der einige für den elohistischen Dekalog benutzt worden sind.

Ferner kann man auf die Aufzählungen in Jos 7 11 und Lev 19 11 hinweisen, die wie Hos 4 2 »stehlen« und »lügen« miteinander verbinden und von denen Lev 19 11 mit »betrügen« außerdem an Jer 7 9 anklingt. Das ist um so beachtenswerter, als die Anordnungen in Lev 19 3 ff. überwiegend vom Dekalog in Ex 20 abhängig zu sein scheinen (s. u. V, 1); sollte in »betrügen« oder »betrügerisch schwören« ein weiteres Glied der anzunehmenden apodiktischen Reihe vorliegen?

c) Zwei Gebote schließlich stammen aus einer apodiktischen Reihe von Sätzen mit je drei Hebungen:

Treffender scheint die Definition von A. Jepsen, Du sollst nicht töten! Was ist das?, ELKZ 13 (1959), 384f.: das grundlose Töten eines (an seinem Mörder nicht schuldig gewordenen) Menschen, ob versehentlich oder absichtlich.

[50] Vgl. z. B. Noth a. a. O. 134f.

IV Gedenke an den Tag des Sabbats[51].
V Ehre deinen Vater und deine Mutter.

Daß man noch in späterer Zeit um die herkunftsmäßige Zusammengehörigkeit dieser beiden Gebote gewußt hat, läßt sich vielleicht aus der im wesentlichen von Ex 20 abhängigen Gebotsreihe ersehen, die in Lev 19 3-12 verarbeitet worden ist. Sie bringt die beiden Sätze gemeinsam am Anfang (v. 3).

4. Fragt man weiter nach *Alter und Herkunft der Dekalogsätze*, so ist sogleich deutlich, daß die Verbote I—III den Jahweglauben voraussetzen und Anordnungen über ihn erteilen. Sie können erst nach oder frühestens mit der Annahme dieses Glaubens durch die Israeliten oder die Moseschar entstanden sein. Eine genaue zeitliche Fixierung ist nicht möglich. So wenig der Annahme im Wege steht, daß sie auf die Mosezeit selbst zurückgehen, zumal sie zunächst in einem nicht mehr feststellbaren Wortlaut gemeinisraelitisches Gut gewesen zu sein scheinen, so wenig läßt sich dies beweisen. Sind sie einmal gemeinisraelitisches Gut gewesen, wie die Verwendung in Ex 20 und 34 nahelegt, so läßt sich als untere Zeitgrenze nur die ziehen, daß sie längere Zeit vor der Reichsteilung, die nach dem Tode Salomos stattfand, entstanden sein müssen. Gleiches dürfte für die mit ihnen in einer Reihe verbundenen Verbote IX—X gelten. Festzuhalten ist schließlich, daß die Nennung Jahwes in der 3. Person im Verbot III zeigt, daß es sich ursprünglich nicht um von Jahwe gegebene Verbote gehandelt, sondern daß eine andere Autorität die Weisungen erteilt hat.

Für die aus den beiden anderen apodiktischen Reihen entnommenen Verbote und Gebote gibt es keinerlei Hinweise auf Alter und Herkunft. Auch die Erwähnung des Sabbats hilft nicht weiter, weil er offensichtlich schon in vorjahwistischer Zeit bekannt gewesen ist[52]. Die Sätze bzw. ihre Reihen lassen sich ebensogut aus der nomadisch-vorjahwistischen[53] wie aus der palästinisch-jahwistischen Zeit Israels[54]

---

[51] Das anschließende »ihn zu heiligen« ist wohl ein später Zusatz, weil der Sabbat zunächst und für lange Zeit als wöchentlicher Ruhetag galt, vgl. Gen 2 1-4 a. Den obigen Satz mit Reventlow a. a. O. S. 48—56 als eine priesterliche Tora zu verstehen, besteht kein Anlaß; Reventlow, der das Elterngebot in ein Verbot ändert, scheint merkwürdigerweise stillschweigend vorauszusetzen, daß apodiktische Sätze stets negativ formuliert sein müßten, obwohl es durchaus positiv formulierte apodiktische Gebote geben kann.

[52] Vgl. zur ganzen Frage neuerdings G. J. Botterweck, Der Sabbat im Alten Testament, ThQ 134 (1954), 134—136. 448—457; E. Jenni, Die theologische Begründung des Sabbatgebotes im Alten Testament, 1956; H.-J. Kraus, Gottesdienst in Israel, 1962², 98—108.

[53] Dafür vgl. H. H. Rowley, Moses and the Decalogue, BJRL 34 (1951/52), 81—118.

[54] Wenigstens auf palästinische Überarbeitung könnte das Wort »Haus« im zehnten

herleiten, während die verhältnismäßig kurze Zeit der Wanderung der Moseschar nach Palästina schwerlich für das Entstehen mehrerer Gruppen von apodiktischen Reihen in Betracht kommt. Gerade die knappe apodiktische Satzform, in der über die Beweggründe für die Verbote und Gebote nichts verlautet, läßt die Möglichkeit der Beziehung auf verschiedene kulturelle Verhältnisse durchaus offen.

Auch über den Charakter der drei Reihen, denen die Dekalogsätze entstammen, läßt sich insofern nichts Abschließendes sagen, als sie uns lediglich bruchstückweise bekannt sind. Immerhin muß man doch wohl die unter a) genannte Reihe als einen Katalog der Pflichten gegenüber dem Jahweglauben und dem »Nächsten« bezeichnen. Falls die unter b) genannte Reihe in Hos 4 2 ebenfalls benutzt worden ist, zeigen die dort genannten weiteren Stichwörter »fluchen« und »lügen«, daß es sich um eine Lebens- und Verhaltensregel gehandelt hat. Gleiches gilt für die unter c) genannte Reihe, zumal das Elterngebot in seiner positiven Fassung weit über die gesetzliche Formulierung von Ex 21 17 hinausgeht und mit der Forderung des »Ehrens« eine rechtlich gar nicht erzwingbare Regel aufstellt.

5. Erst bei der Zusammenstellung zum Dekalog sind die aus verschiedenen Reihen ausgewählten Sätze mittels des vorangestellten v. 1 zur Jahweordnung, d. h. als von Jahwe selbst gegeben, erklärt worden. Darin wiederholt sich der gleiche Vorgang wie bei der Neuinterpretation der nomadischen Reihe in Lev 18 und der Assimilation des kasuistischen Rechts durch die Israeliten.

Die Frage, wann dies erfolgt ist, d. h. die Frage nach dem *Alter des Dekalogs* als einer neuen Reihe, läßt sich ebensowenig sicher beantworten wie diejenige nach dem Alter der vorgegebenen Reihen und Sätze. Am nächsten liegt freilich die Annahme, daß E es war, der den Dekalog in Ex 20 — wie J denjenigen in Ex 34 — zusammengestellt hat. Hätte beiden ein alter Dekalog vorgelegen, der vielleicht gar aus der Mosezeit stammte, so ist nicht verständlich, warum sie ihn nicht benutzt haben sollten. Für die Hypothese, daß E den Dekalog in Ex 20 aus älterem Material gebildet hat, spricht 1. die Existenz einer der von ihm herangezogenen Reihen noch in der Zeit Hoseas und 2. die für E bestehende Notwendigkeit, für die nach Ex 24 3 ff. erfolgende Verpflichtung der Israeliten am Sinai eine Grundlage zu schaffen, deretwegen es zugleich nötig wurde, die Dekalogsätze Jahwe selber in den Mund zu legen.

Selbst wenn man annehmen will, daß E den Dekalog schon vorgefunden habe, bleibt er ein sekundäres Gebilde. Er ist keine ursprüng-

---

Verbot hinweisen. Denn obwohl es auch »Familie« und »Siedlung (von Blutsverwandten)« bedeuten kann, wäre seine Verwendung für (halb)nomadische Verhältnisse doch ungewöhnlich.

liche, sondern eine nach anderen Beispielen künstlich zusammengestellte Reihe; und seine Gebote und Verbote sind kein ursprüngliches Jahwe- oder Gottesrecht, sondern durch den Vorspruch in v. 1 erst zu göttlichen Anordnungen erklärt worden. Von da aus erheben sich grundsätzlich Zweifel an den Hypothesen über eine kultische Entstehung oder Zweckbestimmung des Dekalogs. Ein solch künstliches Gebilde, das zudem kein »Recht« ist, kann weder die Bedingungen für die Teilnahme am Kult des Neujahrs- und Thronbesteigungsfestes enthalten[55], noch zum Rechtsvortrag am Laubhüttenfest jedes 7. Jahres dienen[56], geschweige denn auf die Weise entstanden sein, daß die Verkündigung eines postulierten Festes die bereitliegenden apodiktischen Stoffe aufgegriffen und in ihren Kreis einbezogen hätte[57] oder daß die hetitischen Vasallenverträge das Modell geliefert hätten[58], zumal nach dem Wegfall des erst später zugefügten Verses 20 2 praktisch nur die Parallelität der Verbots- und Gebotssätze mit den Vertragsbestimmungen als einer von mehreren Vergleichspunkten übrigbleibt.

Vielmehr ist der Dekalog als ganzer wie die Reihen, denen die ihn bildenden Verbote und Gebote entnommen sind, als eine Lebens- und Verhaltensregel gedacht, so daß er in dieser Hinsicht der ursprünglichen Reihe in Lev 18 ähnlich ist. Diese Zweckbestimmung apodiktischer Reihen scheint demjenigen, der den Dekalog geschaffen hat — nach der oben dargelegten Ansicht: dem Elohisten — durchaus geläufig gewesen zu sein. Denn nach Ex 24 3-8 wird ja nicht ein »Bund« zwischen Gott und Volk geschaffen, dessen Bedingungen im Dekalog niedergelegt wären, sondern das Volk verpflichtet sich umgekehrt dazu, »alle Worte, die Jahwe geredet hat«, zu befolgen und zu tun, und bekräftigt diesen Entschluß. Damit proklamiert E seinen Dekalog aufs deutlichste als eine Lebens- und Verhaltensregel für Israel, wie es dem ursprünglichen Sinn solcher Reihen apodiktisch formulierter Sätze entspricht; nur begründet er ihre Geltung nicht mehr mit der Autorität der Sippe oder ihres Hauptes, sondern führt sie als gottgewollte Regel ein. Dies letztere ist wiederum der gewan-

---

[55] S. Mowinckel, Le décalogue, 1927.
[56] Alt, Die Ursprünge des israelitischen Rechts, 324—328. Damit sind die vielfältigen Überlegungen hinfällig, wer denn das sog. genuin israelitisch-jahwistische apodiktische Recht verkündet habe: die »kleinen Richter«, Priester oder Propheten. Hat es kein solches Recht gegeben (sondern höchstens kasuistisches Recht in apodiktischer Formulierung, s. u. V, 3) und also auch kein »Gottesrecht«, so war nichts zu verkünden und daher kein Verkündiger nötig, von dem das Alte Testament ohnehin nichts berichtet.
[57] Reventlow a. a. O. 94.
[58] Beyerlin a. a. O. 59—78; vgl. auch Baltzer a. a. O. 37 Anm. 1.

delten Situation in der Zeit des E gemäß, in der Jahwe längst alle anderen aus der Rolle der gebietenden Autorität verdrängt und sie selbst übernommen hatte.

In der gleichen Weise hat der spätere Redaktor oder Bearbeiter des Sinaikomplexes den Dekalog aufgefaßt. Indem er die bei E vor dem Dekalog stehenden Verse an ihre jetzige Stelle in 20 18-21 umgestellt und ihnen das sogenannte »Bundesbuch« angeschlossen hat, stellt er dessen Gesetze als die rechtlichen Ausführungsbestimmungen zur Grundregel des Dekalogs hin. Und schließlich bestätigt die hauptsächlich aus dem Dekalog abgeleitete Gebotssammlung in Lev 19 3-12 dessen Auffassung als Lebens- und Verhaltensregel, indem sie infolge der Voranstellung des Eltern- und Sabbatgebots geradezu wie ein häuslicher Katechismus erscheint.

6. Zusammenfassend können wir feststellen, daß der Dekalog in Ex 20 1-17 zehn — später mehrfach erweiterte — apodiktische Sätze in verbietender und gebietender Form enthält, jedoch keine ursprüngliche und in sich geschlossene Reihe bildet, sondern aus Sätzen zusammengestellt ist, die drei ursprünglichen Reihen angehört haben. Gemäß der eigentlichen Herkunft solcher Reihen apodiktischer Formulierungen aus dem Nomadentum, in dem sie nicht Recht, sondern vor allem das Zusammenleben schützende Anordnungen und nicht Kult-, sondern Lebensregeln darstellten, sind sowohl die ursprünglichen Reihen, die die Dekalogsätze geliefert haben, als auch der Dekalog selber als Lebens- und Verhaltensregel zu verstehen. Während die ersteren teilweise aus der Mosezeit, teilweise sogar aus der nomadisch-vorjahwistischen Zeit stammen können und zwei von ihnen sich noch an anderer Stelle nachweisen lassen (J, Hos 4 2), ist der letztere von E aus ihnen zusammengefügt und der göttlichen Autorität unterstellt worden.

IV.

Ein Blick auf eine bereits erwähnte andere Reihe bestätigt einige der gewonnenen Einsichten. Gemeint ist der Dekalog des Jahwisten (J), der dem elohistischen Dekalog parallel steht. Er liegt in Ex 34 14-26 vor und weist gleichfalls zahlreiche spätere Erweiterungen auf. Zudem ist er sowohl mit einer Einleitung, die im Grundbestand von 34 10-13 enthalten ist (v. 10aα. 11-12), als auch mit einer Schlußbemerkung in 34 27-28 versehen, die auf den vorhergehenden Dekalog als die »Zehn Worte« hinweist[59]. Überblickt man den Text von 34 14-26, so

---

[59] Die Erwähnung der »Zehn Worte« ist keineswegs sekundär, wie H. Kosmala, The So-Called Ritual Decalogue, ASTI 1 (1962), 31—61, annimmt, der den Text aufteilt

scheinen sich bei der Anordnung der Gebote und Verbote sogar 12 Sätze zu ergeben, obwohl der Jahwist ausdrücklich einen Dekalog meint. Jedoch liegt v. 19 a gar keine apodiktische Anordnung, sondern ein einfacher Aussagesatz vor, der mit seiner Erweiterung nachträglich in den Textzusammenhang eingefügt worden ist; und ferner weicht die Anordnung von v. 23 nach Form und Umfang so stark von den anderen Sätzen ab, daß man sie ebenfalls als späteren Zuwachs betrachten muß.

Die dann verbleibenden 10 Sätze weisen zwei Grundformen auf, die im einzelnen variieren. Einmal finden sich vier positiv formulierte apodiktische Anordnungen, die sich auf das Massotfest (III: v. 18 aα), den Sabbat (V: v. 21 a), das Wochenfest (VI: v. 22 aα) und die Erstlinge der Ackerfrüchte (IX: v. 26 a) beziehen. Sie befassen sich mit besonderen Tagen des Jahres, da ja auch die Darbringung der Erstlingsgarben nach Lev 23 9 ff. nicht am Erntefest, sondern »am Tag nach dem Sabbat«, also wohl am ersten Tag der Erntezeit, erfolgen sollte — zumindest in der älteren Zeit. Daher ist es durchaus möglich, daß sie einer Satzreihe mit Anordnungen für die besonderen Tage des Jahres entnommen sind, dann allerdings nicht mehr im ursprünglichen Wortlaut vorliegen:

    III Das Massotfest sollst du halten[60].
    V Sechs Tage sollst du arbeiten, aber am siebten Tage ruhen.
    VI Das Wochenfest sollst du dir halten.
    IX Das Beste der Erstlinge des Ackers sollst du in das Haus Jahwes bringen.

Ferner lassen sich sechs negativ formulierte apodiktische Anordnungen erkennen, von denen vier sich mit Fragen des Opferwesens befassen. Es handelt sich um die Verbote, vor Jahwe mit leeren Händen zu erscheinen (IV: v. 20 bβ), Schlachtopferblut zusammen mit Gesäuerten darzubringen (VII: v. 25 a), das Fleisch des Passa über Nacht aufzubewahren (VIII: v. 25 b) und ein Böckchen in der Milch seiner Mutter zu kochen (X: v. 26 b). Wieder liegt die Annahme am nächsten, daß die Verbote einen Auszug aus einer Reihe darstellen, in diesem Falle über die Darbringung von Opfern:

---

auf v. 10-16. 27. 28 b als Bericht über den Bund im Blick auf die Landnahme und v. 18-24 als alten Festkalender mit vier zusätzlichen Bestimmungen über das Passa in v. 25-26. Doch diese Aufteilung ist unrichtig, weil sie die Verbote in v. 14 a und 17 übergeht oder ausscheidet, in v. 18 ff. die ursprünglichen Anordnungen und die späteren Erweiterungen nicht auseinanderhält und die Verbote VII, IX und X auf das Passa bezieht. Ebensowenig gehört v. 28 mit der Erwähnung der »Zehn Worte« der Quellenschicht E an, wie von E. Sellin—L. Rost, Einleitung in das Alte Testament, 1959[9], 52, angenommen wird; vgl. auch Eißfeldt a. a. O. 159*.

[60] Das Gebot liegt vielleicht unvollständig vor.

IV 'Du sollst nicht' mit leeren Händen vor mir erscheinen[61].
VII Du sollst nicht schlachten das Blut meines Opfers zu Gesäuertem.
VIII Es soll nicht über Nacht bleiben das Schlachtopfer.
X Du sollst nicht kochen das Böckchen in der Milch seiner Mutter.

Die beiden ersten Verbote des jahwistischen Dekalogs entsprechen den beiden ersten Verboten in Ex 20. Es wurde bereits die Vermutung ausgesprochen, daß sie einer älteren gemeinisraelitischen Reihe, die sich im Süd- und Nordreich verschieden entwickelt hat, entstammen:

I Du sollst nicht niederfallen vor einem anderen Gott.
II Gegossene Gottesbilder sollst du dir nicht machen.

Abgesehen von diesen beiden Verboten ist demnach der jahwistische Dekalog aus anderen Reihen als der elohistische zusammengestellt worden, nämlich aus zwei Reihen über die besonderen Tage des Jahres und über Opferbestimmungen. Man bezeichnet sie am besten als judäische Heiligtumsregeln, die der Belehrung der Laien dienten. Da sie ursprünglich kanaanäische Feste oder Begehungen aufnehmen (III, VI, IX) und sich gegen kanaanäische Opferbräuche wenden (X), sind sie zweifellos erst in Palästina an einem Jahweheiligtum entstanden. Doch wirkt der ursprüngliche Charakter der apodiktischen Reihen als Lebens- und Verhaltensregeln eben darin weiter, daß sie Verhaltensmaßnahmen — wenn auch kultischer Art — darlegen. Es ist höchst beachtenswert, daß dieser Grundsinn der apodiktischen Reihen bis in die palästinischen Heiligtumsregeln hinein bewahrt geblieben ist.

Doch wenn J auch weithin andere Reihen als E für seinen Dekalog benutzt hat, ist beiden die Methode des Zusammensetzens gemeinsam. Denn das Bild, das sich in Ex 34 14-26 enthüllt hat, bekräftigt wiederum das für Ex 20 erzielte Ergebnis. Ja, es stützt sogar die dort dargelegte Annahme, daß E es gewesen ist, der seinen Dekalog zusammengestellt hat, wie sich dies in analoger Weise für J nahelegt. Ein Gebilde wie Ex 34 14-26 kann auch in seiner ursprünglichen Form ohne die späteren Erweiterungen schwerlich als selbständige Größe existiert haben und überliefert worden sein.

Schließlich erweist sich die These einer kultisch-liturgischen Verkündigung des Dekalogs an Ex 34 14-26 nochmals als irrig. Für diesen Dekalog wäre eine solche Verkündigung ein geradezu absurdes Unterfangen, wie ein Versuch des lauten, feierlichen Verlesens der Reihe sogleich deutlich machen dürfte. Derartige Anordnungen sind zum Erlernen und Merken bestimmt.

---

[61] In diesem Fall ist es durchaus möglich, daß die Verbform der 3. pers. pl. infolge des Anschlusses an die Bestimmungen in v. 20 a.bα aus der ursprünglichen 2. pers. sg. hergestellt worden ist.

V.

Mit der ursprünglichen oder primären Reihe, die in Lev 18 7-17 a zu erfassen ist, und den beiden sekundären Reihen, als die sich die Dekaloge in Ex 20 1-17 und 34 14-26 erwiesen haben, sind die für das Verständnis derartiger Satzreihen mit apodiktischen Formulierungen wichtigsten Texte behandelt. Immerhin gibt es außer ihnen einige weitere Reihen mit 10 oder 12 apodiktisch formulierten Sätzen. Wenn sie auch teilweise von einem oder mehreren der genannten drei Dekaloge abhängig oder aus anderen Gründen als jünger denn diese zu beurteilen sind, bezeugen sie doch das Weiterleben und vor allem die Weiterentwicklung der apodiktisch formulierten Sätze in Reihenform. Daher ist ein kurzer Blick auf sie nicht ohne Interesse.

1. In Lev 19 3-12 läßt sich ein pluralistischer Dekalog erkennen oder vermuten[62]. Seine vier ersten und letzten Sätze sind mühelos zu erkennen; ihre verschiedenartigen Formen zeigen zugleich, daß es sich nicht um eine ursprüngliche und echte Reihe handelt. Inhaltlich ist festzustellen, daß die Sätze im Anschluß an solche des Dekalogs von Ex 20 gebildet sind. Schwierig bleibt lediglich der Versuch, die beiden mittleren Sätze in v. 5-8 und 9-10 zu erfassen. Folgt man grundsätzlich, wenn auch mit Abweichungen in Einzelheiten, der von S. Mowinckel vorgeschlagenen Lösung, so entdeckt man in den mittleren Sätzen wie in der Formulierung eines Teils der anderen acht Sätze den Geist der sozialethischen Forderungen des Deuteronomiums, auf dem der Nachdruck liegt. Vor allem aber ergibt sich aus der Abhängigkeit von Ex 20, daß es sich um eine tertiäre Reihe handelt, die jünger als das Deuteronomium ist. Sie bildet eine Lebens- und Verhaltensregel, die wegen des vorangestellten Elterngebots vielleicht als ein häuslicher »Katechismus« bezeichnet werden kann.

Eine weitere tertiäre Reihe liegt in den apodiktischen Sätzen vor, die in Ex 23 10-19 begegnen. Die Verse bilden im jetzigen Textzusammenhang den Abschluß des sogenannten Bundesbuchs. Man kann aus ihnen zunächst einen Dodekalog erarbeiten, wenn man v. 10-11, die vom Sabbatjahr handeln, auf einen kurzen apodiktischen Satz zusammendrängt, der dem Sabbatgebot in v. 12 a parallel ist. Allerdings ist dies nicht ganz leicht. Wenn man zudem feststellt, daß v. 14 mit dem Gebot, für Jahwe jährlich dreimal ein Fest zu halten, inhaltlich mit v. 17 identisch ist und daß dieser Vers, der das jährlich dreimalige Erscheinen vor Jahwe fordert, genauso wie Ex 34 auf das bzw. die Festgebote selber folgt, dann wird man einen älteren Dekalog an-

---

[62] S. Mowinckel, Zur Geschichte der Dekaloge, ZAW 55 (1937), 218—235. Einen anderen Weg zur Erfassung eines Dekalogs in Lev 19 geht J. Morgenstern, The Decalogue of the Holiness Code, HUCA 26 (1955), 1—27.

nehmen müssen, der später um die stärker kasuistisch gehaltene Bestimmung über das Sabbatjahr und das Gebot der dreimaligen Festfeier erweitert worden ist. In diesem Dekalog befassen sich die drei ersten Sätze mit dem Sabbat (v. 12 a), dem Verbot anderer Götter (v. 13 bα) und dem Massotfest (v. 15 a), die weiteren sieben Sätze folgen genau in der Ordnung des jahwistischen Dekalogs in Ex 34, der darüber hinaus die drei ersten Sätze ebenfalls enthält. So ergibt sich folgendes Bild:

Ex 23:   I Sabbat (v. 12 a)   Ex 34:   V (v. 21 a)
        II andere Götter (v. 13 bα)   I (v. 14 a)
       III Massot (v. 15 aα)   III (v. 18 aα)
                                            vgl.   VI (v. 22 aα)
        IV Kornernte (v. 16 aα)   v. 22 a
         V Lese (v. 16 bα)   v. 22 b
        VI Dreimaliges Aufsuchen Gottes (v. 17)   v. 23
       VII Opfer ohne Gesäuertes (v. 18 a)   VII (v. 25 a)
      VIII Opferfett (v. 18 b)   VIII (v. 25 b)
        IX Erstlinge des Ackers (v. 19 a)   IX (v. 26 a)
         X Böckchen (v. 19 b)   X (v. 26 b)

Daß Ex 23 darin vom Dekalog des J in Ex 34 abhängig ist, ergibt sich ganz eindeutig daraus, daß die Reihenfolge in Ex 23 sich nicht an den ursprünglichen, sondern an den bereits erweiterten Text von Ex 34 anschließt und zumindest die Auffüllung in 34 22-23 voraussetzt. Daß es sich nicht umgekehrt verhält und etwa Ex 34 nach Ex 23 erweitert worden ist, folgt einmal aus der jüngeren Ausdrucksweise »erscheinen vor dem Herrn Jahwe« in 23 17 gegenüber der im Konsonantenbestand zu lesenden älteren Fassung »das Angesicht Jahwe schauen« in 34 24 und ferner aus der Voranstellung des für die Spätzeit so wichtig gewordenen Sabbatgebots. So ist in Ex 23 10-19 eine von Ex 34 abhängige tertiäre Reihe verwendet und wieder um allerlei weitere Anordnungen und Bemerkungen ergänzt worden[63].

2. Ein viertes Stadium in der Geschichte der apodiktischen Reihen begegnet zunächst in dem sogenannten singularischen Dekalog in Lev 19 13-18[64]. Er ist das Beispiel einer Reihe, die in recht junger Zeit nach dem Muster älterer Reihen gebildet worden ist. Seine sozialethischen Forderungen zum Schutz des Schwachen und des »Nächsten« überhaupt vor Übergriffen im täglichen Leben und vor Gericht gründen sich auf die prophetische und die deuteronomistische Theologie. So bildet die Reihe eine Art von frei verfaßtem »Katechismus« über das rechte Leben und Verhalten.

---

[63] Das schließt ein, daß es sich um einen jungen Nachtrag zum sog. Bundesbuch handelt, das ursprünglich mit Ex 23 9 geendet hat.
[64] Mowinckel a. a. O.

Derartige Reihen scheinen ebenso in einigen weiteren Fällen verwendet worden zu sein. Sie gehören gleichfalls einer jungen Zeit an, in der sie neuen Zwecken dienen mußten. Dennoch ist unverkennbar, daß man darin die ursprüngliche Zweckbestimmung als Lebens- und Verhaltensregel weiterentwickelt hat. Eine priesterliche Tora liegt der Aufzählung in Ez 18 5-9 zugrunde[65], ein »Beichtspiegel«, der die Zulassung zum Kultus regelt[66], den Aufzählungen in Jes 33 14-16 Ps 15 und 24 3-6 (34 13-15), während es sich in Hi 31 um die Verwendung einer aufgrund solcher Vorbilder zusammengestellten Belehrung der Lebensweisheit und in Ez 22 6-16 Neh 10 31-40 um bunt gemischte Nachahmungen handelt.

3. Schließlich hat man die apodiktische Formulierung und die Reihenbildung noch für einen weiteren Zweck benutzt, wie zwei Beispiele zeigen: für die kurze eindrückliche Zusammenfassung von kasuistischen Rechtsfällen.

Das erste Beispiel liefert die Mot-jumat-Reihe, die aufgelöst worden ist und vor allem im Bundesbuch und Heiligkeitsgesetz verstreut vorliegt (Ex 21 12. 15-17 22 18 f. Lev 20 2. 9-13. 15-16. 27 24 16, dazu Einzelsätze in Ex 31 15 Lev 27 29). Da die Sätze sich nicht nur ergänzen, sondern teilweise auch überschneiden, läßt sich nicht sicher feststellen, welche zur ursprünglichen Reihe gehören und welche nach diesem Muster später gebildet worden sind. Vielleicht haben die von Ex 20 beeinflußten ersten fünf Sätze in Ex 22 19 Lev 24 16 Ex 21 12. 16. 17 und die von Lev 18 beeinflußten zweiten fünf Sätze in Lev 20 10-13. 15 einmal als geschlossene Reihe vorgelegen. Ihre apodiktische Formulierung darf freilich nicht darüber hinwegtäuschen, daß sie eine andere Gattung als die bisher betrachteten Gebote und Verbote darstellen. Sie bestehen aus einem Vordersatz im Partizipialstil, der ein Vergehen beschreibt und aus einem gleichbleibenden verbalen Nachsatz, der die darauf stehende Todesstrafe ansagt:

Wer seinen Vater und seine Mutter verflucht, soll unbedingt getötet werden.

Das ist eine Rechtsbestimmung. Dennoch kann man auch bei dieser Reihe nicht von »apodiktischem Recht« sprechen. Vielmehr handelt es sich um kasuistisches Recht in apodiktischer Formulierung[67], das

---

[65] Vgl. G. Fohrer, Ezechiel, 1955, 98.

[66] K. Galling, Der Beichtspiegel, eine gattungsgeschichtliche Studie, ZAW 47 (1929), 125—130.

[67] So auch Gese a. a. O. 148f.: Die Sätze der Reihe sind nach ihrer sprachlichen Form eine verkürzende Nachahmung der Konditionalsatzperiode, d. h. der kasuistischen Rechtsformulierung, so daß es sich um eine Umgestaltung kasuistischer Rechtssätze handelt. Daß dies zutrifft, zeigt ein Vergleich der apodiktischen Form Ex 21 12 »Wer einen Mann (er)schlägt, daß der stirbt, soll unbedingt getötet werden« mit

einzelne Lebens- und Verhaltensregeln, wie sie aus Ex 20 und Lev 18 bekannt sind, in Recht und Gesetz umwandelt[68].

Das zweite Beispiel bildet die Fluchreihe in Dtn 27 15-26. In ihren Sätzen steht die Strafandrohung »Verflucht ist« voran und die Beschreibung des Vergehens folgt im Partizipialstil. Ein Teil der Sätze schließt sich an Lev 18 und die Mot-jumat-Reihe an; die übrigen sind stark sozialethisch bestimmt. Die Reihe, die wieder kasuistisches Recht in apodiktischer Formulierung enthält, ist daher in der deuteronomistischen Zeit entstanden und in den Rahmen des Buches Deuteronomium für die Darstellung eines fingierten kultischen Aktes eingearbeitet worden.

4. Außer den bisher behandelten großen Reihen mit durchweg 10 Gliedern gibt es mehrere Kurzreihen in apodiktischer Formulierung, für deren Eigenarten im einzelnen auf die Ausführungen von Alt, Rabast und Elliger verwiesen werden muß[69]. Für die meisten von ihnen gilt ohne weiteres das von den sekundären und tertiären großen Reihen Gesagte; ja, der »Königsspiegel« in Dtn 17 16f. beruht wohl auf bloßer Nachahmung apodiktischer Redeweise. Nur bei den Sätzen über die Tabu-Personen in Ex 22 17-20f. 27 und über die Befreiung vom Kriegsdienst in Dtn 20 5-8 könnte es sich anders verhalten. Im ersteren Falle wirkt die Nebeneinanderstellung von Gott, der Zauberin und dem Stammesführer als Tabu-Personen recht altertümlich, so daß eine Herleitung der Sätze aus der nomadischen Zeit nicht ausgeschlossen scheint — vorausgesetzt, daß die jetzige Fünfgliedrigkeit ursprünglich ist und nicht weitere Sätze, die das Bild sogleich verändern könnten, weggefallen sind. Die Bestimmungen in Dtn 20 5-8

---

der kasuistischen Form Lev 24 17 »Wenn einer irgendeinen Menschen erschlägt, soll er unbedingt getötet werden«. Vgl. ferner Kilian a. a. O. 188—194, der dann allerdings annimmt, daß solche Bestimmungen nicht mit profaner Rechtsprechung, sondern mit einem rituellen oder kultisch-sakralen Akt zusammenhängen — aber mit welchem ? Die Parallele des ägyptischen magischen Rituals der Ächtungstexte scheint für Israel nicht zwingend. Vor allem ist die Mot-jumat-Reihe eine formgeschichtlich späte und künstliche Bildung, für die man nach einem »Sitz im Leben« ebensowenig fragen kann wie für die sogleich zu nennende Fluchreihe in Dtn 27, die für einen fingierten und nicht wirklich ausgeführten Kultakt gebildet worden ist.

[68] Zu einem anderen Ergebnis gelangt H. Schulz, Das Todesrecht im Alten Testament, 1969, worauf an dieser Stelle nur kurz hingewiesen werden kann: Die genannten Rechtssätze stellen eine eigene Rechtsform dar, die man am besten als Todesrecht bezeichnet. Sie basiert auf grundlegenden Prohibitivnormen und ist eine Weiterbildung des Prohibitivrechts. In der Frühzeit war der durch das Stammesoberhaupt repräsentierte Stamm der Träger des Todesrechts, in den späteren Ortsgemeinden war die kultische Gerichtsgemeinde zuständig; die Spätzeit entwickelte durchgegliederte kultische Gerichtsverfahren.

[69] Alt a. a. O. 315f.; Rabast a. a. O. 23—25; Elliger a. a. O. (Anm. 13) 14—17.

sind in ihrer jetzigen Form mit fragenden Vorder- und jussivischen Nachsätzen sicherlich jungen Datums. Jedoch gehen sie letztlich auf dämonistische Vorstellungen zurück, aufgrund deren bestimmte Tabu-Personen vom Heerbann ausgeschlossen wurden. So ist es möglich, daß die Sätze aus einer älteren Fassung entwickelt worden sind, die eine kurze apodiktische Bestimmung aufwies. Auch in diesem Fall können sie freilich erst aus der palästinischen Zeit Israels herrühren, weil sie das Bauen eines Hauses und das Anlegen eines Weinbergs erwähnen.

*

Insgesamt ergibt sich, daß die Bezeichnung »Lebens- und Verhaltensregel in apodiktischer Formulierung« dem Sachverhalt näherkommt als »apodiktisch formuliertes Recht«. Nur selten und erst in der Weiterentwicklung der apodiktischen Reihen in verhältnismäßig junger Zeit treffen wir auf Rechtssätze. Und dann sind es kasuistische Bestimmungen, die eine apodiktische Form erhalten haben — in der Mot-jumat-Reihe offenbar deswegen, weil sie apodiktische Verhaltensregeln in Gesetze umprägen. Meist aber handelt es sich eindeutig um Lebens- und Verhaltensregeln, die wenigstens in der ursprünglichen Form von Lev 18 noch auf ihre Herkunft aus dem (halb)nomadischen Lebensbereich hinweisen und sodann in mehreren Entwicklungsstadien und in breiter Fächerung die Regeln für das religiös bestimmte Verhalten auf dem Boden des Jahweglaubens einprägen sollen. Waren es zunächst Sippenregeln (Lev 18), so treffen wir weiter auf Reihen, die die Verpflichtung der Israeliten gegenüber Jahwe beschreiben sollen (Ex 20 34) und die Kult- oder Heiligtumsregeln (Ex 23 34), »Katechismen« (Lev 19) und »Beichtspiegel« darstellen oder gar bloße Nachahmungen der Form sind. Diese Geschichte der apodiktischen Reihenform entspricht denn auch einer Eigenart des Jahweglaubens, der nicht eine Religion des Rechts, sondern eine solche des Lebens und Verhaltens nach den geheiligten, gottgewollten Regeln ist.

»Priesterliches Königtum« (Ex 19 6)

Der Satz in Ex 19 6 a »Und ihr werdet mir sein *mămlækæt koh͞anîm w͞egôj qadôš*« scheint auf den ersten Blick für Übersetzung und Verständnis keine Schwierigkeiten zu bieten. Wenigstens der Ausdruck *gôj qadôš* ist insofern eindeutig, als er durch »heiliges Volk« oder »heilige Nation« wiederzugeben ist und sich auf Israel bezieht: Wenn es auf die Stimme Jahwes hört und seine Verpflichtung einhält, wird es aus allen Völkern sein Eigentum und daher ein »heiliges«, d. h. ausgesondertes und ihm geweihtes, Volk sein. Allerdings bleibt zu überlegen, warum Israel als *gôj* und nicht als *'ăm* bezeichnet wird. Anders verhält es sich mit dem Ausdruck *mămlækæt koh͞anîm*, der verschieden gedeutet werden kann und gedeutet worden ist.

Das weitaus häufigste Verständnis betrachtet den Ausdruck als volle sachlich-inhaltliche Parallele zu *gôj qadôš*: dem Volke Israel wird im Falle des Gehorsams außer der Heiligkeit zugesagt, daß es eine *mămlækæt koh͞anîm* sein soll. Fragt man nach dem Sinn dessen, so gehen die Ansichten darüber freilich auseinander. Nahezu jeder Exeget verleiht dem Ausdruck seine eigene Nuance, obschon sich mehrere Grundauffassungen erkennen lassen: Israel als ein von Jahwe regiertes Gemeinwesen, dessen sämtliche Bürger Priester sind[1]; Israel oder die einzelnen Israeliten als solche, die Jahwe wie Priester nahen und ihm unmittelbar dienen können[2] oder ihm näher stehen als die anderen Nationen[3]; die Israeliten als Verehrer Jahwes[4]; die Israeliten als die Jahwe unmittelbar zur Verfügung stehenden Diener, die seine direkte Herrschaftssphäre bilden[5], oder Israel als Volk, dessen Glieder in trautem Umgang mit Jahwe leben und über das er als König herrscht[6]; Israel in der Rolle eines Priesters oder Mittlers in der Welt der heidnischen Völker[7].

---

[1] H. L. Strack, Gen, Ex, Lev, Num, 1892, 223.
[2] B. Baentsch, Exodus-Leviticus, 1903, 173; G. Beer, Exodus, 1939, 97.
[3] P. Heinisch, Das Buch Exodus, 1934, 146; weiterführend J. B. Bauer, Könige und Priester, ein heiliges Volk (Ex 19 6), BZ NF 2 (1958), 283—286: Das Gottesvolk erhält Teilhabe an der göttlichen Herrschaftsgewalt über alle Welt und hat eine Art Priesterwürde oder -eigenschaft an sich.
[4] K. Galling, Die Erwählungstraditionen Israels, 1928, 27; R. B. Y. Scott, A Kingdom of Priests (Exodus XIX 6), in: OTSt VIII, 1950, 213—219.
[5] M. Buber, Moses, 1952², 125.
[6] H. Wildberger, Jahwes Eigentumsvolk, 1960, 7. 80ff.
[7] H. Holzinger, Exodus, 1900, 67; J. C. Rylaarsdam, The Book of Exodus, in: The

Die Vielzahl der Deutungen ist geeignet, Mißtrauen zu wecken. In der Tat hat W. L. Moran kürzlich mit Recht und völlig überzeugend dargelegt[8], welche Schwierigkeiten die Deutung des Ausdrucks *mămlækæt kohᵃnîm* auf Israel als Volk oder auf alle einzelnen Israeliten mit sich bringt und worin die Schwächen dieser Auffassung liegen, die zu seltsamen Auslegungen geführt hat — nur um zu zeigen, inwiefern und in welcher Weise ganz Israel oder alle Israeliten Priester sein können oder sollen. Es ist nicht erforderlich, dies im einzelnen zu wiederholen; dafür sei auf die Ausführungen Morans verwiesen.

Noch einen zweiten Schritt, dem wir folgen können, hat Moran getan. Er hat den zweifachen Nachweis geführt, daß *mămlakā* und *gôj* nicht inhaltlich parallele oder gar identische, sondern verschiedenartige Begriffe sind und daß *mămlakā* nicht »Königreich« bedeuten muß, sondern häufig im Sinne von »Königtum« oder »König« gebraucht wird. Daher bezeichnen *mămlakā* und *gôj* den Herrscher und die Beherrschten, das Königtum bzw. den König und die regierte Nation: »we can now point to a greater number of passages in which *mamlākā* most probably means 'king, royalty', and among them there are some in which *mamlākâ* together with a *gôy* constitutes a state.«[9] Moran geht dabei von W. Caspari aus, der zuerst diesen Weg eingeschlagen hat[10], und führt aus dem Alten Testament eine Reihe von Stellen an, in denen *mămlakā* das Königtum bzw. den König bezeichnet, während daneben das Wort *gôj* als Ausdruck für die in solcher Weise verfaßte und regierte »Nation« erscheint. Bei einer Überprüfung aller Stellen auf ihre Tragfähigkeit hin ergibt sich einerseits das Nebeneinander von *gôj* und *mælæk* in Gen 17 6 35 11 Ez 37 22 Hag 2 22 (pl.) Ps 46 7, andererseits der zusammenfassende Ausdruck (*hă-*)*gôj* *wᵉ*(*hă-*)*mămlakā* in I Reg 18 10 Jes 60 2 Jer 18 7 27 8 II Chr 32 15. Es ist nicht unwichtig zu beachten, daß es sich um relativ junge Stellen handelt; da die beiden Vorkommen in der Genesis zur Priesterschrift gehören, stellen diejenigen in I Reg 18 10 und im Jeremiabuch die ältesten dar[11].

Interpreter's Bible, I 1952, 972f.; H. Schneider, Exodus, in: Echter-Bibel, 1952, 42; A. Clamer, Exode, 1956, 169; M. Noth, Das zweite Buch Mose, Exodus, 1959, 126; G. Auzou, De la servitude au service, 1961, 251.

[8] W. L. Moran, »A Kingdom of Priests«, in: The Bible in Current Catholic Thought, 1962, 7—20.

[9] Moran a. a. O. 17.

[10] W. Caspari, Das priesterliche Königreich, ThBl 8 (1929), 105—110. G. von Rad, Das formgeschichtliche Problem des Hexateuch, 1938, 35f., hat den Vorschlag grundsätzlich angenommen; W. Beyerlin, Herkunft und Geschichte der ältesten Sinaitraditionen, 1961, 85, hat den Unterschied zwischen beiden Begriffen in der gleichen Art definiert.

[11] Dabei ist zu beachten, daß die Eliaerzählungen, zu denen I Reg 18 10 gehört, nicht

Abgesehen von dieser nicht sehr alten Verbindung von *mămlakā* bzw. *mælæk* mit *gôj* läßt sich die Bedeutung »Königtum, König« für *mămlakā* allein zunächst an Hand außerbiblischer Belege in ältere Zeit zurückverfolgen. Die Belege finden sich in den Karatepe-Inschriften, in der Jeḥomilk- und der Ešmunʽazar-Inschrift und sind nunmehr in dem von J. Hoftijzer nach den durch Ch.-F. Jean gemachten Anfängen bearbeiteten Lexikon der westsemitischen Inschriften gesammelt. Aus ihnen ergibt sich völlig eindeutig der Sinn »prince, roi« für *mămlakā*[12]. Überprüft man daraufhin die alttestamentlichen Vorkommen des Worts, so legt sich die gleiche Bedeutung mit großer Wahrscheinlichkeit für folgende Erwähnungen nahe: I Sam 10 18 I Reg 5 1 (im Vergleich mit II Chr 9 26) 10 20 Jes 13 4 Jer 1 15 25 26 Am 7 13 Ps 68 23 135 11 Thr 2 2 II Chr 12 8 17 10.

Nach alledem ist es künftighin schwerlich möglich, den Ausdruck *mămlækæt koh^anîm* in Ex 19 6 a als sachlich-inhaltliche Parallele von *gôj qadôš* zu verstehen und auf Israel als Volk oder Gesamtheit der Israeliten zu beziehen. Es bleibt die Frage zu beantworten, was er denn neben *gôj qadôš* ausdrücken soll. Moran kommt im Anschluß an Caspari zu der Folgerung, daß eine priesterliche Herrschaft über die heilige Nation gemeint sei, zumal Ex 19 3-6 eine alte, unabhängige Tradition der israelitischen Amphiktyonie mit kultischem Hintergrund bilde[13]. Diese Auffassung wirkt nach der klaren Definition des Begriffs *mămlakā* überraschend und ist durch nichts begründet.

Bevor man zu derartigen kultischen Hypothesen übergeht, hat doch wohl die Grammatik und Syntax ein Anrecht darauf, beachtet zu werden. Und da ist es evident, 1. daß *mămlækæt koh^anîm* zwar nicht eine sachlich-inhaltliche, wohl aber eine sprachliche Parallele zu *gôj qadôš* bildet und 2. daß *koh^anîm* in der gleichen Weise eine nähere Bestimmung oder ein Attribut zu *mămlakā* enthält wie *qadôš* zu *gôj*: Wie die Nation heilig sein wird, so seine *mămlakā*, d. h. sein Königtum bzw. sein König, priesterlich. Es liegt also einer der vielen Fälle vor, in denen ein im Hebräischen fehlendes Adjektiv durch ein im Genitivverhältnis hinzugesetztes Substantiv ersetzt worden ist, so daß eine Art von Genitiv epexegeticus entsteht[14]. Das ist für Übersetzung und

---

in der jetzigen Formulierung geschlossen aus dem 9. Jh. stammen, sondern mannigfache Spuren späterer Bearbeitung aufweisen; vgl. G. Fohrer, Elia, 1968², bes. 50—55.

[12] Ch.-F. Jean—J. Hoftijzer, Dictionnaire des inscriptions sémitiques de l'Ouest, 1965, 155.

[13] Moran a. a. O. 20, ebenso von Rad und Beyerlin. Moran weist auch auf H. Cazelles hin, der zwar *mămlakā* als »Königreich« versteht, aber den Ausdruck in Ex 19 6 auf die priesterliche Tätigkeit bezieht; vgl. jetzt Cazelles in: A. Robert—A. Feuillet, Einleitung in die Heilige Schrift, I 1963, 369, dazu seine Bemerkungen in VT 10 (1960), 93.

[14] Vgl. u. a. W. Gesenius—E. Kautzsch, Hebräische Grammatik, 1902²⁷, § 128 o, p; 135 n; G. Beer—E. Meyer, Hebräische Grammatik, II 1955, 114. Auch Bauer a. a. O.

Verständnis zu berücksichtigen. Daher besagt Ex 19 6 a, daß Jahwe eine heilige, ihm geweihte *Nation* mit einem priesterlichen Königtum bzw. *König* schaffen wird. Wie der *gôj* — die verfaßte und regierte Nation — heilig, ausgesondert, gottgeweiht sein wird, so der jeweilige Herrscher priesterlich, d. h. heilig in gesteigerter Weise und in hervorragendem Maße: »Und ihr werdet mir ein priesterlich(-heiliger) König (bzw. ein priesterlich-heiliges Königtum) und eine heilige Nation sein«.

Handelt es sich in Ex 19 6 a außer der bedingten Zusage an die Nation um eine solche an das Königtum bzw. an den König und läßt sich das Nebeneinander von *gôj* und *mămlakā* erst für die jüngere Zeit nachweisen, so kann die Formulierung wohl nur in der ausgehenden judäischen Königszeit entstanden sein. Man könnte sogar an die exilische Zeit denken, in der manche Kreise offenbar ein künftiges neues Herrschertum erhofften; so verhält es sich ja bei Ezechiel, der den Herrscher allerdings nicht mehr *mælæk*, sondern — einschränkend und degradierend — *nasî'* nennt[15]. Dem genannten Ansatz entspricht einerseits der seit langem bemerkte deuteronomistische Spracheinfluß in Ex 19 3b-8[16], obschon man ihn nicht überschätzen darf[17], andererseits der noch viel engere Zusammenhang mit Sprache und Gedanken des Heiligkeitsgesetzes (Lev 17—26)[18], das zwar erst im Exil seine endgültige Form erhalten hat, jedoch auf vorexilische jerusalemische Priestertraditionen zurückgeht[19]. So legt sich die Annahme nahe, daß

284f. legt dar, daß einerseits *mămlakā* dem *gôj*, andererseits *kohănîm* dem *qadôš* entspricht, und meint, daß im Ausdruck *mămlækæt kohănîm* eine Art von Hendiadyoin vorliegt. Jedoch bezieht er *mămlakā* dann wieder auf das Volk und bezeichnet es (nach E. König, Stilistik, Rhetorik, Poetik, 1900, 65) als abstractum pro concreto, als qualitative Bezeichnung einer Gesamtheit; jedoch wird dies durch die obige Sinnerfassung von *mămlakā* in Frage gestellt.

[15] G. Fohrer, Ezechiel, 1955, 124 Anm. 1.

[16] R. Klopfer, Zur Quellenscheidung in Exodus 19, ZAW 18 (1898), 201f.; Holzinger a. a. O. 64; Baentsch a. a. O. 171; C. F. Whitley, The Prophetic Achievement, 1963, 28f.

[17] Die von Beyerlin a. a. O. 83 Anm. 1 zusammengestellten Einwände gegen eine Abhängigkeit vom Deuteronomium überhaupt scheinen freilich nicht stichhaltig. Abgesehen davon, daß es sich mehr um eine sprachliche Beeinflussung durch den infolge der deuteronomistischen Theologie aufgekommenen theologischen »Jargon« als um eine stilistische Abhängigkeit handelt, ist die mit zweifelhaftem Recht sogenannte paränetische Stilform des Deuteronomiums nicht wesentlich älter als dieses und zudem nicht mit dem Kult verbunden, der diese Stilform schwerlich geboren hat.

[18] W. Staerk, Zum alttestamentlichen Erwählungsglauben, ZAW 55 (1937), 8f.; Whitley a. a. O. 29. Staerk weist u. a. mit Recht darauf hin, daß Ex 19 5 inhaltlich auf einer Linie mit Lev 20 26 (Druckfehler: 19 26) steht, wo der Heiligkeitsbegriff mit dem Erwählungsglauben verbunden wird.

[19] Vgl. G. Fohrer, Die Hauptprobleme des Buches Ezechiel, 1952, 144—148.

Ex 19 3b-8 weder den Quellenschichten des Jahwisten oder Elohisten angehört, noch ein ihnen vorangehendes älteres liturgisches Formular darstellt, sondern mit der Formulierung von v. 6 a von deuteronomistisch beeinflußten und in den Traditionen des späteren Heiligkeitsgesetzes lebenden Priesterkreisen im Jerusalem der ausgehenden Königszeit stammt.

4QOrNab, 11QTgJob und die Hioblegende

1. Der von J. T. Milik im Jahre 1956 veröffentlichten fragmentarischen Qumran-Handschrift 4QOrNab »Gebet des Nabonid«[1] hat R. Meyer eine ausführliche Untersuchung gewidmet, die ernsthafte Beachtung erfordert und weitgehende Zustimmung verdient. Nach dem Inhalt der Handschrift ist der König Nabonid auf Befehl des »höchsten Gottes« sieben Jahre lang von einem bösen Geschwür gepeinigt worden, obwohl er nicht als ein überheblicher und zu Recht bestrafter Tyrann, sondern als ein frommer Mann erscheint. Demgemäß trägt er sein Leiden, dessentwegen er seinen Thron verlassen und sich absondern muß, als von den Göttern verhängt und bemüht sich um Sühnung und Rettung. Freilich begeht er unwissentlich die Sünde, sich dazu an die Götter zu wenden, bis er sich aufgrund der Mahnung eines jüdischen Sehers zu jenem höchsten Gott bekehrt. Dies hat unter anderem seine Heilung und Rückkehr auf den Thron zur Folge.

Höchst wahrscheinlich hat Meyer darin Recht, daß der geschichtliche Haftpunkt von 4QOrNab im historischen Inhalt der neuen Nabonid-Inschriften von Harran[2], insbesondere im Text Nabon H 2, zu suchen ist, die Darstellung jedoch nicht mehr dem geschichtlichen Sachverhalt entspricht, sondern als »Weisheitserzählung« gestaltet worden ist, die sich wiederum von der bisher durchweg zum Vergleich herangezogenen Erzählung Dan 3 31—4 34 deutlich abgrenzt und daher nicht zu einem schon um 4QpsDan^a-c erweiterten Danielzyklus[1] zu rechnen ist. Vielmehr weist Meyer auf mancherlei Berührungspunkte hin, die zwischen 4QOrNab und der für die Rahmenerzählung des Buches Hiob verwendeten alten Hioblegende — jedoch nicht der Hiobdichtung selber! — bestehen. Während er nun zu dem Schluß gelangt, daß 4QOrNab in dem Sinne von Nabon H 2 abhängig ist, daß eine volkstümliche Variante jener Inschrift Nabonids vorliegt[3], ferner im Zusammenhang mit den Berührungen mit der Hioblegende für 4QOrNab die Gattung der Weisheitserzählung nachweist[4] und diese

---

[1] J. T. Milik, »Prière de Nabonide« et autres écrits d'un cycle de Daniel, Fragments araméens de Qumrân 4, RB 63 (1956), 407—415.
[2] C. J. Gadd, The Harran Inscription of Nabonidus, AnSt 8 (1958), 35—92; vgl. auch E. Vogt, Novae Inscriptiones Nabonidi, Bibl 40 (1959), 88—102.
[3] R. Meyer, Das Gebet des Nabonid, 1962, 67.
[4] Meyer a. a. O. 101—104.

schließlich inhaltlich in die orthodoxe Leidenstheologie des Judentums eingliedert[5], scheinen darüber hinaus weitere Beobachtungen möglich und weitere Folgerungen erwägenswert zu sein.

Auffällig ist bereits, daß Nabonid wie Hiob (2 7) durch ein »böses Geschwür« gepeinigt wird und 4QOrNab Text A, Z. 2 dafür den Ausdruck *bšḥn' b'jš'* gebraucht, der dem targumischen *bšḥn' bjš'* Dtn 28 35 für den hebräischen Ausdruck *bšḥjn rʿ* Hi 2 7 entspricht[6]. Abgesehen davon finden sich eine ganze Reihe von Gemeinsamkeiten, auf die auch Meyer aufmerksam macht[7]: Wie der ursprüngliche Nichtisraelit Hiob zu den Ostleuten gehört, ist der babylonische König Nabonid östlich von Palästina beheimatet. Beide sind fromme Männer; wie Hiob in dieser Weise geschildert wird (1 1), so ist auch Nabonid fromm und seinen Göttern ergeben. Beide werden plötzlich mit Unheil geschlagen, als sie auf der Höhe des Glücks oder des Lebens stehen, bei beiden spielt die gleiche Krankheit die ausschlaggebende Rolle, und beiden ist die Ursache ihres Leidens unbekannt. Beide müssen sich infolge ihrer verunreinigenden Krankheit von der Gemeinschaft absondern, lehnen sich aber nicht gegen ihr Geschick auf, sondern bleiben fromme Dulder, wobei Nabonid sich betend an seine Götter wendet (4QOrNab Text A, Z. 5—8), und beide erleben schließlich die Wiederherstellung ihres früheren Glücks, wobei die Wende im Falle Hiobs vielleicht nach sieben Tagen (2 13), im Falle Nabonids nach sieben Jahren eintritt.

Ein weiterer Punkt verdient Beachtung: Nach 4QOrNab Text A, Z. 2 wird Nabonid »durch böses Geschwür auf Befehl des [höchst]en Go[ttes]« geplagt. Man könnte darin eine wesentliche Unterscheidung von der Hioblegende erblicken, in der der Satan es ist, der das Unglück Hiobs wünscht und es — wenn auch mit Genehmigung Jahwes — über ihn bringt. Jedoch habe ich an anderer Stelle wahrscheinlich zu machen gesucht, daß die Satangestalt erst im frühnachexilischen Stadium des Werdens der Hioblegende in diese eingeführt worden ist, während in der älteren Überlieferung die Gottheit selbst das Unheil verhängt[8]. Genau diesem älteren Stadium entspricht 4QOrNab; es ist außerhalb von Palästina noch bewahrt worden, als dort schon die jüngere Form mit der Satangestalt umlief.

Darüber hinaus veranlaßt 4QOrNab zu einer weiteren Überlegung, wenn man Text B, Z. 1, 3—4 liest: »1 ... und überdies (?) träumte ich ..., 3 es s[eufz]te mein Inneres, ich vermochte nicht ...

---

[5] Meyer a. a. O. 97—101.
[6] A. Sperber, The Bible in Aramaic, I 1959, 338. Vgl. den Hinweis bei Meyer a. a. O. 19.
[7] Meyer a. a. O. 97f.
[8] G. Fohrer, Überlieferung und Wandlung der Hioblegende, in: Baumgärtel-Festschrift, 1959, 41—62 (= G. Fohrer, Studien zum Buche Hiob, 1963, 44—67).

4 Wie gleichst du dem ...!«[9] Danach erscheint ein Traum als der Anlaß, der dem leidenden König den Weg weist, auf dem sein Unglück behoben werden kann. Im Traum tritt ein nach Milik als himmlischer Bote zu deutendes Wesen auf, das den König — wie der Ausruf »Wie gleichst du dem ...!« lehrt — an den ihm bereits bekannten und in Text A, Z. 4 erwähnten jüdischen Seher erinnert, worauf die Bekehrung und Wiederherstellung Nabonids erfolgt[10]. Es ist nicht auszuschließen, wenn auch wiederum nicht nachzuweisen, daß die Traumerscheinung des Himmelswesens eine durch die abweichende Situation in 4QOrNab bedingte Abwandlung der Theophanie Jahwes darstellt, die einmal zur alten Hioblegende gehört hat und deren Spuren trotz der Verarbeitung durch den Hiobdichter noch nachweisbar sind[11]. Insbesondere hängt die Erinnerung an den Seher mit dem noch zu nennenden Bekehrungsmotiv zusammen. Dagegen stehen weder die nächtliche Erscheinung, von der Eliphas in Hi 4 12 ff. spricht, noch der Traum, den Elihu in Hi 33 15 ff. anführt, in einer Beziehung zu 4QOrNab oder einer Traumerscheinung in der Hioblegende, falls man eine solche aufgrund des oben angeführten Textes B von 4QOrNab annehmen wollte. Denn Hi 4 12 ff. schildert zwar die Erscheinung eines Himmelswesens, jedoch nicht in einem Traum, sondern in einer Vision[12]; und Hi 33 15 ff. meint zwar einen Traum, läßt aber nicht einen Engel erscheinen, sondern einen Schrecktraum den Menschen warnen. So weist 4QOrNab Text B höchstens wieder eine Parallele zur Hioblegende auf.

Eine wirkliche Abweichung von der Hioblegende liegt darin, daß 4QOrNab lediglich die Krankheit als das verhängte Leid nennt, dagegen die dieser vorangehenden Schicksalsschläge, die Hiob seines Besitzes und seiner Kinder berauben, nicht erwähnt. Doch diese Beschränkung erklärt sich daraus, daß die Darstellung sich an die Inschriften Nabonids angeschlossen hat oder von ihnen ausgegangen ist und ungeachtet aller volkstümlichen Variation einer gewissen Bindung an sie nicht entraten konnte. Auf jeden Fall ist die Grundlage zu gering, um von ihr aus die ursprüngliche Zugehörigkeit der Darstellung jener ersten Schläge zur Hioblegende anzuzweifeln oder in Frage zu stellen.

Der Hauptunterschied zwischen 4QOrNab und der Hioblegende besteht hinsichtlich der Ursache und des Sinns des Leidens[13]. Das

---

[9] Zur Übersetzung vgl. Meyer a. a. O. 30—32.
[10] Vgl. Meyer a. a. O. 40f. 51f.
[11] G. Fohrer, Zur Vorgeschichte und Komposition des Buches Hiob, VT 6 (1956), 249—267 (= G. Fohrer Studien zum Buche Hiob, 1963, 26—43).
[12] Zur Begründung, auch gegenüber der anderen Auffassung von F. Horst, Hiob, Lieferung 1, 1960, 71ff., vgl. G. Fohrer, Das Buch Hiob, 1963, 141ff.
[13] So auch Meyer a. a. O. 99.

Unglück Hiobs dient seiner Prüfung und Bewährung, dasjenige Nabonids dagegen der Erziehung und Bekehrung des unwissenden Heiden, der sich in seinem Unglück fälschlich an seine Götter wendet und endlich zur Erkenntnis des »höchsten Gottes« geführt werden soll. In dieser Zielsetzung macht sich neben den Berührungen mit der Hioblegende ein zweites Motiv bemerkbar, das bei der Ausgestaltung der Weisheitserzählung 4QOrNab verwendet worden ist: das Bekehrungsmotiv.

Insgesamt sind die Übereinstimmungen zwischen 4QOrNab und der Hioblegende zu vielfältig und zu charakteristisch, um auf einem Zufall zu beruhen oder sich auf freischwebende und von beiden benutzte Motive zurückführen zu lassen. Zudem ist die Erzählung vom frommen Hiob, die auch Ez 14 12 ff. als Überlieferung über einen Mann der Frühzeit als bekannt voraussetzt, sehr alt und nicht erst in der exilischen oder nachexilischen Zeit geschaffen worden. So bleibt wohl nur die Schlußfolgerung, daß sie auf die Formung von 4QOrNab eingewirkt hat. Dieser Text ist demnach einerseits zwar von der Inschrift Nabonids (Nabon H 2) ausgegangen, andererseits aber ist deren Inhalt nach dem Muster der Hioblegende und unter Verwendung des Bekehrungsmotivs um- und ausgestaltet worden. Dabei ist die Hioblegende bei der sie anwendenden jüdischen Diaspora in Babylonien oder eher in Nordarabien in einer älteren Form umgelaufen, als sie dem Hiobdichter bekanntgeworden ist, nämlich ohne die Satangestalt. 4QOrNab bezeugt demnach noch für das 5. Jh. v. Chr., in dem 4QOrNab wahrscheinlich entstanden ist[14], 1. das Bekanntsein der Hioblegende als selbständige Erzählung ohne die den Hauptteil des jetzigen Buches Hiob ausmachende Dichtung und 2. ihre Konservierung in einer älteren als der vermutlich in Palästina durch die Einführung der Satangestalt entstandenen und vom Hiobdichter verwerteten jüngeren Form.

2. Anders verhält es sich mit den Aufschlüssen, die das 1956 gefundene Hiobtargum 11QtgJob über die Hioblegende liefern kann. Da seitens der beiden Bearbeiter, J. van der Ploeg und A. S. van der Woude, bisher nur vorläufige Mitteilungen gegeben werden konnten[15], lassen sich noch keine endgültigen Feststellungen machen, für die die Textedition abzuwarten bleibt. Immerhin ist soviel deutlich, daß die hauptsächliche Bedeutung von 11QtgJob darin liegt, daß es das älteste bekannte Targum darstellt; denn während die Handschrift aus dem 1. Jh. n. Chr. stammen dürfte, geht der Text wahrscheinlich bis in die

---

[14] Meyer a. a. O. 105—107.
[15] J. van der Ploeg, Le Targum de Job de la Grotte 11 de Qumran (11QTgJob), 1962; A. S. van der Woude, Das Hiobtargum aus Qumran Höhle XI, in: VTSuppl IX, 1963, 322—331.

zweite Hälfte des 2. Jh. v. Chr. zurück[16]. Auf jeden Fall ist es wesentlich älter als das bislang bekannte Hiob-Targum[17], das seinen Vorgänger nicht gekannt und benutzt zu haben scheint. Legt sich darum die Annahme nahe, daß das ältere Targum — sei 11QtgJob nun das Original oder eine Abschrift — der rabbinischen Zensur zum Opfer gefallen ist, so vergrößert sich damit zugleich die Wahrscheinlichkeit, daß es das Werk darstellt, das Gamaliel einst verurteilt hat[18]. Der zusammenhängende Teil der Rolle 11QtgJob enthält große Partien der Übersetzung von Hi 37 10—42 11; weitere Fragmente bieten Ausschnitte der Übersetzung von 17 14—36 33[19]. Der zugrunde liegende hebräische Text ist offenbar dem MT ähnlich gewesen, obschon der Übersetzer in manchen Fällen einen davon abweichenden Text vor sich gehabt haben kann[20].

Aus diesen Mitteilungen ergibt sich zunächst, daß aus 11QtgJob keinerlei neue Erkenntnisse für den im Prolog (Hi 1 1—2 13) verarbeiteten Hauptteil der Hioblegende erwartet werden dürfen, da der Text bis Hi 17 13 endgültig verloren zu sein scheint. Dagegen enthält die Rolle den Epilog, der einmal den Schluß der Hioblegende gebildet hat. Allerdings endet sie abrupt mit Hi 42 11, so daß sich die Frage nach dem Verbleib von 42 12-17 erhebt. Nach der Mitteilung von van der Ploeg[21] ist die Handschrift an dieser Stelle zwar beschädigt, v. 11 aber schließt in der Mitte einer Zeile, wie es anderwärts nur am Ende eines großen Abschnitts (nach den Reden Hiobs und seiner Freunde) der Fall ist, und die folgende Kolumne ist leer. Gewiß würde der verlorene Teil der beschädigten Kolumne (9 Zeilen) es zur Not erlaubt haben, Hi 42 12-17 als neuen Abschnitt nach v. 11 unterzubringen, doch ist es wahrscheinlicher, daß die Handschrift die Verse gar nicht enthalten und den Epilog mit v. 11 beschlossen hat. Es fragt sich, ob 11QtgJob darin einer älteren Tradition folgt, so daß Hi 42 12-17 nicht von Anfang an zum Buche Hiob gehört und keinen Teil der alten Hioblegende gebildet hätte, sondern eine spätere Erweiterung darstellte, oder ob das Targum die Verse ausgelassen hat.

Dazu ist zu bedenken, daß gerade Hi 42 12-17 mehrfach als zu einer recht alten Überlieferungsschicht gehörig betrachtet werden. So hat L. W. Batten den Epilog in drei Teile gegliedert: Hi 42 7-9 sei vom

---

[16] Van der Ploeg a. a. O. 4—7.
[17] Von P. de Lagarde in seine Hagiographa Chaldaice, 1873, aufgenommen; vgl. auch W. Bacher, Das Targum zu Hiob, MGWJ 21 (1871), 208—223. 283f.
[18] Vgl. die Darstellung im »Traktat der Schreiber« (übersetzt von H. Bardtke in: WZ Leipzig 3, 1953/4, 31—49) und in TSchabbat 115a.
[19] Van der Ploeg a. a. O. 3f.
[20] Van der Ploeg a. a. O. 11.
[21] Van der Ploeg a. a. O. 12 (und Abb.).

Prolog und von 31 1—41 6 unabhängig; 42 10-11 kenne die Himmelsszenen des Prologs noch nicht; 42 12-17 kenne die Krankheit Hiobs noch nicht, stelle statt der Söhne die Töchter in den Vordergrund und bilde das älteste Stück der Tradition[22]. A. Alt hat die beiden Erzählungsschlüsse 42 7-9. 10 und 42 11. 12-17 unterschieden, deren erster den ganzen Prolog voraussetze und dessen Einzelthemen in umgekehrter Reihenfolge erledige, deren zweiter dagegen nur 1 1-22 voraussetze und zu Ende führe und also die älteste Fassung des Epilogs bilde[23]. Vor allem aber ergibt eine literarische, traditionsgeschichtliche und sprachliche Analyse des Epilogs ein Zweifaches: 1. daß v. 12-17 untrennbar mit den vorhergehenden Versen verbunden sind und dem Epilog einen ähnlichen Aufbau wie dem Prolog verleihen[24] und 2. daß gerade v. 13-15 sehr alte Elemente enthalten, die sich bis in die ugaritischen Texte zurückverfolgen lassen[25]. Es ist schwer vorstellbar, daß darin Zutaten aus der späten nachexilischen Zeit vorliegen sollten.

Endlich ist zu beachten, daß 11QtgJob den übersetzten Text gelegentlich gekürzt hat, wenn auch bei weitem nicht in dem Ausmaß der LXX. Immerhin wird Hi 42 3 ausgelassen und durch 40 5 ersetzt. An einigen anderen Stellen, für deren Untersuchung man die Textedition abwarten muß, findet man ein oder zwei Verse mehr oder weniger als im MT[26]. So liegt doch wohl die Annahme am nächsten, daß 11QtgJob die Bemerkungen in Hi 42 10-11 als passenden Schluß des Buches erachtet und die folgenden Verse als bloße Ausführung des Erzählten weggelassen hat.

Unter dieser Voraussetzung ist 11QtgJob — ebenso wie LXX mit ihren umfangreichen Kürzungen und manchmal eigenartigen Übersetzungen des Buches Hiob — ein Zeuge dafür, daß der Text des Buches noch lange Zeit nicht als unantastbar gegolten hat und, falls die Datierung durch van der Ploeg sich als zutreffend erweist, sogar in der zweiten Hälfte des 2. Jh. v. Chr. zumindest in der Übersetzung erweitert oder verkürzt werden konnte. Vielleicht ist die Verwerfung des Hiob-Targums durch Gamaliel aus einer anderen Wertung des Textbestandes und der Ablehnung von derartigen Eingriffen zu erklären.

---

[22] L. W. Batten, The Epilogue of the Book of Job, AThR 15 (1933), 125—128.
[23] A. Alt, Zur Vorgeschichte des Buches Hiob, ZAW 55 (1937), 265—268.
[24] Nachweis in der in Anm. 11 genannten Untersuchung.
[25] Nachweis in der in Anm. 8 genannten Untersuchung (59—61).
[26] Van der Ploeg a. a. O. 11f.

II. Theologie

Das Gottesbild des Alten Testaments

I.

1. Von Anfang an, seit der Annahme des Jahweglaubens durch Israeliten zur Zeit Moses, ist das geschichtliche Gottesbild vom ersten Gebot des Dekalogs in Ex 20 3 bestimmt. Es setzt noch keinen sogenannten Monotheismus in dem Sinne voraus, daß es nur den einen Gott gebe und alle anderen Götter lediglich Wahngestalten und Nichtse seien. Vielmehr geht es gerade davon aus, daß die fremden Götter als wirkliche Mächte bestehen und daß ihre Existenz eine ständige Versuchung dazu bildet, vom eigenen Gott abzufallen und ihnen zu dienen. Das gilt insbesondere von dem umfassenden Vitalismus der kanaanäischen Religion, die die Fruchtbarkeit des Ackers, die Zeugung neuen Lebens und die Bezwingung des Schicksals durch begeisternden Rausch und gesteigertes Lebensgefühl versprach. Vielleicht hat das Alte Testament darin recht, daß es eigentliche Gottlosigkeit nicht gibt, daß der Mensch sich nicht zwischen Gott und Gottlosigkeit, sondern zwischen Gott und den Götzen als wirklichen Lebensmächten zu entscheiden hat. Und sicher hat es darin recht, daß diese Entscheidung nicht in verstandesmäßigem Abwägen fällt, so daß Götzendienst nur Aberglaube und Dummheit wäre, sondern in einem ganz persönlichen Entschluß, der das ganze Dasein des Menschen umfaßt und bestimmt. Zu einem solchen Entschluß fordert das erste Gebot auf, das geradezu das Vorbild eines Verbots des Götzendienstes darstellt. In ihm spricht sich aus, was für das alttestamentliche Gottesbild stets grundlegend war: der ausschließliche Herrschaftsanspruch Gottes, der an dieser Stelle mit der Rettung Israels aus Ägypten begründet wird.

Seitdem durchzieht der Widerstreit zwischen der unbedingten Forderung auf die alleinige Anerkennung des göttlichen Herrn und ihrer Bedrohung, die aus der andersartigen politischen und kulturellen Wirklichkeit Palästinas folgt, die innere Geschichte Israels. Der Jahweglaube ist ja bald vom Gottesberg in der Wüste nach Palästina verpflanzt und damit den Einwirkungen der kanaanäischen Kultur und der übrigen altorientalischen Kulturkreise ausgesetzt worden. Das hat sowohl zu einer geschichtlich bedingten Entfaltung und Ausweitung des Gottesbildes als auch zu schweren Gefährdungen geführt. Uns geht in diesem Zusammenhang nur die erste Seite dieses Vorgangs an. An ihr können wir sehen, daß das Gottesbild nicht ein für allemal fertig vorlag, sondern in der Geschichte gewachsen ist und sich gewandelt hat.

Einmal wird Gottes herrscherliches Walten stärker betont, indem man ihn als Herrn der Zebaot (»Heerscharen«), der ihm zu Diensten stehenden göttlichen Wesen der göttlichen Sphäre, bezeichnet. Diese Wesen dienen ihm unmittelbar wie die Sarafen und Keruben oder führen seinen Willen in der Welt aus wie die sogenannten Engel (»Boten«), sie bilden den Hofstaat und die Ratsversammlung Gottes oder ziehen als Kriegsheer aus. Nach dem Tempelbau Salomos wird für Gott der Königstitel verwendet, wie es vorher für die kanaanäischen Götter El und Baal der Fall war. Und wie El wird er aus einem Gott, der zeitweilig auf dem Gottesberg in der Wüste erscheint, zum Himmelsgott und im weiteren Verfolg dessen zum Schöpfer des Himmels und der Erde.

Damit war der Ansatzpunkt für eine andere Ausweitung des Gottesbildes gegeben: die Erkenntnis des göttlichen Wirkens im Bereich der natürlichen Fruchtbarkeit. Die Verfügungsgewalt darüber wird dem zweiten bedeutenden kanaanäischen Gott Baal entrissen. Nicht der Baal spendet Regen und Fruchtbarkeit, so daß man ihm deswegen dienen müßte, sondern allein Jahwe! Das ist der große und wichtige Schritt, den anscheinend der Prophet Elia erstmalig getan hat.

In solcher Weise wird das Gottesbild im Lauf der Jahrhunderte immer wieder nach dieser oder jener Seite hin schärfer geprägt und zugleich gegen fremde Auffassungen abgegrenzt. Das deuteronomische Gesetz (gegen Ende des 7. Jh.) wendet sich gegen die Aufspaltung der einen Gottesgestalt im Kultus der vielen Heiligtümer im Lande und betont die Einheit Gottes, der stets und überall der gleiche ist. Im Gegensatz zur babylonischen Vielgötterei verkündet im Exil der von uns Deuterojesaja genannte Prophet, daß nur dieser eine Gott von Ewigkeit zu Ewigkeit da ist und daß alle anderen, die man Götter nennt, künstliche Gebilde und Erfindungen des Menschen sind. Und in der nachexilischen Zeit steigert die Priesterschrift die Erhabenheit Gottes zu einer völligen Jenseitigkeit. So ließe sich noch manches aufzählen, denn eigentlich hat jede theologische Richtung und Strömung auch zur Ausformung des Gottesbildes beigetragen. Wir beobachten einen langen geschichtlichen Vorgang.

2. Offenbarung und Glaube ereignen sich nicht nur in der Geschichte, sondern auch unter den Vorstellungen, die man sich jeweils von der Welt macht. Die Bibel setzt das damalige Weltbild ganz selbstverständlich voraus; wie manches andere ist ihr Gottesbild in einzelnen Aussagen dadurch bestimmt. Es ist für uns notwendig, dies zu erkennen, damit wir nicht mit dem Glauben an Gott zugleich irgendein Weltbild zum Gegenstand des Glaubens erheben.

Dies gilt besonders für all das, was das Alte Testament über den Aufenthalt Gottes sagt und wonach er etwa auf dem Sinai, in Palästina (dort wieder in Jerusalem) und im Himmel fest ansässig wäre. Tatsächlich bedeuten diese vom Weltbild mitbestimmten Aussagen etwas ganz anderes. Der Sinai ist kein dauernder Wohnsitz, sondern eine zeitweilige Offenbarungsstätte, zu der Jahwe sich begibt, von wo aus er nach Palästina kommt oder wo Elia ihn als den Kommenden aufsucht. Ebenso glaubt man ihn in Palästina an den Heiligtümern als den sich Offenbarenden gegenwärtig. Er ist nicht an der Kultstätte stationiert, sondern nur im Augenblick seiner jeweiligen Kundgabe gegenwärtig. Dieser Glaube an die Offenbarungsgegenwart Gottes an den dafür bestimmten und vom Menschen aufgesuchten Stätten steht an Stelle des theoretischen und abstrakten Satzes von seiner Allgegenwart und — vom Menschen aus gesehen — seiner Allerreichbarkeit.

Von der späteren Königszeit an wird immer klarer und eindeutiger gesagt, daß Gott im Himmel weilt, in jenem tempelgleichen Palast, der sich in oder über dem Himmelsozean oberhalb der halbkugelförmigen Feste erhebt, die die Erdscheibe überwölbt. Dort thront Gott, von dort redet er und erhört Gebete. Aber nur scheinbar handelt es sich um eine Lokalisierung Gottes, tatsächlich dienen diese in den Formen des alten Weltbildes ausgedrückten Vorstellungen einem praktischen Glaubensinteresse: Einmal sieht Gott alles, und nichts im Menschen bleibt ihm verborgen, weil er über der Erde thront und alles überblickt. Und ferner gebraucht der über dem Erdkreis Thronende, dem die Menschen wie Heuschrecken und die Völker wie der Tropfen am Eimer erscheinen (Jes 40 22. 15), von dort aus seine Macht. So drückt Gottes Wohnen im Himmel nach unseren Begriffen seine Allwissenheit und seine Allmacht aus.

3. Außer mit der Geschichte und mit dem Weltbild ist der Glaube mit den Denk- und Vorstellungsformen des Glaubenden verknüpft. Der Mensch ist in seinen Aussagen und seinem Verstehen an die Denk- und Vorstellungsformen je seiner Zeit gebunden. Dies gilt auch für das, was das Alte Testament über Gott sagt und was Gott zum Israeliten sagt.

Nun ist das Denken und Vorstellen des Israeliten zunächst subjektiver oder personbezogener Art. Wenn daher so häufig von Gottes Güte oder Liebe, Treue oder Wahrheit, Zorn oder Rache gesprochen wird, sind damit nicht seine Eigenschaften gemeint, die man zusammenstellen könnte, um daraus sein Wesen abzulesen. Vielmehr ist es subjektiv zu verstehen: Gott ist gütig oder zornig vom jeweiligen Sprecher oder Erzähler aus gesehen. Oder besser gesagt: in seiner jeweiligen Lage erscheint ihm Gottes Handeln gütig oder zornig; wenn die Lage sich ändert, sieht er Gott wieder anders handeln. So liegen korrelative Aussagen vor, die das Verhältnis zwischen Gott und Mensch in einer bestimmten Lage umschreiben.

Freilich gibt es auch Aussagen über Gottes Eigenschaften — überall dort, wo in den anthropomorphen Redewendungen von Körperteilen Gottes die Rede ist. Sie sind nicht Zeichen einer primitiven Religion, denn in der körperlichen Gestalt sieht der Israelit etwas Wesentliches und Wesenhaftes, ja das Wesen selbst und darum in den Körperteilen einen Teil des Wesens. So bedeuten Hand und Arm die Kraft, Stärke und tatkräftige Hilfe, das Auge das Auffassen, Sehen und Erkennen, die Nase wegen des heftigen Atmens den Zorn. Dabei ist dies alles wieder subjektiv zu verstehen: Es sind Eigenschaften Gottes, die sich in solchen Handlungsweisen ausdrücken, die der Mensch erlebt hat. Sie beschreiben sein Wesen nicht so, wie es an sich ist, sondern wie es dem Menschen zugänglich geworden ist. Dieses dem Menschen zugänglich gewordene Wesen wird auch als der »Name« Gottes zusammengefaßt, weil der Name nach alter Auffassung das Wesen seines Trägers bestimmt oder beschreibt; im letzteren Fall wird das Wesen eben durch den Namen bekanntgemacht.

Gott selbst in seiner Gänze und Fülle kann und darf der Mensch nicht schauen. Als Mose am Sinai darum bittet, Gottes Herrlichkeit schauen zu dürfen (Ex 33 18 ff.), antwortet dieser: »Ich will all meine Güte an dir vorübergehen lassen und den Namen Jahwes vor dir ausrufen« — also mein Wesen kundtun, soweit es den Menschen betrifft und ihm bekanntwerden soll — »nämlich: daß ich Gnade erzeige, wem ich gnädig bin, und Barmherzigkeit, wem ich sie zuwende«. Jedoch: »Von Angesicht kannst du mich nicht schauen, denn der Mensch schaut mich nicht und bleibt am Leben« — der Mensch schaut mich nicht, wie ich an sich bin und wie die eigentliche Persönlichkeit sich im Gesicht offenbart. Der Mensch sieht immer nur etwas vom Wesen Gottes, nur irgendeine Erscheinungsform, die ihm enthüllt wird und ihm etwas von Gott kundtut.

Das israelitische Denken und Vorstellen ist ferner dynamisch bestimmt. Daher ist das »Sein« etwas Lebendiges, Tätiges und Wirksames. Daß Gott »ist«, bedeutet von da aus, daß er als Gott handelt und sich durchsetzt, wie es Israel besonders nachdrücklich in der Rettung aus Ägypten erfahren hat. Das »Sein« Gottes meint sein Wirken, wie der Mensch es durch seine Taten erfährt. Existenz ist gleich Wirksamkeit, die man erfassen und erleben kann. Gott ist für das Alte Testament die Summe aller dynamischen Existenz, die Quelle und der Urheber alles Wirkens. Sein Name wird in Ex 3 14 erläutert: »Ich bin, der ich bin«. Demgemäß ist er die tatkräftige und wirksame persönliche Existenz und der ständig Wirkende. Genau so ist das »Wort« Gottes Ausdruck nicht von Gedanken, sondern eines wirkenden Willens. Es ist eine dynamische Macht — wie ein Feuer und wie ein Hammer, der Felsen zerschmettert (Jer 23 29), und geradezu gleichbedeutend mit der Tat.

II.

1. Seine Theologie des Alten Testaments beginnt L. Köhler mit dem Satz: »Daß Gott da ist, dieser Satz ist die große Gabe des Alten Testaments an die Menschheit.« Aber das trifft in dieser Form nicht ganz zu, wenn man nicht über Köhler hinaus das Sein als Wirken auffaßt. Daß Gott da ist, setzt das Alte Testament als selbstverständlich voraus. Seine Gabe aber ist die, daß Gott für uns da ist, daß er sich mit uns einläßt und wir uns mit ihm einlassen sollen, daß er mit uns zu tun hat und wir mit ihm zu tun haben in Gericht und Heil, daß er dazu über Welt und Menschen herrscht und alleinige Anerkennung als Herrscher beansprucht. Ps 8 2 drückt dies beispielhaft so aus:

> Jahwe, unser Herr,
> wie mächtig ist dein Name
> auf der ganzen Erde,
> daß man deine Hoheit
> über dem Himmel preist!

Das Weltall — Himmel und Erde — steht unter dem Eindruck der Hoheit oder Majestät Gottes, der als der »Herr« bezeichnet wird, um das Herrscherliche in Hoheit und Macht hervorzuheben. Und genauso gilt überall sein »Name«, der sein dem Menschen kundgemachtes Wesen umschreibt. Gottes für den Menschen erkennbares Wesen ist also sein Herrschertum über alle Welt. Oder — da der Name in späterer Zeit auch die Bedeutung »Ruhm« erhalten kann — Gottes Ruhm infolge seines majestätischen Herrschertums ist machtvoll.

In etwas anderer Weise wird Gottes Herrschertum im Berufungserlebnis des Propheten Jesaja unter dem Oberbegriff der Heiligkeit nach drei Seiten hin beschrieben (Jes 6). Zwei von ihnen hebt der Gesang der Sarafen hervor:

> Heilig, heilig, heilig
> ist Jahwe Zebaot!
> Alle Welt ist seiner Herrlichkeit voll!

Einmal bekundet dieser Gesang wie auch das ganze Verhalten der Sarafen die Unnahbarkeit des göttlichen Herrschers, seine Verschiedenheit von allem Geschöpflichen und seine Erhabenheit über es, den unvergleichlichen Wert des göttlichen Wesens und seine bezwingende Anbetungswürdigkeit. Doch ist dies nicht bloß als Steigerung dessen zu verstehen, was man in abgeschwächter Art vom Menschen sagen könnte, sondern als völlige Andersartigkeit Gottes gemeint. Die immerwährende Wiederholung des »heilig« soll auf die Unbedingtheit und Ausschließlichkeit des Heiligen hinweisen. Das heilige Herrschertum Gottes wird ferner dadurch erläutert, daß seine Herrlichkeit die ganze Welt erfüllt. Eigentlich besagt der Ausdruck כָּבוֹד, daß Gottes

»Schwere« oder »Wucht« die irdische Wirklichkeit durchdringt, so daß sein Heiligsein sich schlechthin als Weltmächtigkeit entfaltet.

Jesaja persönlich wird der dritten Seite dessen inne:

> Weh mir, ich bin verloren,
> denn ich bin unreiner Lippen,
> und unter einem Volk unreiner Lippen
> lebe ich;
> denn den König, den Herrn Zebaot,
> habe ich mit meinen Augen geschaut.

Gottes Heiligkeit bedeutet auch seine Herrschaft über den Menschen, so daß Jesaja sie als sittliche Willensmacht erfährt. Gott besitzt den unverbrüchlichen Willen und die erforderliche Macht, um im ganzen menschlichen Lebensbereich zu herrschen. Je nach den Umständen äußert sich dies bald in heilschaffenden Wundertaten, bald in Unheil und Vernichtung. Vor diesem unbedingten Sichdurchsetzenwollen kann der Mensch nicht entrinnen oder anderswo Sicherheit finden. Das tritt bei Jesaja immer wieder zutage: Ist Gott der Weltenherr und sein Wille unabdingbar darauf gerichtet, seine königlichen Herrschaftsansprüche durchzusetzen, so wird seine Hoheit beleidigt und sein Zorn erregt, wenn Menschen seinen Willen nicht erfüllen und seine Gebote übertreten. So erfährt es sogar Jesaja selbst, der sich daraufhin der Verurteilung zum Tode durch die vernichtende Wirkung der Heiligkeit Gottes preisgibt, sich dann aber durch einen der Sarafen entsühnt sieht.

2. Zur Herrschaft Gottes als erstem grundlegenden Zug des alttestamentlichen Gottesbildes tritt als zweiter Gottes heilvolle und helfende Verbundenheit mit dem Menschen; aus beiden folgt schließlich Gottes strafendes Richten über den Abtrünnigen und Frevler. Dies alles ist auch in den Bildern des Königs und des Hirten beschlossen. Denn für den altorientalischen König sind nicht nur seine despotische Macht und seine absolute Verfügungsgewalt über den, der sich gegen ihn auflehnt, bezeichnend, sondern auch der Schutz und die Fürsorge, die er seinen Untertanen angedeihen lassen soll wie jeder Herr seinem Sklaven. Und der Hirt sorgt nicht nur für seine Herde und schützt sie vor Überfällen, sondern scheidet auch die unbotmäßigen Böcke aus.

Gott ist dem Menschen verbunden — das ist also der zweite Grundzug seines für den Menschen erkennbaren Wesens. Er steht in einem unmittelbaren Verhältnis zur Welt und begegnet dem Menschen in vielerlei Weise. So beschreibt es Ex 34 6: barmherzig und gnädig, langmütig und voller Verbundenheit und Treue. Gott ist »barmherzig« in dem Sinne, wie nach dem hebräischen Wort eine innige Verbindung zwischen einer Mutter und ihrem Kind besteht. Er ist »gnädig« als derjenige, der dem Menschen Gunst und Geneigtheit erweist. Er ist »langmütig« als einer, der voller Geduld nicht gleich zürnt. Er ist voller »Verbundenheit« im Sinne der Gemeinschaftspflicht oder Solidarität als Verhalten gegenüber anderen, zu denen man in einem engen Verhältnis steht. Und er erweist sich in alledem als »treu«, weil er darin fest und beständig ist. Der ganze alttestamentliche Glaube wird von dieser Erfahrung einer Gemeinschaft getragen, die zwischen Gott und Mensch besteht oder bestehen sollte und die von seiten Gottes ermöglicht oder begonnen wird. Man kann dies auch als Gottes Güte bezeichnen. Zu ihr nimmt der Mensch in schwierigen Lagen Zuflucht (Gen 24 12 I Reg 3 6). Dem Scheidenden oder als treu Befundenen wünscht man, daß er sie dauernd erfährt und dadurch in Gottes Gemeinschaft bleibt (II Sam 2 6 15 20). Ja, ihre Erwähnung wird zur liturgischen Formel in Gebeten (Ps 106 1 107 1):

> Dankt Jahwe, daß er gütig ist,
> daß seine Verbundenheit ewig währt!

Das bezieht sich nicht allein auf Israel, obwohl davon natürlich am meisten die Rede ist. Vor allem in der prophetischen Verkündigung finden sich sehr umfassende Aussagen. So sagt Am 9 7, daß Gott für Philister und Aramäer in der gleichen Weise wie für Israel sorgt. Die Bücher Jona und Ruth wollen gegenüber theologischer Engherzigkeit zeigen, daß auch die Völkerwelt außerhalb Israels unter Gott lebt. Am tiefsten ist sich wohl Deuterojesaja dieser Weite der göttlichen Verbundenheit mit der Menschheit bewußt gewesen. Er hat seine prophetische Aufgabe darin erblickt, gerade auch den Nichtisraeliten die Heilsbotschaft zu bringen (Jes 49 6):

> Es ist mir zu gering, daß du mein Knecht bist,
> nur um die Stämme Jakobs aufzurichten
> und die Bewahrten Israels zurückzuführen!
> Ich mache dich vielmehr zum Licht der Völker,
> damit mein Heil reiche
> bis an das Ende dieser Erde!

Im einzelnen zeigt sich die Verbundenheit Gottes in mehrfacher Hinsicht, zunächst an seinem Handeln in der jeweiligen Gegenwart der Welt. Man spricht dabei oft nicht ganz zutreffend von seinem Handeln in der »Geschichte«; doch einen solchen Begriff oder eine solche Vorstellung kennt das Alte Testament nicht. Es meint vielmehr, daß Gott ständig handelt oder handeln kann und nicht etwa nur in der Weltschöpfung oder im alljährlichen Aufleben der Natur nach der Art der kanaanäischen Götter und daß dies existentiell-grundsätzlich zu verstehen ist. Stets geht es um Gottes Handeln in der jeweiligen Gegenwart. Von seinem Handeln in einer früheren und nun vergangenen Gegenwart erzählt man nicht aus historischem oder dogmatischem

Interesse, sondern um zu bekunden, daß er auch jetzt in solcher Weise handeln kann. Aus den Erzählungen spricht die Hoffnung auf oder die Furcht vor einem entsprechenden Handeln hier und jetzt.

Ein anderer Aspekt der Verbundenheit ist die Vorstellung von einem engen Verhältnis zwischen Gott und Israel. Wo das Alte Testament es erwähnt, drückt es zugleich aus, daß das Verhältnis zwischen Gott und Israel nicht von Natur aus gegeben, sondern von Gott besonders hergestellt worden ist. Es ist ein Gemeinschaftsband, eine Art Kreis, der beide Partner umfaßt und in dem sie gemeinsam in eine Gemeinschaft aufgenommen sind. Nun ist es immer Gott, der die Gemeinschaft herstellt, auf diese Weise Israel in seinen Lebenskreis aufnimmt und es heiligt, indem er ihm bestimmte Lebensregeln gibt. So entsteht ein ewiges Lebensverhältnis, das im Wesen Gottes begründet ist, das Israel zwar verletzen, aber nicht aufheben kann und in das nach der universalen prophetischen Verkündigung alle Menschen einbezogen werden sollen.

Einen Ansatzpunkt dazu von der Schöpfung her bildet die Vorstellung von der Ebenbildlichkeit des Menschen mit Gott. Sie drückt einerseits die Gewißheit der Gemeinschaft des Schöpfergottes mit dem Menschen als seiner Schöpfung aus und wehrt andererseits jede Gleichheit oder Vermischung beider ab. Mit dem Letzteren hängt es zusammen, daß das Alte Testament fast nie von Vater und Kind spricht, wenn es das Verhältnis zwischen Gott und Mensch beschreiben will. Es redet davon eigentlich nur bildhaft in bezug auf das Volk Israel als ganzes, um die Liebe Gottes und sein Vertrauensverhältnis mit Israel einprägsam mit etwas Bekanntem vergleichen zu können. Den Menschen allgemein aber bezeichnet es, um den Abstand zu Gott nicht zu verwischen und die altorientalische Vorstellung von der Zeugung oder Geburt des Menschen durch die Gottheit auszuschließen, nicht als Kind, sondern als »ähnliches Bild« Gottes (Gen 1 27). Dadurch wird sowohl die Verschiedenheit von Gott und Mensch als auch die dem Wesen Gottes entsprechende Verbundenheit beider festgehalten.

Daß Gott seinem Wesen nach dem Menschen verbunden ist, zeigt sich schließlich in der alttestamentlichen Auffassung der Propheten. Sie sind dazu berufen, durch den Empfang von Geist oder Wort an Gottes Wollen und Handeln teilzunehmen und es den anderen wieder zu deuten. Daher wird im Alten Testament das göttliche Handeln in der jeweiligen Gegenwart von der prophetischen Offenbarung und Verkündigung begleitet. Ein Zusatz zum Amosbuch sagt, daß Gott nichts tue, ohne es vorher den Propheten, seinen Knechten, zu enthüllen (Am 3 7). Damit wird die allgemeine Überzeugung von der Eigenart des Propheten klar umrissen. Beides gehört zusammen: die außerordentliche Begebenheit im irdischen Geschehen, die als wundersam erfahren wird, und der außerordentliche Mensch, der sie als göttliches Handeln deutet. Er vermag sie zu deuten, weil er in einer Verbundenheit mit Gott lebt, die für dessen Wesen bezeichnend ist.

3. Doch darf der letzte Zug des für den Menschen erkennbaren Wesens Gottes nicht übersehen werden: sein strafendes Richten. Gottes heilige Herrschermacht offenbart sich als Gericht über den Menschen in seinem Zorn gegenüber Israel und auch anderen Völkern. Er zürnt, weil der Mensch seine Gebote nicht beachtet, seinen Willen nicht befolgt und damit seinen Herrschaftsanspruch nicht anerkennt.

Freilich wird dieser Zorn manchmal nicht mit dem Versagen des Menschen begründet, sondern meint ganz allgemein den spürbaren Unwillen des Herrschers als Gegensatz zum Wohlwollen. Wie dieses sich in ungestörtem Glück äußert, so der Zorn in jedem unerwarteten Unglück, das als »Schlag« und Zeichen des göttlichen Unwillens hingenommen und nicht religiös-ethisch als Sündenstrafe oder Heimsuchung erklärt wird. Wenn im Kriege das Schwert bald diesen, bald jenen frißt (II Sam 11 25), so ist das weder ein dämonisch-satanisches Geschehen noch in das rationale Schema von Lohn und Strafe einzugliedern, sondern bedeutet für diejenigen, die es trifft, eine Unwillensäußerung des unerforschlichen Herrschers. Im allgemeinen geht man beim Versuch, dergleichen zu verstehen, sowohl dem Dämonismus als auch dem rein verstandesmäßigen Abwägen mit nahezu nachtwandlerischer Sicherheit aus dem Wege.

Weitaus überwiegend wird der göttliche Zorn mit religiös-ethischen Motiven verknüpft: Er hat seine Ursache in der Sünde und bewirkt die Strafe. Gott ist die Quelle von Heil und Leben für denjenigen, der in Gemeinschaft mit ihm lebt. Unheil und Untergang folgen aus dem Bruch dieser Gemeinschaft mit Gott; denn er läßt solchen Bruch nicht ungestraft. Dabei sind wieder zwei verschiedene Auffassungen zu unterscheiden.

Die zeitlich zuerst geäußerte Auffassung sieht den zürnenden Gott überwiegend in einzelnen Strafhandlungen wirken. Sie sind etwas Vorübergehendes, während Gottes Güte das eigentlich Bleibende ist. Das wird sehr deutlich, wenn das Verhängen oder Beendigen der Strafe mit der »Reue« Gottes verbunden wird. Damit ist eine plötzliche Wendung im Verhalten Gottes gemeint, zu der ihn das Verhalten des Menschen nötigt oder bewegt. Entweder nötigt ihn ein Frevel des Menschen, sich von der bisherigen Güte zum Zorn zu wenden, oder bewegt ihn Klage oder Buße des Menschen, sich von der Strafe wieder zur Güte zu wenden. Überall, wo von solcher »Reue« die Rede ist, fühlt der Mensch sich in einem Dasein gottgegebenen Heils, das durch gelegentliche Zornesausbrüche Gottes wegen einer menschlichen Verfehlung unterbrochen wird, aber auch wiederhergestellt werden kann, wenn die Verfehlung bestraft oder vom Täter gesühnt worden ist.

Anders die prophetische Auffassung! Sie geht von einem grundsätzlichen Zorneszustand wegen der sündigen Existenz des Menschen aus. Es ist beachtenswert, daß gerade diejenigen Propheten, die den stärksten Nachdruck auf Gottes liebenden Willen zur Verbundenheit legen, auch in der Beschreibung des göttlichen Zorns am weitesten gehen (Jer 13 12-14 Hos 5 12. 14). Am schlimmsten aber erscheint es, wenn der Mensch in seinem Wahn behauptet, daß Gott nicht zürnen könne (Jes 5 18 ff. Am 9 10 Zeph 1 12). Denn damit wird seine Majestät überhaupt geleugnet. Gerade in der tiefsten und wahrsten Ausprägung des alttestamentlichen Glaubens, bei den großen Einzelpropheten, wird nicht nur die gewaltige Majestät des göttlichen Herrschers und die alles übertreffende Liebe und Treue seiner Verbundenheit erkannt, sondern auch der unauflösliche Zusammenhang dessen mit dem strafenden Richten betont. Ihm entspricht der ebenso unauflösliche Zusammenhang zwischen Sünde und Gericht, Schuld und Unheil, Bosheit und Untergang als Frucht des Zornes Gottes über die Sünde, die das Dasein des Menschen beherrscht. Von da aus betrachten die Propheten die Weltgeschichte, das Wohl und Wehe der Völker und das Geschick ihres eigenen Volkes. Sie betrachten es als ein religiös bedingtes Geschehen, in dem etwas zwischen Gott und Mensch vor sich geht: Die tief enttäuschte Liebe wirkt sich als Zorn aus. Es ist Gottes Unwille nicht über den Menschen überhaupt, sondern über das Sündige seines Daseins. Denn eigentlich hat Gott kein Gefallen am Tode des Frevlers, sondern daß er umkehrt und leben bleiben kann (Ez 18 23). Der grundsätzliche Zorneszustand mit dem strafenden Richten Gottes besteht nur wegen der Unwilligkeit des Menschen zur Umkehr von der Sünde zu Gott. Nur deswegen erfährt er jenes strafende Richten als einzelnen Wesenszug des göttlichen Herrschers.

Daß der Mensch aber das Wesen Gottes auch als strafendes Richten erfährt, ist für das Verständnis seines eigenen Lebens wichtig. Leiden und Tod folgen überwiegend weder aus dem Übelwollen der Götter wie für den Babylonier noch aus ihrer Unvollkommenheit wie für den Griechen, sondern sind Gericht Gottes über die Sünde des Menschen. Gottes Urteil über den Menschen als Sünder entspringt nicht seiner bösen Launenhaftigkeit oder seinem Unvermögen, die Dinge anders zu gestalten, sondern seinem heiligen Zürnen. Gottes heilige Herrschaftsmacht ist ein verzehrendes Feuer und kann die Sünde des Sünders nicht bestehen lassen. Darum folgt, falls es nicht zur Entsühnung oder Entsündigung kommt, aus dem Sündigen das Gericht, weil es dem Wesen Gottes gemäß ist.

III.

Daß Gott seinem Wesen nach der Herr und Herrscher und daß er dem Menschen verbunden ist, aber auch strafend-richtend einschreitet, schließt einige weitere Züge des Gottesbildes ein, die wenigstens in aller Kürze beleuchtet werden müssen.

1. Gott ist ein lebendiger Gott. Für das Alte Testament bedeutet das zunächst, daß er die Fülle des Lebens und die Quelle allen Lebens ist. Von ihm kommt, was Leben hat und Leben gibt. Wo immer Leben ist, erscheint es als eine Gabe Gottes. Der Nachdruck, mit dem er als der Lebendige geglaubt wird, ist auffällig. Am ehesten ist diese Auffassung als Gegensatz zum kanaanäischen Glauben an die dahinwelkenden und wiederauflebenden Götter zu verstehen. Ihnen gegenüber ist Jahwe nicht an Zeit oder Raum gebunden, sondern »lebendig«. Und da lebendiges Sein ein stetes Wirken bedeutet, wirkt er immer und nicht nur zu bestimmten Zeiten, kann er vom Menschen immer aufgesucht und erreicht werden und ist er wirklich Herr über alles Leben, nicht aber etwa von diesem als etwas noch Höherem abhängig.

Wie sich dies auswirkt, zeigt sich am prophetischen Erleben. Der Prophet erfährt, daß Gott unmittelbar zu ihm spricht, ja sich geradezu in Rede und Gegenrede mit ihm auseinandersetzt. Da ist ein persönlicher, unmittelbarer und lebendiger Kontakt und nicht nur eine Beziehung auf dem Wege über die verschiedenen Techniken des unpersönlichen Orakels. Aber niemals ist es Gott selbst, der in den Menschen eingeht, in ihm wohnte und in mystischer Gemeinschaft mit ihm verschmölze. Vielmehr ereignet sich die Beziehung durch die Hand, den Geist oder das Wort Gottes, die über den Menschen kommen und ihn durchdringen, dabei jedoch durchaus Hand, Geist oder Wort Gottes bleiben. Daher führt die Beziehung zu dem lebendigen Gott nicht zur mystischen Einwohnung oder Verschmelzung, sondern zur Inspiration.

2. Gott ist ein mächtiger Gott. Die Macht Gottes begegnet dem Israeliten zuerst am sinnenfälligsten im kriegerischen Handeln Jahwes, das er in den ältesten Liedern besingt (Ex 15 21 Jdc 5). Gott ist ein Kriegsheld, gewaltig und hoch erhaben, furchtbar und herrlich in Heiligkeit, machtvoll und ein Wundertäter — so sprechen es manche Psalmen aus. Alles dies gehört zur Ausübung und Durchsetzung des göttlichen Herrscherwillens, der sich vor allem in der Rettung Israels betätigt hat. Immer wieder wird auf die göttlichen Rettungstaten bei der Flucht aus Ägypten, der Wanderung durch die Wüste, der Landnahme und Ausbreitung in Palästina verwiesen. Es sind Rettungstaten, die jeweils wieder gegenwärtige Erfahrung werden können.

Gott wirkt ferner mit segnender Wunderkraft in der Natur. Besonders nach der Ansiedlung in Palästina erblickt man den Beweis seiner Macht nicht mehr nur in kriegerischen Taten, sondern im steten Spenden von Segen und Fruchtbarkeit. Er waltet in der stillen Regelmäßigkeit der Naturvorgänge, im Wechsel der Jahreszeiten, im Lauf der Gestirne und in der Entstehung des Lebens.

Daran schließt sich der Glaube an, daß Gott mächtig ist als Schöpfer. Die Welt, wie man sie damals kennt, wird erkannt als durch Gott geschaffen und gegeben. Das ist zwar auf das altorientalische Weltbild bezogen, kann aber natürlich davon abgelöst und auf jedes andere Weltbild übertragen werden. Die Bedeutung dessen liegt darin, daß die Welt als eine Einheit betrachtet und in einer engen Beziehung zu Gott gesehen wird. Und ferner können unter dieser Voraussetzung Weltall und Erde keine dem Menschen feindlichen Mächte sein und die natürlichen Gaben und Kräfte nicht als solche verurteilt und verdammt werden. Die Sünde liegt dann auch nicht in der Natur der Dinge, sondern im Willen des Menschen beschlossen; das Unheil rührt nicht von den Dingen an sich her, sondern aus ihrem sündigen Mißbrauch durch den Menschen. Damit ist jede tragische Lebenshaltung ebenso wie jeder Dualismus und Dämonismus als heidnisch ausgeschlossen.

Schließlich ist Gott mächtig als derjenige, der Israel, die anderen Völker und die ganze Welt erhält. Das ist für das Alte Testament außerordentlich wichtig. Vor allem Mensch und Tier bestehen durch den göttlichen Lebensatem, der sie am Leben erhält. Beim Tode kehrt er zu Gott zurück, so daß das Leben überhaupt nur durch diesen Lebensatem und also durch Gott erhalten wird. Gott selbst aber geht in Mensch und Tier nicht auf, sondern ist Herr über alles Leben. Darum darf der Mensch das Blut seines Mitmenschen nicht vergießen; er vergriffe sich sonst an einem Leben, das ihm nicht gehört. Darum ist das Leben des Tiers heilig und muß Gott in Form des Blutes zurückgegeben werden, das nicht genossen werden darf.

3. Gott ist ein »einiger« Gott. Das deuteronomische Gesetz proklamiert in Dtn 6 4: »Höre, Israel! Jahwe, unser Gott, ist ein einziger Jahwe!« Gemeint ist dies im Sinne der Einheit des Wesens Gottes. Sie wird gegenüber der Vielheit und Aufspaltung betont, die sich im Lauf der Jahrhunderte an den verschiedenen Heiligtümern im Lande ergeben hatte. Überall wurden verschiedene Seiten seines Handelns oder Wesens hervorgehoben, so daß die Gefahr einer Aufsplitterung in einzelne Lokalgötter drohte. Aber es gilt ja gerade, die große und umfassende Einheit festzuhalten, der die Einzelzüge unterzuordnen sind. Und weil Gott einheitlich von Wesen ist, wird gefolgert, daß man ihn lieben soll mit ganzem Herzen, ganzer Seele und aller Kraft und nicht nur mit einem Teil dessen wegen eines Einzelzuges seines Wesens.

In Dtn 6 4 wird dieses Gebot mit dem Abschwören an andere Götter in Verbindung gebracht. Das zeigt den Zusammenhang mit der Einzigkeit Gottes als seiner Einheit der Art nach. In der älteren Geschichte Israels bemerken wir freilich nur einen praktischen Eingottglauben — aufgrund der Erfahrung der einzigartigen Wirklichkeit und Wirksamkeit, die praktisch alle anderen Gottheiten ausschließt. Die Überzeugung von der einzigartigen Wirklichkeit und Wirksamkeit Gottes hat sich trotz aller Gefährdungen von außen her mit einer unwiderstehlichen Gewalt und verzehrenden Intensität durchgesetzt, die für anderes einfach keinen Raum ließ. Erst Jeremia spricht den heidnischen Göttern durch die Ausdrücke, die er verwendet, jede Existenz ab. Er nennt sie »Nichts (Hauch, Täuschung)« und »Nichtgötter«. Deuterojesaja hat dies dann in Auseinandersetzung mit der heidnischen Auffassung ausdrücklich in These und Gegenthese formuliert (Jes 44 6):

> Ich bin der Erste und der Letzte,
> außer mir gibt es keinen Gott!

Er verneint nicht nur die Existenz anderer Götter, sondern bekennt auch den einen, einzigen Gott.

4. Gott ist ein ewiger Gott. Auch wo das Alte Testament es nicht sagt, setzt es die Ewigkeit Gottes als selbstverständlich voraus. Der bloße Gedanke an eine Entstehung und Abkunft Gottes ist schon widersinnig. Nicht er, wohl aber die Welt hat einen Anfang. Gerade der Schöpfungsglaube schließt die Ewigkeit Gottes ein (Ps 90 2):

> Ehe noch Berge geboren,
> Erde und Festland hervorgebracht wurden,
> bist du, Gott, von Ewigkeit zu Ewigkeit.

Wie beim Glauben an die Einzigkeit Gottes läßt sich auch hier der Weg allmählicher Entfaltung erkennen. Am Anfang steht die lebendige Überzeugung, daß die einzigartige Wirklichkeit und Wirksamkeit Gottes nicht zeitlich begrenzt, sondern ewig ist; und erst allmählich erfolgt das erkenntnismäßige Durchdringen dessen. Ungeachtet dessen liegt darin eine notwendige Ergänzung des bisher gezeichneten Gottesbildes: Gott ist Herr und Herrscher durch alle Zeiten hindurch. Er ist dem Menschen verbunden und strafender Richter, er ist lebendig, mächtig und »einig« von Ewigkeit zu Ewigkeit.

Theologische Züge des Menschenbildes im Alten Testament

I. Grundlagen

Zu Beginn ist eine Vorbesinnung nötig. Es hat Zeiten gegeben, in denen man die sog. Urgeschichte in Gen 1—11, soweit sie sich auf die Welt als ganze bezieht, als eine Art göttliches oder gottgegebenes Naturkundebuch betrachtet hat. Aus ihm suchte man alle wünschenswerten Kenntnisse über Werden und Entstehen der Welt herauszulesen. Die neuere Forschung macht diese Auffassung, die viel Unheil angerichtet hat, unmöglich. Denn sie zeigt, daß im Pentateuch und wohl noch im Buche Josua mehrere Erzählungsschichten miteinander vereinigt worden sind, die sämtlich große Geschichtsbetrachtungen bis zur Landnahme Israels in Palästina darstellen. Auch die Urgeschichte will keine naturwissenschaftlichen Fragen behandeln, sondern bildet einen Teil dieser Geschichtsbetrachtungen.

Man könnte fragen, ob damit die früheren Schwierigkeiten nicht bloß verschoben werden und an anderer Stelle auftauchen. Sollen wir etwa alles, was erzählt wird, als wirkliche geschichtliche Ereignisse verstehen? Erweist sich nicht, wenn wir dem nachgehen, vieles als geschichtlich fragwürdig oder unzutreffend? Das träfe sicherlich zu, wenn wir diese alttestamentlichen Bücher einfach als Geschichtsberichte oder als Geschichtsbuch betrachteten. Eine solche Auffassung aber wäre falsch, weil es sich nicht um Geschichtsberichte, sondern um theologische Geschichtsbetrachtung handelt, wie wir sie im Alten Testament durchweg antreffen. Geschichte wird meist nicht objektiv darzustellen gesucht; geschichtliche Ereignisse als solche wären für den alttestamentlichen Menschen bedeutungslose Abstraktionen. Sie erscheinen vielmehr als Grundlage einer religiösen oder theologischen Deutung und in Beziehung zu ihr. Das geschichtliche Ereignis und seine Deutung sind untrennbar miteinander verbunden und voneinander abhängig. Daher kann die Geschichte immer neu gedeutet werden, ohne daß eine Deutung unglaubwürdig wirkt oder als endgültig betrachtet wird. Man erzählt die Geschichte also eigentlich nicht um ihrer selbst willen, sondern wegen der in der Darstellung gegebenen Deutung, die denselben Offenbarungsanspruch erheben kann wie das gedeutete geschichtliche Ereignis selbst.

Daß man solche Geschichtsdeutung betreibt, hat seinen Grund in der Art des israelitischen Vorstellungsvermögens. Der Israelit denkt 1. nicht theoretisch oder dogmatisch, sondern konkret und praktisch und 2. in rein zeitlicher Weise. Jede grundsätzliche Aussage muß daher konkret und zeitlich umschrieben und ausgedrückt werden. Auch die augenblickliche Gesinnung, Absicht oder Haltung eines Menschen kann nur mit Hilfe konkreter Einzelbeispiele erläutert oder grundsätzlich in zeitlichen Vorstellungsakten als ein Gewordensein dargelegt werden. Alles, was über den Menschen grundsätzlich oder in bezug auf sein Hier und Jetzt zu erkennen und zu sagen ist, enthüllt sich aus der Deutung bestimmter geschichtlicher Ereignisse.

Dies gilt in vollem Umfang für die Ur- und Patriarchengeschichte. Die Urgeschichte soll etwas theologisch Grundlegendes erläutern, das für alle Menschen gilt; daher steht es am Anfang vor der Aussonderung Israels. Das Thema lautet: der Mensch als geschichtliches Wesen — was und wie der Mensch ist. Die Patriarchengeschichte soll an den Ahnen Israels etwas erläutern, was den mit Gott verbundenen Menschen gilt: Typen des Menschen vor Gott und in der Welt — wie der von Gott beanspruchte Mensch sein soll. Daß der Mensch tatsächlich einen solchen Typus nicht verwirklicht, sondern der Sünde verfällt und dem Untergang zusteuert, ist der Ausgangspunkt der prophetischen Verkündigung. Sie sieht eine mögliche Rettung nur in einer grundsätzlichen Wandlung oder Umwandlung des Menschen, in der er sein Eigentliches erlangt und seiner eigentlichen Aufgabe dienen kann.

II. Der Mensch als geschichtliches Wesen

1. In Gen 1—3 liegen zwei Erzählungen vor, die Grundlegendes über das Wesen des Menschen aussagen, wie denn der alttestamentliche Schöpfungsglaube überhaupt durchweg auf den Menschen bezogen ist und weniger etwas über Gott aussagen will. Die erste Erzählung in Gen 1 1—2 4 a schildert äußerlich die Schöpfung der Welt nach damaligem Verständnis, sachlich handelt sie vom Festsetzen der geschichtlichen Existenz des Menschen. Auf seine Erschaffung am sechsten Tage zielt die ganze Erzählung hin. Er ist das Ziel und die Spitze einer Pyramide, die Krönung der Schöpfertätigkeit Gottes und die Krone alles Geschaffenen: »Und Gott schuf den Menschen nach seinem Bilde, nach Gottes Bilde schuf er ihn; und schuf sie als Mann und als Weib« (1 27). Eigentlich ist diese Übersetzung Luthers ungenau. Wie vorher nicht jeweils ein einzelnes Tier, sondern die Tiere geschaffen werden, so besagt der hebräische Ausdruck *'adam*, der an dieser Stelle zur Bezeichnung einer Gesamtheit verwendet wird: Gott schuf die Menschen oder die Menschheit, und zwar männlich und weiblich. Einige Näherbestimmungen dieser Menschheit brauchen wir in diesem Zusammenhang nur kurz zu beachten: Die geschlechtliche Verschiedenheit der Menschen ist schöpfungsmäßig, d. h. göttlicher Wille; und der Mensch erhält die Kraft, die ihn zur Fortpflan-

zung und Vermehrung befähigt, gesondert aus der Hand Gottes und nicht schon mit der Ebenbildlichkeit (1 28). Grundlegend wichtig ist aber, daß die Menschheit nach dem Bilde Gottes geschaffen ist. Im Hebräischen finden wir an dieser Stelle zwei Ausdrücke, die »Bild« und »Ähnlichkeit« bedeuten. Sie bezeichnen die völlige und die nur annäherungsweise Gleichheit eines Bildes oder einer Statue mit dem lebendigen, urbildlichen Modell. So ist der Mensch nach dem Modell oder Muster Gottes oder der diesen umgebenden Himmelswesen geschaffen, ihnen aber doch nicht völlig gleich, sondern ähnlich. Auf diese Weise wird die besondere Würde des Menschen umschrieben, ohne daß dabei die Erhabenheit Gottes angetastet wird. Der Mensch ist Geschöpf wie die Tiere und nicht selber Schöpfer. Er stellt aber auch eine andere Art als die Tiere dar, über die er zum Herrn eingesetzt wird. Er ist weder Gott noch Tier, sondern steht zwischen ihnen als nach Gottes »Bild« geschaffen. So erhält er sein eigenes Gepräge, das nicht aufhört, sondern nach Gen 5 1. 3 9 6 in der Menschheit fortdauert.

Die Folge der Ebenbildlichkeit ist die Beauftragung der Menschen mit der Herrschaft in der Welt (1 28). Es ist die Aufgabe, die aus der Gabe folgt. Daher kann und darf der Mensch sich ihr nicht entziehen, sondern muß sie ausüben. Aber er muß sie als Ebenbildlicher ausüben — in seiner Sonderstellung zwischen Gott und Tier. Verläßt er sie, will er sich Gott gleichsetzen oder zum Tier absinken, so kann er seine Herrschaft nicht mehr recht ausüben. Sie wird zur Gewalt und Despotie des sich göttergleich wähnenden Menschen, der nicht mehr im Auftrag handeln will, oder zum bloßen Machtkampf auf der tierischen Triebebene im Streben nach dem Sieg des Stärkeren. Daß dem Menschen dann pflanzliche Nahrung zugewiesen wird (1 29), soll die recht ausgeübte Herrschaft als einen paradiesischen Frieden kennzeichnen, der Töten und Schlachten nicht kennt. Freilich weiß der Erzähler, daß es sich in Wirklichkeit nicht so verhält, wie das Ende der Sintfluterzählung sagt (9 1-7). Die tatsächlichen Lebensordnungen sind nicht einfach die schöpfungsmäßigen, sondern von diesen wegen der menschlichen Bosheit in einigen Punkten unterschieden. Der Mensch zwar ist und bleibt Ebenbild und soll nach wie vor herrschen. Aber er ist ein böse gewordenes Ebenbild, in dessen Herrschaft immer wieder die Bosheit durchzubrechen sucht. Desto nötiger ist es, daß er sich über sich selbst klar wird. Er ist ein geschichtliches Wesen, das nach Gen 1 durch Viererlei gekennzeichnet ist: Er muß sich als abhängiges Geschöpf verstehen — mit besonderer Beziehung zu Gott, nach dessen geschichtswirkendem Wesen und Modell er geschaffen ist — mit einer Sonderstellung in der Welt — und mit der geschichtlichen Aufgabe der Weltbeherrschung. Daher kann der Mensch die Welt nur recht beherrschen und sich als das geschichtliche Wesen erweisen, das er ist, wenn und sofern er sich selbst als unter der Herrschaft Gottes lebend weiß.

2. In Gen 2 4 b—3 25 ist der Mensch nicht das Ziel und die Spitze einer Pyramide, sondern der Mittelpunkt eines Kreises — das erste und einzelne Geschöpf, um das herum die ihm nahe Welt aufgebaut wird. Was die erste Erzählung in fast theologischer Begrifflichkeit als Ebenbildlichkeit bezeichnet, wird in dieser älteren und urtümlicheren Erzählung anders und konkreter ausgedrückt: Der Mensch ist an sich Staub oder »staubern« und also geringwertig. Erst daß er am göttlichen Lebensodem Anteil erhält, macht ihn lebendig und hebt ihn hervor. Aber es ist ihm gegeben worden; was am Menschen Besonderes ist, hat er von Gott. Jedoch ist er noch kein geschichtliches Wesen, sondern lebt in einer geschichtslosen Existenz als Betreuer des göttlichen Baumgartens. Zum geschichtlichen Wesen wird der Mensch durch das, was die Erzählung vom Sündenfall besagt. Er erliegt der an ihn herangetragenen Versuchung und ißt vom Baum des Erkennens von gut und böse. Dabei ist »gut und böse« ein formelhafter Ausdruck für »alles« — vom Guten bis zum Bösen. »Erkennen« ist das Erfahren und Vertrautwerden und wird mit Bezug auf die Person des Erfahrenden gebraucht. Die dort essenden Menschen werden restlos mit sich selbst vertraut. Das menschliche Erfassen weitet sich über die ursprünglichen Schranken hinweg aus. Eine vorher ungeahnte Lebenssteigerung beginnt, da der Mensch jener Geheimnisse vertraut und mächtig wird, die jenseits seiner Möglichkeiten lagen. Es ist der erschütternde Augenblick, in dem der Mensch seiner selbst voll bewußt wird — nicht als historische Erinnerung erzählt, sondern als Grundlegendes, das sich in jedem Menschenleben wiederholt. Der Mensch tut den Schritt vom Kind zum Erwachsenen oder vom instinktgebundenen Naturwesen zum geschichtlichen Wesen. Daher wird er sich nicht nur der eigenen Geschlechtlichkeit und der Fähigkeit zur Schaffung neuen Lebens bewußt, sondern sieht sich auch Nöten gegenüber, die er vorher nicht gekannt hat (3 14-19). Er lebt nicht mehr unbewußt in dem großen Ganzen der Welt und des Lebens, sondern steht dem als bewußter Mensch und Geschichtswesen gegenüber. Er muß ständig mit der in der Schlange verkörperten versucherischen Macht in sich selber ringen. Die Frau muß bestimmte Bedingungen auf sich nehmen, um zu ihrem Sein als Frau und Mutter zu finden, und Gefahren wagen, um ihr Sein zu leben. Der Mann sieht sich der Forderung der oft erfolglosen Arbeit und der Sorge für den Lebensunterhalt als seiner geschichtlichen Lebensbedingung gegenüber. Und das Wissen um den am Ende der Lebensgeschichte des einzelnen wartenden Tod überschattet alles. Der Mensch wird aus dem Garten seiner geschichtslosen Kindheit in die geschichtliche Welt

geschickt (3 20-24). Das Finden der Zeit, der geschichtlichen Dimension, ist gleich dem Verlieren des Paradieses. Die gefundene geschichtliche Existenz ist das verlorene Paradies. Entsprechend ist im endzeitlichen oder apokalyptischen Glauben die verlorene Zeit, das geschichtslose Dasein der Endzeit, gleich dem wiedergewonnenen Paradies.

3. Die Urgeschichte erzählt aber nicht nur in dieser Weise vom Menschen als einem geschichtlichen oder seine Geschichtlichkeit im fast notwendigen Sündigwerden gewinnenden Wesen, sondern auch von immer wieder aufbrechenden titanischen Gelüsten, die damit verbunden sind. In Gen 2—3 scheinen einige Bruchstücke verarbeitet zu sein, nach denen der Mensch den Zugang zum Lebensbaum suchte, aber vertrieben wurde, damit die göttliche Lebenskraft in ihm nicht übermächtig werden könne und er ewig lebe. Nach 6 1-4 strömt durch die Ehen der Himmelswesen mit Menschenfrauen die göttliche Lebenskraft in die Menschheit ein, so daß die Riesen entstehen. Damit diese Vermischung zwischen göttlicher und menschlicher Natur nicht ewig dauert und der Mensch nicht größere Macht besitzt, als ihm zusteht, wird seine Lebensdauer begrenzt. Schließlich erzählt 11 1-9 von dem gigantischen Unternehmen des Turm- und Stadtbaus, der der Entfaltung von Macht und Ruhm in ungeahntem Ausmaß dienen soll; und wieder weist Gott den Menschen in seine Schranken. In diesen Erzählungen wird als ein Grundzug der Menschen als geschichtlicher Wesen erkannt, daß sie die ihnen gesetzten Schranken zu sprengen drohen. Sie drohen Anteil an der göttlichen Natur zu erhalten und größere Macht zu erwerben, so daß die Grenzen zwischen Gott und Mensch zu verwischen beginnen und Gott sein ungebärdiges Geschöpf immer wieder zähmen muß.

4. Endlich müssen wir uns den beiden, jetzt in Gen 6 5—8 22 zusammengefaßten Sintfluterzählungen zuwenden, die äußerlich den Übergang von der glücklichen Vorzeit in die jetzige leidvolle Zeit erklären und die begründen sollen, warum es jetzt anders als früher ist. Es verhält sich eben so, wie die jüngere der beiden Erzählungen es darstellt: Die erste »paradiesische« Welt ist untergegangen und eine andere Welt begründet worden, in der wir leben. So wollen die Sintfluterzählungen von einer Krise erzählen, die zum Ende der glücklichen Vorzeit geführt hat — von einer Krise, die nicht zur Genesung, sondern zu Tod und Verderben geführt hat, aus denen nur wenige heil entkommen sind, um ihr Leben in einer veränderten Welt unter anderen Lebensbedingungen zu gestalten. Auch das gehört zum Menschen als einem geschichtlichen Wesen. Er muß immer wieder die Erfahrung des Am-Ende-Seins und des Zunichteseins durchleben. Mit seiner Welt, die er beherrschen soll und will, und mit seiner Kultur, die er

aufgebaut hat, sieht er sich je und dann am Ende und vor dem Nichts. Er sieht mächtigere Gewalten am Werk, die seine Herrschaft als eine Illusion enthüllen und seine Kultur vernichten. Und er selbst ist diesen Gewalten auf Gedeih und Verderb ausgeliefert und ein Spielball in ihrer Hand. Diese Erfahrung drückt die Sintfluterzählung aus. Sie will dem Menschen sagen, daß derartige Krisen mit dem menschlichen Sein unauflöslich verbunden sind, daß man ihnen nicht entgehen kann und daß sie unausweichlich von Gewalten über den Menschen gebracht werden, auf die er keinen Einfluß hat.

Die Ursache der Krisen aber liegt beim Menschen. Sie sind die strafenden Folgen seiner Schuld. Am besten ist dies wohl in der älteren Erzählung ausgedrückt: »Als Jahwe sah, daß die Bosheit der Menschen auf der Erde groß war und alles Gebilde ihrer Herzensgedanken nur noch böse allezeit, da reute es Jahwe, daß er die Menschen auf der Erde gemacht hatte, und es bekümmerte ihn in seinem Herzen. Da sprach Jahwe: Ich will die Menschen vom Erdboden vertilgen, denn es reut mich, daß ich sie gemacht habe.« (Gen 6 5-7). In diesem Urteil von äußerster Schärfe ist doch wohl die eigentliche Ursache für alle Krisen, in die die Menschheit geraten ist und gerät, in geradezu klassischer Weise angegeben. Alles Elend des Menschengeschlechts, alle Krisen der Menschheit und ihrer Kultur haben ihren letzten Grund in der menschlichen Sünde.

Als aber Noah nach der Flut das Opfer darbringt, spricht Gott: »Ich will die Erde nicht noch einmal um des Menschen willen verfluchen, denn die Gebilde des menschlichen Herzens sind doch böse von Jugend an; ich will nicht noch einmal alles Lebendige schlagen, wie ich es getan habe. Solange die Erde steht, sollen nicht aufhören Saat und Ernte, Frost und Hitze, Sommer und Winter, Tag und Nacht« (Gen 8 21-22). Daß Gott sich zu einer Selbstbeschränkung seiner strafenden Heiligkeit entschließt, beruht auf einem letztlich unauflöslichen Gegensatz: Der gleiche Befund, der vorher das Gericht begründet hat, läßt nunmehr die göttliche Nachsicht und Gnade wach werden. Erfahren wird diese Gnade in dem unbegreiflichen Bestand der Dinge trotz der menschlichen Sünde. Vor allem liegt darin die Mahnung, daß der Mensch der göttlichen Zusage sein Vertrauen schenken soll. So müssen wir sagen: Was die Krise überwinden läßt, ist das Vertrauen auf die Zusage Gottes. Wenn die Menschheit sich durch ihre Schuld immer wieder in geschichtliche Krisen stürzt, braucht sie in ihnen doch nicht ganz unterzugehen und als geschichtliche Erscheinung zu verschwinden. Aber Rettung und Überwindung liegen allein im glaubenden Vertrauen auf den Gott, dessen Zusage unverbrüchlich ist. Es gilt weder Resignation und Verzweiflung noch Heroismus und Kampf, sondern zuversichtliches Vertrauen auf die ewige Gnade.

III. Typen des Menschen vor Gott und in der Welt

Mit den Patriarchenerzählungen in Gen 12—50 verfolgen die Erzähler eine andere Absicht als mit der Urgeschichte. Während sie in ihr erläutern wollen, was der Mensch ist — ein geschichtliches Wesen —, suchen sie nun darzulegen, wie der Mensch sein soll. Dies geschieht dadurch, daß sie jeden der vier Patriarchen einen Menschentyp verkörpern lassen, der in seiner positiven Ausprägung beispielhaft sein soll.

1. Die Geschichten um Abraham dienen den Erzählern dazu, den Typ des glaubenden Menschen darzustellen. Darauf muß man bei der Erläuterung dieser Erzählungen das Augenmerk richten, unabhängig von der Frage, welche historischen Erinnerungen ihnen zugrunde liegen.

Einige Erzählungen fassen das Gegenüber von Glaubendem und Nichtglaubendem ins Auge. Grundlegend ist Gen 12 1-9 über den Auszug Abrahams aus seiner Heimat. Von ihm wird verlangt, was für den Menschen der alten Zeit am schwersten war: sich aus den lebenfördernden Bindungen der Heimat, Sippe und Familie zu lösen und sich aus ihrem Schutz heraus rechtlos auf die Wanderung ins Ungewisse zu begeben — in ein Land, von dem er lediglich erfährt, daß Gott es ihm zeigen will. Kein Grund wird angegeben, sondern Gehorsam verlangt; denn der Glaubende fragt nicht nach Gründen, sondern gehorcht. Darin sagt die Erzählung etwas, was für das Dasein des glaubenden Menschen überhaupt gilt. Er wird aus allen bestehenden Bindungen seines Lebens herausgerufen und auf eine Wanderung geschickt, die von ihm aus gesehen ins Ungewisse führt; denn ihr Ende und Ziel liegen in Gottes Hand. Inzwischen ist er vogelfrei in der Fremde. Er geht immer einen anderen Weg als die übrigen und sieht dabei diesen Weg selber nur von Schritt zu Schritt. Er steuert nicht auf ein wohlbekanntes Ziel zu, das leuchtend aus der Ferne winkt, sondern muß sich seinen Weg führen lassen. Und daß das Ziel nicht ein unentrinnbarer Abgrund ist, in dem er zerschellt, weiß er nur daraus, daß Gott selbst es ist, der ihn auf die Wanderung schickt. Als Abraham nun gehorcht, wird ihm über den anfänglich zugesagten Segen hinaus eine weitere Verheißung gegeben: »Deinen Nachkommen will ich dies Land geben« (12 7). Da Abraham gehorcht und der Segenszusage geglaubt hat, erhält er Größeres und Umfassenderes als vorher. Dem Glaubenden wird mehr zuteil, als er erhoffen durfte.

In anderer Weise stellt ein zweiter Erzähler den Auszug Abrahams dar; es geschieht in der Geschichte von der Gefährdung der Sara in Ägypten in 12 10-20. Abraham wandert nicht auf Befehl Gottes und im Glauben, sondern wegen einer Hungersnot, vor der er sich mit seiner Frau zu retten sucht. Und er handelt nicht als der Glaubende, sondern wie ein kluger und vorausschauender Orientale, der nicht vor dem Hunger flieht, um in das Schwert derer zu laufen, die die Frau des rechtlosen Fremden begehren. Er handelt wie einer, der sein Leben um jeden Preis retten und dabei noch Geschäfte machen will. Das gelingt ihm auch — aber nur, weil Gott insgeheim in seinem Leben wirkt und waltet, ohne daß Abraham ahnt und erfährt, worauf alles beruht. Er glaubt, sich und sein Leben retten zu können; aber es gelingt ihm nur, damit er später Gott begegnen kann. Er handelt nach den Auffassungen seiner Zeit klug und weitsichtig, indem er Sara als seine Schwester ausgibt; aber er gibt damit Gott nur Gelegenheit, noch klüger und weitsichtiger zu handeln, indem er eingreift und Sara aus dem Harem des Pharao rettet, damit sie später den Erben der Verheißung zur Welt bringen kann.

Wie Abraham zum Glaubenden wird, stellt der gleiche Erzähler in 15 1 b-2. 7-12. 17-18 dar. Bei ihm begegnet Abraham nun erstmalig Gott; das zeigt die Vorstellungsformel: »Ich bin Jahwe« (15 7). Und den leidvollen oder zweifelnden Fragen Abrahams (15 2. 8) steht die feierliche Selbstverpflichtung Gottes gegenüber, aufgrund derer Abraham nun auch bei diesem Erzähler glaubt. Gott gibt Abraham eine feste Zusicherung, die nach altem Ritus bekräftigt wird: Aus einander gegenübergelegten Tierteilen und Vögeln bildet Abraham eine Gasse, durch die man hindurchgeht und sich für den Fall des Bruchs einer Verpflichtung verwünscht. Aber das Weitere, das das Schauerliche und Grauenvolle der Szene andeutet, schildert nur, wie Gott zwischen den Fleischstücken hindurchfährt — mit Feuer und Rauch als den Anzeichen der Gotteserscheinung, der Theophanie. Er verpflichtet und bindet sich ganz allein — nicht auch Abraham — in einer als besonders heilig und unverbrüchlich geltenden Form. Und auf diese Selbstverpflichtung Gottes vertraut Abraham nunmehr.

Demgegenüber steht die Erzählung von Sodom und Gomorra in 18 16—19 29, die das Geschick des nichtglaubenden Sünders zeigen soll. Dabei müssen wir in diesem Zusammenhang die an sich wichtige Fürbitte Abrahams beiseite lassen (18 22b-33); immerhin macht sie deutlich, daß es weder allein um die Rettung Lots geht, der in der Fürbitte gar nicht erwähnt wird, noch um Sodom-Gomorra als nichtisraelitische, heidnische Städte. Was für sie gilt, ist vielmehr auf Israel und alle anderen menschlichen Gemeinschaften anwendbar; Sodom-Gomorra sind ihr Typus. Sie sind im ganzen Alten Testament das stets gültige Beispiel für die in der Sünde beharrenden Menschen und für das vollständige und umfassende Strafgericht Gottes über sie (eine andere Überlieferung nennt die Städte Adma und Zeboim: Hos 11 8 Dtn 29 23; alle vier sind in Gen 14 2 verbunden).

Was bedeutet »glauben«? Ein Erzähler hatte Abraham in 12 1-9 als Glaubenden dadurch gekennzeichnet, daß dieser gehorsam war.

Ein anderer Erzähler sagt in 15 6: »Abraham glaubte Jahwe, und das rechnete er ihm zur Gerechtigkeit«. Daß Abraham glaubt, bedeutet im Hebräischen wörtlich: Er macht sich fest in Gott. Er vertraut Gott und verhält sich wie ein frommer und treuer Anhänger Gottes. Dieses Vertrauen rechnet Gott als Gerechtigkeit an. Er hat den deutlichen Beweis, daß Abraham vertraut, und kann ihn daher als gerecht »beurteilen« — wie ein Priester die dargebrachten Opfer beurteilt. Gott beurteilt Abraham als »gerecht«: als rechtbeschaffen, fromm und treu im Verhältnis zu Gott; er wird den Anforderungen gerecht, die sich aus dem Verhältnis zwischen Gott und Mensch ergeben. Der Erzähler sagt also, daß das persönliche Verhältnis des Glaubenden zu Gott richtig ist, wenn er — wie Abraham — Gott vertraut, ihn ernst nimmt und sich ganz auf ihn verläßt.

Auf etwas anderes weist die Einsetzung der Beschneidung in 17 9-14 hin. Bei diesen Bestimmungen liegt der Nachdruck darauf, daß vom Hausvater jeder einzelne erfaßt wird, die Beschneidung als Zeichen annehmen und sich zu Gott bekennen soll. Es geht demnach um die persönliche Glaubensentscheidung des Israeliten für sich selbst und um seine Glaubensverantwortung für seine Hausgenossen.

Freilich zeigt die Erzählung von der Gefährdung der Sara in der Kanaanäerstadt Gerar in 20 1-18, daß der Glaube kein Monopol ist und der Glaubende kein Recht hat, einen Ausschließlichkeitsanspruch für seinen Glauben zu erheben. Abraham gibt Sara als seine Schwester aus — für den Erzähler in halber Lüge und halber Wahrheit, da sie als seine Halbschwester betrachtet wird —, weil er annimmt: »Vielleicht ist keine Gottesfurcht an diesem Ort, und sie werden mich um meiner Frau willen erschlagen« (20 11). Aber dann muß er feststellen, daß auch in Gerar Gottesfurcht herrscht und daß es nicht nur einen einzigen Glaubenden gibt, sondern daß man Glaube und Gehorsam manchmal sogar dort findet, wo man sie nicht erwarten zu können meint. Das ist eine echt prophetische Erkenntnis, die in späterer Zeit noch die Bücher Ruth und Jona aufnehmen und die dem nationalen und religiösen Stolz Israels sehr widerstrebt. In dieser Frage hat auch Abraham versagt und muß nun umlernen. Der Glaubende muß wissen, daß es auch bei den sogenannten Heiden ein religiöses Verhalten (Gottesfurcht) geben kann, das den grundlegenden göttlichen Geboten entspricht.

Wie verhält sich der Glaubende im Leben? Einen Zug dessen schildert die Erzählung von der Trennung Abrahams und Lots in 13 1-13. Als sich durch das Anwachsen ihrer Herden Schwierigkeiten ergeben, schlägt Abraham die Trennung vor und ist sogar bereit, sich in der Auswahl der Wohngegend nach dem jüngeren Lot zu richten. Der Streit wird nicht mit den Waffen ausgetragen, wie andere Völker dergleichen entscheiden lassen. Vielmehr ist Abraham friedfertig und unkriegerisch, wie der Glaubende es sein soll, und wünscht friedliche Trennung statt Kampf. Darin erscheint er als Beispiel und Vorbild. Es ist leicht, sich mit anderen zu streiten und, wenn man sich festgefahren hat, zur Waffe zu greifen. Weil es leicht ist, tut man es so oft. Es ist schwerer, friedfertig zu sein, einmal nachzugeben und auf eigene Vorteile zu verzichten; aber es ist richtiger. Der Glaubende zieht die Versöhnung und den Frieden vor, weil Gott ein Gott des Friedens ist. Lot ist freilich im Gegensatz zu Abraham eigennützig und wählt für sich die fruchtbare Gegend des Jordangaus, so daß der friedfertige Abraham übertölpelt scheint. Aber im Jordangau wohnen jene verderbten Leute, die im Strafgericht über Sodom-Gomorra untergehen, so daß der glaubende Abraham letztlich besser gewählt hat als der eigennützige Lot, der seinen Besitz verliert. Die Entscheidung des wahrhaft Glaubenden führt für ihn eben dennoch zum Guten. (In der späten nachexilischen Zeit, wahrscheinlich im Zeitalter der Makkabäerkämpfe, empfand das werdende Judentum jenes Bild Abrahams und also des Glaubenden als ergänzungsbedürftig und hat ihm in Gen 14 widersprechende Züge beigegeben: kriegerisch gegen diejenigen, die den Verwandten bzw. den Glaubensgenossen bedrohen; stolz gegen Fremde, aber edelmütig gegen Bundesgenossen; demütig gegen Jerusalem und seinen Hohenpriester.)

Auf einen anderen Zug weist die Erzählung von Abrahams Vertrag mit dem (schon in 20 1-18 genannten) Stadtkönig Abimelech in 21 22-34 hin. Im Anschluß an die Ereignisse um die Gefährdung und Rettung der Sara schlägt nach 21 22-24 der etwas beunruhigte König einen Freundschaftsvertrag vor. Äußerlich ist Abraham als rechtloser Fremder zwar der schwächere Teil, aber er steht unter dem Schutz und Segen seines machtvollen Gottes. Der Staatsmann weiß hinter dem Glaubenden eine Macht, die ihn letztlich unangreifbar werden läßt. Obwohl Abraham rechtlich auf die Freundlichkeit und den Schutz Abimelechs angewiesen sein sollte, ist er tatsächlich von den äußeren Verhältnissen unabhängig und hat sein Leben auf anderes gegründet als die Freundlichkeit Abimelechs. Daher erscheint er dem König, der umgekehrt auf Abrahams Fürbitte angewiesen war, als ungewöhnlich, ja unheimlich. Dieser glaubende Abraham, für den die gewöhnlichen staatsrechtlichen Maßstäbe nicht passen, erscheint ihm unberechenbar. Er ist seiner Loyalität im staatspolitischen Sinne (hebräisch: ḥæsæd mit dem allgemeinen Sinn »Solidarität, Verbundenheit«, Luther: Barmherzigkeit) nicht sicher und wünscht daher eine einwandfreie rechtliche Grundlage. Abraham will sich dem nicht entziehen und stimmt zu. Er ist als Glaubender zwar unabhängig von Abimelech und Gerar, von rechtlichen Zusicherungen und Verträgen. Aber er ist auch kein Revolutionär und Anarchist, der unberechenbar sein will; das ist er nur gezwungen durch seinen Glauben. So will er sein Verhältnis zu dem Staatswesen, in dessen Grenzen er lebt, gern in klarer Weise regeln, wie es dann nach 21 27. 31 geschieht. Mit dieser Darstellung hat der Erzähler in 21 25-26. 28-30. 32 eine andere Geschichte verflochten, in der Abraham sein Recht auf einen Brunnen geltend macht, den seine Knechte gegraben und den die Leute von Gerar in Besitz genommen haben. Der in seinem Recht gekränkte Abraham ist nicht gesonnen, das hinzunehmen, sondern wünscht klare rechtliche Verhältnisse, die seine Existenz ermöglichen. Doch der zur Rede gestellte Stadtkönig behauptet, von nichts zu wissen; das ist eine höflich ausgedrückte Ablehnung. Abimelech will von der Sache nichts wissen, damit er sie nicht zu untersuchen braucht und der Brunnen im Besitz von Gerar bleibt. Da nötigt Abraham ihm sieben Lämmer als Geschenk auf und bekundet damit nach alter Sitte seinen Rechtsanspruch, der durch die Übergabe der umstrittenen Sache als Gegengeschenk oder durch einen Vertrag anerkannt zu werden pflegte. So soll diese Erzählung die Kritik Abrahams an der selbstgefällig betonten Freundlichkeit Abimelechs darstellen. Von solcher Art ist die Loyalität des Staates gegenüber dem Glaubenden, von dem eben dieser Staat wirkliche Loyalität wünscht! Beide miteinander verbundenen Erzählungen stellen die bloß staatsrechtliche und staatspolitische Loyalität mit ihrer gleichzeitigen Betrugsmöglichkeit der echten Loyalität des Glaubenden gegenüber. Der Glaubende ist zu ihr bereit, obwohl er zugleich die letzten Rechtsmittel anwenden muß, damit der seine Loyalität fordernde Staat nicht seine Existenz vernichtet.

Daß derartige Rechtsmittel nicht immer am Platze sind, zeigt die Erzählung von Hagars Flucht und Ismaels Geburt in 16 1-16: Sie können Glaube und Vertrauen auf Gott nicht ersetzen und Probleme des Glaubens nicht lösen! Das Problem ist dasjenige der Kinderlosigkeit der Sara, die sie nicht nur persönlich betrifft, sondern die ganze Verheißung Gottes an Abraham in Frage stellt — wobei merkwürdigerweise das drohende Scheitern ebenso von Gott kommt wie die Verheißung (16 2). In dieser Schwierigkeit schlägt Sara den rechtlich möglichen Weg der Kindeszeugung mittels ihrer eigenen Sklavin Hagar vor. So könnte das Problem nach Recht und Sitte gelöst werden, wenn sich nicht die Frage stellte, ob sich das glaubende Vertrauen auf Gott durch rechtliche Maßnahmen ersetzen und das Wahrwerden der Verheißung durch sie erzwingen läßt. Tatsächlich beginnen sich nun die Dinge immer mehr zu verwickeln: Überheblichkeit der Hagar, Verlangen der Sara nach Genugtuung, Rückgabe der Hagar in ihre Gewalt, Degradierung zum früheren Sklavendasein, Flucht der Hagar. Man greift zu einem Rechtsmittel nach dem anderen, doch die Lage wird dadurch stets verfahrener — nicht nur für Abraham und Sara, sondern auch für Hagar, die in dieses Getriebe hineingeraten ist und darin langsam zerrieben wird. Rechtlich ist alles klar und einwandfrei, tatsächlich aber alles unklar und höchstes Unrecht. So geht es, will der Erzähler sagen, wenn ein Glaubensproblem mit Rechtsmitteln gelöst werden soll! Rechtliche Maßnahmen können das fehlende Vertrauen des Glaubenden nicht ersetzen und tragen nichts zu einer Sicherung bei. Man kann auf solche Weise nicht nachhelfen. Das gewünschte Ergebnis — der ersehnte Erbe — stellt sich doch nicht ein; und man stürzt darüber höchstens andere Menschen ins Unglück und vergiftet die Beziehungen zu ihnen durch die Berufung auf das Recht. Demgegenüber erbarmt sich Gott der geflohenen Sklavin, die das Opfer des Rechts geworden ist, indem er ihr eine Verheißung gibt (16 10-12). Bei ihm ist anderes und mehr als Recht; bei ihm ist das, was Abraham und Sara nicht zu kennen schienen. Ihm gegenüber ist sogar das menschlich verständliche Lachen der altgewordenen Sara über die Verheißung eines Kindes in 18 12 voreilig und unüberlegt, weil es seine Allmacht nicht berücksichtigt.

Schließlich zeigt die Erzählung vom Opfergang Abrahams in 22 1-19, was und wie das rechte Opfer des Glaubenden sein müßte. Die Bereitschaft Abrahams verdeutlicht ein Zweifaches: daß man Gott als ein Opfer, das seiner würdig ist, eigentlich nur den erstgeborenen Sohn und Erben der Verheißung darbringen könnte und daß man dies in ehrfürchtiger Hingabe tun müßte, zu der man sich gehorsam entschließt. Freilich wird das Menschenopfer als schwerste Prüfung und Erprobung des Glaubenden gerade nicht dargebracht und soll auch von niemandem mehr dargebracht werden. Aber die Forderung danach bedeutet eine neue Beurteilung des Opfers und eine Entwertung des herkömmlichen Tieropfers. Indem dargelegt wird, was und wie ein Opfer für diesen Gott eigentlich sein müßte — nicht ein Tier als kleiner Teil des Eigentums, sondern das Liebste und Wichtigste, was der Mensch besitzt —, wird das Tieropfer innerlich überwunden. Zwar wird es nach der Erzählung noch dargebracht (22 13); aber der Höhepunkt ist schon erreicht, als Gott den hingebenden Glauben Abrahams erkennt, und das Tieropfer nur der beibehaltene Abschluß der überlieferten und vom Erzähler verwendeten Legende. Wesentlich ist, daß das rechte Opfer des Glaubenden als Tat des radikalen Glaubensgehorsams erscheint, in der das Liebste und Wichtigste hingegeben wird.

2. Wie Abraham der Typ des glaubenden Menschen, so ist Isaak der Typ des duldend hinnehmenden Menschen. Dieses Erdulden zeigt sich schon in den Erklärungen seines Namens mit Hilfe des Wortes »lachen«, die sich nicht wie sonst üblich auf ihn persönlich beziehen, sondern stets in Zusammenhang mit dem Verhalten eines seiner Elternteile stehen (Gen 17 17 Abraham lacht; 18 12 ff. und 21 6 Sara lacht). Der eigentliche Sinn seines Namens »Gott möge (gnädig oder freundlich) lachen« wird ihm genommen. Ferner ist er in den Ismaelgeschich-

ten (16 1-16 21 8-21) derjenige, für oder gegen den einfach verfügt wird und der dies hinzunehmen hat. Ebenso verhält es sich in der Erzählung von Abrahams Opfergang (22 1-19), nach der er erdulden muß, was über ihn beschlossen wird, obwohl es um Leben und Tod geht. Der Segen Gottes wird ihm nicht um seinetwillen, sondern um seines Vaters willen zugesagt (26 3). Auch nach 26 12-17 wird über ihn verfügt: Er wird reich, weil Gott ihn segnet; er gerät in Bedrängnis, weil man ihn beneidet; und er muß Gerar verlassen, weil Abimelech ihn mit dürren Worten fortschickt. Noch als alter Mann wird er durch seine Frau und ihren Lieblingssohn Jakob um die Erteilung des Segens an den dafür ausersehenen Sohn betrogen.

Die gleichen Grundzüge weist die Erzählung von der Brautwerbung um Rebekka in Gen 24 auf. Isaaks Frau darf nicht frei gewählt werden, sondern nur aus dem engeren Bereich der aramäischen Sippe; und Isaak darf nicht selber wählen und werben, sondern ist auf den im Auftrag seines Vaters suchenden Sklaven angewiesen. Er muß wieder hinnehmen, was über ihn beschlossen wird. Aber — und das ist ein neuer Zug — dieses Hinnehmen steht doch unter der Führung Gottes. Er waltet unauffällig, aber wirksam in den Ereignissen, worauf die Ausdrücke »glücken lassen«, »begegnen lassen« und »bestimmen« hinweisen. Er lenkt im Anerbieten der Rebekka am Brunnen und dem Einverständnis ihrer Angehörigen zur Heirat die Menschen von innen her. Er führt sie im Herzen zugunsten des duldend hinnehmenden Isaak, der auf diese Weise eine allen Idealen gemäße Frau erhält. So soll gezeigt werden, daß der duldend hinnehmende Mensch nicht hilflos preisgegeben ist, sondern unter der Führung Gottes lebt.

Einen weiteren Zug fügt die Erzählung von der Gefährdung der Rebekka in 26 1-11 hinzu. Auch in ihr ist Isaak der Mensch, über den durch die Abrahamverheißung schon verfügt ist; er darf das zugesagte Land in der Hungersnot nicht verlassen und aufgeben. Das bedeutet aber zugleich, daß Gott ihn schützen und segnen wird (26 2 ff.). Er verliert nichts und büßt nichts ein, wenn er darauf verzichtet, über sich selbst bestimmen zu wollen. Ginge er in eigenem Entschluß nach Ägypten, so könnte er dort vielleicht menschlichen Schutz vor dem Hunger finden. Verzichtet er aber auf sein eigenes Wollen und nimmt hin, was von Gott bestimmt und verfügt ist, so findet er durch den Verzicht mehr als sonst: den Schutz und Segen Gottes selbst. Der Mensch, der Gottes Eingreifen und Verfügen duldet und hinnimmt, findet mehr als andere Menschen. Dem entspricht es, daß Isaak, als er aus seiner Passivität heraustritt und Rebekka als seine Schwester ausgibt, andere in Lebensgefahr bringt, da das Antasten einer verheirateten Frau dem einfachen Stadtbewohner wahrscheinlich die Todesstrafe eingetragen oder Unheil über alle gebracht hätte. Das hält der König dem Isaak vor (26 10). Aber was er selbst nicht erreichen konnte, ohne Rebekka und andere Menschen zu gefährden, fällt ihm dann wieder in den Schoß: Abimelech verfügt seine und der Rebekka Unantastbarkeit (26 11). Das will die Erzählung zeigen: Gottes Schutz und Segen, den man sich weder erringen noch durch Lügen überflüssig machen kann, sondern hinnehmen muß, wenn er verfügt wird.

Den gleichen Grundgedanken hat die Erzählung vom Brunnenstreit im Tal von Gerar in 26 18-22. Anders als Abraham setzt Isaak seinen Rechtsanspruch auf seine Brunnen nicht durch, sondern gibt duldend nach, als sie ihm streitig gemacht werden, und zieht schließlich von dort weg in die Steppe. Aber gerade als Duldender steht er unter Gottes Schutz und Segen. Denn er findet einen neuen Brunnen, den er »freie Plätze, Weite« nennt und als Gottes Geschenk versteht. Gott schafft ihm auf diese Weise Raum genug, so daß er im Lande wachsen kann (26 22). Genauso fällt ihm endlich nach 26 23-33 der Vertrag mit dem Stadtkönig Abimelech von Gerar zu. Dieser Vertrag ist eine glatte Kapitulation Abimelechs; er bittet um ihn und darum, daß Isaak ihm und Gerar nichts Böses antut. Und wegen des Vertrages wagt es dann auch niemand mehr, dem Isaak seinen neuen Brunnen streitig zu machen. Ihm, der alles hingenommen hat, ist zugleich alles wie von selbst zugefallen!

3. Wieder anders verhält es sich mit Jakob, der den Typ des hoffenden und harrenden Menschen verkörpert. Dabei sucht er zunächst das Erhoffte mit sehr fragwürdigen Mitteln zu erreichen. Er betrügt Esau um das Recht des Erstgeborenen (25 29-34) oder den Segen des Vaters (27 1-45). Besonders bei dieser zweiten Begebenheit hat er nach der Erzählung ein schlechtes Gewissen und wie seine Mutter das Empfinden, daß ihr Tun eigentlich nicht den Segen, sondern den Fluch verdient. Aber das hindert ihn doch nicht daran, sich das Erhoffte betrügerisch anzueignen. Auch in den Laban-Erzählungen ist Jakob der Mann, der die Hoffnungen, mit denen er ausgezogen ist, durch wenig einwandfreie Mittel zu verwirklichen sucht — besonders in der Art, wie er seinen Viehreichtum durch Anwendung magischer Praktiken erlangt (30 37 ff.).

Wie dieses sein Handeln ist seine Frömmigkeit geartet. Das zeigt die Erzählung vom Traum in Betel in 28 10-22, in der er durch den Traum und die Verheißung merkt, daß er an einer heiligen Stätte nächtigt. Da tut er ein Gelübde, d. h. gibt Gott ein bedingtes Versprechen: »Wenn Gott wird mit mir sein und mich behüten auf dem Wege, den ich reise, und mir Brot zu essen geben und Kleider anzuziehen und mich mit Frieden wieder heim zu meinem Vater bringen, so soll Jahwe mein Gott sein; und dieser Stein, den ich aufgerichtet habe zu einem Mal, soll ein Gotteshaus werden; und von allem, was du mir gibst, will ich dir den Zehnten geben« (28 20-22). Jakob stellt Gott eine ganze Reihe von Bedingungen und gibt dann sein Versprechen für den Fall, daß Gott die Bedingungen erfüllt. Er kann auch Gott für seine Pläne brauchen; es kann nicht schaden, wenn dieser noch mithilft. Freilich soll er nur das tun, was Jakob wünscht. Dazu, aber zu nichts anderem, ist er ihm willkommen. So wird Jakob als Vertreter einer eigennützigen Frömmigkeit dargestellt, wie sie für den Menschen vielfach typisch ist.

Doch dann findet in Jakob eine tiefgreifende innere Wandlung statt, die ihn in ganz anderer Weise zum Typ des Hoffens und Harrens macht: zu dem auf Gott hoffenden und harrenden Menschen. Das besagt die Erzählung vom nächtlichen Ringen Jakobs in 32 25-33. Als er da am Jabbok mit dem »Mann« ringt, beginnt er ein anderer zu werden. Der Erzähler meint keineswegs mehr einen körperlichen Kampf wie in der zu vermutenden ältesten Form der Erzählung. Der Ausruf: »Ich lasse dich nicht, du segnest mich denn« (32 27) weist darauf hin, daß das äußere Geschehen symbolhaft als inneres Ringen verstanden werden soll: als Gewissens- und Gebetskampf. Nachdem Jakob viele seiner Wünsche mit schlechten Mitteln verwirklicht hat, nun aber dem betrogenen Esau entgegengeht und Gefahr läuft, alles und selbst sein Leben zu verlieren, ringt er in dieser kritischen Lage mit Gott und sich selber auf Leben und Tod. Und darin wandelt er sich und geht mit einem neuen Namen (Israel) — d. h. nach altem Verständnis mit einem neuen Wesen — und dem erbetenen Segen — d. h. mit einer in und an ihm wirkenden Kraft — aus dem Ringen hervor. Zugleich trägt er eine Verletzung davon, wie man sie in solchem Kampf davonzutragen pflegt; sie wird ihn ständig an diese Stunde erinnern. In anderer Weise hat ein zweiter Erzähler in 35 6 a. 9-13. 15 die Wandlung Jakobs dargestellt: Nicht als Folge seines heftigen Ringens, sondern durch eine ausschließliche Tat Gottes erhält Jakob ein neues Wesen und zugleich eine reiche Verheißung, die ihm alles zusagt, was er begehren könnte. Worauf sich sein Hoffen richtet, dies alles erhält er von Gott, so daß er es nicht mehr auf eine typisch menschlich-unanständige Art erschleichen soll.

Die Wirkung dieser Wandlung Jakobs zeigt sich in 35 1-4. 6 b-7 über den Altarbau in Betel. Er erscheint in einem anderen und neuen Licht. Er soll gewiß sein Gelübde erfüllen und tut es auch. Doch dazu hätte der Bau des Altars mit der kultischen Verehrung Gottes ausgereicht. Tatsächlich geht Jakob weit darüber hinaus: In feierlicher Weise schafft er die anderen, fremden Götter aus seinem Hause und bekennt sich zu dem Gott, der ihm begegnet ist. Mit der Hinwendung seiner ganzen Familie zu diesem Gott bekennt Jakob, daß er seine Hoffnungen und Wünsche nicht mehr selbst verwirklichen will, erst recht nicht auf krummen Wegen, sondern auf Gott hofft und harrt.

Das wird besonders deutlich, wenn wir bedenken, daß sich unter den vergrabenen Dingen auch die Teraphim, die Hausgott-Symbole, befinden, die Rahel ihrem Vater Laban gestohlen und mit denen sie nach altem Recht dem Jakob den Anspruch auf das Erbe Labans gesichert hatte. Nun wird der Erbanspruch beiseite getan! Dieser Verzicht ist für den neuen Jakob bezeichnend. Und in alledem soll er Beispiel und Vorbild sein: Der eigennützige Mensch soll sich dahin wandeln oder wandeln lassen, daß er darauf verzichtet, typisch menschliche Hoffnungen (Reichtum) durch typisch menschliche Mittel (Betrug) zu verwirklichen, und allein auf Gott hofft und harrt.

4. Nur einen kurzen Blick brauchen wir auf die Gestalt Josephs zu werfen, da die große, einheitliche Erzählung sich als ganze erfassen läßt. Auch an ihm vollzieht sich durch Gottes Walten etwas, freilich nicht durch solch ein plötzliches und fast gewaltsames Eingreifen wie bei Jakob. Gott wird in der Josephgeschichte kaum erwähnt und als die im Stillen wirkende Macht verstanden, die die bösen Handlungen der Menschen in gute verwandelt, so daß sie den göttlichen Absichten dienen. So wird es in 50 20 gesagt, das sozusagen den theologischen Leitspruch angibt: »Ihr gedachtet es böse mit mir zu machen; aber Gott gedachte es gut zu machen, um zu tun, was jetzt vorliegt: viele Menschen am Leben zu erhalten.« Dies wirkt sich für die Darstellung der Gestalt Josephs aus. Bei ihm ist, vielleicht noch deutlicher als bei Jakob, eine Änderung zu erkennen: vom hochmütigen Menschen, wie er in seinen ersten Träumen in 37 1-11 erscheint, zu dem demütigen Menschen, der als solcher jenen Leitspruch 50 20 sagt. Das erfolgt nicht durch eine plötzliche Wandlung, sondern durch eine allmähliche Änderung, die sich in Monaten und Jahren vollzieht. So steht Joseph schließlich als der Typ des demütigen Menschen vor uns. Und zugleich weist die Erzählung darauf hin, daß eine solche Änderung zum gottgewollten Leben sich nicht unbedingt durch eine jähe, erschütternde und umwälzende Bekehrung von einer Stunde auf die andere vollziehen muß, sondern sich ebenso gut in einem langsamen und fast unmerklichen Werden ereignen kann.

IV. Das Erlangen der eigentlichen Existenz des Menschen

Die Erzählungen der Genesis erläutern, was der Mensch ist und welchen Weg er gehen soll: Er ist ein Wesen mit einer geschichtlichen Existenz, aufgrund seiner Gaben mit dem geschichtlichen Auftrag der Weltherrschaft unter der Oberherrschaft Gottes versehen und dazu aufgefordert, den Weg des glaubenden, des duldenden, des hoffenden oder des demütigen Menschen zu gehen. Dies ließe sich noch ergänzen und vervollständigen, wenn wir andere Bücher des Alten Testaments heranzögen. Wir sähen den gehorsamen Menschen unter dem Gesetz, den betenden Menschen in den Psalmen und den klug und kundig handelnden Menschen in den Weisheitsbüchern. Wichtiger aber ist die Beobachtung, die sich besonders an der Urgeschichte und den Jakoberzählungen machen ließ, daß das Alte Testament die Lage nicht so einfach und einlinig sieht. Es ist noch anderes im Spiel. Der geschichtliche Mensch ist das böse gewordene Ebenbild Gottes, von titanischem Streben getrieben und von Krisen geschüttelt. Es ist nötig, daß er sich auf sein eigentliches Wesen besinnt und um es ringt und daß er daraus als ein gewandelter, neuer Mensch hervorgeht. Damit stoßen wir auf eine andere Schicht, die am Beispiel Hiobs und der prophetischen Theologie zu klären bleibt.

1. Gewöhnlich gilt als das Ziel des Menschen das »Leben« selbst, dessen vollbewußter Besitz in den grundlegenden Lebensäußerungen von Essen und Trinken bis zu Liebe und Haß als höchstes Gut empfunden wird und als Voraussetzung aller übrigen Güter und Werte gilt. Das Eigene des Menschen ist mit dem Lebensvollzug selbst gegeben. Es scheint alles gesagt, wenn das Leben lange und glücklich genannt werden kann und der Mensch alt und lebensgesättigt wird, ohne daß der Gedanke an eine Entwicklung auftaucht, die erst zum eigentlichen Wesen des einzelnen Menschen hinführte.

Demgegenüber sucht und findet Hiob den Weg, der zum Eigentlichen des Menschen jenseits des bloßen Lebensvollzuges führt. Er muß dieses Eigentliche erst gewinnen und kann es in der Gottesgemeinschaft finden. So sehen wir es nach der Gottesrede in Hi 40 3-5 42 2-3. 5-6. In tiefster Erschütterung seiner Existenz wird Hiob der eigenen Nichtigkeit inne, so daß er nicht mehr ohnmächtig-zähneknirschend vor dem angeblichen feindlichen Gott steht, sondern demutsvoll schweigt:

> Sieh, ich bin zu gering; was könnte ich dir erwidern?
> Ich lege meine Hand auf meinen Mund.
> Einmal habe ich geredet, doch tu ich's nicht noch einmal,
> ein zweites Mal, doch tu's nicht mehr.

Außer der eigenen Nichtigkeit hat Hiob zugleich die Allmacht Gottes erfahren und erkannt. In Zusammenhang mit der Gottesrede sieht er, daß die Rätsel des Lebens bloß für den Menschen bestehen, dem Gottes Wollen und Tun uneinsichtig sind, daß sie jedoch in Wirklichkeit ein sinnvolles Handeln Gottes darstellen:

> Ich habe nun erfahren, daß du alles vermagst
> und dir kein Gedanke unmöglich ist.
> So habe ich denn ohne Einsicht geredet
> von Dingen, die mir zu wunderbar und unbekannt sind.

Das Leiden ist für Hiob der Anlaß dafür geworden, daß er Gott nicht mehr vom bloßen Hörensagen, sondern aus persönlicher Begegnung kennt. Er »schaut« ihn im Sinn der Begegnung, die eine vertraute Gemeinschaft bewirkt. Denn Gott schauen bedeutet im Alten Testament: seinem Vertrautenkreis angehören und sich ihm vertrauensvoll hingeben. Daher sagt Hiob:

> Vom Hörensagen hatte ich von dir vernommen,
> nun aber hat mein Auge dich geschaut.

So hat sich mit Hiob eine grundlegende Wandlung vollzogen, die ganz deutlich wird, wenn man diese Worte mit seinen früheren heftigen Reden vergleicht. Bei ihm ist das Leid das Mittel, durch das er dazu geführt worden ist, das Eigentliche seines Lebens in der Gottesgemeinschaft zu gewinnen. Und daß dies jenseits des bloßen Lebensvollzuges liegt, zeigt sich daran, daß er nicht gleichzeitig seine Gesundheit wiedererlangt, sondern erst zu einem späteren Zeitpunkt.

2. Die Propheten weisen auf ein Weiteres hin. Sofern der alttestamentliche Mensch das Ziel im Leben selbst erblickt, glaubt er auch, daß die Möglichkeit zu einem langen und glücklichen Leben weitgehend in seine Hand gelegt ist. Er kann dieses Ziel durch den Gehorsam gegen die göttlichen Gebote erreichen und etwaige Verfehlungen, die er begeht, durch entsprechende Buß- und Sühnemaßnahmen gutmachen und den Heilszustand wiederherstellen. Demgegenüber erkennen die großen Einzelpropheten die völlige und grundsätzliche Sündhaftigkeit und Schuldverfallenheit des Menschen, die seine Existenz bedroht. Sie sehen ihn in einer grundlegenden Unheilssituation und stellen angesichts dessen nicht mehr die Frage der Patriarchenerzählungen, wie denn der Mensch sein solle, sondern diejenige, ob das schuldige Dasein überhaupt zu retten ist.

Eine Möglichkeit dazu erblicken sie in der inneren und äußeren Wandlung des Menschen. Sie mahnen zu ihr, indem sie die Umkehr fordern, und kündigen sie an, indem sie die Erlösung verheißen. Nur auf diesem Weg über Umkehr und Erlösung kann der Mensch das Eigentliche seines Lebens erlangen, in der Gemeinschaft mit Gott leben und in seinem Leben die Gottesherrschaft verwirklichen. Von den vielen Prophetenworten, die genannt werden können, sei nur das Wort von der neuen Verpflichtung in Jer 31 31-34 angeführt:

> Es kommt die Zeit,
> daß ich Israel
> eine neue Verpflichtung geben werde.
> Nicht eine solche wie ihren Vätern,
> als ich sie bei der Hand nahm
> und aus Ägypten führte,
> und die sie dann gebrochen haben.

> Sondern so wird die Verpflichtung sein,
> die ich nach dieser Zeit
> Israel geben will:
> Ich lege meine Weisung in ihr Inneres
> und schreibe sie in ihre Herzen.
> Dann will ich ihr Gott sein
> und sie sollen mein Volk sein.
>
> Dann brauchen sie einander
> nicht mehr gegenseitig zu belehren:
> Erkennt den Herrn!
> Denn alle werden sie mich kennen
> vom Kleinsten bis zum Größten.
> Denn ich vergebe ihnen ihre Schuld,
> gedenke ihrer Sünde nicht mehr.

Der Inhalt dieser neuen Verpflichtung wird der gleiche sein wie in der Mosezeit. Es geht nach wie vor darum, den göttlichen Willen zu tun und ein Dasein vor Gott zu leben. Aber dies wird in Zukunft wirklich möglich sein, weil Gott seinen Willen nicht äußerlich als Gesetz aufschreiben läßt, sondern ihn ins Herz und Innere des Menschen legt. Gottes Weisung trägt der Mensch dann im Herzen, so daß sie ein Teil seines Daseins und er innerlich mit ihr eins wird. Dann fallen das Wissen um den göttlichen Willen und das Tun zu einer Einheit zusammen. Alle ohne Ausnahme in der Gemeinde Israel sollen Gott kennen und erkennen, d. h. in Vertrautheit und Gemeinschaft mit ihm leben. Und als Zeichen dafür, daß das Alte wirklich vorbei ist, vergibt Gott die Sünde. Unter das Alte wird damit ein Schlußstrich gezogen, ein neues Dasein mit Gott beginnt. Gott selbst schafft das Neue. Dann allerdings kann und muß es vom Menschen bejaht, ergriffen und gelebt werden. Die Wandlung des Menschen verwirklicht sich durch die erlösende Gnade Gottes, die der Mensch sich aneignen darf. Das gilt heute wie damals.

Zion-Jerusalem im Alten Testament[1]

I. Vorkommen, Etymologie, Bedeutung

1. Zion und verwandte Begriffe

Im Alten Testament wird צִיּוֹן 154mal gebraucht, freilich in sehr unregelmäßiger Verteilung[2]. Ferner steht es in fast einem Drittel der Vorkommen ohne weiteren Zusatz oder parallelen Ausdruck, besonders in Jes, Jer und Ps. Häufiger ist es allerdings mit einem Zusatz verbunden, darunter 20mal mit der geographisch-topographischen Bezeichnung הַר *Berg*. Dazu zählen noch der Plural הַרְרֵי *Berge* (Ps 133 3, aber textlich unsicher) und der kombinierte Zusatz הַר בַּת *Berg der Tochter* (Jes 10 32 cj. 16 1). Auch מְצָדָה (II Sam 5 7 I Chr 11 5) scheint *Zion* eher als einen *unzugänglichen Ort* denn als eine Festung

---

[1] H. Vincent—F. M. Abel, Jérusalem, I 1912; II 1914—1926; H. Vincent, Les noms de Jérusalem, Memnon 6 (1913), 88—124; A. Causse, Le mythe de la nouvelle Jérusalem du Deutéro-Esaïe à la IIIe Sibylle, RHPhR 18 (1938), 377—414; J. Simons, Jerusalem in the Old Testament, 1952; J. Klausner, Geschichte des zweiten Tempels, 1954² (neuhebr.); H. Vincent, Jérusalem de l'Ancien Testament, I—III 1954—1956; M. Avi-Yonah, Sepher Jeruschalajim, I 1956 (neuhebr.); Judah and Jerusalem, The Twelfth Archaeological Convention, 1956 (neuhebr. mit engl. Zusammenfassung); M. Noth, Jerusalem und die israelitische Tradition, OTSt VIII, 1950, 28—46 (= Gesammelte Studien zum Alten Testament, 1957, 172—187); M. Join-Lambert, Jérusalem israélite, chrétienne, musulmane, 1957; J. S. Wright, The Building of the Second Temple, 1958; S. Zimmer, Jerusalem als Tochter, Frau und Mutter, Diss. München 1959; J. Schreiner, Sion-Jerusalem, Jahwes Königssitz, 1963; E. Vogt, Das Wachstum des alten Stadtgebietes von Jerusalem, Bibl 48 (1967), 337—358; Kathleen M. Kenyon, Jerusalem, die heilige Stadt von David bis zu den Kreuzzügen, 1968; Jerusalem through the Ages, The Twenty-Fifth Archaeological Convention, 1968 (engl. und neuhebr. mit engl. Zusammenfassung).

[2] Häufigere Vorkommen sind in folgenden Büchern festzustellen: Jes (47), Jer (17), Joel (7), Mi (9), Sach 1—8 (6), Ps (38) und Thr (15). In II Sam, I—II Reg, Am, Ob, Zeph, Cant und I—II Chr begegnet der Name ein- bis zweimal. In den übrigen Büchern findet er sich überhaupt nicht. LXX hat *Zion* noch an weiteren Stellen: statt ירושלם III Βας 8 1 und statt קדשך Dan 9 24; als erläuternden Zusatz ohne hebräisches Äquivalent III Βας 3 15 Jes 1 21 52 1 ψ 72 28 Dan 9 19; im Mißverständnis hebräischer Namen und Ausdrücke Jes 9 10 22 1. 5 25 5 32 2 Ιερ 38 (31) 21; ferner in B: Jos 13 21 19 26; in S*: Jes 23 4; in anderen Handschriften: Jes 23 12; in verschiedenen Handschriften offenbar als innergriechischen Fehler B: Jos 13 19 II Chr 32 30; S*: II Εσδρ 23 4.

zu bezeichnen. Zahlreiche andere Zusätze beziehen sich auf die Bevölkerung: בַּת *Tochter* (23mal) oder בְּתוּלַת בַּת *Jungfrau Tochter* (II Reg 19 21 Thr 2 13), eindeutiger יוֹשֶׁבֶת *Einwohnerschaft* (Jes 12 6 Jer 51 35) und בְּנֵי oder בְּנוֹת צִיּוֹן *Söhne* oder *Töchter Zions* (Jes 3 16f. 4 4 u. ö.). Außerdem finden sich die Ausdrücke *Tore Zions* (Ps 87 2), *Zion des Heiligen Israels* (Jes 60 14) und *Zionslied* (Ps 137 3).

Eine Reihe von Ausdrücken steht parallel mit *Zion*, dessen verschiedenartige Bedeutung daraus teilweise ersichtlich wird. Nur selten wird es durch die Bezeichnung *Davidstadt* mit dem davidischen Stadtteil gleichgesetzt (II Sam 5 7 I Reg 8 1 I Chr 11 5 II Chr 5 2), sehr oft dagegen mit *Jerusalem* (mehr als 40mal), einmal mit *Salem* (Ps 76 3). Andere Parallelausdrücke kennzeichnen die religiöse und kultische Funktion: Es ist die *Stadt Jahwes* (Jes 60 14), zu der man sich begibt (Jer 31 6), die *Stadt unseres Gottes* (Ps 48 2), sein *heiliger Berg* (Joel 2 1 Ps 48 2) und sein *Heiligtum* (Ps 20 3). Sachlich gleichbedeutend sind die Apposition *mein heiliger Berg* (Joel 4 17 Ps 2 6) und die Parallele *Tempelberg* neben *Jerusalem* (Mi 3 12; vgl. Jer 26 18). Schließlich ist *Zion* parallel mit *Israel* (Jes 46 13 Zeph 3 14 f. Ps 149 2), *Jerusalem* und *Jakob* (Thr 1 17), den *vom Frevel Umkehrenden in Jakob* (Jes 59 20) und der *Gemeinde der Frommen* (Ps 149 2). Ebenso ist die synthetische Nebeneinanderstellung aufschlußreich. Neben *Zion* stehen *Juda* (Jer 14 19), *das Land* (Jes 66 8), die *Städte Judas* (Ps 69 36 Thr 5 11) und *Töchter Judas* (Ps 48 12 97 8). Neben den *Söhnen* Zions finden sich *Juda* und *Ephraim* (Sach 9 13), neben dem *Zionsberg* der *Stamm Juda* (Ps 78 68)[3].

Die Etymologie des Namens Zion hat bisher kein klares Bild ergeben[4]. Er ist als Eigenname ohne Artikel überliefert und rührt zweifellos aus vorisraelitischer Zeit her. Von früheren Deutungen abgesehen[5], hat man manchmal an nichtpalästinischen Ursprung gedacht: an das aus einem sumerischen Lehnwort erklärte elamitische *čijām Tempel*[6] oder an das hurritische *šej^a Wasser, Fluß*, so daß מצדת ציון *die Festung*

---

[3] Aus den angeführten Ausdrücken ergibt sich, daß gleichfalls Zion gemeint ist, wenn andere Bezeichnungen verwendet werden. Als politische Bezeichnung findet sich *Davidstadt* für das davidische Jerusalem II Sam 6 10 ff. oder den alten Stadtteil I Reg 3 1 u. ö., besonders in Zusammenhang mit der Erwähnung der Königsgräber I Reg 2 10 u. ö. Sonst beziehen sich die Ersatzausdrücke auf Zion als Tempel- oder Kultstätte, besonders unter Verwendung der Bezeichnung *Berg* Ex 15 17 Jes 26 5 f. 27 13 30 29 Ez 17 22 20 40 Sach 8 3 Ps 3 5 68 17, daneben als *mein Heiligtum* Ez 24 21 und *Gottesstadt* Ps 46 5.

[4] Vgl. Vincent, Jérusalem, III 632; Simons a. a. O. 61—64.

[5] P. de Lagarde, Onomastica sacra, 1870, 39. 43. 198; F. Wutz, Onomastica sacra, 1914/15, 81. 96f. 120. 193f. 312. 409.

[6] G. Hüsing, Zur Ophir-Frage, OLZ 6 (1903), 370; Nachträgliches zur Ophirfrage, ebd. 7 (1904), 80; Semitische Lehnwörter im Elamischen, Beiträge zur Assyriologie 5 (1906), 410; auch: Elamisches, ZDMG 56 (1902), 791f.

des Wassers bedeuten sollte, d. h. die Burg, die die Wasserversorgung Jerusalems gewährleistet[7]. Statt dessen scheint es richtiger, nach einer palästinisch-semitischen Wurzel zu fragen[8]. So ging man von *צִיר* *schützen* (= *Burg*)[9] oder von צוּב *aufstellen* mit צִוּן als Übergangsform aus[10], wobei man an eine Verwandtschaft mit צִיּוֹן *Säule* dachte, so daß der Name einen aufspringenden Bergstock bezeichnete[11]. In ähnlicher Weise schloß man aus arabischen Parallelen auf die Bedeutung *Gipfel einer Anhöhe* und weiterhin *Burg, Zitadelle*[12]. Ferner leitete man den Namen aufgrund des Syrischen von *צהה* = *ציה* *dürr, trocken sein* ab und verstand ihn als Zusammenziehung von צָיוֹן im Sinne von *kahler, dürrer Hügel*[13]. Oder man glaubte ihn aus צִיָּה *Trockenlandschaft* bzw. צִיּוֹן *wasserloses Land* mit der Bedeutung *Dürrland* erklären zu können[14]. Eine eindeutige und einleuchtende Erklärung ist jedoch einstweilen nicht möglich. Nur dies läßt sich sagen, daß der Name Zion vorisraelitischer Herkunft ist und sich auf die Eigenart des Geländes bezogen haben dürfte, an dem er haftete.

Ursprünglich ist *Zion* anscheinend eine topographische Bezeichnung, die für den Südosthügel des späteren Stadtgebietes verwendet wurde, auf dem sich die kanaanäische Siedlung befand. Ihr entspricht der Name *Ophel* für die nördlich davon gelegene Kuppe des Nordosthügels, auf der Salomo seine Residenz errichtete (vgl. Jes 32 14 Mi 4 8)[15]. Die Siedlung selbst, die sich auf dem Hügel Zion befand, führte seit alters den Namen *Jerusalem*. Unter David erhielt sie statt dessen den Namen *Davidstadt*, aber von Salomo an erscheint für das erweiterte

---

[7] S. Yeivin, The Sepulchres of the Kings of the House of David, JNES 7 (1948), 41, unter Verweis auf E. A. Speiser, Introduction to Hurrian, 1940/41.

[8] Die Ableitung von biblisch-aramäisch צִיּוּן *Kenntlichmachen* (der Grabstätten) dürfte ebenso ausscheiden wie diejenige von צִי *Wildkatze* durch A. Šanda, Die Bücher der Könige, I 1911, 212.

[9] J. G. Wetzstein in: Frz. Delitzsch, Commentar über die Genesis, 1872[4], 578. Vgl. P. Haupt, Critical Notes on Micah, AJSL 26 (1909/10), 219: protection, protected place.

[10] Frz. Delitzsch, Commentar über die Psalmen, I 1873[3], 70.

[11] H. Hupfeld, Die topographische Streitfrage über Jerusalem, namentlich die Ἄκρα und den Lauf der zweiten Mauer des Josephus vom Alten Testament aus beleuchtet, ZDMG 15 (1861), 224f.

[12] G. A. Smith, Jerusalem, I 1907, 145.

[13] W. Gesenius, Thesaurus linguae hebraicae et chaldaicae, 1835ff., s. v.; P. de Lagarde, Übersicht über die im Aramäischen, Arabischen und Hebräischen übliche Bildung der Nomina, 1889, 198.

[14] G. Dalman, Jerusalem und sein Gelände, 1930, 126.

[15] עֹפֶל begegnet für den Nordosthügel in Jes 32 14 und Mi 4 8 (exilisch) ohne Artikel als Eigenname, dagegen mit Artikel beim Chronisten II Chr 27 3 33 14 Neh 3 26 f. 11 21 an Stelle des sonst auf den Tempelberg übertragenen Namens *Zion*, der sich nur I Chr 11 5 II Chr 5 2 für die jebusitische Stadt findet. Der Name geht von der Geländeform aus und bezeichnet eine *Anschwellung*, einen *Buckel* der Erdoberfläche, vgl. II Reg 5 24 und Mesa-Inschrift Z. 22 (als medizinischer Ausdruck Dtn 28 27 I Sam 5 6 ff. 6 4 f.); vgl. Simons a. a. O. 64—67; A. Schwarzenbach, Die geographische Terminologie im Hebräischen des Alten Testaments, 1954, 21.

Stadtgebiet wieder der Name *Jerusalem*, während *Davidstadt* für den nunmehrigen alten Stadtteil erhalten blieb. Dagegen tritt *Zion* als topographische Bezeichnung und zunächst sogar als Name in der Folgezeit gänzlich zurück. Erst in der späteren Königszeit findet es sich wieder, jedoch von jetzt an mit einer Bedeutungserweiterung oder -verschiebung. Der Name wird auf den ganzen Osthügel bzw. die ganze Stadt erweitert oder in seiner Bedeutung auf den Nordosthügel als den Tempelberg verschoben.

Einmal wird *Zion* in übertragener Bedeutung verwendet. Am 6 1 setzt die *Sorglosen in Zion* mit den *Vertrauensseligen auf dem Berge Samarias* parallel. Auf sie, die zum *Haus Israel* gehören, bezieht sich das ganze Schelt- und Drohwort. Demnach ist *Zion* in diesem Falle ein Fachausdruck für die Lage der Hauptstadt, die sich im Nordreich Israel auf dessen »Zion«, dem Berg Samarias, befindet.

2. Jerusalem und verwandte Begriffe

Gegenüber dem selteneren ציון findet sich der Name ירושלם *Jerusalem* im Alten Testament 660mal. In einigen Büchern wird er häufig gebraucht[16], in anderen sind die Vorkommen wesentlich geringer[17]. Sehr oft steht *Jerusalem* ohne weiteren Zusatz oder parallelen Ausdruck. Es bezeichnet den ursprünglichen kanaanäischen Stadtstaat (Jos 10 1 u. ö.), die Hauptstadt des davidisch-salomonischen Reiches (II Sam 5 5—I Reg 11 42 und Parallelen in I—II Chr) oder des Südreichs Juda (I Reg 12 18—II Reg 24 18 und Parallelen in II Chr u. ö.), die von Jahwe erwählte Stadt (I Reg 11 36 u. ö.) als kultischen Mittelpunkt (I Reg 12 27 u. ö.) oder in einfachen chronologischen Angaben (Jer 1 3 u. ö.). Ferner ist *Jerusalem* mit verschiedenartigen Zusätzen versehen. Sie beziehen das Gebiet des früheren Stadtstaates ein: *Umgebung Jerusalems* (Jer 17 26 32 44) oder sind topographischer Art: *Hügel* (Jes 10 32), *Mauern* (Ps 51 20), *Tore* (Jer 1 15 u. ö.), *Gassen* (nur Jer 5 1 u. ö.), *Plätze* (Sach 8 4) und *Mitte Jerusalems* (Jer 6 1 Sach 8 8). Andere Zusätze nennen die Einwohner der Stadt: בַּת *Tochter* (II Reg 19 21 Mi 4 8 u. ö.), יוֹשֵׁב (Jes 5 3 8 14) oder יוֹשְׁבֵי *Bewohner*

---

[16] Häufige Vorkommen in II Sam (30), I—II Reg (90), Jes (49), Jer (102), Ez (26), Sach (39), Esr (48), Neh (38) und I—II Chr (151).

[17] Seltenere Vorkommen in Jos (9), Jdc (5), I Sam (1) durch die geschichtliche Situation bedingt; Joel (6), Am (2, Auftreten im Nordreich), Ob (2), Mi (8), Zeph (4), Mal (2), Ps 51—147 (17), Cant (8), Koh (5), Thr (7), Est (1) und Dan (10). In den in Anm. 16—17 nicht genannten Büchern findet sich der Name überhaupt nicht. LXX hat Jerusalem noch an weiteren Stellen: statt ישראל Gen 36 31 A Jes 1 24 A u. ö., בנימן II Chr 25 5, אריאל Jes 29 7 B und שלום IV Bας 22 20, ohne Äquivalent in MT, teilweise durch den umfangreicheren Text der LXX bedingt. Umgekehrt hat LXX mehrfach ירושלם ersetzt: durch Ισραηλ III Bας 15 4 (Origenes außer Σ) IV Bας 8 26 BA u. ö., Δαυιδ II Chr 28 27 und Σιων III Bας 8 1.

(vor allem Jer Ez II Chr), בְּנֵי *Söhne* (Joel 4 6), בְּנוֹת *Töchter* (nur Cant), בְּתוּלֹת *Jungfrauen* (Thr 2 10) und *Propheten Jerusalems* (Jer 23 14f.). Mit dem Schicksal der Stadt hängt die Erwähnung des *Restes* (Jer 24 8) und der גָּלֻת *Deportierten Jerusalems* (Ob 20) zusammen.

Einige Ausdrücke stehen mit *Jerusalem* parallel: *Bergrücken der Jebusiter* (Jos 15 8), *Jebusiterstadt* (Jos 18 28 Jdc 19 11) und *Jebus* (Jdc 19 10f.), häufiger *Zion* (außer Mi 3 10. 12 an jüngeren Stellen), *Zionsberg* (an jüngeren Stellen: II Reg 19 31 Jes 10 12 u. ö.), *Tochter Zion* (an jüngeren Stellen: Jes 52 2 Zeph 3 14) und *Bewohnerschaft Zions* (Jer 51 35), wobei diese Parallelisierung sich fast nur in der exilischen oder nachexilischen Zeit findet. Parallelen sind ferner: *Tor meines Volkes* (Mi 1 9), *dieses Volk* (Jer 4 11) und *mein Volk* (Jes 65 19), aber auch der *Berg des Jahwe Zebaot* (Sach 8 3) und der *Tempel* (Jer 26 6. 9. 12)[18], so daß die *Vorhöfe des Hauses Jahwes* die *Mitte Jerusalems* sind (Ps 116 19).

Eine synthetische Nebeneinanderstellung findet sich in sehr verschiedenen Formen. Die staatsrechtliche oder landschaftliche Gliederung wird aus den in III, 2 aufgeführten Wendungen ersichtlich. Mehr eine Gegenüberstellung liegt in der Nennung von *Samaria* und *Jerusalem* vor (Ez 23 Mi 1 5). Je einmal findet sich *Jerusalem und all seine Städte* (Jer 19 15) und *Jerusalem* neben *Tempel und Palast* (Jer 27 18). Zahlreiche Arten der Nebeneinanderstellung sind angewendet, wenn von den Einwohnern der Stadt die Rede ist. Nur in wenigen Formeln steht *Jerusalem* an erster Stelle (Jes 5 3 22 21 Sach 8 15 II Chr 21 11); meist wird *Juda* zuerst genannt (Jer 17 20 Zeph 1 4 II Chr 20 15 u. ö.). Später werden beide gelegentlich enger zusammengefaßt (Esr 4 6 II Chr 20 27). Schließlich ist vom *Haus Davids und den Bewohnern Jerusalems* die Rede (Sach 12 10 13 1). Aufschlußreich für die Auffassung Jerusalems sind außerdem die zugefügten Appositionen: *heilige Stadt* (Jes 52 1 Neh 11 1), *heiliger Berg* (Jes 27 13) und *Thron Jahwes* (Jer 3 17 14 21 17 12); es ist *deine Stadt Jerusalem, dein heiliger Berg* (Dan 9 16). Bezeichnenderweise handelt es sich dabei nur um exilische und spätere Stimmen[19].

Als Namensform findet sich im MT fast ausnahmslos der Konsonantentext ירושלם; er ist als Qere perpetuum יְרוּשָׁלַם (für יְרוּשָׁלַיִם)

---

[18] Ähnlich ist wohl Ez 21 7 zu lesen: *Jerusalem* und *sein Heiligtum* (statt *Heiligtümer*).

[19] Den genannten Ausdrücken und Redewendungen entsprechend ist Jerusalem gleichfalls gemeint, wenn andere Bezeichnungen verwendet werden: die einfache Bezeichnung *die Stadt* (häufig bei Ez), die etwas verächtliche Bezeichnung *diese Stadt* (oft in den Jeremia-Erzählungen Jer 19 11. 15 21 1-10 u. ö., ähnlich Ez 11 2. 6), die *Stadt der Blutschuld* Ez 22 2 24 6a, die *Stadt, die Blut vergießt* Ez 22 3, *diese große Stadt* Jer 22 8, die *fröhliche Stadt* Jes 22 2 32 13, die *heilige Stadt* Jes 48 2 und *Stadt Jahwes* Ps 101 8.

vokalisiert worden und danach $j^e r\hat{u}šal\check{a}jim$ auszusprechen[20]. Nur an fünf jungen Stellen, die eine masoretische Bemerkung zu Jer 26 18 aufzählt, findet sich die der Lesung des Qere entsprechende Konsonantenform ירושלים (Jer 26 18 Est 2 6 I Chr 3 5 II Chr 25 1 32 9)[21]. Sie kommt neben der üblichen Konsonantenform noch auf jüdischen Münzen aus der Zeit Simons (142—135 v. Chr.) oder des ersten Aufstandes gegen Rom (66—70 n. Chr.)[22] und gelegentlich in der rabbinischen Literatur vor[23]. Die darin angenommene Endung -ăjim beruht weder auf einem alten Namen, noch war sie für die feierliche gottesdienstliche Schriftlesung bestimmt. Vielmehr trifft die herkömmliche Deutung zu, nach der es sich um eine künstliche Dualbildung handelt, die die Doppelheit der oberen und unteren oder der auf dem Ost- und Westhügel gelegenen Stadt ausdrücken sollte. Die ältere und richtigere Aussprache ist zweifellos diejenige des Ketib: יְרוּשָׁלֵם. Sie ergibt sich aus den Konsonanten des Worts und wird bestätigt durch die Erwähnung bei dem aristotelischen Philosophen Clearchus von Soli Ιερουσαλημη[24], die Transkription Ιερουσαλημ in LXX und im Neuen Testament (von der wiederum die koptische und armenische Version ausgehen[25]) und die biblisch-aramäische Form יְרוּשְׁלֵם (daneben auch יְרוּשְׁלֶם)[26].

Außerdem findet sich eine scheinbare andere Namensform, die eine lange Tradition hat. Sie beginnt vielleicht in der bisher ältesten Erwähnung Jerusalems in den ägyptischen Ächtungstexten vom Anfang des 2. Jahrtausends[27] (' $wš'mm$ = Uršalem

---

[20] In Pausa יְרוּשָׁלָיִם (gleiche Form ohne Pausa Ps 79 3 137 5), mit ה locale יְרוּשָׁלַיְמָה (statt יְרוּשָׁלַיְמָה in I Reg 10 2 II Reg 9 28 Jes 36 2 Ez 8 3, wobei in I Reg 10 2 von 27 Handschriften יְרוּשָׁלַיְמָה geschrieben wird).

[21] In I Chr 3 5 wird teilweise auch ירושלים gelesen, in II Chr 32 9 findet sich die volle Form mit ה locale. Im Qumranschrifttum findet sich in 1QpHab dreimal ירושלם, dagegen in 1QM fünfmal ירושלים.

[22] M. Lidzbarski, Handbuch der nordsemitischen Epigraphik, 1898, 290; Smith a. a. O. 251.

[23] So z. B. Tosefta Ketubbot 4; gewöhnlich wird ירושלם geschrieben, z. B. Sebachim 14, 8; Menachot 10, 2. 5; Arakin 9, 6.

[24] Clearchus (um die Wende des 4./3. Jh.) wird von Josephus, Contra Apionem, 1, 179f., zitiert. Er fügt dem Namen die griechische Endung η an, während Josephus selbst Ἱεροσόλυμα verwendet.

[25] Vgl. Vincent, Les noms, 91.

[26] Im Alten Testament 26mal: Dan 5 2f. 6 11 Esr 4 8. 12. 20. 23f. 5 1f. 14-17 6 3. 5. 9. 12. 18 7 13-17. 19. Vgl. ferner A. Ungnad, Aramäische Papyrus aus Elephantine, 1911, 1, 18.

[27] K. Sethe, Die Ächtung feindlicher Fürsten, Völker und Dinge auf altägyptischen Tongefäßscherben des Mittleren Reiches, 1926; G. Posener, Princes et pays d'Asie et de Nubie, 1940. In den Texten Sethes, die aus dem 20. Jh. stammen können, wird Jerusalem in e 27—28 und f 18 erwähnt, in den Texten Poseners aus dem 19. Jh.

oder Rušlem-Rušalem[28]). Deutlich liegt sie vor in der sumerischen Ideogrammform ^{ál}DI-ma = Urusilimma auf einer wahrscheinlich dem 18. Jh. entstammenden Götterliste[29], in der babylonischen Form Urusalim (U-ru-sa-lim oder Uru-sa-lim) in den Amarnabriefen des 14. Jh.[30] und in der auf dem Prisma Sanheribs verwendeten assyrischen Form Ursalimmu (*Ur-sa-li-im-mu*) aus dem beginnenden 8. Jh.[31]. Sie begegnet im syrischen Urišlem (hebräisch transkribiert אוּרִשְׁלֵם) wieder[32]. Der Unterschied zwischen der Ketib-Form und diesen hauptsächlich mesopotamischen Formen beruht auf der durch die Umsetzung ins Akkadische bedingten Veränderung, so daß die mesopotamischen Formen das genaue Äquivalent zu יְרוּשָׁלֵם bilden.

Die Etymologie des Namens יְרוּשָׁלַ͏ִם, zu der das Alte Testament selbst nichts beiträgt, war bis nahezu in die Gegenwart ein Gebiet, das allen Spekulationen offenstand[33]. Ernsthafte neuere Erklärungsversuche, die wenigstens den ersten Teil des

---

in E 45. Vgl. ferner R. Dussaud, Nouveaux renseignements sur la Palestine et la Syrie vers 2000 avant notre ère, Syria 8 (1928), 216—233; W. F. Albright, The Egyptian Empire in Asia in the Twenty-first Century B. C., JPOS 8 (1928), 223—256; The Land of Damascus between 1850 and 1750 B. C., BASOR 83 (1941), 30—36; A. Alt, Herren und Herrensitze Palästinas im Anfang des zweiten Jahrtausends v. Chr., ZDPV 64 (1941), 21—39 (= Kleine Schriften zur Geschichte des Volkes Israel, III 1959, 57—71); H. Vincent, Les pays bibliques et l'Égypte à la fin de la XIIe dynastie égyptienne, RB 51 (1942), 187—212. Die Bedenken von A. Jirku, Bemerkungen zu den ägyptischen sog. »Ächtungstexten«, ArOr 20 (1952), 167—169, gegen die Bezeugung Jerusalems sind schwerlich stichhaltig.

[28] Vincent, Jérusalem, III 612 Anm. 4.

[29] O. Schröder, Keilschrifttexte aus Assur verschiedenen Inhalts, 1920, Nr. 145 Rs 6 (zusammengehörig mit dem Bruchstück Nr. 73, vollständigeres Duplikat in: Cuneiform Texts from Babylonian Tablets in the British Museum 24, 1908, 20—46) mit Namen der Göttin Ischtar verschiedener Länder und Städte. So nach F. M. Th. de Liagre Böhl, Älteste keilschriftliche Erwähnungen der Stadt Jerusalem und ihrer Göttin ?, AcOr 1 (1922), 76—80, während H. Schmökel, Heilige Hochzeit und Hoheslied, 1956, 98, die Lesung des Ideogramms als Urusilimma für unmöglich hält.

[30] J. A. Knudtzon, Die El-Amarna-Tafeln, II 1908, Nr. 285—290; Übersetzung eines Briefes bei K. Galling, Textbuch zur Geschichte Israels, 1968², 25f. (1950, 23—29: fünf Briefe). Die Briefe des Jerusalemer Stadtkönigs werden um 1360 angesetzt.

[31] H. C. Rawlinson, The Cuneiform Inscriptions of Western Asia, I 1861: sog. Taylor-Prisma; D. D. Luckenbill, The Annals of Sennacherib, 1924: Prisma des Oriental Institute Chicago. Vincent, Les noms, 91 Anm. 4, weist auf die anderwärts vorkommende Variante Ur-sa-li-im-ma hin.

[32] Man glaubte zeitweilig, אוּרִשְׁלֵם auch in einer nabatäischen Inschrift entdeckt zu haben (Corpus Inscriptionum Semiticarum, I 1881, 294 Nr. 320 B und Tafel 41); so noch Smith a. a. O. 252 und R. Schütz in ZNW 11 (1910), 169 Anm. 2. Jedoch ergab sich aufgrund der Nachprüfung von A. Jaussen—R. Savignac, Mission archéologique en Arabie: Médâin Ṣâleḥ, 1909, 245 und Tafel 29 Nr. 183, daß אדר שלם zu lesen ist.

[33] J. Grill, Beiträge zur hebräischen Wort- und Namenerklärung, 1. Über Entstehung und Bedeutung des Namens Jerusalem, ZAW 4 (1884), 134—148; I. Marquart, שִׁבֹּלֶת = ephraimitisch סִבֹּלֶת = שִׁבֹּלֶת, ebd. 8 (1888), 152; P. Haupt in: T. K. Cheyne, Isaiah, 1899, Exkurs zu 19 1; F. Prätorius, Über einige Arten hebräischer Eigen-

Namens als יְרוּשׁ *possessio (pacis)*³⁴ oder יְרוּ (von ירה) *fundatum, fundatio (pacis)*³⁵ deuteten, wurden nach der Entdeckung der Amarnabriefe mit der babylonischen Form Urusalim von der Auffassung abgelöst, Jerusalem sei kein palästinischer oder kanaanäischer, sondern ein babylonischer Name³⁶. Von den möglichen Erklärungen des Namens auf palästinisch-kanaanäischer Grundlage scheiden aus mannigfachen Gründen die als *Stadt Salems* (יְרוּשָׁלִַם = אֲרוּשָׁלֵם = עִר[וּ]שָׁלֵם) und als *Licht Salems* aus³⁷. Vielmehr enthält der Name als erstes Element das Wort *יְרוּ *Gründung* (von ירה), das wohl weder als pf.³⁸ noch als jussivisches impf.³⁹, sondern als Nomen st. cs. zu verstehen ist⁴⁰. Als zweites Element ist der Name des Gottes Šlm verwendet, der in Syrien-Palästina offensichtlich eine gewisse Rolle gespielt hat⁴¹. Er wird in den ugaritischen Texten (17, 12; 52, 12 f.; 107, 8) genannt⁴² und begegnet teilweise zusammen mit dem Gott Šḥr »Morgendämmerung«, so daß er die »Abenddämmerung« (genauer die »Vollendung des Tages«) repräsentiert⁴³. Šḥr und Šlm, die beiden Zwillingssöhne Els, stellen als Stern der Morgendämmerung und Tagesvollendung wahrscheinlich zwei Hypostasen oder Aspekte des (männlichen) Morgen- und Abendsterns ʿAṭṭar dar⁴⁴. Der gleiche Gott Šlm liegt wohl auch dem Gottesnamen Šal-majāti in den Amarnabriefen des

---

namen, ZDMG 57 (1903), 782; G. A. Smith, The Name Jerusalem and other Names, Exp 6, 7 (1903), 122—135; E. Nestle, Zum Namen Jerusalem, ZDPV 27 (1904), 153—156; J. A. Montgomery, Paronomasias on the Name Jerusalem, JBL 49 (1930), 277—282; Vincent, Les noms, 87—124; Jérusalem III 611—613.

³⁴ A. Reland, Palaestina ex monumentis veteribus illustrata, 1714.

³⁵ Gesenius a. a. O.

³⁶ Besonders Haupt a. a. O. trat für diese Auffassung ein; weiteres darüber bei Smith a. a. O. 258; Vincent, Les noms, 97—99.

³⁷ Vgl. im einzelnen Vincent, Les noms, 99—105.

³⁸ W. F. Albright in JPOS 8 (1928), 248 (s. o. Anm. 27).

³⁹ W. F. Albright, Palestine in the Earliest Historical Period, JPOS 15 (1935), 218 Anm. 78.

⁴⁰ J. Lewy, Les textes paléo-assyriens et l'Ancien Testament, RHR 110 (1943), 61 f.

⁴¹ Vgl. darüber in älterer Zeit KAT 224. 474—477. A. Jeremias, Das Alte Testament im Lichte des Alten Orients, 1916³, 291. 426; H. S. Nyberg, Studien zum Religionskampf im Alten Testament, ARW 35 (1938), 352—364, führt mit Šlm zusammengesetzte Namen aus den Kültepe-Texten und dem phönizischen Bereich, die Vorkommen in den ugaritischen Texten sowie normale und abweichende Formen des Gottesnamens an, um daraus weitreichende religionsgeschichtliche Folgerungen für das Alte Testament zu ziehen. Vgl. ferner S. Yeivin, The Beginnings of the Davidids, Zion 9 (1944), 53 Anm. 30 und 33 mit Lit. (neuhebr.). Doch ist Šlm gegen Lewy a. a. O. 61 f. keinesfalls mit אֵל עֶלְיוֹן identisch.

⁴² Nach der Zählung von C. H. Gordon, Ugaritic Textbook, 1965.

⁴³ Vgl. auch Lewy a. a. O.; Nyberg a. a. O. Šḥr findet sich in dem theophoren Namen Kšḥrʾibʾi in den ägyptischen Ächtungstexten (vgl. Posener a. a. O. 74), Šlm im Namen des moabitischen Königs Šalamanu im 8. Jh. (KAT 475) und im Namen ʾapšlm auf einem Ostrakon von *tell el-ḫlēfi* (Ezion-Geber) im 5./4. Jh. (N. Glueck, Ostraca from Elath, BASOR 82, 1941, 3—11).

⁴⁴ Vgl. J. Gray, The Desert God ʿAṭṭr in the Literature and Religion of Canaan, JNES 8 (1949), 73—83.

Abimilki von Tyrus zugrunde⁴⁵. Man hat in den Jerusalemer Amarnabriefen sogar einen Hinweis auf einen dem Šlm geweihten Tempel in Jerusalem zu finden geglaubt⁴⁶. Außerdem enthält wahrscheinlich eine assyrische Götterliste mit den Namen der Göttin Ischtar in verschiedenen Ländern und Städten⁴⁷ die Angabe, daß die Ischtar von Urusilimma den Namen Šul-ma-ni-t(u) trage. Dieser Göttin Šulmītu oder (in erweiterter Form) Šulmanītu, die in ideographischer Umschreibung mehrfach genannt wird⁴⁸, galt offenbar als weibliche Entsprechung des Gottes Šalmānu oder Šulmānu⁴⁹, der in der kanaanäischen Form Šlm in niedrigerer Stellung im Pantheon begegnet⁵⁰. Ungeachtet der Frage, ob man in Jerusalem neben Šlm (und dem davon zu unterscheidenden kanaanäischen Gott El) auch die entsprechende weibliche Gottheit verehrt haben mag, ist man bei der Benennung der Siedlung jedenfalls der verbreiteten Anschauung gefolgt, den Ursprung des Ortes auf die ausdrückliche Willensbekundung oder die besondere Gegenwart einer Gottheit zurückzuführen und seinen Namen danach zu bestimmen. Jerusalem ist die *Gründung* (bzw. *Stadt*) *des* (*Gottes*) *Šlm* (*Šalim, Šalem*)⁵¹.

Die Bedeutung der Bezeichnung *Jerusalem* liegt fest und ist stets gleich geblieben. Anders als *Zion* hat sie nicht gewechselt, sondern sich von Anfang an auf die ganze Siedlung bezogen. Sie ist an dieser haften geblieben, als sie wuchs, so daß der Gesamtname *Jerusalem* von den Teilbezeichnungen *Zion* oder *Davidstadt* gelegentlich ausdrücklich unterschieden wird (I Reg 3 ₁ 8 ₁ 11 ₂₇).

3. Seltene Begriffe

Nur zweimal findet sich der Name שָׁלֵם *Salem*. In Ps 76 ₃ meint er in Parallele zu *Zion* eindeutig Jerusalem und soll im Anklang an das gleichlautende Adjektiv die Stadt als *unversehrt, friedlich* kennzeichnen. Daher hat LXX *in Salem* mit ἐν εἰρήνῃ übersetzt. Umstritten ist die Erwähnung in der Melchisedek-Episode (Gen 14 ₁₈)

---

⁴⁵ Vgl. Knudtzon a. a. O. 1254—1256; C. Lindhagen, The Servant Motif in the Old Testament, 1950, 8—10.
⁴⁶ J. Lewy, The Šulmān Temple in Jerusalem, JBL 59 (1940), 519—522, deutet Brief Nr. 290 in Z. 14—17: »die Hauptstadt der Gegend von Jerusalem, deren Name Bīt Šulmani ist, ... ist abtrünnig geworden«. Zwar läßt sich das dortige Bīt Ninib so deuten, da der Gott Šalmānu oder Šulmānu offenbar eine Bezeichnung des Gottes Ninurta = Ninib und die Gleichsetzung verständlich ist. Aber es fragt sich doch, ob nicht eine Ortschaft des Jerusalemer Territoriums statt der Hauptstadt des königlichen Briefschreibers selbst gemeint ist.
⁴⁷ Schröder a. a. O. Nr. 145 Rs 6.
⁴⁸ Schröder a. a. O. Nr. 42 col. II 20; 72 Vs 10 und Rs 19; 78 Vs 12.
⁴⁹ Vgl. zum Ganzen de Liagre Böhl a. a. O.
⁵⁰ Diese Form findet sich im assyrischen Königsnamen Salmanassar = *Šulmānu asaridu Šulmānu ist der erste an Rang* (unter den Göttern).
⁵¹ Eine Parallele bildet der Name des Ortes יְרוּאֵל II Chr 20 ₁₆ (vgl. auch יְרִיאֵל I Chr 7 ₂). Anders F. Rundgren in der Besprechung von Semitica 2 in Oriens 11 (1958), 287 f.: *Urw/j-Šalim* »Schalems Krippe« wird zu hebräisch *ʾarî*- oder *ʾărî-šalem* und dies zu Jerusalem.

(LXX Σαλημ). Da *Salem* nicht näher bestimmt wird, wenn man von der Nähe des Tales שוה — *das ist das Königstal* — absieht[52], hat man die Angabe auf andere Orte als Jerusalem deuten wollen[53]. Jedoch spricht außer Ps 76 3 und der Etymologie von Jerusalem die Verbindung Melchisedeks mit der davidischen Dynastie in Ps 110 4 für die Deutung auf Jerusalem, die denn auch mehrfach bezeugt ist[54]. In diesem Falle ist *Salem* offenbar ein Deckname. Den vollen Namen der Stadt hat man bewußt vermieden, da er in der Entstehungszeit der Erzählung (Gen 14) in der vorliegenden Form schon theologisch eindeutig geprägt war.

Nur in Jes 29 1f. 7 findet sich der Ausdruck אֲרִיאֵל (LXX Αριηλ)[55]. Er bezeichnet in Ez 43 15f. den *Opferherd* im Heiligtum, auf dem man zum Verbrennen der Opfertiere ein Feuer unterhält[56], dagegen in II Sam 23 20 I Chr 11 22 *Krieger, Kriegsheld* (gegen LXX in II Sam und LXX L in I Chr, die ihn als Eigennamen verstanden haben)[57] und in Esr 8 16 einen Eigennamen. Jesaja hat zweifellos Jerusalem gemeint, *die Stadt, wo David Lager bezog* (29 1). Der *Opferherd* steht für den salomonischen Stadtteil mit dem Palast- und Tempelbezirk und dieser für die Gesamtstadt[58].

Schließlich wird die Stadt in Jdc 19 10f. I Chr 11 4 יְבוּס *Jebus* genannt (LXX Ιεβους, ebenso Jos 18 28 für הַיְבוּסִי), obwohl sie diesen Namen niemals getragen hat. Die falsche Ansicht, daß sie Jebus geheißen habe, beruht darauf, daß sie von den kanaanäischen Jebusitern bewohnt war.

4. Zur Verwendung der Namen Zion und Jerusalem

Es fällt auf, daß die Begriffe Zion und Jerusalem ungleichmäßig verwendet werden. Gegenüber *Jerusalem* tritt *Zion* völlig zurück in

---

[52] Nach Josephus, Antiquitates, 7, 243f., lag es in der Nähe von Jerusalem.
[53] Teils folgte man Hieronymus, Epistulae, 73, 7 (MPL XXII 1845, 680), der zeitweilig im Anschluß an Σαλίμ Joh 3 23 an diesen südlich von Skythopolis (Besan) gelegenen, freilich ganz unbedeutenden Ort dachte. Teils dachte man im Anschluß an Eusebius, Onomasticon, 290, 55ff. (GCS XI 150, 1ff.) an eine Gleichsetzung mit einem Salem östlich von Sichem. Vgl. im einzelnen P. Winter, »Nazareth« and »Jerusalem« in Luke chs. I and II, NTSt 3 (1957), 136—142.
[54] So identifiziert das Genesis-Apokryphon in Col. XXII 13 durch die Bemerkung היא ירושלם Salem ausdrücklich mit Jerusalem. In dieser Bemerkung wie P. Winter, Note on Salem-Jerusalem, NT 2 (1957), 151f., einen Zusatz erblicken zu wollen, ist nicht einleuchtend. Ebenso setzen Targum und Josephus, Antiquitates, 1, 180, τὴν μέντοι Σολυμᾶ ὕστερον ἐκάλεσεν Ἱεροσόλυμα beide gleich.
[55] Vielleicht ist außerdem in dem nachexilischen Jes 33 7 statt des verderbten אראלם entweder אֲרִיאֵל oder אֲרִיאֵלִים Leute des Ariel zu lesen.
[56] Ableitung und weitere Einzelheiten bei K. Galling in: G. Fohrer, Ezechiel, 1955, 239f.
[57] Vgl. im einzelnen W. Rudolph, Chronikbücher, 1955, 98f.
[58] Zur Auseinandersetzung darüber vgl. im einzelnen Vincent, Les noms, 111—115; Jérusalem III 613f.

Ezechiel, Maleachi, Esra und Nehemia, praktisch auch in II Samuel, I Regum und I—II Chronik, da *Zion* in diesen Büchern nur 4mal für die jebusitische Kanaanäerstadt gebraucht wird. Verhältnismäßig oder sehr wenig findet es sich in II Regum, Jeremia, Sacharja und Canticum. Umgekehrt tritt es gegenüber *Jerusalem* in Psalmen und Klageliedern in den Vordergrund.

Diese Sachlage erklärt sich aus der Verwendung von *Zion* (teilweise parallel mit *Jerusalem*) für die verschiedenen Begriffsaspekte. Am häufigsten begegnet es für die Stadt der eschatologischen Heilszeit, d. h. in erster Linie in den exilischen und nachexilischen Prophetenworten (Zusätze in Jes 1—39 und Jeremia, ferner Deutero- und Tritojesaja, Joel, Mi 4 und Sach 1—9). Sehr häufig bezeichnet es auch Gottessitz und -stadt, außer in einigen Prophetenworten besonders in den Psalmen. Eine zweite Gruppe mit einer geringeren Zahl von Vorkommen bilden die Begriffsaspekte: Königsresidenz und Hauptstadt, Symbol des Volkes oder der Gemeinde (besonders Deuterojesaja, in den Psalmen und Klageliedern), Kultusort und Tempelstadt (besonders in den Psalmen und Klageliedern). Noch seltener findet sich *Zion* für die Begriffsaspekte: Stadt der Sünde und des Gerichts (hauptsächlich von Jeremia an), höfisch-sakrale (Psalmen) und mythische Aspekte. Ganz selten wird es für Nebenbedeutungen und überhaupt nicht für die Stadt der Theokratie gebraucht, vielleicht wegen seiner stark eschatologischen Prägung.

In den vorexilischen Prophetenworten meint *Zion* genauso wie *Jerusalem* fast immer die Königsresidenz und Hauptstadt, die zugleich die Stadt der Sünde und des Gerichts ist. Die übrigen Vorkommen in den Prophetenbüchern gehören überwiegend der exilischen und nachexilischen Eschatologie an; teilweise verwendet Deuterojesaja *Zion* als Symbol der Gemeinde. In den Psalmen bezeichnet der Name vor allem Gottessitz und -stadt, ferner Volk oder Gemeinde und Kultus- oder Tempelstätte; gelegentlich weist er auf höfisch-sakrale, mythische und eschatologische Aspekte hin. In den Klageliedern findet sich *Zion* ebenfalls für Volk oder Gemeinde und Kultus- oder Tempelstätte, selten für Jerusalem als Stadt der Sünde und des Gerichts. Dagegen konzentriert sich die Verwendung des Namens *Jerusalem* nicht auf bestimmte Bedeutungsaspekte; vielmehr wird er für alle ziemlich gleichmäßig gebraucht.

II. Das geschichtliche Werden der Bedeutung von Zion-Jerusalem

Jerusalem hat seine Bedeutung nicht infolge der natürlichen Gegebenheiten seiner Lage erlangt. Diese wirkten vielmehr im abträglichen Sinn und hätten die Stadt eher zu einem Winkeldasein verurteilt als zu Aufschwung und Entfaltung verholfen[59]. Die natürliche Lage hätte andere Orte für die Rolle einer Hauptstadt Palästinas mehr begünstigt als Jerusalem, das weder in einem Schwerpunkt des Landes liegt noch auf dem judäischen Gebirge leicht zugänglich ist. Es bildet nicht einmal den natürlichen Mittelpunkt seiner engeren Landschaft Juda. Zwar liegt es nahe der Wasserscheide des Gebirges und damit an der wichtigsten Straße in der Nordsüdrichtung; aber die entsprechende Verbindung in der Westostrichtung fehlt, die es erst zu einem Knotenpunkt gemacht hätte. Denn wichtiger und bedeutender als der südliche Aufstieg von Jericho ins Gebirge, der in die Nähe Jerusalems führt, ist der nördliche über Betel in die Küstenebene. Dem südlichen Aufstieg fehlt es in der Nähe Jerusalems an einer guten Fortsetzung nach Westen über die Stadt selbst zur Küstenebene. Nicht der Natur, sondern dem geschichtlichen Geschehen verdankt Jerusalem seinen Aufstieg zu der Bedeutung, die es gewonnen hat. Dieser Aufstieg vollzog sich im Lauf vieler Jahrhunderte und nicht in gleichmäßiger Art, sondern mit öfteren und langen Perioden des Rückgangs.

1. Vor- und frühisraelitische Zeit

In der vorisraelitischen Zeit bildet Jerusalem wie die zahlreichen anderen Städte mitsamt seinem Territorium[60] einen der für das bronzezeitliche Palästina kennzeichnenden Stadtstaaten. Es wird — wenigstens in der späteren Zeit — von den Jebusitern bewohnt[61] und von einem Stadtkönig beherrscht. Soweit ersichtlich, hat es stets nur eine lokale Rolle gespielt und ist nie die Hauptstadt eines umfassenden Staatsgebildes oder Palästinas gewesen. Als selbständiges Herrschaftsgebilde läßt es sich mit Hilfe der ägyptischen Ächtungstexte aus dem 19./18. Jh. bis nahe an den Anfang des 2. Jt. zurückverfolgen. Jedoch

---

[59] Zum Folgenden vgl. A. Alt, Jerusalems Aufstieg, ZDMG 79 (1925), 1—19 (= Kleine Schriften zur Geschichte des Volkes Israel, III 1959, 243—257).

[60] Dieses Territorium ist sicher nicht sehr groß gewesen; bei manchen Stadtstaaten bestand es nur aus deren Feldflur. Die natürliche Flur Jerusalems bildet eine in den Gebirgsrücken eingesenkte Fläche von etwa 3 km Durchmesser zwischen dem nahezu halbkreisförmig nach Westen ausgebuchteten Höhenzug der Wasserscheide und der ähnlich halbkreisförmig im Osten liegenden Kette des Ölbergs.

[61] Sie begegnen in den Reihenaufzählungen palästinischer Völkerschaften gewöhnlich an letzter Stelle: Gen 15 21 Ex 3 8. 17 Dtn 7 1 Jos 3 10 Jdc 3 5 I Reg 9 20 II Chr 8 7 u. ö., an vorletzter Stelle: Jos 11 3, mitten unter den anderen: Num 13 29 Esr 9 1 Neh 9 8; die Quellenschichten des Hexateuchs verwenden in der Aufzählung offenbar ein geläufiges Schema. Als Abkömmlinge Kanaans werden die Jebusiter Gen 10 16 I Chr 1 14 bezeichnet, als Bewohner des alten Jerusalem Jos 15 63 Jdc 1 21; nach II Sam 5 6. 8 bewohnen sie nicht nur die Stadt, sondern auch die Gegend. Auch aus der Stadtbezeichnung Jos 15 8 18 16. 28 sind sie als Einwohner ersichtlich.

zeigt der archäologische Befund der Ausgrabungen in verschiedenen Teilen der Jebusiter- oder Davidstadt[62], daß der Beginn der Ansiedlung in wesentlich früherer Zeit anzusetzen ist[63]. Die 6 Amarnabriefe, die der Stadtkönig Abdi-Ḫepa[64] um 1360 an den Pharao gerichtet hat, befassen sich mit den gleichen Sorgen wie die übrigen Briefe und sind für die besondere Geschichte Jerusalems wenig ergiebig. Ein anderer Stadtkönig von Jerusalem ist der in der alttestamentlichen Tradition weiterlebende Melchisedek (Gen 14 18 Ps 110 4), an dem ersichtlich wird, daß der König priesterliche Funktionen wahrgenommen hat[65].

Nach der Darstellung des Jahwisten hat Jerusalem in der vorstaatlichen Zeit Israels zum Interessengebiet des Stammes Benjamin gehört; die Priesterschrift übernimmt diese Auffassung (Jos 15 8 18 16). Zutreffender als diese theoretische Zuweisung ist die ausdrückliche Feststellung, daß die Stadt zunächst nicht eingenommen werden konnte, so daß die Jebusiter in der Nachbarschaft der Benjaminiten (Jdc 1 21) oder Judäer (Jos 15 63) wohnen blieben. Jerusalem galt als eine fremde Stadt, in der ein Israelit nicht übernachtete, weil in ihr keine Stammesgenossen wohnten (Jdc 19 11f.). So blieb Jerusalem nach der Landnahme Israels weiterhin ein selbständiger Stadtstaat, der die Judäer und die ihnen verwandten Gruppen im Süden von der Masse der nördlicher angesiedelten Israeliten so stark trennte, daß sie sich dem Königtum Sauls anscheinend nicht unterstellten und eine Sonderentwicklung durchmachten. Die spätere Entstehung der eigenständigen

---

[62] R. Weill, La cité de David, I Campagne de 1913—1914, 1920; II Campagne de 1923—1924, 1947; R. A. S. Macalister—J. G. Duncan, Excavations on the Hill of Ophel, Jerusalem 1923—1925, 1926; J. W. Crowfoot—G. M. Fitzgerald, Excavations in the Tyropoeon Valley, Jerusalem 1927, 1929. Vor allem sind die jüngsten Ergebnisse der Ausgrabungen von Kathleen M. Kenyon zu beachten, vgl. die Vorberichte in PEQ 94 (1962), 72—90; 95 (1963), 7—21; 96 (1964), 7—18; 97 (1965), 9—20; 98 (1966), 73—88; 99 (1967), 65—71.

[63] Schon vor Jahrzehnten wurde bei einer Ausgrabung besonders frühe Keramik gefunden; vgl. H. Vincent, Jérusalem sous terre: les récentes fouilles d'Ophel, 1911, 30—32 und Tafel 7—12.

[64] Der Stadtkönig trägt den hetitischen oder hurritischen Namen ARAD-ḫepa, der als Abdi-Ḫepa oder Puti-Ḫepa aufgelöst wird. In Ez 16 3 scheint die Erinnerung an die amoritisch-hetitische Frühgeschichte nachzuwirken.

[65] E erwähnt Jos 10 1. 3 einen Stadtkönig Adonisedek von Jerusalem; die deuteronomistische Erweiterung dieser Notiz in 10 3. 5. 23 ist geschichtlich ebenso wertlos wie die Liste der besiegten Könige in Jos 12 10, unter denen der Jerusalemer König erscheint. Da der von N in Jdc 1 6 f. genannte Adonibesek nicht als König bezeichnet wird, bleibt sein Verhältnis zu Adonisedek unklar. Der spätere Zusatz in Jdc 1 8, nach dem die Judäer Jerusalem erobert und eingeäschert haben sollen, ist vielleicht aus einer falschen Deutung des Schlusses von 1 7 entstanden und entspricht nicht den Tatsachen.

und getrennten Staatswesen Juda und Israel beruht hauptsächlich auf der Existenz der kanaanäischen Jerusalem.

2. Zeit des davidischen Königtums bis Josia

Nachdem David das Königtum über Juda (II Sam 2 4) und Israel (5 3) erhalten hatte, sah er sich vor der Notwendigkeit, den kanaanäischen Sperriegel zwischen beiden Staaten zu beseitigen und sich eine Residenz zu wählen, die beiden genehm war. Er löste das doppelte Problem durch die überfallartige Eroberung Jerusalems. Allerdings ist der kurze Bericht darüber in II Sam 5 6-8 textlich und sachlich sehr schwierig, so daß man in Einzelheiten nicht zu voller Gewißheit gelangt[66]. Wichtig ist, daß David die Stadt in einem privaten Unternehmen durch seine Söldner einnehmen ließ. Die Folge war, daß er sie keinem der beiden israelitischen Staatsgebilde einverleibte, sondern mitsamt ihrem Territorium in seinen Eigenbesitz überführte, wie es der Name »Davidstadt« ausdrückt. Seither ist Jerusalem während der ganzen Dauer der davidischen Dynastie deren Eigenbesitz und staatsrechtlich in einer Sonderstellung neben Juda und Israel geblieben. Darauf beruht zu einem Teil die wachsende Bedeutung Jerusalems; das Ansehen und die Wertschätzung, die die davidische Dynastie in Juda besaß, wurden gleicherweise auf die Königsstadt übertragen. David scheint keine wesentlichen Veränderungen an der eroberten Stadt vorgenommen zu haben. Er errichtete lediglich mit Hilfe phönizischer Bauleute und Materialien einen neuen Palast für sich und seinen Hofstaat und bezog einen geringen Teil des bisherigen Vorgeländes auf der Nordseite in die ummauerte Stadt ein (II Sam 5 9-11).

Da Davids Herrschaft über Jerusalem auf dem Recht der Eroberung beruhte, trat er einfach in die Nachfolge der bisherigen Stadtkönige des kanaanäischen Stadtstaates ein. Er übernahm deren Rechte und Pflichten, darunter auch die in der kanaanäischen Tradition wurzelnden priesterlichen Funktionen (vgl. Ps 110 4). In Zusammenhang damit scheint es geradezu zu einer Verschmelzung des El-Kultus mit dem Jahweglauben gekommen zu sein. Dafür spricht vielleicht schon die Tatsache, daß gegenüber den Namen der dem David in Hebron geborenen Söhne diejenigen der 11 oder 12 in Jerusalem geborenen in keinem Falle *Jahwe*, dagegen in mehreren Fällen *El* als theophores Element aufweisen (II Sam 5 14-16)[67] und daß Davids Sohn

---

[66] Vgl. im einzelnen die ausführliche Untersuchung von H. J. Stoebe, Die Einnahme Jerusalems und der Ṣinnôr, ZDPV 73 (1957), 73—99, mit Erörterung der verschiedenen Ansichten, wobei freilich außerdem die Ausgrabungsergebnisse von Kathleen M. Kenyon zu berücksichtigen sind (s. o. Anm. 62).

[67] Darauf weist besonders nachdrücklich Nyberg a. a. O. 373f. hin.

Jedidja »Liebling Jahwes« den Namen Salomo (שְׁלֹמֹה) erhält oder annimmt, der ungeachtet des Anklangs an שָׁלוֹם ebenso mit dem im Namen *Jerusalem* enthaltenen Gottesnamen Šlm zusammenhängt wie der Name des Davidsohnes Absalom. Ein unübersehbarer Hinweis liegt darin vor, daß die kanaanäische Priesterfamilie des El, deren Haupt damals Zadok war, von nun an — zunächst neben dem Jahwepriester Abjatar, später allein — als Jahwepriester amtierte[68]. Vor allem erklärt sich aus dieser Verschmelzung, aus der schließlich Jahwe siegreich hervorging, die Übertragung wichtiger Elemente der kanaanäischen El-Religion auf Jahwe.

Jedoch lagen in solchen kanaanäischen Einflüssen zugleich schwere Gefahren, die Art und Erbe Israels auf die Dauer völlig in den Hintergrund zu drängen vermocht hätten. David hat ihnen entgegengewirkt, indem er die heilige Lade, die einst in Silo beheimatet gewesen war[69], nach den dies ermöglichenden Siegen über die Philister nach Jerusalem überführte (II Sam 6). Auf diese Weise übereignete David die mit der Lade verknüpften Traditionen an Jerusalem und leitete die in Silo verkörperten national-religiösen Werte Israels nach Jerusalem über (Erweiterung und Entfaltung des Jahweglaubens, in dem Namenszusatz »Zebaot, der Kerubenthroner« ausgedrückt[70]).

Die Bedeutung Jerusalems gründete sich demnach auf die Erhebung zur Residenz der Davididen, die Übertragung der Gegenwart des Jahwe Zebaot, des Kerubenthroners, dorthin und auf die Erweiterung des Jahweglaubens durch Aneignung kanaanäischen Gedankenguts. Dagegen bleibt die Annahme eines Weiterwirkens amphiktyonischer Vorstellungen besser außer Betracht[71]. David hat mit

---

[68] Vgl. dazu vor allem H. H. Rowley, Zadok and Nehushtan, JBL 58 (1939), 113—141; Melchizedek and Zadok (Gen 14 and Ps 110), in: Bertholet-Festschrift, 1950, 461—472.

[69] Vgl. besonders J. Maier, Das altisraelitische Ladeheiligtum, 1965.

[70] Vgl. dazu auch O. Eißfeldt, Jahwe Zebaoth, Miscellanea Acad. Berol. II 2, 1950, 128—150 (= Kleine Schriften, III 1966, 103—123). Während die Vorstellung des Kerubenthroners kanaanäisch ist, werden die »Zebaot« verschieden gedeutet. Eißfeldt a. a. O. versteht das Wort als Abstraktpl. »Mächtigkeit, Mächtiger«; Eichrodt, Theologie des Alten Testaments, I 1959⁶, 120f.: Inbegriff aller irdischen und himmlischen Wesen, vgl. auch A. L. Williams, The Lord of Hosts, JThSt 38 (1937), 56; W. F. Albright, Von der Steinzeit zum Christentum, 1949, 286: die Heere Israels; V. Maag, Jahwäs Heerscharen, Schweiz. Theol. Umschau 20, 3—4 (1950), 27—52: die depotenzierten und Jahwe untergeordneten mythischen Naturmächte Kanaans. Vgl. im einzelnen G. Fohrer, Geschichte der israelitischen Religion, 1969, 159f.

[71] Zur Kritik an der Amphiktyonie-Hypothese vgl. G. Fohrer, Altes Testament — »Amphiktyonie« und »Bund«?, s. o. 84—119. Ferner ist zu beachten, daß man sich zu Sauls Zeiten um die Lade anscheinend nicht gekümmert hat (I Chr 13 3) und daß sie nach der Überführung in den salomonischen Tempel keine wesentliche Rolle mehr gespielt, also zur Bedeutung Jerusalems nicht mehr beigetragen hat. Die Be-

alledem eine Entwicklung eingeleitet, die durch den Tempelbau Salomos zu einem ersten Abschluß gelangte.

Salomo hat den Entschluß zu einer bedeutenden Vergrößerung des in »Davidstadt« umbenannten Jerusalem gefaßt und ausgeführt. In unmittelbarem Anschluß an die bisherige Stadt und mit ihr durch eine gemeinsame Umfassungsmauer verbunden, hat er nördlich von ihr einen neuen Stadtteil errichtet. Die Vergrößerung der Stadt erfüllte einen doppelten Zweck: Sie ermöglichte den Bau einer neuen Residenz, die dem Repräsentationsbedürfnis des Beherrschers eines Großreiches entsprach und behob zumindest weitgehend die Raumnot, da neben den Residenzbauten noch Platz für die wachsende Bevölkerung blieb. Für die geschichtliche Bedeutung Jerusalems sind die Residenzbauten von größter Wichtigkeit geworden. In einem einheitlichen Baukomplex nach der Art der Residenztempel des ägyptischen Neuen Reiches wurden Palast- und Tempelbauten zusammengefaßt. Das Ganze wurde mangels einer eigenen israelitischen Bautradition wie schon der Palast Davids mit phönizischer Hilfe nach kanaanäischem Vorbild errichtet.

Der Bau des Tempels erwies sich in der Folgezeit als von allergrößter Bedeutung für Jerusalem[72]. Da Palast und Tempel in der gleichen Stadt angelegt und von einer Mauer umschlossen waren, kam deutlich zum Ausdruck, daß der Tempel Eigentum der herrschenden Dynastie[73] und Staatsheiligtum war, in dem sowohl die privaten Opfer des Königs als auch der offizielle Staatskultus dargebracht wurden. Dadurch wurde Jahwe zur Staatsgottheit und Jerusalem zur obersten und hervorragendsten Kultstätte erklärt. Da ferner der Bau dem kanaanäischen Tempeltyp folgte und sich mit seiner Errichtung die im Kulturland herrschende Sitte fester lokaler Kult-

---

fürchtung Jerobeams nach der Reichsteilung, daß seine Untertanen aus dem Nordreich weiterhin zum Jerusalmer Tempel ziehen könnten (I Reg 12 26 ff.), ist eine deuteronomistische Darstellung und läßt sich weder für eine Anerkennung Jerusalems bei den Nordisraeliten noch für eine im 10. Jh. vollzogene Scheidung zwischen politischer und kultischer Geltung der Stadt anführen. Ebensowenig setzt Jer 41 5 die dauernde Anerkennung des Jerusalemer Heiligtums voraus, sondern beruht auf der weitgehenden Angliederung des früheren Nordreiches an Juda durch Josia; da außerdem durch die deuteronomische Reform der Jerusalemer Tempel zum alleinigen Heiligtum erklärt worden war, begann gleichzeitig die Scheidung der kultischen von der politischen Bedeutung Jerusalems.

[72] Zum Verständnis des Baus vgl. im einzelnen K. Möhlenbrink, Der Tempel Salomos, 1932; C. Watzinger, Denkmäler Palästinas, I 1933, 88—95; W. F. Albright, Die Religion Israels im Lichte der archäologischen Ausgrabungen, 1956, 159—173; G. E. Wright, Biblische Archäologie, 1958, 133—143; M. Noth, Könige, 1964 ff., 95—193.

[73] Vgl. K. Galling, Königliche und nichtkönigliche Stifter beim Tempel von Jerusalem, ZDPV 68 (1951), 134—142.

stätten durchsetzte, wurde das Heiligtum selbst zur eigentlichen heiligen Stätte, die als solche ein Eigengewicht erhielt und die Möglichkeit zum Einströmen weiterer kanaanäischer Vorstellungen und Bräuche bot. Daher verlor die Lade sehr schnell ihre frühere Bedeutung, während umgekehrt der Tempelkultus weithin nach kanaanäischem Vorbild ausgestattet wurde. Damit setzt — von Jerusalem ausgehend — ein neuer Gestaltwandel des Jahweglaubens ein, der sich vor allem in einer kultischen und einer national-religiösen Richtung ausprägte und im Bereich des Staatskultus sogar zum gewollten Synkretismus führte.

Der Bau des Tempels und die Verlegung des Kultus aus der Davidstadt dorthin bedeuteten gegenüber den Anfängen unter David eine umwälzende Neuerung und Steigerung, auf die sich die weitere geschichtliche Rolle Jerusalems vor allem gründet. Die Gegenwart Jahwes, der als »König« nun über ein »Haus« verfügte, wurde auf den Tempel übertragen. Vom Tempelweihspruch Salomos an (I Reg 8 12f.) findet sich der Gedanke vom »Wohnen« Jahwes in Jerusalem. Er haftet zunächst am Tempel selbst, dann auch am Tempelberg (Jes 8 18: *der auf dem Zionsberg wohnt*).

Nachdem schon unter Salomo einzelne Randgebiete des Großreiches abgebröckelt waren, zerbrach nach seinem Tode sogar die Personalunion zwischen Israel und Juda, so daß zwei getrennte Staaten weiterbestanden. Jerusalem geriet in eine besondere Krise, da die hart an der Grenze des Staates Juda gelegene Stadt von den Davididen als Residenz hätte aufgegeben werden können. Doch der Nimbus Jerusalems und das eingespielte Regierungswesen wirkten stärker als alle Schwierigkeiten[74]. Sowohl die Davididen als auch die Judäer haben wie selbstverständlich an Jerusalem festgehalten. Es ist unwahrscheinlich, daß Jerusalem sich in der weiteren Königszeit stark vergrößert haben sollte; die allgemeine Lage des Staates entsprach dem nicht. Immerhin werden mehrfach Arbeiten an der Stadtmauer (II Chr 26 9 27 3 32 5 33 14)[75] und die Namen neuer Stadtteile genannt (II Reg 22 14 Zeph 1 10f.)[76]. Dagegen dürfte der breitere und höhere

---

[74] Um die Nachteile der Grenzlage zu beheben, waren die Davididen ständig bemüht, die Nordgrenze vorzuschieben und einen möglichst großen Teil des Stammesgebietes von Benjamin zu besetzen. Wenigstens zeitweilig verlief die Grenze fast eine Tagereise nördlich von Jerusalem, so daß hinreichende Sicherheit vor einem plötzlichen Überfall gegeben war. Vgl. im einzelnen K.-D. Schunck, Benjamin, 1965.

[75] Davon dürften die in II Chr 26 9 erwähnten Arbeiten noch der Behebung der Schäden gedient haben, die die Schleifung der Nordmauer durch Joas von Israel nach II Reg 14 13 verursacht hatte.

[76] Am wichtigsten dürften die »Neustadt«, die sich schon durch ihren Namen als jüngeres Stadtviertel zu erkennen gibt, und der »Mörser«, anscheinend der bevorzugte Sitz der Kaufmannschaft, gewesen sein. Manchmal werden beide als identisch betrachtet.

Westhügel in vorexilischer Zeit noch nicht in die ummauerte Stadt einbezogen worden sein[77]. Besonders wichtig war die Verbesserung der Wasserversorgung durch Hiskia, der das Wasser der Gichonquelle im Kidrontal durch den Siloatunnel in das Innere der Stadt leitete und sie auf diese Weise für längere Zeit belagerungsfähig machte (II Reg 20 20 II Chr 32 30)[78]. Die Notwendigkeit dessen wird daraus ersichtlich, daß beim Ausbruch des syrisch-ephraimitischen Krieges der König Ahas persönlich die Wasserleitung inspizierte (Jes 7 3). Der Tempel in Jerusalem spielte weiterhin die Rolle, die Salomo ihm zugedacht hatte. Als das den Davididen gehörige Staatsheiligtum wurde er wie von selbst zur bedeutsamsten heiligen Stätte des judäischen Staates.

Von allen Ereignissen der Königszeit bis zum Tode Josias (609) haben nur zwei die Stellung Jerusalems wesentlich berührt[79]. Sanherib hatte im Jahre 701 vergeblich versucht, Jerusalem in seine Gewalt zu bringen; wider Erwarten wurde es vor ihm durch seinen plötzlichen Abzug gerettet (II Reg 18f.; vgl. Jes 36f.). Obwohl die geschichtlichen Einzelheiten nicht klar zu durchschauen sind, da mehrere Gründe für den Abzug angegeben werden oder anklingen[80], diente das Ergebnis dazu, die Bedeutung Jerusalems mit seinem Tempel mächtig zu steigern: An ihm war der fast allmächtige Assyrer gescheitert und hatte sich fluchtartig zurückziehen müssen. Die Jesajalegenden mitsamt den in ihnen enthaltenen angeblichen Worten des Propheten zeigen, daß die erlebte Rettung bald zu dem schließlich wie ein Dogma geltenden Glauben an die Unantastbarkeit und Uneinnehmbarkeit Jerusalems geführt hat (Jer 7 4).

Das zweite entscheidende Ereignis war die politisch-religiöse Reform des Königs Josia in den Jahren des beginnenden Zerfalls des assyrischen Großreichs (nach 626). Zu ihr gehörte außer der Säuberung des Jerusalemer Tempels und Kultus vor allem die Aufhebung aller

---

[77] Gegen Simons a. a. O. 227—281 und Vincent, Jérusalem, I 90—113. Erst recht ist die Annahme von Dalman a. a. O. unzutreffend, daß Jerusalem spätestens schon zur Zeit Davids eine Doppelstadt auf dem Ost- und Westhügel gewesen und von Salomo durch eine neue Umfassungsmauer zusammengeschlossen worden sei.

[78] Vgl. dazu Simons a. a. O. 178—188. 222—225; Vincent, Jérusalem, I 269—279; zur Siloainschrift vgl. K. Galling, Textbuch zur Geschichte Israels, 1968², 66f. (mit Lit.), und G. Levi Della Vida, The Shiloah Inscription Reconsidered, in: In Memoriam P. Kahle, 1968, 102—106.

[79] Außer acht bleiben können die Plünderung durch Pharao Sisak (I Reg 14 25f.), die Schleifung der Nordmauer (II Reg 14 13) und der syrisch-ephraimitische Krieg (II Reg 16 5) sowie die mißlungenen Versuche, die davidische Dynastie zu beseitigen (II Reg 11 1 21 23 Jes 7 6). Der in II Chr 21 16f. erwähnte Angriff von Philistern und Arabern hat Jerusalem entgegen der Meinung früherer Exegeten nicht berührt; der Notiz können Erinnerungen an Grenzzwischenfälle zugrunde liegen.

[80] Gerüchte aus Assyrien (II Reg 19 7), Herannahen eines ägyptischen Hilfsheers für Hiskia (19 8f.) und Seuche im ägyptischen Lager (19 35).

übrigen Heiligtümer im Lande. Es gab nur noch das Heiligtum in Jerusalem, das Jahwe erwählt hat, um seinen Namen dort wohnen zu lassen. Dieser Begriff der »Erwählung« für Jerusalem und seinen Tempel ist von der deuteronomischen Theologie eingeführt und mit dem des »Wohnens« verbunden worden; er hängt mit der Beschränkung des Kultus auf Jerusalem zusammen[81]. Die deuteronomische Theologie erreichte mit dieser Sonderstellung der als Stätte des Heiligtums erwählten Stadt ein bis dahin nicht angestrebtes Ziel: Jerusalem wird für jeden gläubigen Israeliten zum kultischen Mittelpunkt und wichtigsten Ort überhaupt. Gesteigert wurde dies durch die überraschenden politischen Erfolge Josias, der sich aus der palästinischen Erbmasse des untergehenden Assyrerreiches weite Gebiete aneignen konnte, so daß er schließlich anscheinend die Landschaften der früheren Teilreiche Juda und Israel beherrschte. Auf diese Weise wurde Jerusalem nach David und Salomo nochmals für einige Jahre die Hauptstadt eines großen Teils von Palästina.

3. Zeit der letzten judäischen Könige und des Exils

Das Ende des judäischen Staates vollzog sich unter den Eingriffen der Babylonier in zwei Jahrzehnten. Während die judäische Landschaft an die Provinzen Edom und Asdod angegliedert wurde, verfügten die Babylonier über Jerusalem anders[82]. Es bestand weiter, bildete aber nur mehr den Vorort eines sehr kleinen territorialen Gebildes, das eigentlich einen größeren Stadtstaat darstellte, und war im übrigen ein verwaltungsmäßig gesondertes Anhängsel der nördlichen Nachbarprovinz Samaria. Wider Erwarten hat Jerusalem diesen vernichtenden Schlag überstanden. Zwar war die erwählte davidische Dynastie abgesetzt, aber die »Erwählung« Jerusalems als des alleinigen Kultortes durch Jahwe hatte sich in kurzer Zeit so fest im Glauben verankert, daß nach seiner Zerstörung sogar Leute aus den von Josia angegliederten israelitischen Gebieten mit Opfergaben dorthin pilgerten (Jer 41 5). Zwar hatten die Babylonier den Tempel als heiliges Symbol der Selbständigkeit des Volkes zerstört und den Glauben an die Uneinnehmbarkeit der Stadt schwer erschüttert, aber die Deutung dessen als Strafgericht Jahwes für die Sünde Judas und die sich allmählich bildende eschatologische Hoffnung auf eine künftige Heilszeit ließen dies ertragen.

---

[81] Vgl. ThW IV 148—173; ferner Th. C. Vriezen, Die Erwählung Israels nach dem Alten Testament, 1953, besonders 46f.; teilweise anders K. Koch, Zur Geschichte der Erwählungsvorstellung in Israel, ZAW 67 (1955), 205—226.

[82] Zum Folgenden vgl. A. Alt, Die Rolle Samarias bei der Entstehung des Judentums, in: Procksch-Festschrift, 1934, 3—28 (= Kleine Schriften zur Geschichte des Volkes Israel, II 1953, 316—337).

Aufs Ganze gesehen ist während des Exils die Bedeutung Jerusalems zumindest für weite Kreise der Deportierten noch gewachsen und hat sie zu inbrünstiger Sehnsucht (vgl. Ps 137) und kühnen Erwartungen (Deuterojesaja und andere exilische Prophetenworte) geführt[83]. Erleichtert wurde die eschatologisch bedingte Steigerung der Wertschätzung Jerusalems dadurch, daß nach dem Zurücktreten der Lade hinter den Tempel als Ort der Gegenwart Jahwes auch das Tempelgebäude durch die heilige Stätte Jerusalem selbst als den örtlich festliegenden und alleinberechtigten Kultort ersetzt werden konnte, so daß die Stadt mit ihrem »heiligen Berg« zum Mittelpunkt der gläubigen Israeliten in Palästina und in der Diaspora werden konnte. In der Folgezeit ist über den nachexilischen Tempel hinaus Jerusalem selbst mit dem Tempelberg entscheidend wichtig. Gegenüber der Königszeit kehren sich nunmehr die Verhältnisse um: Das Ansehen Jerusalems beruht nicht mehr in erster Linie auf seinem äußeren Glanz als Königsstadt, die seine innere Bedeutung als Stätte des Tempels hebt, sondern auf seiner inneren Glaubensbedeutung, die seine äußere Stellung erhöht. So vollzog sich eine Wandlung, die Jerusalem aus einem überwiegend politischen zu einem religiös-geistlichen Mittelpunkt machte.

4. Nachexilische Zeit

In der frühnachexilischen Zeit steigerte sich die religiös-geistliche Bedeutung Jerusalems nochmals[84]. Zwar übernahm die persische Regierung von den Babyloniern die provisorische Regelung, die für Juda getroffen war. Aber es kam zur Rückführung der deportierten jerusalemisch-judäischen Oberschicht, durch die der frühere Bestand der Bevölkerung mit Ausnahme des Königtums annähernd wiederhergestellt wurde, und zur Verleihung der Kultusrechte an Jerusalem, das auf diese Weise für die ganze Bevölkerung im restlichen Juda, in Samaria und Galiläa mit derartigen Privilegien ausgestattet wurde. Dies hatte zwei Folgen. Einerseits bildete sich angesichts des völligen Verlustes der Souveränität und der politischen Eigenrechte in und um Jerusalem notgedrungen eine Gemeinschaft, die im wesentlichen eine Kultus- und später eine Tempelgemeinde war. Andererseits führte die Gewährung der Kultusrechte zum Neubau des Tempels in Jerusalem, wenn er auch erst nach dem Eingreifen der Propheten Haggai und Sacharja 515 eingeweiht werden konnte. Dann aber erlangte er,

---

[83] Die Lage in Palästina hat E. Janssen, Juda in der Exilszeit, 1956, erneut untersucht. Doch sind im einzelnen mannigfache Einwände zu erheben, vgl. F. Maass in ThLZ 82 (1957), 685f.

[84] Vgl. zum Folgenden vor allem Alt a. a. O.; W. Rudolph, Esra und Nehemia, 1949, XXVIf. Die frühnachexilische Zeit beurteilt anders K. Galling, Studien zur Geschichte Israels im persischen Zeitalter, 1964.

der nicht mehr königliches, sondern Volkseigentum war[85], die allergrößte Bedeutung. Er bildete nicht nur den Kristallisationspunkt der Jerusalemer Gemeinde, sondern entwickelte sich auch mehr und mehr zum religiösen Mittelpunkt des werdenden Judentums in der Zerstreuung.

Die allmählich und in großen zeitlichen Abständen sich vollziehende Errichtung einer eigenen Provinz Juda fand ihren äußeren Abschluß durch die Tätigkeit des vom babylonischen Diasporajudentum unterstützten Nehemia[86]. Er bezeichnet sich selbst als den vom Großkönig »im Lande Juda« eingesetzten Statthalter (Neh 5 14); für das Jahr 408 ist dann durch die Elephantine-Papyri die Existenz eines besonderen Statthalters in Juda neben dem in Samaria bezeugt[87]. In Zusammenhang mit diesen Maßnahmen erfolgte die Wiederherstellung der Stadtmauern, außerdem der offenbar schon vorher in nachexilischer Zeit errichteten Tempelburg (Neh 2 8; vgl. 3 1 7 2)[88]. Obwohl die Provinz nur mehr einen Teil der Landschaft Juda umfaßte[89], wurde Jerusalem nochmals zu einer Hauptstadt — allerdings geringeren Ranges — erhoben. Im Vergleich mit der überwiegend kanaanäischen Bevölkerung in der vorexilischen Zeit war es nunmehr eine fast ausschließlich israelitisch besiedelte Stadt. Auch diese nach dem Exil begonnene Entwicklung fand unter Nehemia ihren Abschluß.

Der politischen Konstituierung, die zugleich eine gewisse Absonderung bedeutete, folgte die Errichtung einer konstitutiven Gemeindeordnung, die die schon von Hag 2 10-14 geforderte religiöse Absonderung einschloß. Sie ist das Werk Esras. Indem er eine um den Tempel gescharte Gottesgemeinde unter der Führung der priesterlichen Hierarchie schaffen wollte, hat er das eigentliche Judentum begründet und

---

[85] Vgl. Galling in dem in Anm. 73 erwähnten Aufsatz.

[86] U. Kellermann, Nehemia—Quellen, Überlieferung und Geschichte, 1967. Zu der schwierigen Frage des gegenseitigen Verhältnisses von Nehemia und Esra sowie ihrer chronologischen Einordnung vgl. die Überblicke von H. H. Rowley, Nehemiah's Mission and its Background, BJRL 37 (1954/55), 528—561 (= Men of God, 1963, 211—245); U. Kellermann, Erwägungen zur Esradatierung, ZAW 80 (1968), 55—87.

[87] E. Sachau, Aramäische Papyri und Ostraka aus einer jüdischen Militärkolonie zu Elephantine, 1911, Nr. 1/2, vgl. Nr. 3 und 4; A. E. Cowley, Aramaic Papyri of the Fifth Century B. C., 1923, Nr. 30—33.

[88] Gewöhnlich versteht man sie als Vorläufer der von Hyrkan erbauten Burg, an deren Stelle später Herodes die Antonia errichtete, während Dalman a. a. O. beide unterscheidet.

[89] Zur Provinz Juda gehörte die Landschaft zwischen Betlehem und nördlich von Hebron und der Ostteil des Hügellandes um Kegila, d. h. von den früheren Gauen außer Jerusalem: Jericho, Beerseba, Bet-Zur, Betlehem und Kegila. Die südlichen Gaue Debir, Hebron und Maon bildeten die Provinz Arabien (später Idumäa), die westlichen Gaue Ekron, Adullam und Lachis gehörten zur Provinz Asdod.

zugleich Jerusalem die letzte Weihe gegeben. Daher kann trotz der bestehenden Unterschiede etwas später der chronistische Erzähler in der konkreten jüdischen Gemeinde das Ideal der Theokratie verwirklicht sehen. Demgegenüber konstituierte sich ein Teil der Bevölkerung von Samaria als eine von Jerusalem unabhängige Religionsgemeinschaft. Es handelt sich um die Lostrennung der Samaritaner von Jerusalem und den Bau eines neuen Tempels auf dem Garizim. Ursache dafür war nicht der Gegensatz zur Tora oder zum Tempel, sondern derjenige zum Führungsanspruch Judas und Jerusalems in politischer und religiöser Hinsicht, zu David als dem nationalen und religiösen Helden und zum priesterlich-levitisch ausgestalteten Kultus. Doch konnte diese Einbuße der Bedeutung Jerusalems keinen Abbruch mehr tun.

Auf den persischen Maßnahmen bis zur Zeit Nehemias beruht es letztlich, wenn Jerusalem unter der Herrschaft der Ptolemäer (von 301 an) und Seleukiden (von 198 an) seinen Charakter im wesentlichen bewahren konnte. Denn Juda mit Jerusalem galt nicht als Königs-, sondern als Volksland, als das in sich geschlossene Wohngebiet des ἔθνος τῶν Ἰουδαίων, das normalerweise nicht mehr von einem Statthalter des Königs, sondern vom einheimischen Adel in Form einer Gerusie verwaltet und gegenüber dem König vertreten wurde. Nur Antiochus IV. Epiphanes hat den Versuch gewagt, Jerusalem in eine hellenistische πόλις umzuwandeln. Spätestens in der hellenistischen Zeit ist der breitere und höhere Westhügel Jerusalems, der in der vorexilischen Zeit unbesiedelt geblieben war, in das Stadtgebiet einbezogen und durch eine Erweiterung der Stadtmauer gesichert worden. Das ist die sog. zweite Mauer[90].

5. Niederschlag in literarischen Formen und Bildern

Im Unterschied von anderen Heiligtümern ist die heilige Stätte von Jerusalem nicht durch die Übernahme einer kanaanäischen Kultsage legitimiert worden. Vielleicht erwies sich dieses Verfahren im Fall Jerusalems als ungeeignet, weil es nicht nur außerhalb jeder Jahweüberlieferung stand, sondern auch als kanaanäischer Stadtstaat mit entsprechenden Heiligtümern und Kulten den Israeliten besonders fremd sein mußte. Statt dessen liegt in II Sam 24 der israelitische ἱερὸς λόγος von Jerusalem vor, der die Errichtung des ersten Jahwealtars dort begründet. Nachdrücklich wird betont, daß der Ort der Tenne noch kein Heiligtum war, sondern dadurch eins wurde, daß der Jahwebote erschien und David so auf den Ort hingewiesen wurde

---

[90] Vgl. dazu H. Guthe, Die zweite Mauer Jerusalems und die Bauten Constantins am heiligen Grabe, ZDPV 8 (1885), 245—287; H. Vincent, La deuxième enceinte de Jérusalem, RB 11 (1902), 31—57; Jérusalem I 90—113; Simons a. a. O. 282—343.

und daß der Seher Gad die Weisung zum Altarbau erteilte. Der Ort wird ordnungsgemäß angekauft und nicht von einem Heiden geschenkt; daß er Jahwe wohlgefällig war, soll das Aufhören der von ihm verhängten Plage nach der Errichtung des Altars verdeutlichen.

Demgegenüber können weder Gen 22 noch die Ladeerzählung als ἱερὸς λόγος von Jerusalem gelten[91]. Wohl aber dürfte in der Erzählung von der ehernen Schlange (Num 21 4-9) eine ätiologische Kultsage vorliegen, die das nach II Reg 18 4 bis in die Zeit Hiskias in Jerusalem (wahrscheinlich im Tempelbezirk) verehrte eherne Schlangenidol durch die Herleitung von Mose legitimierte.

In der als ganzer jungen, midraschartigen Erzählung Gen 14 wird in v. 17-20 durch die Verbindung des sicherlich kanaanäischen Traditionselements von Melchisedek mit der Person Abrahams der Anspruch Jerusalems weit in die Vorzeit zurückgeführt. Sollte dies schon in vorexilischer Zeit erfolgt sein, so diente es der Legitimierung der Davididen, denen Abraham schon in Melchisedek gehuldigt und denen er sich durch dessen Segen verpflichtet gewußt hätte. In nachexilischer Zeit diente es dem Nachweis der berechtigten Ansprüche des Jerusalemer Tempels und seines Hohenpriesters gegenüber dem sich manchmal regenden Widerstand, der sich in der Trennung der Samaritaner deutlich ausdrückte: War Jerusalem als Heiligtum nicht von einem der Patriarchen gegründet, so doch als Stätte der Verehrung des wahren Gottes anerkannt worden!

In der religiösen und kultischen Poesie sprach sich die Bedeutung Jerusalems als einer heiligen Stätte gleichfalls aus. Allerdings bleiben die sog. Thronbesteigungspsalmen außer acht, da sie besser als monotheistische Hymnen aus der Zeit nach Deuterojesaja verstanden werden. Doch findet sich unter den Hymnen des Psalters eine kleine Gruppe, die zweckmäßig als Wallfahrtslieder bezeichnet werden. Gewiß dürfte es sie auch sonst gegeben haben, aber nur auf Jerusalem bezügliche Wallfahrtslieder sind erhalten geblieben (Ps 84 122). Man hat sie vom Antritt bis zum Erreichen des Ziels der Wallfahrt gesungen und in ihnen den Gefühlen und Vorstellungen Ausdruck gegeben, die die Pilger erfüllten.

Eine andere Unterabteilung der Hymnen bilden die Zionslieder (Ps 46 48 76 87), die sich mit Formen und Motiven der Wallfahrtslieder berühren und in denen Lob und Preis der heiligen Stätte im Mittelpunkt stehen. In besonderem Maße sind sie mit eschatologischen Erwartungen verknüpft; so spielt die Hoffnung auf den endgültigen

---

[91] Der in Gen 22 2 als »Moria« bezeichnete Ort der befohlenen Opferung Isaaks wird in II Chr 3 1 auf den Tempelberg in Jerusalem gedeutet; doch ist der Name in Gen 22 sekundär oder verderbt, wie schon das mit ihm verbundene ältere Wort »Land« zeigt; vgl. dazu H. Gunkel, Genesis, 1964⁶, z. St.

Sieg Jahwes über die anstürmenden Feinde eine große Rolle. Aus alledem ergibt sich ein eindrückliches Bild des Glauben, wie er in wenigstens einem großen Teil des werdenden Judentums in nachexilischer Zeit lebendig war[92].

Vorher hatte die Eroberung und weitgehende Zerstörung Jerusalems die Klagelieder (Thr 1—5) hervorgerufen. Sie klagen über die eingetretene Katastrophe und die dadurch bedingte trostlose Lage der Stadt. Diese erscheint vorwiegend als politische Größe, nur innerhalb dieses Rahmens wird das Heiligtum genannt. Daher sind die Lieder 1 2 und 4 politische Leichenlieder, 3 ein Klagelied des einzelnen und 5 ein Volksklagelied. Sie sind in Erinnerung an den Fall Jerusalems gedichtet worden, am ehesten als Äußerungen persönlichen Schmerzes über die Katastrophe, während die Sammlung für den Zweck kultartiger Trauerfeiern der Gemeinde zustande gekommen sein dürfte, bei denen man sie vorgetragen hat.

Schließlich hat man Bedeutung und Schicksal Jerusalems mit allerlei Bildern zu verdeutlichen gesucht. Die Stadt ist das Tor des Volkes (Mi 1 9), da sie für das ganze Volk die Rolle spielt, die dem Tor einer Ortschaft für diese zukommt. Sie ist als Jahwes Aue sein Eigentum (Jer 25 30), stand in engem Verhältnis zu ihm während der Liebe der Jugend und Brautzeit (Jer 2 2) oder wie eine Ehefrau (Ez 16) und wird wiederum zur prächtigen Krone und zum königlichen Kopfbund (Jes 62 3) und zu seiner Braut werden (Jes 62 5), für alle, die sie lieben, zur tröstenden Mutter (Jes 66 11f.), für die Heidenvölker aber zu Taumelschale und Hebestein (Sach 12 12f.). Sie ist ein sicheres Zelt (Jes 33 20), die Krone der Schönheit (Ps 50 2 Thr 2 15), sie selbst oder ihre Jungmannschaft wie Gold und Feingold (Thr 4 1f.).

Demgegenüber steht das schroffe Urteil, daß die Jerusalemer wie das wertlose Holz des Weinstocks sind (Ez 15 6), die Stadt selbst eine untreue Dirne (Jes 1 21 57 7-13 Jer 4 31 Ez 23) und Ehebrecherin (Ez 16 15ff.), deren Strafe sie treffen wird (Jer 13 22. 26f.). So muß sie dem Strafgericht zitternd wie eine Gebärende entgegensehen (Mi 4 10), wie ein rostiger Topf ausgeglüht (Ez 24 9-13) und wie ein Schmelzofen zur Vernichtung seiner Bewohner benutzt werden (Ez 22 19-21). Bleibt sie zunächst wie eine Laubhütte und ein Gestell für den in der Nacht Wache haltenden Feldhüter übrig (Jes 1 8) und kann sie auch nach der Katastrophe noch als kleiner Turm betrachtet werden, wie ihn Hirten zum Bewachen der Herde errichteten (Mi 4 8), so erscheint der Schaden gewöhnlich als wesentlich größer — unermeßlich, wie das Meer weit ist (Thr 2 13). Jerusalem ist die vom Zornesbecher Trunkene (Jes 51 17ff.), die des Verbandes und der Heilung bedürftige

---

[92] Vgl. G. Wanke, Die Zionstheologie der Korachiten in ihrem traditionsgeschichtlichen Zusammenhang, 1966.

Verwundete (Jer 30 17), die in Fronpflicht geratene Witwe (Thr 1 1), die klagende Mutter, die ihre Kinder verloren hat (Thr 2 19ff.), glanzlos und dunkel gewordenes Gold (Thr 4 1). Die Jungmannschaft ist in der Katastrophe wie unansehnliches irdenes Geschirr behandelt worden (Thr 4 2); und die übriggebliebenen Frauen sind zum Säugen weniger fähig als Schakale und grausam wie Strauße (Thr 4 3).

III. Aspekte und Bedeutungen der Begriffe Zion-Jerusalem

1. Königsresidenz und Hauptstadt

Eine große Zahl der Vorkommen des Namens *Jerusalem*, seltener des Namens *Zion*, betrifft die Stadt als politischen Begriff: als kanaanäischen Stadtstaat (Jos 10 1ff. u. ö.), als Haupt- und Residenzstadt Davids (II Sam 5 5ff. u. ö.) oder des davidisch-salomonischen Großreichs (II Sam 8 7—I Reg 11 42), danach häufig als Haupt- und Residenzstadt des Reiches Juda (I Reg 12 18—II Reg 24 18 u. ö.). Hierher gehört gleichfalls die amtliche persische Formulierung *Jerusalem in Juda* (Esr 1 2f.), d. h. Jerusalem, das in Juda liegt. Entsprechend trifft Nehemia Maßnahmen zur Sicherung der Hauptstadt der neuen Provinz Juda (Neh 7 1-3) und zur Vermehrung ihrer Bevölkerung (Neh 7 4-72a.).

Häufig findet sich Jerusalem in längeren oder kürzeren staatsrechtlichen Formulierungen, in denen neben der Hauptstadt das übrige Staatsgebiet oder andere Gebiete aufgezählt werden. So nennt Jes 8 14 *Jerusalem*, das sich in königlichem Eigenbesitz befand, neben Juda und Israel als den *beiden Häusern Israels*. In Jer 17 26 32 44 33 13 wird der Staat Juda nach seiner landschaftlichen und seiner staatsrechtlichen Gliederung beschrieben. Außer den Städten Judas und dem Land Benjamin gehört die Stadt Jerusalem mit ihrem Territorium, das als סְבִיבוֹת oder סְבִיבִים *Bezirk* angeführt ist, zum Staatswesen. Meist findet sich die kürzere Formulierung, die den Stadtstaat *Jerusalem* (Jer 14 19 Zion[93]) und den Stammes- oder Stämmestaat *Juda* anführt (Jes 3 1. 8 Jer 2 28 u. ö.) — die beiden wichtigsten Bestandteile des Reiches —, neben denen das kleine benjaminitische Gebiet vernachlässigt wird. Auch in der Redewendung *Jerusalem und all seine Städte* (Jer 34 1) sind nach Jer 19 15 mit letzteren die judäischen Landstädte gemeint. Die Nachwirkung dieser staatsrechtlichen Unterscheidung findet sich noch in den anders gearteten politischen Verhältnissen der exilischen und nachexilischen Zeit, in der man ebenfalls

---

[93] In ähnlicher Weise unterscheidet Jer 4 31 das ironisch betrachtete Zion von dem mit Mitleid bedachten Land.

Jerusalem und *Juda* bzw. die *Städte Judas* (Sach 1 12 Esr 4 6 u. ö.) oder *Zion* und die *Städte Judas* (Ps 69 36 Thr 5 11) nebeneinander stellt.

Als Hauptstadt kommt Jerusalem und seinen Bewohnern eine hervorgehobene und Vorzugsstellung gegenüber dem Lande zu (Jes 22 21 Thr 2 15), wie sie die Frauen der Oberschicht in ihrem Auftreten verkörpern (Jes 3 16f.). Es ist die am stärksten befestigte Stadt, in die man vor dem Feinde flieht (Jer 4 6 35 11), der Brennpunkt des öffentlichen, sozialen, kulturellen und religiösen Lebens (Mi 1 9), wo die für das Volk Verantwortlichen leben (Mi 1 5) und an dem das Volk mit Liebe und Freude hängt (Ps 122 2f. 6). In der späteren nachexilischen Zeit bildet Jerusalem wieder den politischen Mittelpunkt des palästinischen Judentums (Esr 4 8 u. ö. Neh 1 2f. u. ö.), in dem politische Versammlungen des Volkes stattfinden (Neh 5 7 7 5).

Daher steht *Jerusalem* als Vorort und Hauptstadt Judas für das ganze Land und Reich und wird in einigen Prophetenworten als pars pro toto erwähnt (Jes 10 11 Ez 16 1-3. 23-25 23 4 b Mi 1 1). Oder es wird als noch nicht eroberter Rest des Landes während eines feindlichen Feldzugs genannt (Jes 1 8).

Während ein späterer Zusatz die zur Deportation Bereitstehenden klagen läßt, daß sie Zion als Heimat und Wohnstätte verlassen müssen (Jer 9 18), wird zu Beginn des Exils angesichts der Bedeutung des Tempels zwischen der »Stadt« und dem Tempelbezirk in Jerusalem unterschieden (Jer 52 24f.) und später in Verbesserung Ezechiels die räumliche Trennung der Stadt als eines profanen Gebiets vom Tempel gefordert (Ez 48 9-22. 30-35).

2. Höfisch-sakrale Aspekte

Im Zusammenhang mit der Bedeutung Jerusalems als Königsresidenz und Hauptstadt finden sich Ansätze zu einer höfisch-sakralen Theologie, in der die Stadt ebenfalls eine gewisse Rolle spielt. Dazu gehören sowohl die Erzählung von der Errichtung des ersten Jahwealtars in Jerusalem (II Sam 24) als auch die Ladeerzählung, die sich mit den Schicksalen der Lade vom Philisterkrieg bis zur Überführung nach Jerusalem befaßt (I Sam 4—6 II Sam 6 7 1-7. 17). Die Verbindung von Königtum und priesterlicher Aufgabe leitete man aus der Melchisedek-Tradition her, die die Hoftheologie ausdrücklich für die davidische Dynastie anerkannte (Ps 110 4). Daneben finden sich als wesentliche Elemente der Inthronisierung eines Königs seine in *Zion*, auf dem *heiligen Berg* Jahwes, vollzogene Legitimation durch Jahwe (Ps 2 6) und die sakral-symbolische Verleihung des Zepters als Übernahme der von Jahwe verliehenen Macht (Ps 110 2). Die spät- oder nachsalomonische Begründung und Legitimierung der davidischen Dynastie als ganzer in II Sam 7 8-16. 18-29 verleiht dem Königtum in

Jerusalem eine besondere Weihe. Ihren letzten Ausdruck findet diese höfisch-sakrale Theologie während der Königszeit in der deuteronomischen Aussage von der göttlichen Erwählung der Davididen und Jerusalems (I Reg 11 13. 32), die die offizielle Auffassung in neuer Weise umschreibt und steigert[94]. Ebenso verbindet Ps 132 den göttlichen Schwur an David (v. 11f.) mit der Erwählung Zions als Wohnsitz und Ruhestätte Jahwes (v. 13f.); die offizielle Theologie erwartet daraus reichen materiellen Segen (v. 15), inneres Glück der Gemeinde der Frommen (v. 16) sowie Macht und Bestand des Königtums (v. 17). Auch der jüngere Ps 78 enthält die Sätze von der Erwählung Zions als des Kultortes und Davids als des frommen und klugen Königs (v. 68-72). Insgesamt darf man die Bedeutung dieser Hoftheologie, die Jahwe — Königtum — Jerusalem miteinander verband, nicht überschätzen.

3. Symbol des Volkes oder der Gemeinde

Einige Male findet sich der Begriff Zion-Jerusalem in einer Übergangsform von der Bezeichnung der Stadt zur Symbolisierung ihrer Bewohner. Sie ist die Stadt des Tempels und der *Knechte Jahwes*, der Gemeinde (Ps 79 2), die als *Zion* mit den judäischen Städten Jahwe zujubelt (Ps 97 8). Sie kann auch personifiziert gedacht sein und als solche sprechen (Mi 7 8-20), leiden (Jes 51 17-23) oder gerettet werden (Jes 46 13), da sie die Gottesgemeinde in sich hat (Ps 147 12). Besonders im chronistischen Werk, das oft die Bewohner Jerusalems ausdrücklich nennt (z. B. II Chr 32 26. 33), wirkt nicht nur in der Nebeneinanderstellung von *Juda* und *Jerusalem* die frühere staatsrechtliche Gliederung des Reiches nach, sondern bezeichnen die beiden Ausdrücke auch Land und Stadt, die von der Gottesgemeinde Israel bewohnt sind. Die Begriffe symbolisieren die Wohnorte der theokratischen Gemeinde (I Chr 5 41 II Chr 2 6 u. ö.). In all diesen Fällen ist eine Annäherung an die Gleichsetzung mit dem Volk oder der Gemeinde selbst zu beobachten.

Neben der besonderen Bezeichnung der Bewohner von Zion-Jerusalem begegnen von Jeremia an die Bezeichnungen der Stadt als Symbol des Volkes oder der Gemeinde. Die *Wegführung Jerusalems* (Jer 1 3) meint diejenige der Jerusalemer. Nebeneinander stehen *Jerusalem* und *dieses Volk* (Jer 4 11 8 5), *Juda, Jerusalem* und *dieses schlimme Volk* (Jer 13 9f.), *Juda* und *Zion* (Jer 14 19), *Jerusalem* und die *Bewohner Zions* (Jer 51 35); oder es ist vom *Rest Jerusalems* als bestimmten Menschengrup-

---

[94] Auch die Chronik spricht von einer Erwählung Davids (I Chr 28 4 II Chr 6 6), Salomos (I Chr 28 5f. 29 1) und der Stadt Jerusalem (II Chr 6 6. 34. 38 12 13 33 7), ebenso aber von einer Erwählung der Priester und Leviten (II Chr 29 11) und des Jerusalemer Tempelgebäudes (II Chr 7 16).

pen die Rede (Jer 24 8). Die Glosse Jer 4 14 richtet die Aufforderung, sich vom Bösen zu waschen, an *Jerusalem*, meint aber die Jerusalemer (vgl. 4 3f.). In Ez 5 5 stellen die für die symbolische Handlung verwendeten Haare nach dem Wortlaut Jerusalem (*dies ist Jerusalem*), tatsächlich jedoch seine Einwohner dar. Ebenso ist in den Klageliedern der Begriff *Zion* teilweise die Verkörperung des Volkes als einer vorwiegend politischen Größe, wobei sogar an Gesamtisrael gedacht werden kann (Thr 1 17): Zion — Jakob — Jerusalem. Der Begriff *Tochter Zion* schillert zwischen der Verkörperung der Stadt und des in ihr lebenden Volkes (Thr 2 1). Der eigentliche Glanz Zions ist seine Jungmannschaft (Thr 4 2). Für Deuterojesaja ist *Jerusalem* nicht allein die palästinische Stadt, sondern auch Symbol für *mein Volk* (Jes 40 1f.), d. h. die israelitische Gesamtgemeinde in aller Welt und zu jeder Zeit, so daß sie nach der Stadt benannt werden (Jes 48 2) und *Zion* die Bezeichnung *mein Volk* erhalten kann (Jes 51 16). Die Parallelität von *Jerusalem* und *mein Volk* in Erwartung der verheißenen Endzeit findet sich noch Jes 65 19-25, während Jes 59 20 *Zion* und *die sich in Jakob vom Frevel abkehren* nebeneinander stellt. Schließlich sind in diesem Zusammenhang einige Psalmenstellen zu erwähnen. In Ps 76 68 stehen *Stamm Juda* und *Berg Zion* parallel, in 126 1 könnte man statt von *Zions Geschick* nahezu von »unserem« sprechen, in 128 5f. ist *Zion-Jerusalem* in etwa Symbol für Israel, in 149 2 sind *Zions Söhne* gleich Israel. Daher gilt Jerusalem ausschließlich als Stadt der Juden, in der niemand anders Teil, Anrecht und Gedächtnis hat (Neh 2 20; vgl. Hag 2 10-14); daher die Tempelreinigung (Neh 13 4-9).

4. Gottessitz und Gottesstadt, Kultusort und Tempelstadt

Die geschichtliche Entstehung des Glaubenssatzes, daß Zion-Jerusalem die eigentliche Stätte der Gegenwart Jahwes sei, läßt sich wenigstens in den Grundzügen erkennen. Zunächst ist mit dem Symbol der Lade die Gegenwart des Jahwe Zebaot, des Kerubenthroners, nach Jerusalem übertragen worden. Vom Bau des salomonischen Tempels an findet sich die Redewendung vom »Wohnen« Jahwes, die zunächst den Tempel (I Reg 8 12f.), dann den Stadthügel und die Stadt selbst zum Gottessitz erklärt[95]. Für diese Ausdehnung und Übertragung des Ausdrucks »wohnen« ist Ps 43 3 bezeichnend, der den

---

[95] Man hat das Verb שׁכן gegenüber dem anderen Ausdruck ישׁב für *sitzen* oder *wohnen* als »zelten« im nomadischen Sinn verstehen wollen, so daß Gott im Himmel »wohne«, das Geheimnis seiner Gegenwart aber auch auf Erden bekannt sei, da er inmitten seines Volkes »zelte«; vgl. F. M. Cross, Jr., The Tabernacle, BA 10 (1947), 65—68; Wright a. a. O. 143. Jedoch ist שׁכן von akkadisch *šakānu hinlegen* = ugaritisch *škn wohnen* abzuleiten und nicht von einem nomadischen Begriff, während ישׁב mit ugaritisch *jṯb* (*jšb*) *sitzen* parallel geht.

Tempel als Jahwes *Wohnung* und den *heiligen Berg* parallel setzt. Ist hier die Verbindung zwischen *wohnen* und *Berg* offensichtlich, so haftet der Ausdruck schon zur Zeit Jesajas am *Zionsberg* (Jes 8 18 Ps 74 2) und wird später auf *Jerusalem* überhaupt ausgedehnt, das als Ganzes die Wohnstatt Jahwes bildet (Joel 4 21 Ps 76 3 u. ö.). Der Gedanke wird auch mit der deuteronomischen Erwählungstheologie verbunden (Ps 132 13f.). Eine gegenteilige Auffassung findet sich I Reg 8 27 Jes 66 1f. Ferner wird Jerusalem, da der Tempel eine Art irdischen Palastes darstellt, der dem himmlischen Palast Jahwes entspricht, die Stadt des Königs Jahwe. In Jer 8 19 14 19 spricht sich zumindest der Glaube des Volkes aus, daß der Tempel der Palast des Königs Jahwe und Jerusalem seine Königsstadt sei. Ez 43 7 verbindet das Königtum Jahwes mit seiner Gegenwart im Tempel; nach Ps 9 12 *thront* er auf Zion. Beide Gedanken sind in dem jüngeren Meerlied Moses miteinander verbunden worden: Jahwe hat sich in Jerusalem eine Wohnung, den Tempel, bereitet, um für immer als König herrschen zu können (Ex 15 17f.). Zugleich wird der Stadthügel als *Berg seines Eigentums* einbezogen und im Zusammenhang mit dem Wohnen und Königsein Jahwes zum Gottesberg erklärt. Die deuteronomische Theologie bestimmt das Verhältnis Jahwes zur heiligen Stätte genauer dahin, daß er seinen Namen dort *wohnen läßt* und bezieht damit die frühere Vorstellung vom Wohnen Jahwes in Jerusalem eindeutig auf seine Offenbarungsgegenwart[96]. Dazu fügt die deuteronomische Theologie den Gedanken der Erwählung, der im Deuteronomium selbst auf die Kultstätte beschränkt ist, jedoch schon von den deuteronomischen Verfassern der Königsbücher auf die Stadt Jerusalem ausgedehnt wird (I Reg 11 13. 32. 36 14 21 II Reg 21 4. 7). Auch die Chronik redet von einer Erwählung sowohl des Jerusalemer Tempelgebäudes (II Chr 7 16) als auch der Stadt Jerusalem (II Chr 6 6 12 13 33 7). Auf diese Weise werden der Jerusalemer Tempel, der Zionsberg und Jerusalem nicht nur die allein legitime Kultstätte, sondern auch das Zeichen der Offenbarungsgegenwart Gottes.

Entscheidend für das steigende Ansehen Jerusalems als Gottesstadt war die stete Erweiterung und Übertragung der Heiligkeit seiner Offenbarungsstätte: von der Lade auf den Tempel — den Tempelberg — die ganze Stadt. Die Gleichsetzung von Tempel und Tempelberg wird in Ps 15 1 24 3 deutlich vollzogen. Der Tempel ist dem *Berg Jahwes* oder dem *heiligen Berg* parallel. Da dieser den Namen *Zion* trägt, ist der Zion der heilige Berg Jahwes (Jes 31 4 Joel 2 1) und können auch Tempel und Zion einander parallel werden. Wie Ps 78 68f. den Bau des Heiligtums mit der Weltschöpfung vergleicht, so wird nach Ps 68 18 der Gottesberg Sinai als Symbol der Offen-

---

[96] Zur abweichenden Übersetzung der LXX vgl. ThW VI 523.

barungsgegenwart mit dem Tempel verknüpft. Weiterhin wird der heilige Berg Jahwes mit *Jerusalem* als seiner Stadt (Jes 45 13) parallel gesetzt (Dan 9 16f.). Weil Gott Zion-Jerusalem als Tempelstadt mehr als alle anderen Orte Israels liebt und also keine anderen Kultstätten will, hat er es selbst auf heiligen Bergen als *Gottesstadt* gegründet; so faßt Ps 87 alle Gesichtspunkte zusammen. Daher ist Jerusalem schließlich die *Gottesstadt* (Ps 46 5), die *Stadt unseres Gottes*, des *Großkönigs* (Ps 48 2f.) und daher die *heilige Stadt* (Jes 48 2 52 1 Neh 11 1). *Nach Zion* bedeutet *zu Jahwe* (Jer 31 6), *aus Zion* bedeutet *von Jahwe* (Ps 14 7).

So ist es allgemeiner Glaube, daß Jahwe, der in Jerusalem wohnt, Gott in Zion ist (Ps 65 2 99 2 135 21). Wenn Ezechiel in seiner Vision Jahwe die Stadt einäschern und verlassen sieht (Ez 9 3a 10 2. 7. 18f. 11 22f.), setzt er die Offenbarungsgegenwart zu Hilfe oder Gericht als selbstverständlich voraus. Und die persische Regierung formuliert amtlich: *das ist der Gott, der in Jerusalem ist* (Esr 1 3; dagegen 7 15 von seiner *Wohnung zu Jerusalem*). Der Offenbarungsgegenwart Jahwes in Jerusalem, dem Gottessitz und der Gottesstadt, entspricht es, wenn sich die Theophanie von dort her als dem neuen Sinai (Ps 68 18) ereignet. So nimmt Ezechiel sie in Babylonien wahr, als Jahwe sich — dem Karawanenweg folgend — vom Norden naht (Ez 1 4). Ein Abglanz dessen fällt wiederum auf Zion, die *Krone der Schönheit*, zurück (Ps 50 2)[97]. Von Zion aus naht Jahwe der späteren Zeit ferner zum Gericht. Das Jeremiawort, nach dem er als Krieger vom Himmel her über seine Aue Jerusalem brüllt (Jer 25 30), ist in Joel 4 16 auf Zion-Jerusalem als den wahren Offenbarungssitz Jahwes umgedeutet und von da aus in Am 1 2 dem Prophetenbuch wie ein Motto vorangestellt worden: Von Zion-Jerusalem als der Gottesstadt geht das Gericht über das Nordreich Israel (Am 1 2) und über die Völkerwelt aus (Joel 4 16). Ebenso aber sind *Zionsberg* und *Jerusalem* auch Symbol des Schutzes Jahwes; ewig wie sie ist die Hilfe Gottes für die, die auf ihn vertrauen (Ps 125 1f.). Daher kann sogar eine neue Segensformel gebildet werden: *Jahwe segne dich von Zion her* (Ps 128 5 134 3), die dem Gesegneten die Kräfte der heiligen Stätte zuspricht.

Obwohl Micha für Jerusalem als Kultstätte keine Zukunft mehr sieht (Mi 3 12) und im Bericht über die Tempelrede Jeremias (Jer 7 1-15) die Drohung gegen den Tempel auf Jerusalem als die Stadt des Tempels erweitert wird (Jer 26 6-12), setzt sich der Glaube an seinen Be-

---

[97] Dagegen ist in Jes 6, dem Bericht über das Berufungserlebnis des Propheten, schwerlich an den Jerusalemer Tempel als Stätte der Schau, sondern an den himmlischen Palast Jahwes gedacht; anders zuletzt I. P. Seierstad, Die Offenbarungserlebnisse der Propheten Amos, Jesaja und Jeremia, 1965², u. a. mehr. Dagegen G. Fohrer, Das Buch Jesaja, I 1966², 95.

stand durch, da Zion — zunächst der Tempel, im weiteren Sinn die Stadt Jerusalem — als Gründung Jahwes (Jes 14 32 Ps 125 1 132 13f.) und die ganze Anhöhe mit dem Tempelgebäude als ihm heilig, d. h. als sein Eigentum gilt (Ez 43 1-9). Obwohl für die große, verstreut lebende, aber immer wichtiger werdende nachexilische Diaspora die Teilnahme am Tempelkultus — von gelegentlichen Wallfahrten abgesehen — unmöglich ist, hält man nicht nur an der unauflöslichen Verbindung von Tempel und Gemeinde und an der entscheidenden Heilsbedeutung der Zugehörigkeit zur Tempelgemeinde fest, der sich sogar Eunuchen und Fremde anschließen können (Jes 56 1-8), sondern betrachtet den Tempel als *Bethaus für alle Völker*, als geistlichen Mittelpunkt der Welt (Jes 56 7). Man unterscheidet zwar einmal zwischen Jerusalem und dem Tempel (Ps 68 30), für den die Bilder des Zeltes (Thr 2 4) oder der Hütte (Thr 2 6) begegnen; aber gewöhnlich gilt aufgrund der Gleichsetzung von Zion und Heiligtum (Ps 20 3) die ganze Stadt Jerusalem als die Tempelstadt (Ps 48 Esr 5 15ff. u. ö.), weil es in seiner Mitte den Tempel birgt (Ps 116 19). Wenn man Gott in Zion schaut (Ps 84 8), ist an den Höhepunkt gedacht, den der Wallfahrer im Kultus erfährt. Zion bedeutet in diesem Zusammenhang sowohl die Kultstätte als auch den sich dort abspielenden Kultus selbst.

5. Stadt der Sünde und des Gerichts

Gegenüber aller positiven Bewertung Jerusalems steht die prophetische Kritik, in der die Stadt keine Ausnahmestellung eingeräumt erhält, sondern inmitten des sündigen Volkes als Stadt der Sünde gilt. Meist trifft die prophetische Scheltrede Juda und Jerusalem in gleichem Maße, so daß nicht die Stadt gegenüber dem Lande als solche verwerflich erscheint. Wenn Micha *Jerusalem* und *Samaria* besonders schilt und bedroht, geschieht es, weil in der Hauptstadt als dem Brenn- und Mittelpunkt des Landes die eigentlich Verantwortlichen leben, die die Hauptschuld für die Sünde des ganzen Volkes tragen (Mi 1 5). Die Hauptstadt stellt für das Land dar, was das »Tor«, in dem sich das öffentliche Leben abspielt, für die Ortschaft bedeutet (Mi 1 9).

Die eigentliche Sünde Jerusalems bzw. der Bewohner Jerusalems besteht wie immer in der prophetischen Theologie im Abfall von Gott und in der Empörung gegen ihn (Jes 3 8. 16f. 22 1-14 28 14). Im Bilde des Treubruchs des zur Dirne herabgesunkenen Jerusalems wird diese religiöse Sünde drastisch beschrieben. Zugleich weist das Bild auf den Abfall von Gott durch die kultische Sünde und den Götzendienst hin, die die prophetische Kritik in Jerusalem genauso wie im Lande Juda und in Israel feststellt (Jes 10 11 65 11 Jer 1 16 2 28 11 13)[98].

---

[98] Zur prophetischen Kritik am Tempel vgl. ThW III 238.

Gleich schwerwiegend ist die ethische und soziale Sünde, die Micha in der mit Frevel und Blut vorgenommenen privaten Bautätigkeit seiner Zeit erblickt (Mi 3 10)[99]. Jeremia weiß zwar von einer früheren Zeit der Liebe zu Jahwe, die er mit der Brautzeit vergleicht (Jer 2 2ff.). In der Gegenwart aber glaubt er in Jerusalem keinen rechtlich denkenden Menschen zu finden (Jer 5 1) und bezeichnet Bedrückung als das Wesen der Stadt, die Bosheit wie Wasser sprudeln läßt (Jer 6 6f.). Ezechiel betrachtet neben den religiösen und kultischen Sünden, die er als »Götzendienst« zusammenfaßt, die ethisch-sozialen Vergehen als so schwerwiegend, daß er Jerusalem kurzerhand als *Stadt der Blutschuld* bezeichnet (Ez 22 2f. 19 24 6). Dazu tritt die politische Sünde: das Werben um die Gunst der Großmächte (Ez 16 23-25; in v. 26-29 auf die Politik der letzten Jahre des Königs Zedekia gedeutet), wobei mit den eingegangenen Bündnissen wieder religiös-kultische Verpflichtungen verbunden waren[100].

Es ist angesichts der prophetischen Kritik verständlich, wenn die Jeremia-Erzählungen durchweg und Ezechiel gelegentlich Jerusalem verächtlich und wegwerfend *diese Stadt da* nennen (Jer 21 1-10 u. ö. Ez 11 2. 6)[101] oder wenn Ezechiel den heidnischen Ursprung Jerusalems aus Amoritern und Hetitern hervorhebt, ihn anders als Jes 1 21 von Anfang an für Jerusalem als maßgeblich betrachtet und die Stadt im Gegensatz zur zeitgenössischen deuteronomischen Theologie zur Welt des Heidentums rechnet (Ez 16 1-3). Die Jerusalemer taugen von Natur aus nichts (Ez 15 6). Wenn aus dem Gericht eine Schar gerettet wird, dann lediglich als Anschauungsmaterial für die Deportierten, die an ihnen die Berechtigung der Strafe erkennen sollen (Ez 14 22). Sie sind ungehorsamer als alle anderen Völker (Ez 5 6; vgl. Jer 2 10f. über Juda allgemein), schlimmer als Samaria und Sodom (Thr 4 6; Zusatz Ez 16 44-58). In deuteronomischem Geist lautet die Anklage etwas anders auf Verwerfung des Gesetzes und Götzendienst (Am 2 4f.) oder auf den heidnischen Greuel der Heirat mit fremden Frauen (Mal 2 11).

---

[99] Zur prophetischen Kritik am Reichtum vgl. ThW VI 322.
[100] Daher kann Ez 16 16-21 das Bild der Untreue in einem Nachtrag wieder auf den Kultus ausdehnen.
[101] Ebenso in Anlehnung daran in den späteren Zusätzen Jer 32 3. 28f. 33 4f. Zum Bild des Zornesbechers für das Gericht vgl. ThW VI 149. Die Glosse Ez 12 10 aβ-b deutet die Drohung auf den Fürsten in Jerusalem und das ganze Haus Israel in ihm. Fälschlich bezieht 12 19 die in 12 17-20 enthaltene Drohung vom ganzen Land nur auf Jerusalem. In Ez 5 10f. werden sekundär Einzelheiten des Gerichts ausgemalt, in 5 3-4a ein übrig bleibender Rest und ein neues Läuterungsgericht vorausgesetzt. Dabei verbindet Ez 24 25 das Ende des Verstummens mit dem Tag der Eroberung Jerusalems, 33 21 dagegen mit dem Eintreffen der Nachricht darüber. Die Glosse 24 26 sucht den Unterschied dadurch auszugleichen, daß sie das Eintreffen des Boten schon für den Tag der Eroberung annimmt.

Weil Jerusalem die Stadt der Sünde ist, wird es die Stadt des Gerichts sein; so lautet die Drohung der Propheten. Die Stadt, die David einmal belagert und eingenommen hat, wird zum Vollzug des göttlichen Strafgerichts wieder belagert werden (Jes 29 1-7); dann wird die fröhliche Stadt veröden (Jes 32 13f.). Jahwe wird sie genau durchsuchen, um alle Schuldigen zur Rechenschaft zu ziehen (Zeph 1 12). Mit Nebukadnezar naht der Vollstrecker des Gerichts (Ez 21 25-27). Dazu sammelt Jahwe die Judäer in Jerusalem wie in einem Schmelzofen — nicht um das Unedle auszuscheiden (so Jes 1 21. 25 Jer 6 27-29), sondern um im Schmelzprozeß alle zu vernichten (Ez 22 19). Da nützt es nichts, wenn Jerusalem die Feinde wie eine Dirne verführen möchte; man hört nur noch den Todesschrei der Gerichteten (Jer 4 30f.). Für den Vollzug des Gerichts denken die Propheten besonders häufig an einen Krieg mit seinen Schrecken (Jer 6 23) und an die folgende Deportation der Einwohner (Ez 12 1-11). Das Gericht wird ohne Mitleid vollstreckt (Jer 15 5). Auf das vollstreckte Gericht blicken Jer 42 18 44 13, der deuteronomistische Geschichtsschreiber (II Reg 24 13. 20) und Thr 1—5 zurück. Ist es für Jeremia klar, daß Gottes Zorn und Grimm sich über Jerusalem ergossen haben (Jer 42 18), so erscheint in Thr 1—5 das Unheil als unerwartete und unfaßbare Katastrophe, obgleich auch die Besinnung darauf spürbar wird, daß der *Tag von Jerusalem* (Ps 137 7) als Gericht wegen der Sünde längst angedroht war. Wie die Sünde Jerusalems hat das Gericht sonst nicht seinesgleichen mehr (Dan 9 12).

6. Stadt der eschatologischen Heilszeit

Die Hoffnung auf eine Wiederherstellung Jerusalems begegnet fast ausnahmslos als eschatologische Naherwartung, sobald während des Exils die prophetische Botschaft vom Entweder des Gerichts über die sündige Stadt und vom Oder einer möglichen Rettung durch radikale Umkehr oder durch Erlösung im zeitlichen Sinne eines Vorher-Nachher interpretiert wird: zuerst Gericht, danach Heil. Da der Untergang Judas und Jerusalems mit dem babylonischen Exil zweifellos das von den Propheten angedrohte Gericht bildete, konnte nunmehr nur noch die Heilszeit kommen, die nach dem beendeten Gericht endgültig und ewig sein und die Verwirklichung der Gottesherrschaft bedeuten wird. Dann wird und bleibt *Zion-Jerusalem* die Stadt dieser eschatologischen Heilszeit.

Der Ansatzpunkt zur eschatologischen Deutung ist in Thr 4 22 zu erkennen: Das Gericht über Zion ist abgeschlossen, doch wird noch keine Wende oder Heilszeit verkündet, sondern lediglich den seither verhaßten Edomitern ihre Strafe angedroht. Dagegen verbinden sich bei Deuterojesaja mit der Feststellung, daß das Gericht beendet ist, die Tröstung Jerusalems angesichts der bevorstehenden Wende (Jes

40 1f.), die Ankündigung der Erscheinung Jahwes (Jes 40 3-5) und der Weckruf an Jerusalem (Jes 51 17). Etwas später stellt Sacharja der abgeschlossenen Zornesepoche den bevorstehenden Umbruch der Zeiten mit der Verheißung der künftigen Heilsepoche für Juda und Jerusalem ausdrücklich gegenüber (Sach 8 15), so daß sich die klagende Frage erheben kann, wann endlich diese Heilszeit für Jerusalem anbrechen wird, nachdem die in Jer 25 11 (später noch 29 10) angekündigten 70 Jahre des Zürnens[102] verflossen sind (Sach 1 12).

Das Erbarmen Jahwes über Jerusalem bedeutet den Anbruch der Endzeit (Sach 1 12). Er hat Jerusalems kommende Erlösung als erster kundgetan (Jes 41 27) und schenkt ihm das nahe bevorstehende Heil (Jes 46 13), da er Zion so wenig vergißt wie eine Frau ihr Kind (Jes 49 14f.). In die augenblickliche entmutigende Lage hinein erklingt die Ankündigung der großen Wende (Zeph 3 16). Ja, im Gegensatz zur früheren prophetischen Drohung erscheint das Exil nur als eine Gelegenheit für Jahwe, seine Macht an Zion erweisen und dessen deportierte Einwohner retten und befreien zu können (Mi 4 10)[103]. Die bevorstehende eschatologische Wende kündigt in nachexilischer Zeit der unbekannte Prophet von Jes 60 für Jerusalem an, das im Mittelpunkt seines ganzen Denkens steht: Jerusalems Heilszukunft, sein »Licht«, wird sich im Aufstrahlen des Lichtglanzes Jahwes erfüllen (v. 1) — als Wiederholung der Weltschöpfung (v. 2), so daß das Weltende dem Weltanfang entspricht. Jerusalem wird in der dunklen Welt wie eine strahlende Lichtburg mit einer unwiderstehlichen Anziehungskraft stehen (Jes 60 2f.). Trotz des gegenteiligen Scheins »eifert« Gott um Zion-Jerusalem, d. h. er nimmt in fürsorglicher Liebe seinen Rechtsanspruch für es wahr (Sach 1 14 8 2). Er wird es von neuem erwählen (Sach 1 17[104] 2 16), so daß *Jahwe, der Jerusalem erwählt*, geradezu als Titel verwendet wird (Sach 3 2). Haggai und Sacharja erwarten die Verwirklichung dieser Verheißungen in Zusammenhang mit dem Bau des zweiten Tempels. Die Heilszeit beginnt mit der neuen Grundsteinlegung (Hag 2 19) oder dem Einsetzen des letzten Steins in den Tempel (Sach 4 6aβ-10a).

Man erwartet die schon von Ezechiel geschaute Rückkehr Jahwes nach Zion (Ez 43 1-9), dessen Ankunft die Freuden- und Siegesboten

---

[102] Zur Umbildung in LXX vgl. ThW V 413.

[103] Mi 4 10, ein Zusatz zu 4 9. 11f., kündigt nach dem Wortlaut das Exil erst an, obwohl es in Wirklichkeit schon vorausgesetzt wird. Für den Verfasser führt der Weg durch Leiden zur Herrlichkeit.

[104] Die Erwartung wird zugleich auf die Landschaft Juda ausgedehnt: »meine Städte sollen von Glück überfließen«. Anders Th. H. Robinson—F. Horst, Die Zwölf Kleinen Propheten, 1954², 220: »sind Städte glücklos in der Zerstreuung«; doch ist dazu die Änderung in עָרִים und die Annahme der Sonderbedeutung des Verbs פוץ (*sich zerstreuen*) *in Zerstreuung sein* (statt *überfließen*) erforderlich.

melden (Jes 52 7ff.) oder eine Heuschreckenplage ahnen läßt (Joel 2 1). Wie bei der Herausführung aus Ägypten wird er herabkommen (Jes 4 5), wenn er den Sieg über seine himmlischen Feinde errungen hat (Jes 24 23). Dann ist er in Jerusalem sichtbar gegenwärtig (Jes 4 5 30 20); seine Hand ruht auf dem Berge (Jes 25 10), und die Jerusalemer wohnen in seinem Angesicht (Jes 23 18). Jahwe, der Fels Israels, ist wieder auf seinem Berg (Jes 30 29). Dadurch wird Jerusalem aufs neue und endgültig zur Gottesstadt — zur Stadt Jahwes (Jes 60 14), zur heiligen Stadt (Jes 52 1) und zum Heiligtum (Joel 4 17). Außer dem Begriff des Erwählens kehren in diesem Zusammenhang weitere alte Begriffe wieder: Jahwe »wohnt« neuerlich auf dem Zion (Sach 2 14 8 3 Joel 4 17), Zion ist die Stätte seines »Namens« (Jes 18 7).

Dort wird Jahwe die endzeitliche Königsherrschaft antreten (Jes 24 23 52 7 Ob 21 Mi 4 7 Zeph 3 15 Sach 14 9 Ps 146 10 149 2). Es ist bezeichnend, daß mit Jerusalem selbst gewöhnlich nur dieser Gedanke an die von Jahwe selbst ausgeübte Gottesherrschaft verbunden wird und die Namen *Zion-Jerusalem* in messianischen Verheißungen lediglich in Sach 9 9f. über den Einzug des messianischen Herrschers[105] erwähnt werden[106]. Freilich setzen Haggai und Sacharja wohl einfach voraus, daß der Messias Serubbabel (Hag 2 20-23) bzw. die beiden Messiasse Serubbabel und Josua (Sach 4 1-6aα. 10b-14 3 8f. 6 9-15[107]) in Jerusalem leben; in anderen Fällen mag es ähnlich liegen[108]. Immerhin gilt Jerusalem viel zu sehr als Stadt Jahwes selbst, als daß man es zur Residenz bloß des Messias als seines irdischen Statthalters hätte erklären können. Die stärker verbreitete nichtmessianische Eschatologie, die eine unmittelbare Gottesherrschaft erwartete, hatte in Anknüpfung an die älteren Vorstellungen von Jerusalem als Gottessitz

---

[105] Für Herkunft aus vorexilischer Zeit spricht sich Robinson—Horst a. a. O. 247f. aus. Auf akkadische Parallelen verweist S. I. Feigin, Babylonian Parallels to the Hebrew Phrase »Lowly, and riding upon an ass«, in: Studies in Memory of M. Schorr, 1944, 227—240.

[106] Man könnte vielleicht noch auf Sach 12 9—13 1 hinweisen, doch ist es nicht sehr wahrscheinlich, daß mit dem »Haus Davids« eine messianische Dynastie gemeint ist.

[107] Der Text von Sach 6 9-15 ist stark geändert und erweitert worden. Der ursprüngliche Wortlaut, für dessen Wiederherstellung nur v. 9. 10b. 11 a.bα. 12 a. 13. 15 aα heranzuziehen sind, hat vom Befehl zur Krönung Serubbabels gehandelt, die Sacharja als symbolische Handlung vornehmen sollte; vgl. im einzelnen G. Fohrer, Die symbolischen Handlungen der Propheten, 1968². Das entsprechende Wort für den Hohenpriester Josua als zweiten Messias liegt in Sach 3 8f. vor.

[108] So dürfte Jer 33 17f., das eine Reihe messianischer Davididen und ein immerwährendes levitisches Priestertum erwartet — in ähnlicher Doppelheit wie Sacharja, aber als feste Institution —, mit dem Hinweis auf den Thron des Hauses Israel an Jerusalem als dessen Stätte denken; der Name der Stadt wird jedoch gerade nicht genannt.

und -stadt bereits die Ansicht durchgesetzt, daß die Stadt die endzeitliche Residenz Gottes selbst sein werde. Er wird dort eine ihm wohlgefällige Regierung einsetzen (Jer 3 15)[109] oder durch seine Gegenwart Schutz und Hilfe bieten (Jes 4 5f. Joel 4 16f. Ps 46), da er wie ein Held den Sieg erringt (Zeph 3 17) oder die Stadt nach außen wie eine Feuermauer abschirmt und im Inneren ihre Herrlichkeit darstellt (Sach 2 9).

Die endzeitliche Herrlichkeit Jerusalems beruht ganz und gar auf dem Heilshandeln Gottes (Jes 62 66 10-15). Der verheißene Wiederaufbau der zerstörten Stadt (Jes 49 16f. Sach 1 16) wird in ungeahnter Pracht und Herrlichkeit erfolgen — mittels Edelsteinen wie eine Märchenstadt (Jes 54 11-17). Sogar der Umfang der neuen Stadt wird an Hand der alten topographischen Merkmale angegeben (Jer 31 38-40 Ez 48 30-35 Sach 14 10). Meist stellt man sie sich wieder mit Stadtmauern vor (Jes 60 10 62 6 Mi 7 11), die zum Schutz erforderlich sind (Jes 26 1)[110], obwohl wiederum die Tore wegen der zahlreichen Karawanen Tag und Nacht offenstehen werden (Jes 60 11). Dagegen lehnt Sach 2 6. 8f. den Bau neuer Befestigungen ab, da Mauern nur der reichen Segensfülle Grenzen setzten und Gott selbst Jerusalem beschützen wird. Zum Neuaufbau gehört selbstverständlich die Wiedererrichtung des Tempels (Jes 44 28 Sach 1 16), zu der dann Haggai und Sacharja antreiben, damit der neue Tempel als Zeichen des Anbruchs der Endzeit dienen kann. Er wird aufs prächtigste ausgeschmückt werden (Jes 60 13 Hag 2 7-9). Jerusalem aber wird wieder (Jes 44 26) und für immerdar bewohnt (Joel 4 28) und sein Land mit großer Fruchtbarkeit gesegnet sein (Jes 4 2 30 23ff.; vgl. Joel 4 18). Wie Edom ihm Tribut zahlt (Jes 16 1), Tyrus seinen Handelsgewinn als Gabe sendet (Jes 23 18) und das von Ägypten und Kusch Erhandelte ihm zufällt (Jes 45 14), so wird überhaupt der ganze Besitz und Reichtum aller Völker in einem nicht abreißenden Zuge (Jes 60 5-11) infolge der eschatologischen Umwälzung (Hag 2 7f.) nach Jerusalem strömen. Dann wird Zion in der Tat zum Paradies und Jahwegarten werden, so daß die Endzeit der wunderbaren Urzeit entspricht (Jes 51 3).

Jerusalem wird zur eschatologischen Hauptstadt (Jes 16 1) und zum religiösen Mittelpunkt (Jes 45 14), daher unantastbar für jeden Feind (Jes 52 1 Joel 3 5 4 17 u. ö.). Wegen seiner Würde wird es einen neuen Namen erhalten (Jes 62 2), der sowohl — da von Jahwe verliehen — dessen Hoheitsrechte als auch das neue Wesen der Stadt ausdrückt. Er lautet: *mein Gefallen an ihr* (Jes 62 4), *Aufgesuchte* und

---

[109] Jer 3 14-18 ist ein nicht von Jeremia stammender, nachexilischer Abschnitt; anders W. Rudolph, Jeremia, 1968³, z. St.
[110] J. Lindblom, Die Jesaja-Apokalypse, 1938, 85—90, deutet Jes 26 1-14 nicht eschatologisch, sondern auf eine geschichtliche Begebenheit.

Stadt, die nicht verlassen blieb (Jes 62 12), *Thron Jahwes* (Jer 3 17 nach 14 21 17 12), *Jahwe unsere Gerechtigkeit* (Jer 33 16), *Jahwe daselbst* (Ez 48 35) oder *die treue Stadt* (Sach 8 3 nach Jes 1 21. 26)[111], während der Tempelberg ausdrücklich *heiliger Berg* genannt werden wird (Sach 8 3 wie Joel 4 17). Darin spricht sich angesichts der prophetischen Schelt- und Drohworte die Erwartung eines neuen und besseren Jerusalem aus, das allein durch das heilvolle und erlösende Handeln Gottes geschaffen werden kann. Sie bildet den Ansatzpunkt für die spätere Vorstellung vom oberen oder himmlischen Jerusalem, die sich im Alten Testament noch nicht findet. Alle alttestamentlichen Stellen beziehen sich auf das irdische Jerusalem, das nur als das neue, zukünftige Jerusalem der eschatologischen Heilszeit geschaut wird. Dabei haben allerlei ältere Gedanken auf diese Schau eingewirkt.

Allerdings machen sich in den eschatologischen Erwartungen für Jerusalem auch menschlich-allzumenschliche Züge bemerkbar. Sie zeigen zwar, daß die Eschatologie mit konkreten geschichtlichen Größen rechnet und nicht beziehungslos sublimiert und spiritualisiert; aber innerhalb dieses Rahmens beginnt bereits mit Deuterojesaja und Haggai die oftmals krasse materielle Ausmalung der Heilszeit. Während Jes 66 13 zunächst die Tröstung durch Gott verheißt, fügt später eine Glosse hinzu: *an Jerusalem werdet ihr getröstet*, d. h. durch seine endzeitliche Pracht und Herrlichkeit statt durch Gott. Nach Mi 4 8 wird in der Endzeit das in der Katastrophe von 587 wie ein kleiner Herdenturm zusammengeschrumpfte und machtlose Zion selbst — nicht Jahwe! — eine weit ausgedehnte Herrschaft ausüben. Demgegenüber verkündet Sach 12 7, daß Jahwe zuerst Juda vor Jerusalem helfen werde, damit die Jerusalemer nicht überheblich werden.

Andere Worte befassen sich mit den Einwohnern des neuen Jerusalem der Endzeit. Ihre Existenz beruht auf der Vergebung und Gnade Gottes, der die von Ezechiel gerügte Blutschuld Jerusalems tilgt und den Schmutz der Sünde abwäscht (Jes 4 4), der schon darauf harrt, sein Volk zu begnadigen (Jes 30 18f.). Daher werden die Erlösten nach Zion heimkehren (Jes 35 10 51 11). Sie sind der heilige Rest (II Reg 19 31 Jes 4 3), mit dem dann Haggai und Sacharja die tatsächlich heimgekehrten Deportierten gleichsetzen. Dazu tritt in nachexilischer Zeit die Erwartung, daß auch die Diaspora zurückkehrt — zunächst die babylonische (Sach 6 8. 15a), dann universal die in der ganzen Welt lebende (Jes 27 13 62 11 u. ö.).

Das Ziel der Heimkehr nach Jerusalem ist die Herstellung eines rechten Verhältnisses mit ewiger Dauer (Jer 50 5), in Treue und Ge-

---

[111] Dabei kennzeichnet die Treue eigentlich die Gottesgemeinde in der Stadt, so daß der Begriff *Jerusalem* dadurch wieder der Symbolisierung der Gemeinde angenähert wird.

rechtigkeit, die Gott den Seinen mitteilt, so daß sie an der Gemeinschaft festhalten (Sach 8 8). Auf diese Weise kommt es zur Geburt eines neuen Volkes in Zion (Jes 66 8), das rechtschaffen und treu (Jes 26 2) und unantastbar ist (Ob 17), so daß die Frommen in Zion-Jerusalem stets aus aller Not gerettet werden (Joel 3 5). Dazu gehört, daß die Volkszahl sich mehrt (Jer 3 16 Sach 2 8 8 5), so daß der Raum zu eng wird (Jes 49 20f.), besonders da das infolge der Sünde gesunkene Lebensalter (vgl. Gen 5 6 1-4) nun wieder ansteigen wird (Jes 65 20 Sach 8 4). Zu dem Ideal quellenden und langen Lebens tritt dasjenige einer heldenhaften Stärke (Sach 12 8) und der wirtschaftlichen Blüte auch ohne den Reichtum anderer Völker (Jes 62 8f. Sach 2 8). Daher wird in Jerusalem eitel Freude über das neue Glück herrschen (Jes 61 3 Jer 33 11 Sach 2 14), dazu aber auch Dank und Lobpreis erschallen (Jes 12 4-6 61 3 Jer 33 11).

Schließlich ergeben sich für die Völker verschiedene Beziehungen zu Zion-Jerusalem als Stadt der eschatologischen Heilszeit. Konkret handelt es sich um die Babylonier und Edomiter, denen wegen der über Juda und Jerusalem heraufgeführten Katastrophe besonderer Haß entgegenschlägt und für den Tag der eschatologischen Wende die göttliche Rache angedroht wird (Jer 51 44 Ob 17f. 21 Sach 1 14f. 2 2 u. ö.). Jedoch erwartet eine Strömung der eschatologischen Prophetie schlimme Geschehnisse. In der Endzeit werden die Heidenvölker einen Eroberungszug und Angriff auf Jerusalem unternehmen — freilich ohne Erfolg (Jes 29 8 Mi 4 11); denn die Völker, die gegen die Stadt zu Felde ziehen, werden angesichts Jerusalems vernichtet (Jes 17 12-14[112] Sach 12 2-6 u. ö.). Auf diese geläufige Vorstellung spielt auch Jes 10 12 an[113], während Joel 4 9-12. 13-17 ausführlichere Schilderungen des Heranziehens und der Versammlung der Völker enthalten, über die Jahwe von Zion-Jerusalem aus das Endgericht hält[114]. Sogar die ganze Erde soll zur Wüste werden, wenn Jerusalem triumphiert (Mi 7 13). Dagegen läßt Zeph 3 14f. eher an eine gegenwärtig im Land weilende oder sonst das Volk bedrückende Feindmacht in nachexilischer Zeit als an die zur letzten Entscheidung vor Jerusalem versammelten Völker denken. Ist es nach alledem gewöhnlich Jahwe, der das Endgericht an den Völkern vollstreckt, so klingen einige Male doch nationalistische Gedanken an. Das Glück der Jerusalemer und die Rache an den Feinden entsprechen einander recht häufig (vgl.

---

[112] Jes 17 12-14 ist deutlich von Ez 38f. abhängig. Damit erledigen sich die Versuche, das Wort für Jesaja in Anspruch zu nehmen.

[113] Unter dem »König von Assur« ist der Erbe der assyrischen Macht in der Zeit des Verfassers des Wortes zu verstehen.

[114] Die Vorstellung des Brüllens Jahwes vom Himmel her, die sich Jer 25 30 findet, wird von Joel 4 16 auf Zion-Jerusalem umgedeutet. Daher ist sie weder aus Am 1 2 übernommen, noch bezieht sie sich auf die Theophanie.

Mi 4 13 Ps 149 6ff.). Besonders gegenüber diesen Auswüchsen ist die andere Strömung der eschatologischen Prophetie bedeutsam, die die Völker in eine positive Beziehung zu Jerusalem setzt (vgl. Jes 18 7 45 14); denn dort bereitet Gott allen Völkern sein eschatologisches Festmahl und entfernt die hindernde Hülle und Decke von ihren Augen, so daß sie ihn erkennen (Jes 25 6f.).

So wird eine große Wallfahrt zum Tempel auf dem Zion stattfinden, wo die Völker sich von Jahwe belehren lassen, um nach seinem Willen zu leben (Jes 2 2-4; vgl. Mi 4 1-3[115]), wo sie ihn aufsuchen und begütigen (Sach 8 22). Sie versammeln sich einmütig im Tempel, um sich zu bekehren (Jer 3 17) und Jahwe zu dienen (Ps 102 23). Auf diese Weise wird jeder Mensch in Jerusalem seine geistige Heimat finden, gleichgültig in welchem Land er geboren ist (Ps 87 5). Die anderen Völker werden durch die Anerkennung Jahwes zu Gliedern des Gottesvolkes werden; das Merkmal der Zugehörigkeit ist das Bekenntnis zu dem einen, wahren Gott (Sach 2 15). Dann findet der Krieg überhaupt ein Ende (Jes 2 4 Ps 46 10). Freilich ist auch diese universale Eschatologie manchmal mit nationalistischen Gedanken durchsetzt (vgl. Jes 25 8 60 3f. 10ff. Jer 33 9 Sach 8 3 14 16-19).

7. Mythische Aspekte

Von der frühexilischen Zeit an sind ursprünglich mythische Vorstellungen — ihres eigentlichen mythischen Charakters entkleidet — als Bilder und Symbole zur Beschreibung der Bedeutung von Zion-Jerusalem verwendet worden. Am häufigsten begegnet die Vorstellung vom höchsten Berg und vom Segens- oder Lebenswasser. So findet sich mehrfach die Anschauung, daß Jerusalem auf dem höchsten Berg liege (Jes 2 2 Mi 4 1 Ez 17 22 40 2 Sach 14 10 Ps 48 3)[116]. Darin klingt sowohl ein mesopotamisches Motiv an, da das südbabylonische Eridu als Gottesgarten und wegen des im kosmischen Eridu thronenden Gottes Ea als Abbild des kosmischen Götterberges betrachtet wurde[117], als auch ein kanaanäisches Motiv, da der Gott El auf einem Gottesberg wohnt[118], als den man wenigstens teilweise den nordsyrischen

---

[115] Das zweimal (mit geringfügigen Unterschieden) überlieferte Wort verrät zu deutlich den Geist der nachexilischen universalen Eschatologie, als daß es sich Jesaja oder Micha zuschreiben ließe; anders zuletzt H. Wildberger, Jesaja, 1963ff., 78—80.

[116] Die ebenfalls der mythischen Bildsprache entnommene Symbolbedeutung des Felsens (vgl. ThW VI 95) findet sich im Alten Testament noch nicht, vgl. H. W. Hertzberg, Der heilige Fels und das Alte Testament, JPOS 11 (1931), 32—42 (= Beiträge zur Traditionsgeschichte und Theologie des Alten Testaments, 1962, 45—53).

[117] Vgl. Jeremias a. a. O. 66f. 77, ferner die Übersicht ThW V 475—478.

[118] ThW V 478. Vgl. ferner die ugaritischen Texte 51 IV 20ff.; 137, 13ff.; 'nt III 21ff.

Berg Zaphon (Mons Casius) betrachtet hat[119]. Beide Motive sind miteinander zur Paradiesvorstellung verschmolzen oder mit ihr verbunden worden, so daß Jerusalem auf dem höchsten, dem Gottesberg zugleich das Paradies darstellt. Von ihm oder vom Tempel geht ein Strom des Segens- und Lebenswassers aus (Ez 47 1-12 Joel 4 18 Sach 14 8 Ps 46 5); Jes 33 21 vergröbert das Bild zu Strömen mit breiten Ufern[120]. Diese Vorstellung konnte gewiß an die tatsächlichen Verhältnisse in Jerusalem anknüpfen und die Gichon- und Rogelquelle meinen[121], durch die das Wasser der unterirdischen Flut an die Oberfläche träte[122]. Doch sind wieder die mythischen Motive entscheidend: Am kanaanäischen Gottesberg entspringen die »(beiden) Ströme« und die »(beiden) Fluten«[123], und vom Paradiesgarten gehen der Segensstrom oder die vier Weltströme aus[124].

Andere mythische Bilder begegnen seltener. Jerusalem liegt in der Mitte der Völker (Ez 5 5), da das wiederbesiedelte Palästina der Nabel der Erde ist (Ez 38 12)[125]. Die es bedrohenden Mächte werden

---

[119] Vgl. O. Eißfeldt, Baal Zaphon, Zeus Casios und der Durchzug der Israeliten durchs Meer, 1932. Daher ist der Zionsberg in Ps 48 3 »der entlegenste Teil des Nordens (Zaphon)«; zu LXX vgl. ThW V 482 Anm. 86.

[120] Daher rührt auch der Vergleich in Jes 66 12, daß Jahwe dem endzeitlichen Jerusalem »den Frieden wie einen Strom« und »den Glanz der Völker wie einen Bach« zuteil werden läßt. Vgl. ferner ThW VI 596.

[121] Das Wasser der Gichonquelle, das Hiskia durch den Felstunnel zum oberen Siloateich geführt hat (II Reg 20 20) und das Jes 8 6f. als Symbol für das Walten Jahwes erscheint, hat in älterer Zeit vielleicht einmal kultische Bedeutung gehabt (vgl. I Reg 1 33. 45). Neh 2 13 nennt die Rogel- oder Drachenquelle. Josephus, Bellum Judaicum, 5, 410, der von »Siloa und all den Quellen außerhalb der Stadt« spricht, scheint nur die erstere gekannt zu haben. Die Annahme einer weiteren Quelle im Tempelbezirk (Aristeasbrief 89; Tacitus, Historiae, V 12) ist unwahrscheinlich. Vgl. Simons a. a. O. 47f. 157—194.

[122] Dagegen geht A. R. Johnson, Sacral Kingship in Ancient Israel, 1967², vom Herbst- oder Laubhüttenfest als Hintergrund zahlreicher Psalmen aus. Es habe nicht nur das Königtum Jahwes in Natur und Geschichte, sondern auch die Erwartung der herbstlichen Regenfälle zum Gegenstand gehabt. Damit bringt er auch die Anspielungen auf einen Quell oder Strom am Zion in Verbindung.

[123] Text 51 IV 21f.

[124] G. Hölscher, Drei Erdkarten, 1949, 35—44.

[125] In Jdc 9 37 bezeichnet Gaal den Garizim als Nabel der Erde, nach Jes 19 24 bildet Israel den Mittelpunkt der Welt. Für die spätere Zeit vgl. äthHen 26 1f. Jub 8 12. 19 bJoma 54b und bSanhedrin 37a. Auch Mohammed betrachtete Jerusalem als Mittelpunkt, bis Mekka und später Bagdad diese Stelle einnahmen. Mittelalterliche Landkarten gruppieren die Länder der Erde um Jerusalem, in dessen Grabeskirche der Erdnabel gezeigt wird. Analoge Vorstellungen finden sich mehrfach: Delphi als ὀμφαλός, Rom als *umbilicus orbis*, China als Reich der Mitte. Vgl. W. H. Roscher, Der Omphalosgedanke bei verschiedenen Völkern, besonders den semitischen, 1918.

mit den Bildern des Chaoskampfes dargestellt, in dem die Stadt fest und unerschütterlich bestehen bleibt (Ps 46 2-4.6 125 1). Die Katastrophe der Stadt scheint mit dem Sturz eines Himmels- oder Paradieswesens, vielleicht des Urmenschen, auf die Erde vergleichbar (Thr 2 1; vgl. Jes 14 12-15 Ez 28 17)[126], während in späterer Zeit der Messias in Jerusalem unter dem Bild des großen Weltenbaums (vgl. Ez 31 1ff.) dargestellt wird, in dessen Schatten alle Völker Platz finden (Ez 17 22-24).

8. Stadt der Theokratie

In anderen, weiteren Kreisen der nachexilischen Zeit trat die eschatologische Erwartung fast völlig hinter einer kultisch-gesetzlichen Haltung zurück. Zu ihnen gehört die Strömung, aus der das chronistische Werk hervorgegangen ist[127]. Dessen Hauptzweck ist der Nachweis, daß allein Juda und in ihm seine Hauptstadt Jerusalem der Sitz der Theokratie ist, weil dort die rechtmäßige davidische Dynastie beheimatet ist und die rechtmäßige Kultstätte Jahwes steht. Die Theokratie gründet sich auf die Aussonderung Israels aus der Völkerwelt, d. h. auf die Erwählung Judas und Jerusalems, wo David seinen Thron und Jahwe seinen Tempel besitzt.

Dadurch rückt Jerusalem viel stärker in den Mittelpunkt der Darstellung als in I—II Reg; denn, so drückt II Chr 6 6 es grundlegend aus, Jahwe hat Jerusalem erwählt, damit sein Name daselbst sei, und David, damit er Israel regiere. Er ist der *Gott von Jerusalem* (II Chr 32 19), der dort für immer Wohnung genommen (I Chr 23 25) und für seinen Namen eine ewige Stätte geschaffen hat (II Chr 33 4. 7). So hat er den Jerusalemer Tempel vor aller Welt durch das vom Himmel gesandte Feuer als Offenbarungs- und Opferstätte anerkannt (II Chr 7 1ff.). Der Tempel ist die alleinige Kultstätte (II Chr 30 5), die auch den Heiden offensteht (II Chr 6 32f.) und zu dem die — allerdings nicht zahlreichen — wahren Jahwegläubigen aus dem in Götzendienst versunkenen Nordreich Israel auswandern (II Chr 11 14. 16 30 11). Dem entspricht es, daß ungeachtet der geschichtlichen Tatsachen ganz Israel Jerusalem erobert (I Chr 11 4) und die Lade dorthin gebracht haben soll (I Chr 15f.), daß David den dort versammelten Oberen von ganz Israel Salomo als seinen von Jahwe erwählten Nachfolger nennt (I Chr 28 1) und daß die Stadt immer wieder als Versammlungsort der den Davididen unterstehenden Israeliten (II Chr 15 10 u. ö.) oder ihrer Ältesten (II Chr 34 29) genannt wird. Hauptzweck des Kultus ist demgemäß Lobpreis und Dank dafür, daß Jahwe Jerusalem zur Stadt der Theokratie erwählt hat.

---

[126] Vgl. im einzelnen G. Fohrer, Ezechiel, 1955, zu 28 17.
[127] Zum Folgenden vgl. Rudolph, Esra und Nehemia, 1949, XXVII—XXX; Chronikbücher, 1955, XVIIf.

Indem auf diese Weise das chronistische Werk die nachexilische Gemeinde darüber belehrte, daß sie das wahre Israel sei, ergibt sich die höchste Würdigung Jerusalems: Nicht in einer ungewissen Endzeit, sondern in der Gegenwart ist in ihm und um es herum die Gottesherrschaft verwirklicht.

9. Nebenbedeutungen

Mehr als geographischer denn als staatsrechtlicher Begriff steht Jerusalem als Stadt neben dem Land (Ez 7 23 9 9). Wie die Stadthügel selbst (Ps 133 3) werden die die Flur Jerusalems umgebenden Höhenzüge genannt (Ps 125 2) und diese geographischen Gegebenheiten bildlich-symbolhaft verwendet. Die Umgebung der Stadt wird bei der eschatologischen Herabkunft Jahwes große Änderungen erfahren (Sach 14 4f.). Für Ezechiel ist das neue Jerusalem als Stadt überhaupt nur ein geographischer Begriff; wichtig an ihm, das im Landgebiet der Priester liegen soll, ist allein der Tempel, während die Flur der Stadt südlich ins frühere Juda verlegt wird (Ez 45 1-8).

Um einen topographischen Begriff handelt es sich, wenn die Davidstadt auf dem Zion oder der salomonische Stadtteil auf dem Ophel genannt werden oder das Stadtgebiet in eschatologischen Ankündigungen des Wiederaufbaus beschrieben wird (Jer 31 38-40 Sach 14 10). Zahlreiche topographische Einzelangaben enthalten die Bücher Jer[128], Esr-Neh[129] und I—II Chr[130], die in erster Linie für die Topographie Jerusalems in der Zeit Jeremias, Nehemias, Esras und des Chronisten wichtig sind. Außerdem werden an Einzelheiten gesondert erwähnt: die Erweiterung oder der Neubau des salomonischen Palastes durch Jojakim (Jer 22 13-19), die Sorge um die Beschaffung des Wassers (Jes 7 3) und die Beisetzung der Könige in den Königsgräbern[131], neben denen der Friedhof der gemeinen Leute im Kidrontal begegnet (II

---

[128] Jer 17 19-21. 24f. 27 19 2 26 10 32 2 33 1 35 4 36 10f. 20. 22 37 13. 16. 21 38 6f. 11. 14 39 3f. 52 7.

[129] Esr 2 13-15 3 Neh 8 1 12 31-39. Vgl. M. Burrows, Nehemiah 3 1-32 as a Source for the Topography of Ancient Jerusalem, in: Annual of the American Schools of Oriental Research XIV, 1933/34, 115—140; Nehemiah's Tour of Inspection, BASOR 64 (1937), 11—64.

[130] I Chr 11 7f. 22 1 II Chr 3 1 23 5. 15. 20 25 23 26 9 27 3 32 3-5. 30 33 14 34 22.

[131] Die Königsgräber in der Davidstadt werden I Reg 2 10 11 43 14 31 15 8. 24 22 51 II Reg 8 24 9 28 12 22 15 7 16 20 und II Chr 9 31 12 16 13 23 21 1 24 16 25 28 27 9 32 33 35 24 genannt. Einige Könige wurden in Jerusalem an anderen, nur teilweise näher bezeichneten Stätten beigesetzt (II Reg 20 21 21 18. 26 23 30 24 6 und II Chr 16 13 21 20 24 25 26 33 28 27 33 20). Alt a. a. O. 42 weist darauf hin, daß die im Süden der Davidstadt nahe ihrem Ostrand gelegenen Felsstollen nicht mit Sicherheit als das Erbbegräbnis des Königshauses gelten können. Vgl. auch Simons a. a. O. 194ff.; Vincent-Abel I 313ff.

Reg 23 6), der nach Jer 26 23 wieder von den Familiengräbern der Oberschicht (Jes 22 15) zu unterscheiden ist[132].

Seltener ist von Jerusalem im soziologischen Sinn die Rede. Sieht man von den allgemeinen Erwähnungen der Einwohner der Stadt ab, so werden nur die *Töchter Jerusalems* als eine Art Chor der Gefährtinnen und der Umwelt (Cant 2 7 u. ö.) oder als die verzärtelten Damen der Stadt bzw. des Hofes im Unterschied zum Landmädchen (Cant 1 5) genannt.

Als historischer Begriff begegnet Jerusalem, wenn der Verfasser des Koh sich als *König in Jerusalem* o. ä. bezeichnet (Koh 1 1 u. ö.) und damit als Salomo erkannt sein will, unter dessen Regierung die Weisheitslehre am Jerusalemer Hof heimisch wurde. Ebenso wird Jerusalem zur Herkunftsbestimmung Mardochais verwendet (Est 2 6), obwohl er schon in der Diaspora geboren ist.

Zu chronologischen Zwecken dient die Erwähnung Jerusalems ebenfalls. Man verwendet es zur Datierung der vorexilischen Zeit (Sach 7 7) oder des Untergangs des Staates Juda und Beginns des Exils (Ps 137 7 Est 2 6 Dan 1 1; vgl. Ez 40 1).

IV. Zion-Jerusalem in der alttestamentlichen Theologie

1. Gott und Zion-Jerusalem

In großer Einhelligkeit geht nahezu das ganze Alte Testament — außer der Weisheitsliteratur, für die Jerusalem keine besondere Rolle spielt — von der engen Beziehung zwischen Gott und Zion-Jerusalem aus. Er hat die Stadt erwählt (Dtn 12 5 I Reg 11 36 Sach 3 2 Ps 68 16f. 132 13 II Chr 6 6 7 12. 16 12 13) und gegründet (Jes 14 32 Ps 87 1). Er erwählt und baut sie in seinem Erbarmen nach der Zerstörung von neuem (Sach 1 17 Ps 147 2), so daß man des Wiederaufbaus gewiß sein kann, der sich in wunderbarer, märchenhafter und paradiesischer Art vollziehen wird (Jes 49 14 54 11ff. 65 17ff. Jer 30 18 33 9ff. Sach 1 14ff. Ps 69 36 78 68). Dann hat die Stadt ewigen, vom Feinde ungestörten Bestand (Joel 4 17. 20 Mi 7 10ff. 16f.). Daß Gott Zion gebaut hat, bedeutet, daß er es zu seiner Wohnung gemacht hat, in der er in seiner Herrlichkeit erscheint (Ps 102 17); dadurch werden Zion und der Tempelberg heilig (Jes 65 11 Joel 2 1 4 17 Sach 8 3 Ps 2 6 48 2f. 68 17). So ist die Stadt oder der Tempel seine Wohnung (I Reg 8 27ff.

---

[132] Die Felskammergräber der Oberschicht befanden sich wenigstens teilweise im Gebiet des heutigen Dorfes *silwān* auf der Ostseite des Kidrontals; vgl. u. a. Ch. Clermont-Ganneau, Archaeological Researches in Palestine, I 1899, 304ff.; K. Galling in PJB 32 (1936), 91ff.; Vincent-Abel I 327ff. Über Reste althebräischer Inschriften vgl. A. Reifenberg in JPOS 21 (1948), 134ff.; N. Avigad in IEJ 3 (1953), 137ff.; 5 (1955), 163ff.; G. Fohrer, Das Buch Jesaja, I 1966², 254 Anm. 56.

Jes 8 18 63 18 Joel 4 17. 21 Sach 1 16 2 14 8 3 Ps 43 3 74 2 132 13ff. 135 21 I Chr 23 25 II Chr 32 19 33 4. 7) und sein Thron (Jer 3 17 14 21 17 12), zu denen er in der Endzeit wie beim Auszug aus Ägypten herabkommen und einziehen wird (Jes 4 5 24 23 52 7ff. Sach 14 5). Dann ist er sichtbar gegenwärtig (Jes 30 20f.), so daß die Stadt wegen seiner Nähe und Gegenwart (Sach 2 9) den Namen »Jahwe daselbst« erhalten wird (Ez 48 35). Er tritt seine eschatologische Königsherrschaft in Zion-Jerusalem an (Jes 33 22 52 7 Jer 8 19 Mi 4 7 Zeph 3 15 Sach 14 9 Ps 48 3 146 10) oder läßt sie durch seinen Messias ausüben (Sach 9 9f.). Von dort aus läßt er seinen Segen ergehen (Ps 128 5 134 3) und zeigt sich in der Theophanie (Ps 50 2).

So steht Zion-Jerusalem im engsten Verhältnis zu Gott (Jes 40 9 62) und kann die sichtbaren Beweise seiner Macht und Gnade preisen (Ps 147 13ff.). Was Zion-Jerusalem war, ist und sein wird, beruht ganz und gar auf der Liebe und dem Erbarmen Gottes (Ez 16 1ff. Sach 1 12. 14. 16 8 2 Ps 78 68 87 2), aufgrund deren er es nicht vergißt (Jes 49 14). Daher werden ihm göttlicher Schutz und Segen zuteil (Jes 31 5 Ps 46 147 12ff.). Gott füllt es mit Recht und Gerechtigkeit (Jes 33 5), gewährt ihm seine Hilfe in der Not (I Reg 19 21. 32-34 20 6 Jes 64 11 Zeph 3 16 Ps 69 36), rettet die Frommen (Joel 3 5) und vergilt den Feinden (Jer 51 24), kündigt die kommende Erlösung an (Jes 41 27) und wird das eschatologische Heil schenken (Jes 46 13). So wankt die Stadt nicht (Ps 125 1), sondern bietet Sicherheit (Jes 33 20). Die eschatologische Heilszeit wird die Vollendung bringen: Glanz und Ruhm durch die Herrlichkeit Gottes (Jes 60 1f. 14f. 61 9 62 1-3. 12), immerwährendes Licht (Jes 30 26 60 19f. Sach 14 7), die Umwandlung in ein Paradies (Jes 51 3) und die Erhebung zum Mittelpunkt der Welt (Jes 2 2-4 Mi 4 1-3), so daß Gott selbst über das neue Jerusalem jubeln wird (Jes 65 19).

Gegenüber diesem zuversichtlichen und manchmal selbstzufriedenen Vertrauen auf die helfende Liebe Gottes und gegenüber diesen hochgespannten eschatologischen Erwartungen aufgrund des behaupteten engen Verhältnisses zu Zion stehen freilich die prophetischen Warnungen und Drohungen. Zion-Jerusalem ist zwar wie ganz Israel, ja wie letztlich alle Welt auf Gott angewiesen und von ihm abhängig; aber umgekehrt ist Gott, dessen Majestät kein Tempel faßt (I Reg 8 27 Jes 66 1f.), nicht auf Zion-Jerusalem angewiesen. Er kann und wird es vielmehr wie ganz Israel zur Rechenschaft ziehen und dem läuternden (Jes 1 21-26 3 1-9 Ez 24 11 Zeph 1 12f.) oder vernichtenden Gericht (Jes 22 14 32 14 Jer 14 16 21 7. 10 32 3 34 2. 22 37f. Ez 9 10 2. 7 Mi 3 12) überliefern, um seine Sünde zu ahnden. Obwohl er sich von der Stadt schwer trennen kann und sich fast losreißen muß (Jer 6 8 Ez 11 22f.), wird er das Gericht an ihr und dem Tempel doch ohne Mitleid vollstrecken (Jer 7 14f. 15 5). So warnt die Prophetie vor dem billigen

Sicherheitsgefühl der herkömmlichen Theologie und stellt dem Glauben an die angeblich von Gott gewährleistete Unantastbarkeit Jerusalems die göttliche Gerichtsdrohung entgegen. Gott wird die Stadt wegen ihrer Sünde genauso wie jeden anderen Ort zur Verantwortung ziehen.

2. Die Menschen in Zion-Jerusalem

Die vorexilische Prophetie kündigt das Gericht über Zion-Jerusalem und seine Einwohner an, das sich später zur Erwartung der täglichen Vertilgung aller Frevler steigert (Ps 101 8). Der Grund liegt in der Sünde der Jerusalemer, die letztlich Abfall von Gott und Empörung gegen ihn ist (Jes 3 1. 8). Sie zeigt sich im einzelnen in der religiösen Sünde des Götzendienstes (II Reg 21 11-15 22 16-20 Jes 65 11 Jer 1 16 2 28 11 13 Ez 7 23) oder in ethischen Vergehen (Jes 1 21-23 Jer 5 1 23 14f. Ez 7 23), die im weiteren Sinne mit sozialen und politischen als »Blutschuld« zusammengefaßt werden (Ez 22 2f.). Diese Sünden der Jerusalemer wiegen besonders schwer, weil in der Hauptstadt die für das Tun und Lassen des ganzen Volkes Verantwortlichen leben, so daß Jerusalem als eigentlicher Sitz und Herd der Sünde des Volkes erscheint (Mi 1 5).

Gegenüber dieser Beschreibung des Verhaltens der Menschen in Zion-Jerusalem, wie es tatsächlich ist, stehen einerseits die Behauptung des chronistischen Werkes, daß die tatsächliche Gemeinde in Jerusalem das Ideal der Theokratie verwirkliche, andererseits die eschatologischen Hoffnungen über das Leben, wie es in Jerusalem nach dem Anbruch der Endzeit sein wird. Zion-Jerusalem ist dann der Ort der Rettung (Joel 3 5 Ob 17), der das Land beherrscht (Sach 14 10f. 20) und den davidischen Messias und das Priestertum in sich birgt (Jer 33 17f. Sach 3 8f. 4 1-6aα. 10b-14 6 9-15). Dort herrschen keine Angst und Furcht (Mi 4 9. 11f.), sondern Stolz über das Bürgerrecht (Ps 87), Jauchzen und Jubel nach dem Endgericht über die Heiden (Jes 12 4-6 Ps 149 2), ein langwährendes und quellendes Leben (Jes 65 20 Sach 8 4f.) und statt Trauer eine Freude, die sich besonders im Kultus Ausdruck verschafft (Jes 61 3 Jer 33 11 Joel 2 23 II Chr 30 26).

Doch mit mehr Recht legen die Propheten dar, wie das Verhalten der Jerusalemer sein soll und muß, damit es dem göttlichen Willen entspricht. Rettung vor dem Untergang, der dem schuldig gewordenen Menschen droht, gibt es nur auf dem Wege der Umkehr oder Erlösung (Jes 1 27 29 4 30 15 Jer 4 14). Dann, in Glauben und Vertrauen, kann Zion-Jerusalem der Rest sein, der übrigbleibt (Jes 7 3. 9), oder doch wenigstens ein Rest von seinen Einwohnern bewahrt bleiben (II Reg 19 31 Zeph 3 12), dem sonst ebenfalls der Untergang bevorstünde (Jer 24 8). Das Volk, das in Zion-Jerusalem lebt, soll demütig und gering (Zeph 3 12), rechtschaffen und treu sein (Jes 26 2).

3. Die Menschen und Zion-Jerusalem

Der Israelit schätzt Zion-Jerusalem je länger desto mehr als kultischen Mittelpunkt, wo der rechte Kultus ausgeübt wird (I Reg 12 26. 28 II Reg 22f. Ez 20 40f. Ps 51 20 65 2-4 84 8 116 19; die Bedingungen zur Zulassung in Ps 15), aber auch als befestigte Stadt in Kriegsnöten (Jer 4 6) und als Stätte der Familiengräber (Neh 2 3. 5). Man steht staunend und bewundernd vor der großen Stadt (Jer 22 8), die so lieblich (Cant 6 4) und eine Krone der Schönheit ist (Ps 50 2). Sie ist Gegenstand der Liebe und Freude (Ez 24 25 Ps 48 13f. 122 1) — insbesondere das Zionslied gilt als heiter und fröhlich (Ps 137 3) —, der Sehnsucht (Ez 24 25 Ps 42f. 137 5f.), der Fürbitte und des Segenswunsches (Ps 51 20 122 6-9 128 5), des Gedenkens und der Trauer angesichts seines Untergangs (Jer 51 50 Ps 102 14f. 137 5f. Thr 1—5) — vorausgesetzt, daß man vor Schmerz und Entsetzen der Trauer überhaupt fähig ist (Ez 21 11f. 24 21). In Zion-Jerusalem findet man Zuflucht bei Gott (Joel 4 16) und bringt die Bitte um Hilfe vor ihn (Ps 3 5). Von dort erwartet man Hilfe (Ps 14 7 20 3 53 7) und Segen (Ps 128 5 134 3). Daher ist der Blick der Deportierten auf Zion-Jerusalem gerichtet (Jer 51 50). Sie lassen sich nur zu gern zur Flucht oder Heimkehr dorthin auffordern oder mit deren verheißender Zusage trösten (Jes 35 9f. 40 9-11 48 20f. 49 22f. 51 11 52 7-12 Sach 2 11). Ja, für die Endzeit darf die ganze Diaspora mit ihrer Heimführung rechnen (Jes 27 13 43 1-7 66 20 Sach 8 7f. Anders Ob 20).

Anders ist das Verhalten vieler Nichtisraeliten. Ihnen wird Zion-Jerusalem als schlimmes Beispiel für den Abfall von Gott vor Augen geführt, dem man nicht folgen soll (Jer 22 8f.). Sie sind voller Rachsucht (Ez 25 12. 15) oder blicken mit Schadenfreude auf seine Katastrophe (Ez 25 3. 6. 8 26 1-6 Thr 2 15f.) und wiederholen immer von neuem die alten Vorwürfe und Anklagen (Esr 4 12. 15. 19). Wegen dieser Angriffe auf die Stadt schlagen ihnen Haß und Rachewünsche entgegen (Jer 51 24. 35 Ob 11 Sach 2 2 Ps 137 7). Eine weitere Steigerung dieses Verhaltens der Völker zu Zion-Jerusalem erwartet man für die Endzeit. Dann erfolgt der letzte Ansturm auf die Stadt, die sich jedoch als unantastbar erweist, so daß die Angreifer vernichtet werden (Jes 29 8 Ez 38f. Joel 4 17 Mi 4 13 Sach 12 1—13 6 14 1-21 Ps 48 2f.). Bei Jerusalem wird sogar das Endgericht über die Heiden stattfinden (Jes 10 12 17 12-14 30 27-33 31 5. 8f. Joel 4 14-17). In dieser Welterschütterung senden die Völker ihre Schätze zu der heiligen Stadt und ihrem Tempel (Jes 45 14 Sach 2 16 8 23). Sie bekehren sich zu dem einen wahren Gott in Zion-Jerusalem (Jes 45 14 Sach 2 16 8 23) und strömen wallfahrend dorthin, um Gott zu erkennen, seine Weisung zu empfangen, ihn anzubeten und zu verehren und in seinem Friedensreich zu leben (Jes 2 2-4 Mi 4 1-3 Jes 18 7 25 6f. 60 5 62 10 Jer 3 17 Sach 8 22

Ps 102 23) oder im Schatten seines Messias als eines Weltenbaums Platz zu finden (Ez 17 22f.).

4. Zusammenfassung

Die Sonderstellung Jerusalems ist in den kultisch, gesetzlich und national bestimmten Ausprägungen alttestamentlicher Theologie und in den hochgespannten eschatologischen Erwartungen sowohl Ausdruck demütigen Glaubensgehorsams unter der erhofften oder gewiß gewordenen Gottesherrschaft als auch Zeichen gottloser Verstocktheit und frivoler Selbstsicherheit gewesen. Der Glaube an die Unantastbarkeit der heiligen Stadt infolge ihres einzigartigen Schutzes durch Gott wurde zu einer Gefahr. Nur zu schnell verkehrte sich die Glaubensgewißheit in religiös-politische Vermessenheit. Mit dem Ruf: »Der Tempel Jahwes, der Tempel Jahwes, der Tempel Jahwes ist dies!« entzog man sich nur zu leicht der Mahnung und bedingten Zusage: »Bessert euren Wandel und eure Taten, dann will ich an dieser Stätte bei euch wohnen!« (Jer 7 3f.). Demgegenüber sind die großen Einzelpropheten weder einem kultisch-nationalen Dogma noch einer theokratischen Illusion noch einer eschatologischen Spekulation nachgejagt. Ihnen galt Jerusalem letztlich nicht mehr als die anderen Städte Israels, da nicht die Offenbarungsstätte, sondern der sich offenbarende Gott wichtig ist. Sie sahen die Jerusalemer unter der gleichen göttlichen Forderung, Drohung und Verheißung wie alle anderen Israeliten oder Nichtisraeliten. Und sie zögerten nicht, der Stadt und ihren Bewohnern das göttliche Gericht anzukündigen, durch das Gott sich als unabhängig von Jerusalem und ihm überlegen erweist. Daß damit die Offenbarungsgeschichte kein Ende findet, hat Ezechiel erfahren. Schon sein Berufungserlebnis (Ez 1 1—3 15) zeigte ihm, daß Gott nicht an Jerusalem und seinen Tempel gebunden ist, sondern dem Menschen auch im fremden Lande begegnen und nahe sein kann. Offenbarung und Heil sind nicht unauflöslich mit Zion-Jerusalem verknüpft; vielmehr kann der Glaubende die Nähe seines Gottes überall erfahren, ohne von ihm durch irdische Verhältnisse räumlich oder zeitlich getrennt zu sein.

Die Weisheit im Alten Testament[1]

I. Terminologie

Da LXX mit σοφία/σοφός gewöhnlich den hebräischen Stamm חכם wiedergibt, braucht im wesentlichen nur dieser betrachtet zu werden. Das Verb חכם kommt 26mal (qal 18, pi. 3, pu. 2, hi. 1, hitp. 2), חָכָם als Adjektiv oder Substantiv 135mal, das Substantiv חָכְמָה 147mal und im pl. חָכְמוֹת viermal[2] vor. Davon finden sich 73 Vorkommen in den Geschichtsbüchern des Alten Testaments (חכם 3, חָכָם 31, חָכְמָה 39), 41 in den Prophetenbüchern (חכם 1, חָכָם 24, חָכְמָה 16), 13 in den Psalmen (חכם 4, חָכָם 2, חָכְמָה 7)[3], 180 in der eigentlichen Weisheitsliteratur (חכם 18, חָכָם 76, חָכְמָה 86)[4] und 5 in den übrigen Büchern. Demnach sind in der Weisheitsliteratur fast drei Fünftel der Vorkommen festzustellen. Bedeutungsmäßig bezeichnen die Begriffe in den Geschichtsbüchern hauptsächlich das hand-

---

[1] Zum Ganzen vgl. J. Meinhold, Die Weisheit Israels, 1908; H. Greßmann, Israels Spruchweisheit im Zusammenhang der Weltliteratur, 1925; H. Ranston, The Old Testament Wisdom Books and their Teaching, 1930; W. Baumgartner, Israelitische und altorientalische Weisheit, 1933; J. Fichtner, Die altorientalische Weisheit in ihrer israelitisch-jüdischen Ausprägung, 1933; G. Boström, Proverbiastudien, 1935; A. Drubbel, Le conflit entre la Sagesse profane et la Sagesse religieuse, Bibl 17 (1936), 45—70. 407—428; H. Duesberg, Les scribes inspirés, I—II 1938/39; R. Gordis, The Social Background of Wisdom Literature, HUCA 18 (1943/44), 77—118; J. C. Rylaarsdam, Revelation in Jewish Wisdom Literature, 1946; H. Ringgren, Word and Wisdom, 1947; J. Kázmér, Wesen und Entwicklung des Weisheitsbegriffes in den Weisheitsbüchern des Alten Testaments, 1950; O. S. Rankin, Israel's Wisdom Literature, 1954[2]; H. Gese, Lehre und Wirklichkeit in der alten Weisheit, 1958; J. Paterson, The Wisdom of Israel, 1960; R. E. Murphy, The Concept of Wisdom Literature, in: The Bible in Current Catholic Thought, 1962, 46—54; H. H. Schmid, Wesen und Geschichte der Weisheit, 1966.

[2] Außerdem ist es in Prov 14 1 statt des Adjektivs zu lesen. Zur Auffassung von חכמות als pl. vgl. im einzelnen E. Brønno, Studien über hebräische Morphologie und Vokalismus, 1943, 187f. Es dürfte sich um eine Art Ausdehnungs-, Intensitäts- und Hoheitsplural handeln, der wohl als Ehrenbezeichnung gemeint ist und die allumfassende, lautere, wahrhaftige und höchste Weisheit bezeichnet.

[3] Die Begriffe des Stammes חכם werden in den Psalmen möglichst gemieden, weil sie schon früh eindeutig festgelegt sind, während inhaltlich-sachlich eine Reihe von Psalmen von der Weisheitslehre beeinflußt oder gar der Weisheitsliteratur zuzurechnen ist.

[4] Dazu sind Hi, Prov und Koh zu rechnen.

werklich-künstlerische Können, die Klugheit und Kenntnis sowie Salomos Weisheit, seltener die Zauberkunst, die Lebenskunst und das ethische oder fromme Verhalten. In den Prophetenbüchern bezeichnen sie das menschliche Können verschiedener Art, die »Weisheit« und die Zauberer anderer Völker; ferner begegnen sie anläßlich der Kritik der Weisheit und sehr selten, aber nur in der Prophetie, in eschatologischen Vorstellungen. In der Weisheitsliteratur beschreiben die Begriffe zwar einige Male die Klugheit und Lebenskunst, vor allem aber werden sie wie auch in den Psalmen für die Verhaltensregeln, das ethische oder fromme Verhalten verwendet. Eine Sonderstellung nimmt Kohelet ein, da er die Begriffe für die lehrmäßig fest umrissene »Schulweisheit« gebraucht. In den wenigen sonstigen Vorkommen ist an Zauber oder Wissenschaft gedacht.

Außerdem findet sich in den aramäischen Teilen des Alten Testaments 14 mal in substantivischer Bedeutung חַכִּימִים *Weiser* zur Bezeichnung von Männern, an die man sich zwecks Deutung von Träumen wendet, und achtmal das Substantiv חָכְמָה, das in Esr 7 25 die Tora und sonst die dem Daniel verliehene Gabe der Traumdeutung meint.

Der Überblick zeigt, daß die übliche Übersetzung *weise, Weisheit* unglücklich und weithin unzutreffend ist. Sie wird weder der Bedeutungsbreite der hebräischen Ausdrücke noch ihrem eigentlichen Sinn gerecht. So sehr im einzelnen eine Kenntnis vorausgesetzt ist, so wenig geht es doch um eine tiefere Erkenntnis in theoretischer Bewältigung der Lebens- und Weltfragen als vielmehr um eine Lösung praktischer Art aufgrund konkreter Anforderungen. Es handelt sich um ein vorsichtiges und überlegtes und daher geschicktes und sachkundiges Vorgehen und Handeln, um sich der Welt zu bemächtigen, die verschiedensten Aufgaben des Lebens und dieses selbst zu meistern. Es hat sich mit dem ganzen Leben zu befassen und auf allen Lebensgebieten zu betätigen. Unter Berücksichtigung aller Einzelaspekte bedeutet חכם das *Klugsein und Kundigsein zum Zweck praktischer Gestaltung*. Wenn dazu öfters das Wort לֵב tritt[5], wird ersichtlich, daß das Kundigsein zwar keine Eigenschaft darstellt, wohl aber aus einem inneren *Sinn* für das kundige Handeln entspringen kann, der durch Kenntnis der Tradition, Erziehung und eigene Erfahrung gefördert wird. Wie es sich beim Menschen findet, so auch bei den Göttern und bei Jahwe, ohne daß man sagen könnte, daß sich eine Vorstellung aus der anderen entwickelt hätte.

Der genannten Bedeutung von חכם entspricht es, daß als parallele Ausdrücke am häufigsten Derivate von בין (unterscheidend) *einsehen*, (zu handeln) *verstehen* er-

---

[5] So Ex 28 3 31 6 35 25 36 1f. 8 Hi 9 4 37 24 Prov 10 8 11 29 16 21; als *Verstand* I Reg 5 9.

scheinen: נָבוֹן *einsichtig, kundig*[6], בִּינָה *Einsicht*[7] und תְּבוּנָה *Einsicht, Geschick* (des Handwerkers)[8]. An zweiter Stelle folgen Derivate von ידע, die z. T. das *Verständigsein*[9], z. T. das *Erfahrensein* (Dtn 1 13. 15) betonen, aber auch das *Geschick* des Kunsthandwerkers oder die Zauber*kunst* bezeichnen[10]. An ein praktisches Verhalten ist gedacht, wenn zu den von חכם hergeleiteten Begriffen als parallele Ausdrücke *Geradheit, Redlichkeit* (Prov 4 11), *das Herz den geraden Weg führen* (Prov 23 19) und צַדִּיק *gerecht, fromm* (Dtn 16 19 Prov 9 9 23 24 Koh 9 1) treten. Die gleiche Verbindung ist bei den gegensätzlichen Ausdrücken zu beobachten: der *Tor* ist weniger dumm als vielmehr zum richtigen Handeln unfähig[11]. Die entsprechenden Ausdrücke beziehen sich weniger auf das Denken und Erkennen, sondern mehr auf das Handeln. Torheit ist Unordnung in der Lebensmitte des Menschen, die sich zunächst in seinem Verhalten, dann allerdings auch in Unbesonnenheit und Überheblichkeit auswirkt[12].

II. Die Weisheit als altorientalische und israelitisch-alttestamentliche Erscheinung

Einerseits sind die Begriffsinhalte von חכם weithin durch eine entsprechende gemeinsame altorientalische Gedankenwelt bestimmt und gehören insbesondere die alttestamentlichen Weisheitsbücher, in denen die Begriffe überwiegend erscheinen, in den Kreis der in ihren Grundzügen wesensgleichen altorientalischen Weisheitsliteratur hinein. Andererseits ist in Israel die Begriffsbildung kräftiger als sonst vorangetrieben und die internationale und überreligiöse eigentliche Weisheitslehre sowohl nationalisiert als auch dem Jahweglauben eingegliedert und angepaßt worden.

1. In Mesopotamien fehlt ein dem hebräischen חכם entsprechender Begriff[13]. Von den überlieferungsmäßig und philologisch schwieri-

---

[6] So Gen 41 33. 39 Dtn 1 13 4 6 I Reg 3 12 Jes 5 21 29 14 Jer 4 22 Hos 14 10 Prov 1 5 17 28 18 15 Koh 9 11.

[7] So Dtn 4 6 Jes 29 14 Hi 28 12. 20 38 36 39 17 Prov 2 3 7 4 9 10.

[8] So Ex 36 1 I Reg 5 9 7 14 Jer 10 12 51 15 Ob 8 Hi 12 12f. Prov 2 2 3 19 5 1 24 3.

[9] So Jer 4 22 Hi 34 2 Koh 6 8; vgl. auch טַעַם *verständig* Prov 26 16.

[10] I Reg 7 14 Jes 47 10. דַּעַת *Einsicht* Prov 5 2 15 2.7 21 11, *Wissen* Koh 1 18, *Erkenntnis* Jes 33 6.

[11] Neben אֱוִיל *töricht, dumm* steht אֱוִלִי *ungeschickt, unbrauchbar*, während אִוֶּלֶת (*unfromme*) *Torheit* mit עשה *unbesonnen handeln* bedeutet. כְּסִיל ist religiös *frech* und in praktischen Dingen *töricht*. לֵץ *Schwätzer, Spötter* ist derjenige, der den Mangel an Kundigsein in seinen Worten zeigt. נָבָל *nichtig, töricht* bedeutet *unverständig* hinsichtlich Verstand und ethischem Verhalten, נְבָלָה neben *Dummheit* euphemistisch die *arge Sünde*. סָכָל ist der *töricht* Handelnde (vgl. das Substantiv סִכְלוּת bei Koh). Von I פתה *unerfahren sein, sich verleiten lassen* ist פֶּתִי als Bezeichnung des jungen, unerfahrenen, leicht verleitbaren, *einfältigen Menschen* hergeleitet.

[12] Vgl. auch W. Caspari, Über den biblischen Begriff der Torheit, NkZ 39 (1928), 668—695.

[13] W. G. Lambert, Babylonian Wisdom Literature, 1960, 1.

gen sumerischen Texten abgesehen[14], hat das Babylonische den Ausdruck *nēmequ* »Weisheit« und mehrere Adjektive »weise« (*enqu, mūdú, ḫassu, etpēšu*). Doch werden sie nur selten im Sinn der alttestamentlichen Weisheitsliteratur verwendet[15]; vielmehr bezieht *Weisheit* sich gewöhnlich auf das Geschick und die Fertigkeit in Kultus und Magie und ist der *Weise* der darin Eingeweihte. In dem Text »Ich will preisen den Herrn der Weisheit«[16] ist der Gott Marduk gemeint, dessen »Weisheit« darin besteht, daß er der Riten des Exorzismus kundig ist. Das akkadische Wort *hakâmu etwas begreifen, verstehen* ist wahrscheinlich ein westsemitisches Lehnwort und, da synonym mit *lamâdu lernen*, wohl schon als fertiger terminus technicus übernommen[17].

Ungeachtet des fehlenden Sammelbegriffs gibt es eine ziemlich umfangreiche mesopotamische Literatur, die inhaltlich den alttestamentlichen Weisheitsbüchern entspricht[18]. Obwohl sie vornehmlich in akkadischer Fassung vorliegt, geht sie weithin auf sumerische Überlieferungen zurück. In alter sumerischer Fassung sind eine größere Zahl von Sprichwortsammlungen erhalten (z. T. auf Schultafeln) und gewöhnlich nach dem ersten Schriftzeichen der Sprichwörter zusammengestellt[19]. Ihre Sammler gehören demnach offensichtlich den gleichen Kreisen an, die die sumerische Listenwissenschaft geschaffen haben; durch diese sollte eine systematische Ordnung der gesamten Gegenstands- und Erfahrungswelt ermöglicht werden[20]. Diese Ordnung ist beim praktischen Gebrauch wohl nicht rational erläutert, sondern durch die Heranziehung von Mythen und anderen Dichtungen, die von der Schaffung oder Wiederherstellung der Ordnung nach chaotischen

---

[14] Zwar glaubt J. J. A. van Dijk, La Sagesse suméro-accadienne, 1953, 17—21, in sumerisch ME den zentralen Begriff im Sinne einer »immanence divine dans la matière morte et vivante, incréée, inchangeable, subsistante, mais impersonnelle« gefunden zu haben; aber angesichts der Kritik daran (T. Fish, Rez. in: JSS 1, 1956, 286—288) erscheint diese Auffassung fragwürdig.

[15] Lambert a. a. O. 24f. nennt als mögliches Beispiel die Weisheitssprüche, Counsels of Wisdom.   [16] AOT 273—281; ANET 434—437.

[17] Vgl. W. Gesenius—F. Buhl, Hebräisches und aramäisches Handwörterbuch zum Alten Testament, 1915[17], s. v. חכם.

[18] AOT 284—295; ANET 410f. 425—430. 434—440; Lambert a. a. O.

[19] S. N. Kramer, Sumerian Wisdom Literature, BASOR 122 (1951), 28—31; van Dijk a. a. O. 5—11 (ausführliche Lit.); ANET 425—427; E. I. Gordon, The Sumerian Proverb Collections, JAOS 74 (1954), 82—85; Sumerian Proverbs: »Collection Four«, ebd. 77 (1957), 67—79; A New Look at the Wisdom of Sumer and Akkad, BiOr 17 (1960), 122—152. Bereits dieser veröffentlichte Bruchteil des gesamten Materials läßt die gleiche Art des Sammelns erkennen, die für Prov angewendet worden ist.

[20] Vgl. im einzelnen L. Matouš, Die lexikalischen Tafelserien der Babylonier und Assyrer in den Berliner Museen, I 1933; W. von Soden. Leistung und Grenze sumerischer und babylonischer Wissenschaft, Die Welt als Geschichte 2 (1936), 411—464. 509—557; Zweisprachigkeit in der geistigen Kultur Babyloniens, 1960.

Verhältnissen erzählten, anschaulich gemacht worden. Im Sinn der Sumerer waren die Listen die systematische Ergänzung zu den bloß paradigmatischen Dichtungen. Indem die Babylonier und Assyrer sie übernahmen und weiterbildeten, ist ein ganzer Zweig der Weisheitslehre in Form der Bildungsweisheit ins Leben gerufen worden, die ihre endgültige Gestalt besonders in der großen Serie ḪAR-ra (*ḫubullu*) mit 24 Tafeln und Tausenden von Eintragungen erhalten hat. Wie sie sich mittels der Ordnung der Namen der Welt bemächtigen will, so wollen die Sprichwortsammlungen die Gesetzmäßigkeit des Lebens erfassen, um es meistern zu können. Andere Texte befassen sich, manchmal in der Form von Weisheitssprüchen, mit ethischen Fragen und erteilen praktische Ratschläge für ein der Weltordnung entsprechendes und daher erfolgreiches Leben[21] oder gehen auf die Probleme ein, die sich aus eben dieser Lebensauffassung ergeben[22], so daß man einige gern als Vorläufer des alttestamentlichen Hiob betrachtet[23]. Schließlich zählt man herkömmlich Fabeln, Dispute und Debatten sowie weitere, z. T. gattungsmäßig schlecht bestimmbare Texte zur Weisheitsliteratur[24].

2. In Ägypten liegt ein deutlicherer Ansatz zur Begriffsbildung vor. Die Norm des Verhaltens, das die Weisheitslehren vermitteln wollen, wird durch den Ausdruck Maat umschrieben[25]. Dieser zentrale Begriff ist freilich nicht eindeutig geprägt und schwer übersetzbar: gewöhnlich *Wahrheit*, besser *Recht, Richtigkeit, Ur-Ordnung, Weltordnung*. Dabei ist zwischen göttlicher und menschlicher, himmlischer und irdischer Richtigkeit und Ordnung nicht zu trennen, da es nur eine einzige Richtigkeit und Ordnung gibt, die in der ganzen Welt gleichermaßen gilt. Ziel der Weisheitslehren ist es, der von der Gottheit stammenden Ordnung (Maat)[26] den Weg dadurch zu ebnen, daß

---

[21] Die bei Lambert a. a. O. in Kap. 4—5 enthaltenen Texte.

[22] Die bei Lambert a. a. O. in Kap. 2—3 enthaltenen Texte.

[23] Vgl. mit weiterer Lit. J. J. Stamm, Das Leiden des Unschuldigen in Babylon und Israel, 1948; A. Kuschke, Altbabylonische Texte zum Thema »Der leidende Gerechte«, ThLZ 81 (1956), 69—76; Gese a. a. O. 51—69. Jedoch sind die Texte formgeschichtlich nicht mit dem Buch Hiob, sondern mit Psalmen vergleichbar und weisen inhaltlich neben mehr am Rande liegenden Parallelen grundlegende Unterschiede gegenüber dem Buch Hiob auf.

[24] Vgl. Kramer a. a. O.; van Dijk a. a. O.; Gordon, New Look a. a. O.

[25] A. de Buck, Het religieus karakter der oudste egyptische wijsheid, NThT 21 (1932), 322—349; H. Frankfort, Ancient Egyptian Religion, 1948, passim; H. Brunner, Die Weisheitsliteratur, in: HdO I 2, 1952, 93—96; R. Anthes, Die Maat des Echnaton von Amarna, JAOS Suppl 14, 1952; Gese a. a. O. 11—21.

[26] Brunner a. a. O. 93: »Als Göttin gehört Maat in das religiöse System von Heliopolis, wo sie als Tochter des Sonnengottes auftritt. Sie kam als rechte Ordnung aller Dinge in der ‚Urzeit' zu den Menschen herab. Durch böse Anschläge des Seth und seiner Genossen wurde diese Ordnung gestört, durch den Sieg des Horus wiederhergestellt.

man sie überliefert. Vorgeblich unter fast völligem Absehen von der eigenen Erfahrung, die in der alttestamentlichen Weisheitslehre eine große Rolle spielt, verstehen sich die weisen Lehrer als getreue Überlieferer einer objektiv wahren, längst vorhandenen und gültigen Richtigkeit[27]. Indem die Erkenntnisse vom Wesen dieser Maat überliefert werden, soll sie durchgesetzt und dadurch ein harmonischer Zustand in Staat und Gesellschaft hergestellt werden. Da die Maat als der »richtige Lebensweg« eine unwandelbare Größe ist, gilt sie für jeden Menschen der jeweils angesprochenen sozialen Gruppe im gleichen Maße und unverändert. Aufgabe des Menschen ist es dann, sich ihr unterzuordnen und darin die Norm weisen Handelns zu erblicken. Das Ideal dieses Menschen ist der »Schweigende« oder — unter Verwendung des Begriffs Maat — der »rechte Schweiger«, der stets Herr der Lage ist und Selbstbeherrschung übt, weil er sich nach der Maat richtet, der sich auch äußerlich und innerlich zurückhält und alle Erregung vermeidet[28]. Sein Gegenbild ist der »Heiße«, der seinen Begierden unterlegene, unbeherrschte Mensch[29]. Dem Verhalten des Menschen entspricht das Ergebnis. So gewiß Erfolg des Handelns und »innere Wahrheit« desselben eine Einheit bilden, ist nicht zu übersehen, daß die Verhaltensregeln teilweise rein utilitaristisch begründet werden; dem Gehorchenden winken Nutzen und Erfolg, dem Übertreter drohen Schaden und Nachteil[30]. Teilweise wird statt dessen einfach hinzugefügt: »denn das ist Gottes Wille« oder »das ist ein Abscheu Gottes«. Beide Begründungen gehören für ägyptisches Denken zusammen, da jeder, der gegen die Maat verstößt, sich zugleich gegen den göttlichen Willen vergeht und daher Schaden leidet.

In stärkerem Maße als der Ansatz zur Begriffsbildung hat die ägyptische Weisheitsliteratur[31] auf Israel eingewirkt[32]. Da der Begriff

---

Als Verkörperung des Horus setzt jeder neue König bei seiner Krönung diese rechte Ordnung erneut ein, ein neuer Zustand der Maat, d. h. des Friedens und der Gerechtigkeit bricht an.«

[27] Dem entspricht es, wenn Jes 19 11 die Ratgeber des Pharao ihr Wissen damit erklären läßt, daß sie Schüler von Weisen und Königen der Vorzeit sind.

[28] Vgl. auch G. Lanczkowski, Reden und Schweigen im ägyptischen Verständnis, vornehmlich des Mittleren Reiches, in: Grapow-Festschrift, 1955, 186—196.

[29] Ähnlich sprechen Prov 15 18 22 24 29 22 unter Verwendung von חֵמָה vom *hitzigen* Mann oder *Hitzkopf* und sagt Prov 29 11, daß der Tor seine Erregung sich austoben läßt, während der Weise sie beschwichtigt.

[30] Daher schießt die völlige Ablehnung eines utilitaristischen Verständnisses durch Gese a. a. O. über das Ziel hinaus.

[31] A. Erman, Die Literatur der Ägypter, 1923, 86—121. 238—302; R. Anthes, Lebensregeln und Lebensweisheit der alten Ägypter, 1933; AOT 23—46; ANET 405—410. 412—425; F. W. von Bissing, Altägyptische Lebensweisheit, 1955.

[32] Besonders W. O. E. Oesterley, The Wisdom of Egypt and the Old Testament, 1927;

Maat die zwei im modernen Denken unterschiedenen Bereiche der Ordnung des Kosmos und der Ordnung des menschlichen Lebens umfaßt, gehören vor allem zwei Literaturgattungen zur Weisheitsliteratur: die Listenwissenschaft der Onomastika[33], die wahrscheinlich von der sumerischen Listenwissenschaft beeinflußt ist[34], und die »Lehren« oder Instruktionen[35], für die sich eine feste Form herausgebildet hat[36] und von denen sieben ganz oder fast ganz erhalten, fünf weitere in Bruchstücken überliefert und sechs oder sieben andere nur dem Titel nach bekannt sind[37]. Außerdem finden sich einzelne Schriften, die nicht unmittelbar belehrender, sondern betrachtender Art oder als Auseinandersetzungsliteratur zu bezeichnen sind und herkömmlich zur Weisheitsliteratur gezählt werden.

3. Obwohl aus dem übrigen Alten Orient keine oder nur geringfügige Weisheitsüberlieferungen vorliegen[38], hat man in Israel nicht nur um die Weisheit in Babylonien (Jer 50 35 51 57; vgl. Jes 44 25 47 10) und Ägypten (I Reg 5 10; vgl. Gen 41 8 Ex 7 11), sondern auch um diejenige anderer Völker gewußt: der Kanaanäer (Ez 28 3. 17: Phönizier allgemein; Ez 27 8: צמר wahrscheinlich Ṣumra, nördlich Tripolis, unweit Arwad; Sach 9 2: Sidon)[39], der Edomiter (Jer 49 7 Ob 8

P. Humbert, Recherches sur les sources égyptiennes de la littérature sapientiale d'Israël, 1929; A. Causse, Sagesse égyptienne et sagesse juive, RHPhR 9 (1929), 149—169; S. Morenz, Die ägyptische Literatur und die Umwelt, in: HdO I 2, 1952, 194—206 (mit Lit.); E. Würthwein, Die Weisheit Ägyptens und das Alte Testament, 1960. K. Galling, Der Prediger, 1940, weist besonders auf die Parallelität mit dem ägyptischen Papyrus Insinger hin.

[33] A. H. Gardiner, Ancient Egyptian Onomastica, 1947; H. Grapow, Wörterbücher, Repertorien, Schülerhandschriften, in: HdO I 2, 1952, 187—193.

[34] A. Alt, Die Weisheit Salomos, ThLZ 76 (1951), 139—144 (= Kleine Schriften zur Geschichte des Volkes Israel, II 1953, 90—99).

[35] Die ägyptische Bezeichnung umfaßt darüber hinaus die Bedeutung »Erziehung, Unterricht« und besonders die theologische Lehre.

[36] So lautet der Titel regelmäßig: »Beginn der Lehre, die X für seinen Sohn (Schüler) Y verfaßt hat«.

[37] Beschreibung im einzelnen bei Brunner a. a. O. 96—110. Vgl. ferner B. Gemser, The Instructions of ʿOnchsheshonqy and Biblical Wisdom Literature, VTSuppl VII, 1960, 102—128.

[38] Das Buch Achiqar dürfte ungeachtet seiner syrischen und aramäischen Version auf eine assyrische Urform zurückgehen.

[39] Vgl. W. F. Albright, Some Canaanite-Phoenician Sources of Hebrew Wisdom, VTSuppl III, 1955, 1—15; Ch. L. Feinberg, Ugaritic Literature and the Book of Job, Diss. Baltimore 1945; C. I. K. Story, The Book of Proverbs and Northwest-Semitic Literature, JBL 64 (1945), 319—337; M. J. Dahood, Canaanite-Phoenician Influence in Qoheleth, Bibl 33 (1952), 30—52. 191—221; Some Northwest-Semitic Words in Job, ebd. 38 (1957), 306—320; Qoheleth and Northwest Semitic Philology, ebd. 43 (1962), 349—365; Proverbs and Northwest Semitic Philology, 1963; North-

Hi 2 11)⁴⁰ und der »Ostleute« in der Safa-Gegend im nördlichen Ostjordanland (I Reg 5 10)⁴¹. Ob die in I Reg 5 11 genannten Weisen — der Esrachit Etan, ferner Heman, Chalkol und Darda als Söhne Machols — Edomiter oder Kanaanäer sein sollen, ist nicht einwandfrei ersichtlich⁴². Über diese Kenntnis und wohl auch Beeinflussung hinaus reicht die Abhängigkeit der israelitischen von der altorientalischen Weisheitslehre bis in die überlieferten alttestamentlichen Texte hinein. Wie Prov 22 17—23 11 Exzerpte aus der ägyptischen Lehre des Amen-em-ope darstellen⁴³ und 23 13-14 aus der Lehre des Achiqar entlehnt sind, so werden wohl mit Recht die »Worte Agurs, des Sohnes Jakes, 'des Massaiten'⁴⁴«, in Prov 30 1-14 und die »Worte Lemuels, des Königs von Massa« in Prov 31 1-9 von Angehörigen eines nichtisraelitischen Stammes hergeleitet⁴⁵.

4. Die in Israel trotz der einheitlichen Begriffswelt vielschichtige Erscheinung der חכמה, ebenso ihr Verflochtensein in die altorientalischen Zusammenhänge und ihre dennoch zu beobachtende Eigenart werden an verschiedenen Stadien der geschichtlichen Entfaltung ersichtlich.

Ein praktisches, auf Erfahrung gegründetes Kundigsein von bestimmten Gesetzen der Welt und Tätigkeiten des Lebens hat es stets gegeben, da der Mensch — unabhängig von seiner Kulturstufe — sich vor der Aufgabe sieht, sich seiner Umwelt zu bemächtigen und sein Leben in ihr zu meistern. Daher ist die Notwendigkeit gegeben, in der Vielfalt der Erscheinungen und Geschehnisse nach einer Ordnung und

---

west Semitic Philology and Job, in: The Bible in Current Catholic Thought, 1962, 55—74.

[40] R. H. Pfeiffer, Edomitic Wisdom, ZAW 44 (1926), 13—25; Wisdom and Vision in the Old Testament, ebd. 52 (1934), 93—101; Introduction to the Old Testament, 1941, 678—683, hat den Einfluß edomitischer Gedanken auf Israel weit überschätzt.

[41] Lokalisierung nach O. Eißfeldt, Das Alte Testament im Lichte der safatenischen Inschriften, ZDMG 104 (1954), 88—118 (= Kleine Schriften, III 1966, 289—317).

[42] Edomiter: E. Meyer, Die Israeliten und ihre Nachbarstämme, 1906, 350; Kanaanäer: W. F. Albright, Die Religion Israels im Lichte der archäologischen Ausgrabungen, 1956, 142f.

[43] Lit. bei B. Gemser, Sprüche Salomos, 1963², 13f.; E. Sellin—G. Fohrer, Einleitung in das Alte Testament, 1969¹¹, 351f. Die manchmal geäußerte Ansicht, daß umgekehrt Amen-em-ope abhängig sei, ist längst gründlich widerlegt worden.

[44] Es ist הַמַּשָּׂאִי statt »der Ausspruch« zu lesen.

[45] Gemser a. a. O. 103. 105 weist auf parallele sabäisch-minäische Namen und andere Einzelheiten hin, die an einen arabischen Stamm denken lassen. Dagegen handelt es sich nach W. F. Albright, The Biblical Tribe of Maśśā and some Congeners, in: Studi Orientalistici Levi Della Vida, I 1956, 1—14, um einen halb seßhaften Aramäerstamm der syrischen Wüste und in den Worten Agurs und Lemuels um leicht hebraisierte, ursprünglich aramäische Texte aus dem 10. Jh. oder noch früherer Zeit. Wieder anders G. Sauer, Die Sprüche Agurs, 1963.

Gesetzmäßigkeit zu suchen, in die man sich einschalten und die man sich zunutze machen kann. Dies vollzieht sich vor allem in volkstümlichen Sprichwörtern, die Erkenntnisse und Erfahrungen einfach feststellen und es dem Menschen überlassen, die Folgerungen für sein Verhalten daraus zu ziehen (I Sam 24 14 Prov 11 2a 16 18 18 12), wobei die Feststellung durchaus paradoxen Charakter tragen kann (Prov 11 24 20 17 25 15 27 7). So stellt man die Einsichten zusammen und nebeneinander, auch wenn sie sich geradezu widersprechen, um den Rahmen und die Grenzen der Ordnungen zu erfassen, aber ohne sie auf einen allgemeingültigen Grundsatz zurückführen und ein System schaffen zu wollen. Die große Bedeutung solcher Sprichwörter zeigt sich daran, daß man sie später oft um eine zweite Zeile erweitert hat, die ein den Menschen betreffendes Entsprechungsverhältnis feststellt (Prov 25 23 26 20 27 20 Sir 13 1).

Ungeachtet der wahrscheinlich schon früh erfolgten Berührungen mit der altorientalischen und besonders der ägyptischen Weisheitslehre ist diese im eigentlichen Sinn während der Regierung Salomos am Königshof und in den Kreisen der zahlreich werdenden Beamtenschaft im Lande heimisch und an der zumindest in Jerusalem anzunehmenden Weisheitsschule gepflegt worden[46]. So ist nicht verwunderlich, daß besonders häufig von der »Weisheit« Salomos die Rede ist[47], von seiner herrscherlichen, richterlichen oder lehrmäßigen Weisheit[48], und wenigstens das Buch Proverbia auf ihn als den Prototyp des »Weisen« zurückgeführt wird[49]. Einen genaueren Rückschluß läßt die alte Notiz über die Weisheit Salomos in I Reg 5 12-13 zu[50]: »Er dichtete 3000 Sprüche und seiner Lieder waren 1005. Er redete über die Bäume — von der Zeder, die auf dem Libanon steht, bis zum Ysop, der an der Mauer wächst — und redete über das Vieh, die Vögel, das Kriechgetier und die Fische«. Zieht man die Übertreibung der höfischen Geschichtsschreibung ab und bedenkt, daß das Gesagte, das Salomo als dem absoluten Herrscher zugeschrieben wird, eigentlich seiner Zeit und Regierung allgemein gilt, so ergeben sich, wenn man die falsche Verbindung der hohen Zahlen mit Sprüchen und Liedern löst,

---

[46] Vgl. K. Galling, Die Krise der Aufklärung in Israel, 1952, 5—10; H.-J. Hermisson, Studien zur israelitischen Spruchweisheit, 1968, 97—136.

[47] I Reg 2 6. 9 3 12. 28 5 9-11. 14. 21. 26 10 4. 6-8. 23f. 11 41 II Chr 1 10. 12 2 11 9 3. 5-7. 22f.

[48] Vgl. M. Noth, Die Bewährung von Salomos »Göttlicher Weisheit«, VTSuppl III, 1955, 225—237.

[49] Obwohl dies auch für das Buch Kohelet meist als Fiktion des Verfassers angenommen wird, scheint es angesichts 1 16 und ähnlicher Einzelheiten nicht völlig gesichert. Dagegen dürften die in I Reg 5 12 erwähnten »Lieder« ein Anlaß gewesen sein, das Hohelied auf Salomo zurückzuführen.

[50] Vgl. Alt a. a. O., der freilich die Sprüche und Lieder mit der Natur- statt der Lebensweisheit in Verbindung bringt.

nach Form und Inhalt zwei Arten von Weisheitslehre: 1. die aus der Bezogenheit dieser Weisheit auf die Erscheinungen der Pflanzen- und Tierwelt sich ergebende Listenwissenschaft, deren jerusalemische Listen anscheinend 1005 bzw. 3000 Stichwörter umfaßten[51] und die man besser als Bildungs- denn als Naturweisheit bezeichnet, weil sie über bloße Naturerscheinungen hinausgreift; 2. die aus der angegebenen Form von Spruch und Lied[52] zu erschließende Lebensweisheit, die kluge, moralische und manchmal auch religiöse Verhaltensregeln erteilt[53]. Demnach finden sich auch in Israel die beiden Hauptzweige der altorientalischen Weisheitslehre, die in Mesopotamien und Ägypten zu beobachten sind. Eine Mittelstellung zwischen ihnen nehmen das in I Reg 10 1 mit der Weisheit in Beziehung gesetzte Rätsel (vgl. auch Prov 1 6), der wahrscheinlich aus ihm entstandene Zahlenspruch und die Fabel ein[54].

Die Lage im 8. Jh. ist einerseits dadurch gekennzeichnet, daß Jesaja sich veranlaßt sieht, gegenüber den »Weisen« mit ihren scheinbar klugen und doch verderblichen Plänen und Maßnahmen kritisch Stellung zu nehmen[55]. Es ist deutlich, daß er die regierende Schicht meint, so daß die »Weisheit« wie z. Zt. Salomos die Bildung und Moral des hohen Beamtentums im weiteren Sinne darstellt. Dem entspricht andererseits, daß nach der glaubhaften Überschrift (Prov 25 1) die ganze Sammlung Prov 25—29 durch die »Männer Hiskias, des Königs von Juda« (also gegen 700 v. Chr.) zusammengestellt worden ist. Allem Anschein nach sind diese Jahrzehnte eine Zeit erhöhter Bedeutung der Weisheitslehre für das öffentliche Leben.

---

[51] Die weitere Verarbeitung zu Sprüchen und Liedern ist nur gelegentlich zu besonderen Zwecken erfolgt, z. B. in den Zahlensprüchen von Prov und der Gottesrede Hi 38ff.

[52] Auch das Weisheitslied oder -gedicht kann מָשָׁל genannt werden, Ps 49 5. Ein Vergleich der beiden in Hi 18 5-21 20 4-29 vorliegenden Gedichte ist insofern aufschlußreich, als sich aus dem zweiten im Unterschied von dem in sich geschlossenen ersten seine Entstehung aus einzelnen Sprüchen oder Spruchgruppen erkennen läßt. In 20 4-29 bildet die Schilderung keine zusammenhängende Komposition. Die Aufeinanderfolge der Strophen ist willkürlicher und der Gesamteindruck uneinheitlicher; mehrfach sind ursprünglich selbständige Weisheitssprüche aufgenommen, aber nicht in den Zusammenhang eingeschmolzen worden, v. 10. 16. 24 f.

[53] In Zusammenhang damit stehen die der Weisheitsliteratur eigentümlichen Heilssprüche, die im Unterschied vom בָּרוּךְ des kultischen Segensspruchs mit אַשְׁרֵי eingeleitet werden.

[54] Vgl. zum Ganzen besonders J. Hempel, Die althebräische Literatur und ihr hellenistisch-jüdisches Nachleben, 1930, 44—56; J. Schmidt, Studien zur Stilistik der alttestamentlichen Spruchliteratur, 1936; A. R. Johnson, מָשָׁל, VTSuppl III, 1955, 162—169.

[55] Vgl. J. Fichtner, Jesaja unter den Weisen, ThLZ 74 (1949), 75—80 (= Gottes Weisheit, 1965, 18—26).

Erst gegen Ende des 7. Jh. erscheint die Basis verbreitert. Zwar beziehen Jer 50 35 51 57 sich nach wie vor lediglich auf die regierende Schicht (in Babylonien), aber in Dtn 1 13. 15 sind auch kleinste Vorgesetzte und in 16 19 alle Rechtspfleger gemeint. Jer 8 8f. nennt den Priester als Verwalter der Tora weise, während 18 18 von einem neben Priestern und Propheten bestehenden Stand von »Weisen« spricht, deren Aufgabe es ist, Rat zu erteilen. Ebenso enthält Jer 10 9 die nach I Reg 7 14 älteste literarische Verwendung von חכם für die handwerkliche Fertigkeit, von der sonst erst in nachexilischer Zeit in gehäufter Weise die Rede ist. Die immer weitere Ausdehnung der Begriffe ist ein Zeichen dafür, daß vom ausgehenden 7. Jh. an und besonders in nachexilischer Zeit die Weisheitslehre aus einer Beamtenbildung und -moral zu einer sozial und soziologisch nicht mehr eingeengten Angelegenheit breiter Kreise wird. Überliefert und gelehrt wird sie von einem Stand der Weisheitslehrer, deren typische Vertreter der Hiobdichter als Vorbild für das Auftreten der Freunde Hiobs benutzt hat und deren einer im Verfasser der Reden Elihus spricht (Hi 32—37). Ebenso charakterisiert der Schüler des Kohelet diesen als solchen Lehrer (Koh 12 9-11), während Koh 2 14. 16 חכם als terminus technicus für den nicht sehr vorteilhaft beurteilten »Schulweisen« benutzt (vgl. später Sir 39 1f. 8 51 23).

Dieser von Salomo bis in die Spätzeit lebendigen, sich allerdings auch wandelnden Weisheitslehre liegt ein Ideal der Bildung und Formung des ganzen Menschen zugrunde. Obwohl sie wie die Sprichwortweisheit ein Klug- und Kundigsein zur Weltbemächtigung und Lebensgestaltung bezweckt, sucht sie nicht mehr nur die Ordnungen und Gesetzmäßigkeiten in Welt und Leben festzustellen, sondern auf dieser Grundlage bewußt den Menschen zu erziehen. Ihr Ideal ist — dem der ägyptischen Lehren ähnlich — der »Kaltblütige« (Prov 17 27) im Gegensatz zum »Hitzkopf«, der »Langmütige« im Gegensatz zum »Jähzornigen« (Prov 14 29)[56], der Mensch mit »gelassenem Sinn«, der der verzehrenden »Leidenschaft« nicht nachgibt (Prov 14 30), sondern seine Affekte und Triebe beherrscht.

Im nachexilischen Israel ist im Zusammenhang mit den tiefgreifenden geistigen Wandlungen der Zeit in Kreisen der genannten Weisheitslehrer der Weisheitsbegriff in starkem Maße theologisch durchdacht und verwendet worden. Die Weisheit wird als göttlicher Anruf an den Menschen, als Offenbarungsmittler, als die große Erzieherin Israels und der Völker und sogar als das der Welt bei der Schöpfung

---

[56] Allgemein wird der Zorn als gefährlich beurteilt, weil er Unheil anrichtet und schlimme Folgen hat (Prov 6 34 15 1 16 14 19 19 27 4), Gottes gerechtes Walten in Frage stellt (Hi 8 3) und die Gottesfurcht zerstört (Hi 5 4); daher ist der Zornige dem Toren gleich (Prov 14 17. 29).

eingegebene göttliche Prinzip verstanden. So wurde das gesamte theologische Denken mehr oder weniger weisheitlich; zumindest wurde es in dem Oberbegriff der Weisheit in einer zuvor nicht bekannten Weise vereinheitlicht und zusammengefaßt[57]. Außer in Prov 1—9 und Hi 28 findet sich dies andeutungsweise in der inspirierten Weisheit Elihus, der sich in ihrem dauernden Besitz durch offenbarende Erleuchtung weiß, aber auch in der Gottesrede des Buches Hiob, in der die natürliche Welt als Schöpfung wenigstens im Ansatz zu der an den Menschen ergehenden Offenbarung in Beziehung gesetzt wird.

Werden durch die Einbeziehung von Schöpfung und Offenbarung in dieses weisheitlich-theologische Denken diejenigen Gebiete erfaßt, die das Klug- und Kundigsein der Bildungs- und Lebensweisheit nicht berührt und beiseite gelassen hatte, und wird nunmehr ein umfassendes theologisches System geschaffen[58], so mußte eben dieses System mit seinen unvermeidlichen Einseitigkeiten und Unzulänglichkeiten fast notwendig die Kritik wachrufen[59].

In dieser Entfaltung wird als erstes Kennzeichen der israelitischen Weisheit ihre Nationalisierung und Einfügung in das israelitische Volkstum sichtbar. Einerseits bedeutet das, daß sie je länger desto weniger standesgebunden ist, sondern das allgemein Menschliche jenseits aller sozialen und soziologischen Grenzen anspricht; ein Zeichen dafür ist die Aufnahme zahlreicher volkstümlicher Sprichwörter in die Sammlungen des Buches Proverbia. Andererseits wird die Weisheit bis in die Einzelheiten der Lage Israels in Palästina angepaßt. So folgt das der Gottesrede im Buch Hiob doch wohl in Auswahl zugrunde liegende Onomastikon nicht dem ägyptischen Schema, sondern war von Weltbild, landschaftlichen, klimatischen und zoologischen Besonderheiten Palästinas bestimmt, so daß die Beispiele der Gottesrede den Eigentümlichkeiten des palästinischen Raumes entsprechen.

Ein zweites Kennzeichen bildet die analoge Konkretisierung auf religiösem Gebiet, durch die die interreligiöse Weisheitslehre dem Jahweglauben angepaßt und zugeordnet wird. Daraus erklärt sich die große Rolle, die gegenüber der bloßen Weltklugheit die ethische Weisung und das ethische oder fromme Verhalten einnehmen, wobei sie zudem sehr stark den Forderungen des Jahweglaubens entsprechen. Vor allem wird nicht nur häufig der Jahwename statt der allgemeinen

---

[57] G. von Rad, Theologie des Alten Testaments, I 1957, 439.
[58] Von Rad a. a. O. 449: »Die späteren Weisheitslehrer müssen nach alledem die Träger einer sehr umfassenden, ja eigentlich enzyklopädischen Theologie gewesen sein«.
[59] Die Kritik entsteht freilich nicht dadurch, daß im System der Kontakt mit dem Wirken Jahwes in der Geschichte verlorenzugehen drohte (von Rad a. a. O. 451), sondern entzündet sich an dessen grundlegenden Behauptungen und letztlich am Vorhandensein eines Systems überhaupt, wie Hiob und Kohelet zeigen.

Bezeichnung »Gott, Gottheit« eingeführt und so die Gleichsetzung des Schöpfer- und Weltengotts mit Jahwe vollzogen, sondern auch die »Jahwefurcht« als Anfang der Weisheit betrachtet.

Das dritte Kennzeichen ist die umfassende Begriffsbildung mit Hilfe von חכם. Alles für das praktische Tun und Lassen erforderliche Klug- und Kundigsein wird bis zu den schwierigsten und verwickeltsten Sachverhalten mittels dieses einen Wortstammes ausgedrückt, sogar der Gegensatz לֹא חָכָם *unweise* (Dtn 32 6).

III. »Weisheit« (Klug- und Kundigsein) des Menschen

1. Magie und Mantik

In einigen Fällen entspricht die Verwendung von חכם der mesopotamischen Ausdrucksweise. Die ägyptischen חכמים sind den »Zauberern« מְכַשְּׁפִים gleich Ex 7 11, die חכמה Babels ist seine Zauberkunst (Jes 47 10 nach v. 9. 12). Die חכמים des Pharao sind ferner den »Wahrsagepriestern« חַרְטֻמִּים gleich (Gen 41 8), d. h. solchen, die die mantische Technik der Erkenntnis des Zukünftigen durch Traumdeutung üben[60]. So können sie neben dem »Wahrsager«[61] und »Orakelbefrager« stehen (Jes 44 25); חכם ist eine Bezeichnung desjenigen, der um die Hintergründe des Weltgeschehens und die künftigen Ereignisse zu wissen vorgibt. Sogar Tiere — Ibis und Hahn[62] — haben das Vermögen, das nahende Gewitter rechtzeitig anzukündigen (Hi 38 36). Ebenso sind noch in später Zeit חכמים diejenigen, »die sich auf die Zeiten verstehen« (Est 1 13), d. h. die Astrologen, die aufgrund ihrer Sternkunde das künftige Geschick ermitteln, wie sie nach dem MT auch Haman unter seinen Freunden hat, so daß er sie über künftiges Ergehen befragen kann (Est 6 13)[63]. So bilden die חכמים von Babel das Kollegium von Wahrsagern, Zauberern, Stern- und Zeichendeutern, das der König zur Deutung von Träumen heranzieht (vgl. Dan 2 27 4 3).

2. Fertigkeit und Können

חכם ist jemand, der sich auf etwas meisterlich versteht — und sei es nur auf das Tun des Bösen (Jer 4 22). So sind die Zauberer ihrer wirksamen Sprüche kundig und mächtig (Jes 3 3 Ps 58 6), bestimmte Frauen der Klagelieder (Jer 9 16) und die Priester des Gesetzes Jahwes, das sie meisterlich nach ihrem Willen verfälschen (Jer 8 8f.). Häufig

---

[60] Vielleicht meint auch Jes 19 12 die Zukunftsdeuter.
[61] Es ist בָּרִים statt des Schreibfehlers »leeres Geschwätz« zu lesen.
[62] Vgl. dazu G. Fohrer, Das Buch Hiob, 1963, z. St.
[63] Allerdings sind beide Stellen textlich nicht ganz sicher. In 1 13 sind vielleicht die Rechtskundigen gemeint, die sich auf »die Gesetze« (הַדָּתִים) verstehen, während in 6 13 wohl nur von den Freunden die Rede war (vgl. die Versionen).

findet sich die Wortgruppe zur Bezeichnung der handwerklich-künstlerischen Fertigkeit. חכם ist der kunstverständige Handwerker und der Künstler (Ex 36 8 II Chr 2 12f.), der das meisterliche Geschick und den Kunstsinn für jede Arbeit aufweist (Ex 31 3 35 10. 31 36 4 I Chr 28 21), insbesondere für die Arbeiten am Heiligtum (Ex 31 6 36 1f.) und zum Herstellen von Götterbildern (Jes 40 20). Dazu gehören der kunstverständige Metallarbeiter (I Chr 22 15 II Chr 2 6), d. h. der Schmied (Ex 35 35) als Erzschmied (I Kön 7 14) oder Goldschmied (Jer 10 9), ebenso der Zimmermann, Weber und Buntwirker (Ex 35 35), der künstlerisch mit Purpurstoffen umgehen (II Chr 2 6) und kostbare Gewänder herstellen kann (Jer 10 9) wie die Kleider Arons (Ex 28 3). חכמה ist die Kunstfertigkeit der Frauen im Spinnen (Ex 35 25f.), die Geschäftstüchtigkeit des Kaufmanns (Ez 28 3f.), das Wissen des Bauern um die jeweils erforderliche Arbeit (Jes 28 23-29) und die Schiffahrtkunst der Seeleute, die nur gegenüber dem noch mächtigeren Sturm versagt (Ps 107 27).

חכם beschreibt ebenfalls häufig die Regierungskunst. Wer über diese verfügt, kann König werden, obwohl er arm ist (Koh 4 13); und wer König ist, bedarf ihrer (II Chr 1 10). Dazu gehört es, daß man das Können des Eroberers besitzt, um Völker zu unterwerfen (Jes 10 13), und diplomatisch geschickt ein Vertragsangebot macht (I Reg 5 21), daß man die Fähigkeit zum Rechtsprechen hat (I Reg 3 28), um die Schuldigen aus der Gemeinschaft auszuscheiden (Prov 20 26), und den einsichtsvollen Entschluß zum Residenzbau faßt (II Chr 2 11). Die hohen Beamten des Königs sind als חכמים in der Regierungskunst erfahren (Jer 50 35 51 57), ob sie nun Verwaltungsaufgaben selbständig ausführen (Gen 41 33) oder politische Ratschläge erteilen (Jes 19 11). Schließlich aber muß jeder, sogar der kleinste Vorgesetzte, über ein entsprechendes Können verfügen (Dtn 1 13.15).

3. Klugheit, Schläue und List

Während den Straußen, deren Dummheit sprichwörtlich ist, die Klugheit fehlt (Hi 39 15. 17), gibt es andere Tiere, die trotz ihrer Kleinheit sinnvoll und auf Erhaltung ihres Lebens bedacht handeln, so daß sie »mit allen Wassern gewaschene«, *gewitzigte Kluge* sind (Prov 30 24-28). Diese Beispiele zeigen, daß חכם ein nicht von Moral bestimmtes Klug- und Kundigsein ausdrücken kann, das man braucht, um im Leben bestehen zu können[64]. Solche Klugheit oder Schläue besitzen die beiden Frauen, deren eine Joab zu David schickt, damit

---

[64] Nicht eindeutig ist Koh 2 19. Es wird als fraglich bezeichnet, ob der Erbe *klug* genug ist, um das ihm hinterlassene Vermögen richtig zu verwalten und zu nutzen, oder ob er über das nötige geschäftliche *Können* verfügt.

sie auf kluge Weise die Begnadigung Absaloms bewirkt (II Sam 14 2), und deren andere mit Joab verhandelt und ihre Ortschaft vor der Eroberung rettet, indem sie den Kopf des Aufrührers Seba anbietet (II Sam 20 16ff.). Dient diese politische Klugheit der Bewahrung vor größerem Unheil, so bringt die politische List der Ägypter Unheil über die unerwünschten Israeliten, indem ihre Lebenskraft durch Fronarbeit geschwächt wird (Ex 1 10); es ist ein Handeln im eigenen Interesse und zum Schaden anderer. Noch eindeutiger von solcher Art ist der listig-verschmitzte Rat, den Jonadab dem Davidsohn Amnon zur Befriedigung seines Begehrens nach seiner Halbschwester Tamar gibt (II Sam 13 3). Ebenso legt David dem Salomo nahe, schlau und listig einzufädeln, was zur Hinrichtung Joabs und Simeis führt; als kluger Mann wird er wissen, wie er sein Ziel erreichen kann (I Reg 2 6. 9). So stehen denn in Hi 5 13 die Schlauen im negativen Sinn den »Verschlagenen« נִפְתָּלִים parallel, die hinterlistige Machenschaften hegen und krumme Wege gehen (vgl. Dtn 32 5 Ps 18 27 Prov 8 8). Ähnlich haben nach Ansicht Elihus die Freunde Hiobs bekümmert festgestellt, daß sie bei Hiob eine חכמה gefunden haben, der sie nicht gewachsen sind und die allein Gott überwinden kann, d. h. offenbar eine negativ zu beurteilende *Schläue*, die ihren Argumenten immer wieder entwischt (Hi 32 13).

4. Lebensklugheit

Die חכמה ist der Klugheit, Erkenntnis und Besonnenheit eng verwandt (Prov 8 12) und in diesem Falle am besten als Lebensklugheit zu verstehen: als die Kunst, das Leben in jeder Beziehung und in allen Lagen meisterlich zu führen. Es ist eine »Steuermannskunst« תַּחְבֻּלוֹת (Prov 1 5 11 14 u. ö.), eine Technik, mit der man sich durch die Fährnisse des Lebens hindurch- und zum angestrebten Ziel hinsteuern kann. Sie weiß um Reichtum und Armut[65], um Freud und Leid, um die Notwendigkeit der Arbeit und den Erfolg von Freundlichkeit, Geschenk und Bestechung (Prov 10 15 12 25 13 7.8 14 10.13.20 15 13. 30 16 26 17 8 18 16 21 14). Sie kennt die richtige Einstellung zum Lebensgenuß und zum Umgang mit anderen Menschen[66]. Solche Klugheit, die am Beispiel der Ameise zu lernen ist (Prov 6 6), ist das, was den Menschen als seine Krone eigentlich auszeichnen kann (Prov 14 24)[67]. Dann versteht man, daß Gott die Welt lenkt (Dtn 32 29), weiß alles, was auf Erden vorgeht, und kann Gutes und Böses unter-

---

[65] Vgl. J. Fichtner, Die altorientalische Weisheit in ihrer israelitisch-jüdischen Ausprägung, 1933, 15—17.
[66] Vgl. im einzelnen Fichtner a. a. O. 17—23.
[67] Es ist עָרְמָה statt »Reichtum« zu lesen.

scheiden — gleich dem Gottesengel, wie es schmeichelhaft heißt (II Sam 14 17. 20), oder ist in allerlei Wissen bewandert (Dan 1 4) und hat Verständnis für die Wissenschaft (Dan 1 17). So lebensklug und -erfahren ist die Hofdame, die der Mutter Siseras dessen Ausbleiben zu erklären sucht (Jdc 5 29), im Gegensatz zu demjenigen Kind, das in der Krise der Geburtswehen den Weg nach draußen nicht zur rechten Zeit findet (Hos 13 13), zu den Edomitern, die nicht merken, was Jahwe mit ihnen vorhat, obwohl die Katastrophe sich schon abzeichnet (Jer 49 7), und zum gewöhnlichen Menschen, der unversehens stirbt, ohne es vorher zu merken und ohne zu wissen, wieso es mit ihm plötzlich zu Ende geht (Hi 4 21).

5. Bildung

Obwohl die höhere Bildung des Menschen nur in I Reg 5 9-14 mit dem Begriff חכמה in Verbindung gebracht wird, hat sie eine wesentlich größere Rolle gespielt, als die daran uninteressierte alttestamentliche Überlieferung erkennen läßt. Jedenfalls hat חכם auch das Kundigsein des Gebildeten beschrieben. Es fand seinen Niederschlag zunächst in den Onomastika der Listenwissenschaft, die später manchmal als Grundlage für Spruchreihen oder Dichtungen benutzt worden sind. Sie konnten die belebte und unbelebte Natur umfassen, wie Ps 104 148 Hi 38 4—39 30 Prov 30 15-33 zeigen, den Bereich der Erd- und Völkerkunde betreffen, worauf die Listen Gen 10 15 19ff. hinweisen, oder bestimmte Menschentypen erfassen, wie aus Hi 24 5-8 24 14-16 a 30 2-8 hervorgeht. An sich liegt dem eine echte Beobachtung zugrunde, die den Erscheinungen in der Welt unter dem Gesichtspunkt ihrer Andersartigkeit gegenüber dem Beobachter und zugleich ihrer sinnvollen Ordnung untereinander nachgeht. Sie erfolgt mit dem praktischen Ziel, sich dieser Welt auf solche Weise zu bemächtigen. Am deutlichsten wird dies in Hi 28 in dem — allerdings vergeblichen — Suchen nach dem letzten Geheimnis der Welt, dessen Besitz nicht nur theoretisches Wissen, sondern auch praktische Verfügbarkeit bedeuten würde. Freilich ist die Bildungsweisheit weithin aus den Schriften des Alten Testaments ausgeschlossen worden. Ein Rückschluß auf dieses Gebiet israelitischer Kultur ist nur aus den verhältnismäßig wenigen Stücken möglich, die Material dieser »Weisheit« benutzt haben (vgl. noch Gen 1 1—2 4a Ps 8 sf. 147 Hi 28 36 27—37 13 37 15-18 40 15-24 40 25—41 26 Cant 2 11-13 a 3 9-10 Koh 1 5-7 Δα 3 52-90)[68].

---

[68] Später Sir 39 26 ff. IV Esr 7 39-42. Vgl. besonders Alt a. a. O.; G. von Rad, Hiob 28 und die altägyptische Weisheit, VTSuppl III, 1955, 293—301; H. Richter, Die Naturweisheit des Alten Testaments im Buche Hiob, ZAW 70 (1958), 1—20; auch die Bedenken von R. B. Y. Scott, Solomon and the Beginnings of Wisdom in Israel, VTSuppl III, 1955, 262—279.

6. Verhaltensregeln

Mehrfach hat חכם die Bedeutung *Verhaltensregeln, Anweisungen* zum rechten Verhalten. Wenn Elihu den Hiob חכמה lehren will (Hi 33 33), möchte er ihm Verhaltensregeln geben und ihn zum rechten Verhalten anleiten. Der Mensch leiht nach Prov 2 2 der חכמה sein Ohr, indem er auf Worte und Gebote, d. h. auf Verhaltensregeln hört. Daher ist es die Aufgabe des Weisheitslehrers, Erkenntnis zu lehren, Sprüche kritisch zu ordnen, so daß sich daraus die חכמה als Anweisung zum rechten Verhalten ergibt, und schöngeformte, wahre Worte zu schreiben (Koh 12 9-11). Wie er selber Erkenntnis und Klugheit besitzt (z. B. Prov 14 24) und sich gern belehren läßt (z. B. Prov 12 15), so vermittelt er anderen die Einsicht (Prov 15 2. 7). Der Narr kann nur als weise gelten, solange er schweigt; sobald er Lebensregeln vermitteln will, verrät er sich. Darin hat das »si tacuisses, philosophus mansisses« sein alttestamentliches Gegenstück (Prov 17 28 Hi 13 5). חכם ist einer, der »Rat« עֵצָה erteilt wie der Priester die תּוֹרָה und der Prophet den דָּבָר (Jer 18 18), aber auch selber auf solchen Rat hört (Prov 12 15), auf den ebenfalls der Unweise angewiesen ist (Hi 26 3). Kommen derartige kluge und belehrende Worte aus dem »Herzen« (Prov 16 23) und vermag jemand in anziehender Weise zu belehren (Prov 16 21), so ist dergleichen im Unterschied vom gewöhnlichen Reden nicht wie »tiefes Wasser« in einer Zisterne, das dem Durstigen nichts nützt, sondern wie eine sprudelnde Quelle, die jedem nützt, der aus ihr trinken will (Prov 18 4). Dann läßt sich sogar der zornige König besänftigen, da man ihm die rechten Verhaltensregeln beibringen kann (Prov 16 14). Im Unterschied vom Toren und Spötter hört der חכם auf Verhaltensregeln und heilsame Rügen (Prov 15 12. 31), läßt seine Erregung sich nicht austoben, sondern beschwichtigt sie (Prov 29 11), erregt keinen Aufruhr, sondern wirkt beruhigend auf andere ein (Prov 29 8), hat also nicht nur für sich selbst genug, sondern »weidet« durch seine Belehrung noch andere, d. h. führt sie auf den Weg zum Leben (vgl. Prov 6 23 10 17 15 24) und nährt sie mit Lebenskraft (vgl. Prov 3 18 10 11 13 14 16 22 mit den ursprünglichen mythischen Bildern des Lebensbaumes und der Lebensquelle).

7. Ethisches Verhalten

Aus der Anweisung und Regel ergibt sich das darin gelehrte rechte ethische Verhalten, das gleichfalls mit חכם bezeichnet wird (Prov 8 33 19 20 28 26). Es verleiht Verstand, doch setzt seine Verwirklichung wiederum Verstand voraus. Ein vergebliches Bemühen wäre es, das rechte Verhalten verwirklichen zu wollen, wenn kein Verstand da ist (Prov 17 16). So muß man sich bereits beim Suchen und Erlangen dieses Verhaltens recht verhalten. Es ist eine Angelegenheit der Ehrfurcht und Hingabe des Herzens, so daß der Spötter das Ziel nicht erreicht (Prov 14 6). Es handelt sich um ein inneres Bestimmtsein des Menschen (Prov 16 23), das man nicht wieder aufgeben soll, wenn man es besitzt (Prov 23 23). Darum ist eine ernste Haltung angemessen (Koh 7 4). Deswegen soll man sich vor alledem hüten, wovor das weise ethische Verhalten bewahren will (Prov 2 9-11) und was es verdirbt, wenn man dem nachgibt oder verfällt[69]: Wein und Rauschtrank (Prov 20 1), Saufen und Prassen (Prov 23 20f.), böse Leute (Prov 2 12-15) und fremde Frauen (Prov 2 16-19 5 1 7 4)[70], Reichtum (Ez 28 16ff.) und unrechter Gewinn (Koh 7 7), heftiges und leidenschaftliches Reden ohne inhaltliche Substanz und Wahrheit (Hi 15 2), Aneignung fremden Gutes, besonders durch Grenzverrückung und Verwendung von falschem Maß und Gewicht[71], Unrecht in der Gerichtsbarkeit durch Parteilichkeit, Geben oder Annehmen von Bestechung und falsche Zeugenaussage[72]. Das rechte Verhalten ist demgegenüber durch Geradheit und Redlichkeit gekennzeichnet (Prov 4 11 23 19). Es bedeutet gerechte und milde Behandlung der Armen, Witwen und Waisen[73] sowie rechtes Verhalten gegenüber den Eltern und dem persönlichen Feind[74]. Es ist gleich dem Recht (Ps 37 30) und befähigt daher zur Unterscheidung von Recht und Unrecht und damit zur Rechtspflege (Dtn 16 19 I Reg 3 12). Es besteht in einem Leben, das durch die Befolgung der weisen Lebensregeln (Prov 2 2) oder die Befolgung der göttlichen Gebote bestimmt ist (Dtn 4 6); ja, das göttliche Gesetz, die Tora, kann als eigentliche Quelle des rechten ethischen Verhaltens gelten (Ps 19 8 119 98)[75].

8. Frommes Verhalten

Ist חכמה als ethisches Verhalten oft mit religiösen Gedanken verknüpft, so bezeichnet der Begriff mehrfach geradezu das fromme Verhalten des Menschen. Wie der Unweise frevlerisch gegen Gott ist (Dtn 32 6), so hat der חכם die innere, fromme Einsicht darin, daß Gott die Welt lenkt (Dtn 32 39), in die Worte des Propheten und die Wege

---

[69] Zum Verführen vgl. ThW VI 236.
[70] Vor illegitimer Liebe, Ehebruch oder Unzucht wird oft gewarnt (Prov 5 6 24. 25-35 7 5-23). Dabei gilt der Ehebruch zunächst als Verletzung der fremden Ehe und Vergehen gegen fremdes Eigentum. Später wirken religiös-ethische Motive ein (Prov 5 21-23); zu ihnen gehört die Bezeichnung des Ehebruchs als »Schandtat« in Hi 31 11. Vgl. Fichtner a. a. O. 27f.
[71] Vgl. im einzelnen Fichtner a. a. O. 25—27.
[72] Vgl. im einzelnen Fichtner a. a. O. 28—30.
[73] Vgl. im einzelnen Fichtner a. a. O. 30—32.
[74] Vgl. im einzelnen Fichtner a. a. O. 33f.
[75] Mit Fichtner a. a. O. 81—90 ist daran festzuhalten, daß das »Gesetz« im eigentlichen Sinn des Wortes in Prov, Hi und Koh nicht genannt wird.

und Gnadentaten Jahwes (Hos 14 10 Ps 107 43), in die eigene Sünde (Ps 51 8) und die Begrenztheit des Lebens von Gott her (Ps 90 12). Diese Einsicht bewirkt Demut (Prov 11 2 13 10), aber auch ein rechtes Glauben und Vertrauen (Ps 90 12)[76].

Öfter wird חכמה mit der »Jahwefurcht« in Verbindung gebracht[77]. Im einzelnen ist die Sachlage unterschiedlich. Nach Prov 9 10 ist die Jahwefurcht der Anfang (תְּחִלָּה) und nach Prov 1 7 Ps 111 10 der Ausgangspunkt (רֵאשִׁית) der חכמה oder nach Prov 15 33 Züchtigung, die zu ihr führt. Nach Hi 28 28 besteht die חכמה in Jahwefurcht, nach Prov 14 16 ist der חכם gottesfürchtig, so daß beide Begriffe einander gleichgesetzt sind. Dagegen versteht nach Prov 2 6 der Mensch durch die von Jahwe verliehene חכמה die Jahwefurcht und gewinnt Gotteserkenntnis, so daß die Jahwefurcht weder die Voraussetzung frommen Kundigseins bildet noch ihm gleich ist, sondern die theologisch bestimmte חכמה den Anspruch erhebt, zu Gott hinzuführen. Immer bezeichnet der in der Weisheitslehre beliebte Ausdruck Jahwe- oder Gottesfurcht das fromme Verhalten. Er meint nicht die Angst vor Gott, sondern die religiöse Verehrung, wie sie Jahwe als Gott und wie sie jedem Gott von seinen Verehrern entgegengebracht wird. Sie äußert sich nicht im Kultus, der in diesem Zusammenhang nur eine ganz geringe Rolle spielt[78], sondern ist praktische Religion im täglichen Tun und Lassen, d. h. im rechten ethischen Verhalten. Wer daher diese Jahwefurcht als praktische Frömmigkeit (חכמה) übt, hat wertvolle Einsicht (Ps 111 10), so daß die wichtigste Erkenntnis des Lebens nicht auf den Gebieten des Kultus oder des Denkens, sondern auf dem Gebiet des rechten Handelns zu gewinnen ist. Daher kann Hi 37 24 sagen, daß Gott die חכמי לב die *Weisheitskundigen* oder *Verstandesweisen* nicht anblickt, während die Menschen ihm, dem Erhabenen,

---

[76] Vgl. A. Weiser, Die Psalmen, II 1959⁵, zu 90 12.

[77] Ebenso findet sich die Bezeichnung »Gottesfurcht«, z. B. Hi 1 1. Der verkürzte Ausdruck יִרְאָה kommt nur in den Reden des Eliphas vor (Hi 4 6 15 4 22 4), das bloße Verb ירא in Prov 14 16.

[78] Zum Kultus und zum Gebet, das im Unterschied vom Kultus in der Weisheit eine große Rolle spielt, vgl. Fichtner a. a. O. 36—46. Die Deutung seitens von Rad, Theologie des Alten Testaments, I 1957, 431, daß der von der Weisheit Belehrte ein Glied der Kultgemeinde war, dessen Leben unter kultischen Bindungen stand, und daß die Weisheit sich darauf beschränkt habe, das Leben außerhalb des Kultus zu ordnen, geht fehl. In Prov nehmen außer 3 9 (aus jüngerer Zeit) die übrigen Sprüche 15 8. 29 20 25 21 3. 27 28 9 30 12 eine mehr oder minder kritische Stellung zum Kultus ein und liegt der Ton nicht auf der kultischen Handlung, sondern auf der Beschaffenheit des kultisch Handelnden; schließlich wird als wertvoll nicht das Opfer, sondern das Gebet genannt, vgl. Fichtner a. a. O. 41f. Im übrigen ist die selbstverständliche Eingliederung des Weisen in kultische Gemeinde und Bindung eine unbewiesene Voraussetzung.

Gottesfurcht entgegenbringen; ähnlich stellt Prov 3 7 dem »sich weise dünken« die Jahwefurcht gegenüber.

Der Jahwefurcht entspricht das Nichttun des Bösen (Hi 1 1 Prov 3 7 14 16). Diese negative Ausdrucksweise geht nicht auf das Urbild des apodiktischen Rechts mit seinen kategorischen Verboten zurück; ebensowenig ist der חכם dem Bösen »feind«, wie es der prophetischen Theologie entspräche. Vielmehr »hält er sich vom Bösen fern«, er geht ihm vorsorglich aus dem Wege. So entspricht es der vorsichtigen und auf das Nützliche bedachten Lebenshaltung und Frömmigkeit dieser Art, die alle Anstöße zu vermeiden und allen Gefahren zu entkommen bestrebt ist.

Von da aus erklären sich die Sprüche, die Gott nach einer ursprünglich ägyptischen Vorstellung als den bezeichnen, der die Herzen wägt und prüft (Prov 16 2 17 3 21 3 24 12), die vom Wohlgefallen oder Mißfallen wissen, das Gott am guten oder schlimmen Verhalten des Menschen hat (Prov 11 1. 20 15 8f. 26 16 5. 7 17 15 20 10. 23 22 11), und die auf die Grenzen hinweisen, die den menschlichen Möglichkeiten durch Gottes Eingreifen gesetzt sind (Prov 16 1. 9 19 21 20 24 21 30f.). Letztlich soll auch dies dazu dienen, »daß dein Vertrauen auf Jahwe steht« (Prov 22 19).

9. Schulmäßige Weisheitslehre

Schließlich bilden die gesonderten Aspekte zumindest in späterer Zeit eine große Einheit. Sie hat in der jüngeren nachexilischen Zeit ein Lehrganzes dargestellt, das theologisch abgerundet wurde. Daß der Ansatz dazu jedoch von Anfang an gegeben war, zeigen die z. T. recht alten Bemerkungen über Salomos »Weisheit«, in denen חכמה schon nahezu ein terminus technicus ist — allerdings im Unterschied von der späteren Zeit ein terminus technicus für das umfassende Klug- und Kundigsein (I Reg 5 9-14 10 4-8. 23 11 41). Mehr im Sinne einer Lebenshaltung spricht Elihu von den »Weisen« (Hi 34 2. 34); er kann damit sowohl den Stand der Weisheitslehrer als auch alle Menschen meinen, die den von diesen gelehrten Grundsätzen folgen. Hiob verhöhnt in 12 2 die selbstsichere Einbildung seiner Freunde, die allein die ganze Weisheit zu besitzen glauben, neben der es keine andere Möglichkeit des Verhaltens gibt, und meint spöttisch, daß sie mit ihnen als ihren alleinigen Vertretern aussterben müßte[79]. Deutlicher wird in Hi 8 8 der Lehrinhalt als das von den Vätern »Erforschte« (חֵקֶר) und in 11 4 der Inhalt der vorhergehenden Hiobrede als »Lehre« (לֶקַח) bezeichnet. Vor allem Kohelet sieht sich einem geschlossenen Lehrganzen gegenüber, so daß bei ihm die Ausdrücke חכמה und חכם geradezu als »schulmäßige Weisheitslehre« und »schulmäßiger Weis-

---

[79] Ähnlich im Redestreit des Aeschylus gegen Euripides bei Aristophanes, Ranae, 868f.

heitslehrer (Weiser)« übersetzt werden können, z. B. Koh 2 12f. 14. 16. 21 8 17. Auch er hat sie erlernt, mit ihr alles ergründen wollen und sich unablässig darum bemüht, mit ihrer Hilfe zu ihrem angeblichen Ziel zu gelangen: der Beherrschung und Sicherung des Lebens durch Lebensklugheit (Koh 1 13. 16). In der Tat hat sie gewisse Vorzüge vor der »Torheit«: Sie reicht aus, um den Menschen davon abzubringen, sein Glück im bloßen Genießen zu suchen (Koh 2 3), und um ihn Anstöße vermeiden zu lassen (2 14). Hauptsächlich aber übt Kohelet Kritik an ihr, so daß die schulmäßige Lehre in dieser Beleuchtung sehr deutlich wird.

10. Eschatologisches Heilsgut und Begabung des Apokalyptikers

An zwei Stellen wird חכמה als eschatologisches Heilsgut genannt. Nach Jes 33 6 werden חכמה und דַּעַת der Heilsreichtum Zions und die Jahwefurcht sein Schatz sein. Dazu treten in v. 5 Recht und Gerechtigkeit, mit denen Jahwe die Stadt füllt. Demnach wird חכמה im Sinne praktischer Frömmigkeit verwendet, die den Reichtum Jerusalems in der eschatologischen Heilszeit ausmachen wird. Nach Jes 11 2 wird sich der Geist Jahwes als dauernder Besitz auf den messianischen Herrscher der Endzeit niederlassen: als Geist der חכמה, der Einsicht, des Rates, der Erkenntnis, der Jahwefurcht, aber auch der Kraft. Es handelt sich also um die Verbindung der durch mehrere Ausdrücke umschriebenen חכמה mit der Kraft, wie sie in Hi 9 4 12 13 von Jahwe selbst ausgesagt wird. Die hervorgehobene dauernde Begabung durch den Geist Jahwes soll angeben, daß die vermittelten Gaben des Kundigseins in seinen verschiedenen Aspekten und der Kraft das normale menschliche Maß übersteigen, so daß der endzeitliche messianische Herrscher den göttlichen Willen, mit dem er sich eins weiß, als irdischer Statthalter Gottes ausführen kann. Was in der endzeitlichen Herrschaft dadurch zustande kommt, schildern die folgenden Verse.

Im Buch Daniel beginnt die Verschmelzung der späten Weisheitstheologie mit der Apokalyptik. Die חכמה Daniels unterscheidet sich von derjenigen, die den Menschen sonst zu eigen ist. Sie übersteigt sie nicht einfach (2 30), sondern ist als ihm verliehene göttliche »Weisheit« grundlegend anders (5 11. 14): Durch sie ist er der Geheimnisse der Zukunft kundig.

IV. »Weisheit« (Klug- und Kundigsein) Gottes

1. Gott besitzt »Weisheit«

Seltener als auf den Menschen wird חכם auf Gott bezogen. Daß der Gottesengel weise ist, sagt zwar schon II Sam 14 20, und Hi 15 8 spricht die Weisheit der himmlischen Umgebung Gottes zu. Daß aber

Gott selbst über sie verfügt, wird ausdrücklich erst verhältnismäßig spät gesagt. Anscheinend hat es längere Zeit gedauert, bis die mesopotamische und ägyptische Vorstellung von Göttern der im einzelnen unterschiedlichen »Weisheit«[80] und die kanaanäische von der »Weisheit« des Gottes El[81] dem Jahweglauben eingeordnet werden konnten. Zunächst hat man stillschweigend vorausgesetzt, daß die חכמה ihren Ursprung in Gott hat und sein Besitz ist, wenn sie als seine Gabe für den Menschen genannt wird; so verhält es sich schon in der Salomogeschichte und der Josepherzählung. Jesaja wird deutlicher: In der Auseinandersetzung mit den angeblich klugen Politikern seiner Zeit sagt er, daß Gott gleichfalls חכם ist (31 1f.), und zeigt am Beispiel des Bauern, daß er je nach der Lage seinem Propheten einen neuen, geänderten Rat (עֵצָה) erteilen kann (28 23-29). Ausdrücklich wird von חכמה als Besitz und Vermögen Jahwes erst in späterer Zeit gesprochen — nicht mit Bezug auf die Geschichte[82], sondern vor allem mit Bezug auf Gott als den Schöpfer, der alles »weise«, d. h. mit handwerklich-künstlerischer Meisterschaft, geschaffen hat (Jes 40 13f. 28 Jer 10 12 51 15 Ps 104 24 Hi 26 12 Prov 3 19f.), der sich darauf versteht, die Wolken in der Luft schweben zu lassen, obwohl sie mit Wasser schwer beladen sind (Hi 37 16; vgl. 36 29), und sie mit kundiger Hand zählt, damit sie in richtiger Menge erscheinen und nicht zuviel oder zuwenig Regen bringen (Hi 38 37). Gottes חכמה ist ebenso sein dem ethischen Verhalten des Menschen entsprechendes geheimnisvolles Handeln an diesem nach dem Grundsatz der vergeltenden Gerechtigkeit (Hi 11 6), die Kodifizierung der Grundsätze des rechten menschlichen Verhaltens im Gesetzbuch Esras (Esr 7 25) und sein Kundigsein der Geheimnisse der Zukunft (Dan 2 20f. 5 11. 14). Weil er mit dergleichen Kundigsein unter den Völkern nicht seinesgleichen findet (Jer 10 7) und zudem über die Kraft und Macht verfügt, das klug Erdachte und kundig Geplante zu verwirklichen — wie der Hymnus (Hi 12 13) preist[83] und Hiob bitter-ironisch beklagt (Hi 9 4)[84] —, kann sich ihm gegenüber kein menschliches Können durchsetzen (Prov 21 30). Er macht alle menschliche Klugheit zuschanden, wenn sie sich seinem Wollen widersetzt (Jes 19 11-15 29 14 31 2f.).

---

[80] Vgl. im einzelnen Fichtner a. a. O. 117f.
[81] C. H. Gordon, Ugaritic Textbook, 1965, Text 51 IV 41; 51 V 65; 'nt V 38; vgl. 126 IV 3.
[82] Vgl. auch J. Fichtner, Zum Problem Glaube und Geschichte in der israelitisch-jüdischen Weisheitsliteratur, ThLZ 76 (1951), 145—150 (= Gottes Weisheit, 1965, 9—17).
[83] Gleiches sagt Prov 8 14 über die personifizierte חכמה selbst.
[84] Hiob will nicht die Ehrfurcht als angemessene Haltung des Menschen gegenüber dem absoluten Recht Gottes hinstellen (A. Weiser, Das Buch Hiob, 1956², z. St.), sondern zur Rechtfertigung seiner Anklage Gottes erklären, warum der Mensch nicht recht haben kann.

2. Gott gewinnt und schafft »Weisheit«

Der Dichter von Hiob 28 bezeichnet mit חכמה das im Welt- und Lebensganzen waltende Prinzip, dessen Kenntnis alles einsichtig macht und bewältigen läßt. Daher bestreitet er im Gegensatz zur üblichen Mahnung, sich חכמה zu erwerben (z. B. Prov 4 5), daß der Mensch über sie verfügen kann[85]. Trotz seines faustischen Triebes zu wissen, was die Welt im Innersten zusammenhält[86], hat lediglich Gott den Weg zu ihr gefunden, sie gewonnen, erforscht und zur Schöpfung der Welt benutzt. Demgemäß bedeutet der Besitz der חכמה nicht ein theoretisches Wissen von der Welt, sondern praktische Verfügbarkeit über sie (v. 25-27). Obwohl die חכמה Gott untergeordnet, in sein Schöpfungshandeln eingegliedert und mit den Geheimnissen der göttlichen Weltschöpfung gleichgesetzt wird, schimmert im Lied ihre ursprüngliche Selbständigkeit durch. Danach war sie eine himmlische, präexistente, neben Gott bestehende eigenständige Größe an einer festliegenden, aber nur Gott zugänglich gewordenen Stätte. Sie erscheint nicht als eine personifizierte Kraft Gottes oder eine selbständig gewordene Größe in Form einer Hypostase[87], sondern als etwas Dingliches, nach dem man wie nach anderen Dingen (Bodenschätzen) sucht und das wie diese örtlich festliegt. Sicherlich ist diese Auffassung nicht ohne Spekulation entstanden, jedoch zugleich im Anschluß an mythische Vorstellungen[88]. Dabei dürfte am ehesten ein gnostischer

---

[85] Ungeachtet dessen, daß das Lied ein späterer Zusatz zum Buch Hiob ist und dem Hiob erst im Verlauf der Umgestaltung des dritten Redegangs in den Mund gelegt worden ist, läßt sich aus seinem negativen Urteil die Absicht der Zufügung erkennen. Das Lied hat die Aufgabe, die Theologie der Freunde Hiobs abschließend und endgültig als falsch zu erweisen und ihre Versuche zur Lösung des Problems des menschlichen Verhaltens im Leide abzulehnen. Allerdings trifft dies zugleich den angeblichen Sprecher Hiob selbst, der seinem Problem zunächst gleichfalls von den Voraussetzungen der Freunde aus nahezukommen sucht. V. 28 mit der Empfehlung der Gottesfurcht ist ein Zusatz zum Lied, so daß er außer Betracht bleiben muß. Vgl. im einzelnen Fohrer a. a. O.

[86] O. Eißfeldt, Religionshistorie und Religionspolemik im Alten Testament, VTSuppl III, 1955, 94 (= Kleine Schriften, III 1966, 359—366).

[87] Vgl. besonders W. Schencke, Die Chokma (Sophia) in der jüdischen Hypostasenspekulation, 1913; J. Goettsberger, Die göttliche Weisheit als Persönlichkeit im Alten Testament, 1919; P. Heinisch, Personifikation und Hypostasen im Alten Testament und im Alten Orient, 1921; Die göttliche Weisheit des Alten Testaments in religionsgeschichtlicher Beleuchtung, 1923; P. van Imschoot, La Sagesse dans l'Ancien Testament est-elle une hypostase?, ColG 21 (1934), 3—10. 85—94; Ringgren a. a. O.; R. Marcus, On Biblical Hypostases of Wisdom, HUCA 23, 1 (1950/51), 157—171; G. Pfeifer, Ursprung und Wesen der Hypostasenvorstellungen im Judentum, 1967.

[88] Baumgartner a. a. O. 28 unter Hinweis auf Achiqar Z. 95 (AOT 438).

Mythos zugrunde liegen, der in anderen und späteren Texten deutlich zutage tritt[89]. Die Anspielung darauf in Hi 28 soll die חכמה, das Geheimnis der Welt, als Gegenstand einer vom Menschen her stets vergeblichen Suche und als der vollen Verfügungsgewalt Gottes unterworfen hinstellen.

Auch andere Wurzeln der Auffassung sind erwogen worden. Schon Ägypten und Babylonien kannten eine ewige göttliche Weisheit, die den Göttern eignet oder von ihnen bzw. von Hypostasen und Personifikationen verkörpert wird[90]. Man hat ferner an iranisch-chaldäischen Ursprung gedacht[91], besonders an die personifizierte »Frömmigkeit« (awestisch *ārmaiti*)[92] oder die personifizierte »Religion« und den »Glauben« (awestisch *daēnā*)[93], an die Gestalt der semitischen Liebes- und Himmelsgöttin (Ischtar, Astarte)[94] oder allgemein an die Umdeutung einer ursprünglich weiblichen Gottheit, die man Gott bei- und unterordnete und als seine Eigenschaft in seinem Wesen aufgehen ließ[95]. Griechischer Einfluß[96] ist sicher nicht anzunehmen.

Der gleiche Mythos steht als eins von mehreren Elementen im Hintergrund des Begriffs חכמה in Prov 1—9, der jüngsten Sammlung des Buches, in der freilich vielfach ältere Sprüche in einem neuen theologischen Rahmen verwendet werden[97]. Die Hauptthemen dieser Sammlung sind die ebenso herzliche wie dringliche Empfehlung der Weisheit und Gottesfurcht in einem (Prov 1 7-9. 20-23 2 3 1-26 4 8 9) und die Warnung vor der fremden Frau (5 6 20-35 7); beide Themen werden mehrfach miteinander verflochten (2 16-19 7 1-5 9). Daß die חכמה, die nach Hi 28 dem Menschen unzugänglich ist, nun als Lehrmeisterin und Offenbarerin zu ihm spricht, ist ebenfalls durch die Vorstellungen des gnostischen Mythos ermöglicht, nach dem diese חכמה eine Wohnstätte unter den Menschen sucht — sie nach dem

---

[89] R. Bultmann, Der religionsgeschichtliche Hintergrund des Prologs zum Johannes-Evangelium, in: Gunkel-Festgabe, II 1923, 3—26.
[90] Baumgartner a. a. O. 28.
[91] R. Reitzenstein, Das mandäische Buch des Herrn der Größe, 1919, 46—58.
[92] Anders W. Bousset—H. Greßmann, Die Religion des Judentums im späthellenistischen Zeitalter, 1926³, 520.
[93] Bousset—Greßmann a. a. O. 520.
[94] Boström a. a. O. 12—14 u. ö. W. F. Albright, Von der Steinzeit zum Christentum, 1949, 367f., denkt an eine ältere kanaanäische Göttin der Weisheit, ähnlich der mesopotamischen Siduri Sabitu. Jedoch ist demgegenüber die abweichende Bedeutung des mesopotamischen Begriffs »Weisheit« zu bedenken (vgl. oben II).
[95] G. Hölscher, Das Buch Hiob, 1952², 68.
[96] R. Kittel, Geschichte des Volkes Israel, III, 2 1929, 731f.; E. Sellin, Geschichte des israelitisch-jüdischen Volkes, II 1932, 181.
[97] Die Behauptung von Albright a. a. O. 365f., daß Prov 8f. kanaanäischen Ursprungs seien, geht über das vertretbare Maß hinaus. Sprachliche Anklänge beruhen auf der Verwendung von mythischen Vorstellungen und Schöpfungsaussagen. Auch die von Christa Kayatz, Studien zu Proverbien 1—9, 1966, vertretene Datierung in die frühe israelitische Königszeit läßt sich nicht halten.

Mythos freilich nicht findet und daher in den Himmel zurückkehrt oder sie wie in Sir 24 8ff. dann doch in Israel und Jerusalem erlangt hat und Sir 24 23ff. mit der Tora gleichgesetzt werden kann. In jedem Falle wird ihr Sprechen zum Menschen verständlich.

Die חכמה ist nach Prov 8 22-31 wie in Hi 28 präexistent vor allen Schöpfungswerken. Aber sie besitzt keine urweltliche Existenz neben Gott, der sie entdecken muß, sondern ist als Erstling von ihm geschaffen worden und hat dann der weiteren eigentlichen Schöpfung beigewohnt — nicht als Helferin, sondern wie ein Kind, das in der Werkstatt seines Vaters spielt[98]. Als Gottes »Hätschelkind, Liebling« (אָמוֹן v. 30) hat sie mit der Schöpfung und dem Menschen gespielt[99]. Sie ist also im Unterschied zu Hi 28 eine persönliche Größe, von Gott geschaffen und an der Schöpfung nicht beteiligt[100]. Gott gewinnt sie nicht, sondern erschafft sie. Der Unterschied ist darin begründet, daß der Einfluß eines zweiten Mythos vorliegt: des Mythos vom Urmenschen, der vor aller Welt geschaffen worden ist und darum über besondere Erfahrungsweisheit verfügt. Mittels dieses Mythos, der in anderer Art auch in Ez 28 1-10. 11-19 und Hi 15 7-8 verwendet wird, ist die חכמה bildhaft personifiziert worden. Der Sinn der Ausführungen liegt darin, daß die חכמה ihren Adelsbrief zeigt[101]. Je älter der Adel, desto höher ist er; je älter die Weisheit, desto maßgeblicher ist sie (vgl. die Argumentation in Hi 15 7f.). So sollen das Gewicht und die Autorität der Anrede an den Menschen gesteigert werden.

Die חכמה wird in Prov 1—9 auch sonst personifiziert vorgestellt: 1 20 als Verkündigerin, 4 6-9 als Braut und Ehefrau, 6 22 7 4 als Lebensgefährtin, 9 1 als Wirtin. Wie andere personhafte Bilder zeigen, ist diese Personifizierung gleichfalls bildlich gemeint (vgl. Jes 59 14 Ps 85 11f. Prov 9 13-18). Auf diese Weise kann sie nicht nur als neutrale Lehre durch die Worte eines Weisheitslehrers an den Menschen ergehen, sondern ihn als Person anrufen und wie ein Prophet an den Stätten des öffentlichen Lebens in den Ortschaften (1 20f.) und an den Kreuzpunkten der Wege (8 2) ihre Stimme erheben. Dieses prophetische Verkündungspathos ist das dritte Element des vorliegenden Weisheitsbegriffs. So spricht sie mit besonderer Autorität, mahnt, lockt und droht und stellt wie ein Prophet den Menschen vor die Entscheidung

---

[98] Gemser a. a. O. 48.
[99] Die spätjüdische Deutung von אמון als »Werkmeister« oder »Handwerker« beruht auf späteren Vorstellungen (vgl. ThW VII 507 Anm. 291). In LXX ist v. 31 mit Gott als Subjekt umgebildet worden.
[100] Die scheinbar abweichende Aussage von Prov 3 19f. beruht darauf, daß in diesen Versen ein älterer Spruch vorliegt, der den Begriff חכמה im handwerklich-künstlerischen Sinn verwendet.
[101] G. Wildeboer, Die Sprüche, 1897, 27.

über Leben und Tod[102]. Denn sie bietet das »Leben«, das im alttestamentlichen Sinn ein vollgültiges, glückhaftes und erfülltes Leben und als solches wahres Heil ist (3 18. 22 4 13. 22f. 8 35). Darin ist sie die Offenbarung des göttlichen Willens an den Menschen. Darum gilt es, ihr nachzuspüren (2 4), sie zu finden (3 13) und zu erwerben (4 7), sich von ihr als Geliebter (4 6ff.), Schwester oder Braut (7 4) zum Gastmahl einladen zu lassen. Denn darin nimmt der Mensch den Willen Gottes an und folgt ihm, so daß ihm dessen Wohlgefallen zuteil wird (8 35). Daß dergleichen nicht nur für Israel, sondern für den Menschen überhaupt und allgemein gilt, zeigen am besten 8 1-21. Dabei ist dies alles in Bildsprache und Ausdrucksweise wiederum von der mythischen Vorstellung von der חכמה beeinflußt, die eine Wohnstatt und ein Einswerden mit dem Menschen sucht[103]. Daß diese Vorstellung nüchtern und vorsichtig gehandhabt wird und dem Jahweglauben nicht abträglich ist, beruht auf der theologischen Grundhaltung, die durch die Einbeziehung des prophetischen Elements gekennzeichnet ist[104].

V. *Ursprung und Quelle des Klug- und Kundigseins*

1. Väterüberlieferung

Zweifellos ist die Tradition eine der Quellen des Klug- und Kundigseins. Die ägyptische Situation wird in Jes 19 11 dadurch gekennzeichnet, daß die Berater des Pharao erklären, sie seien Schüler der Weisen und der Könige der Vorzeit, auf die viele der Lehren zurückgeführt werden; sie schöpfen aus der Väterüberlieferung. Diese wird gleichfalls von den Freunden Hiobs als eine Quelle ihrer Ratschläge angeführt. So entspricht es der üblichen Unterweisung in Israel überhaupt, bei der besonderes Gewicht auf die Einführung in die väterlichen Traditionen gelegt wurde[105]. Bildad beruft sich auf die Lehre der früheren Generationen, weil sie der Erfahrung eines einzelnen oder einer einzigen Generation überlegen ist (Hi 8 8-10), Eliphas auf die bis in seine Gegenwart lebendige und bestätigte Lehrtradition, die wegen der Abwesenheit von Sippen- oder Landesfremden z. Zt. ihrer Entstehung eine reine, unverfälschte Lehre darstellt (Hi 15 19f.).

---

[102] Über Gutes und Schlechtes vgl. ThW III 479.
[103] Von da aus wird deutlich, daß die חכמה nicht die Gegenspielerin der ʼΑφροδίτη παρακύπτουσα darstellt, die durch die ausländischen Frauen den Israeliten zu aphrodisischen Kulten anlockt, wie Boström a. a. O. 127—147 annehmen läßt.
[104] Zu den mannigfachen Berührungen mit Jesaja (besonders Jes 40—66), Jeremia und Dtn vgl. im einzelnen A. Robert, Les attaches littéraires bibliques de Prov I—IX, RB 43 (1934), 42—68. 172—204. 374—384; 44 (1935), 344—365. 502—525.
[105] Vgl. Ex 13 8ff. Dtn 4 9 6 7. 20ff. 11 19ff. Jos 4 6f. 21 Ps 78 5ff. Vgl. L. Dürr, Das Erziehungswesen im Alten Testament und im Alten Orient, 1932, 107f.

2. Eigene Erfahrung

Eine zweite Quelle des klugen Kundigseins ist die eigene Erfahrung, die ein Mensch im Lauf des Lebens sammelt. Daher gelten die Alten gewöhnlich als Träger der weisen Erfahrung und scheinen über genügend Einsicht zu verfügen (Hi 12 12 15 10 32 7; vgl. Ez 7 26). Entsprechend beruft Eliphas sich auf das, was er wahrgenommen oder erforscht hat (Hi 4 8 5 3. 27 15 17) und nun belehrend weitergeben kann, während Hiob seine eigene, entgegengesetzte Erfahrung vorbringt (Hi 21 6). Besonders häufig spricht Kohelet vom eigenen Wahrnehmen und Erfahren oder schildert es z. B. 1 13a. 16-17a 2 1. 3a. 4-8. 12a. 24 3 10f. 16 4 1. 4a. 7. Dieses Moment bildet geradezu ein formgeschichtliches Element vieler seiner Sentenzen, die nach dem Schema Erfahrungsammeln — Ergebnis — Sprichwort zur Begründung oder Bestätigung aufgebaut sind[106].

3. Methoden und Mittel

Die beiden Methoden, die dazu dienen, aufgrund von Tradition und Erfahrung das Klug- und Kundigsein anderen zu vermitteln oder sich vermitteln zu lassen, sind Belehrung und Zucht; so fassen Prov 19 20 21 11 es zusammen. Dabei kann es sich um einfache Belehrung und Unterweisung (Prov 4 11 9 9 13 14 Ps 105 22) im Umgang mit Weisen (Prov 13 20) handeln. Sie kann weiterhin liebreich sein (Prov 31 26), aber auch den Charakter der Zurechtweisung (Prov 9 8), des Tadels (Koh 7 5) und der Rüge (Prov 29 15) annehmen. Sie erfolgt mittels מָשָׁל (Prov 1 1. 6), דָּבָר (Prov 1 6 22 17) und sonstiger Redeweisen (vgl. z. B. Prov 1 6). Und da der Weise schwierige Sentenzen verstehen und dem zu Belehrenden ihre Deutung (פשר) geben kann (Koh 8 1), haben seine Worte antreibende Wirkung wie der Ochsenstachel eines Pflügers und treffen wie Nägel, die man einschlägt (Koh 12 11). Reicht solche Belehrung dennoch nicht aus, so bleiben die Zucht (Prov 8 33 13 1) und die Rute (Prov 29 15). Unter Kummer und durch viele Prügel wächst das Wissen, wie das Sprichwort ursprünglich gesagt haben dürfte, das Kohelet 1 18 in anderer Bedeutung verwendet.

4. Gabe Gottes

Eignet sich der Mensch sein Klug- und Kundigsein gewöhnlich mittels Belehrung oder Zucht aus der Tradition oder Erfahrung an, so findet sich daneben und ergänzend die Möglichkeit einer außer-

---

[106] Koh 1 12-15. 16-18 2 1-11. 12b (in dreifacher Aufeinanderfolge) 2 12a. 13-17 (in zweifacher Aufeinanderfolge, aber etwas abgewandelt) 3 16-17 4 1-3. 4-6. 7f.; mit doppelseitiger Erfahrung in 2 24-26 3 10-15 (in 3 1-15).

ordentlichen Begnadung mit der Gabe der חכמה — einer Begnadung durch Gott, die sich weithin allerdings nur von Fall zu Fall ereignet. So hat er sie einzelnen besonderen Menschen verliehen: Joseph (Gen 41 16. 38f.), Josua durch die Handauflegung Moses (Dtn 34 9), Salomo (I Reg 3 12. 28 5 26 10 24 II Chr 1 12) und Daniel (Dan 1 4. 17. 20 5 11. 14). Ähnlich verhält es sich mit der einzelnen prophetischen Inspiration (Jer 9 11) und dem nächtlichen Offenbarungserlebnis des Eliphas (Hi 4 12-21), aber auch mit der handwerklichen Kunstfertigkeit (Ex 28 3 31 3. 6 35 31 36 1f.) und der Landarbeit (Jes 28 26). Die ältesten Stellen finden sich demnach in der Salomogeschichte, danach in der Josepherzählung und in Jes 28 26, während die übrigen wesentlich jünger sind (vgl. noch Ps 60 8 94 10 119 98 Prov 28 5 Koh 2 26). Auch die Hiobdichtung weiß, daß Gott Weisheit gibt (Hi 11 6 38 36) oder von ihr fernhält (17 4), und vertritt im allgemeinen die Ansicht, daß Gott dem Menschen ein gewisses Maß von חכמה verleiht, dieses sich aber mit der seinigen nicht vergleichen läßt und dem Menschen daher manches als zu wunderbar und unbekannt erscheinen muß (42 3).

Anders verhielte es sich, wenn jemand entsprechend dem Mythos vom Urmenschen (vgl. Ez 28 1-10. 11-19) von sich behaupten könnte, vor der übrigen Schöpfung geboren worden und als der älteste zugleich der weiseste Mensch zu sein; oder wenn er wie der Urmensch zur himmlischen Ratsversammlung zugelassen worden wäre und dadurch etwas von der göttlichen חכמה mitbekommen hätte (Hi 15 7-8; vgl. Jer 23 18. 22). Nur dann könnte er den Lehren der Tradition und der Erfahrung der Alten überlegen sein. Diese Bedingungen treffen für Hiob natürlich nicht zu, so daß Eliphas die ursprünglichen mythischen Vorstellungen als bildhafte Vergleiche verwendet, um das ihm überheblich scheinende Auftreten Hiobs vernichtend zu treffen.

In der jüngeren Weisheitslehre findet sich eine andere Auffassung, die zunächst an den Reden Elihus (Hi 32—37) deutlich wird. Zwar bezeichnet Elihu die Erkenntnis und Lehre, die er besitzt und vermitteln will, als דַּע »Wissen« (32 6. 10. 17 36 3) und einmal mit dem pl. f. דֵּעוֹת (36 4); sachlich aber ist dieser Begriff dem der חכמה gleich. Das seltene Wort meint entweder das Gott eigene (Hi 37 16 I Sam 2 3 Ps 73 11) oder von ihm verliehene Wissen (Jes 28 9 Jer 3 15) und ist für die Reden Elihus absichtlich gewählt worden, um von vornherein durchblicken zu lassen, daß dieser sich im Besitz der Gott eigenen und ihm von diesem verliehenen Erkenntnis weiß[107]. Daher behauptet er, sein Wissen »von fern her«, d. h. angesichts des parallelen Wortes »Schöpfer«, von Gott zu haben (Hi 36 3). Es ist ihm durch den »Geist« und »Atem« Gottes vermittelt worden, so daß er nicht erst im Lauf

---

[107] Dem entspricht es, daß Elihu das geläufigere דַּעַת nur gebraucht, wenn er Hiob oder dem Sünder Klugheit und Wissen abspricht (Hi 34 35 35 16 36 12).

eines langen Lebens Erfahrungen sammeln und die Väterüberlieferung lernen muß, sondern trotz seiner Jugend »weise« ist, weil er die göttliche Weisheit durch Inspiration als dauernden Besitz erhalten hat (Hi 32 7-10). Elihu teilt demnach die Auffassung, daß die חכמה zunächst im Besitz Gottes ist, behauptet dann aber, daß sie dem Menschen weder verborgen bleibt (Hi 28) noch von Fall zu Fall als einzelnes Vermögen vermittelt, sondern ihm überhaupt und als ganze verliehen wird. Was er erhalten hat, ist sein »Teil« (32 17) an der göttlichen Gesamtweisheit, der zu einer vollen Antwort an Hiob und seine Freunde ausreicht. Dieses Wissen ist sündlos (33 3, wahrscheinlich im Anschluß an Zeph 3 9) und vollkommen oder — wie im Verein mit der pluralischen Wortform gesagt werden soll — umfassend und unübertrefflich (36 4). Was Elihu lehrt, ist nach der ernsthaften und keineswegs ironischen Ansicht des Verfassers der Reden der göttlichen Weisheit letzter Schluß. So nimmt Elihu die gleiche Würde der übernatürlichen Erleuchtung und unmittelbaren Eingebung für sich in Anspruch wie der Prophet. Er tritt neben ihn oder an seine Stelle und übertrifft ihn sogar darin, daß der inspiratorische Geist ihn ganz und dauernd erfüllt[108].

In Weiterführung dessen erscheint die bildlich personifizierte חכמה von Prov 1—9 sowohl als Offenbarungsmittler, indem sie mit ihrer Verkündigung wie ein Prophet und mit dem Anspruch höchster Autorität auftritt, als auch als Offenbarung des göttlichen Willens an den Menschen selbst, indem sie dem Menschen das Leben anbietet und ihre Annahme als diejenige des göttlichen Willens versteht. Auch die eschatologisch-messianische und die apokalyptische חכמה sind als dauernd verliehener Besitz gedacht.

VI. Wert, Erfolg und Kritik des Klug- und Kundigseins

1. Wert und Erfolg

Die Belehrung über das Klug- und Kundigsein ist für den Belehrten so nutzbringend wie eine sprudelnde Quelle gegenüber einer Zisterne mit tiefem Wasserstand (Prov 18 4), der Mahner, der Lebensregeln erteilt, für den Hörenden so wertvoll wie Ring und Geschmeide aus Gold (Prov 25 12) und das Klug- und Kundigsein ein köstlicher Schatz (Prov 21 20) oder gar kostbarer als Schätze (Prov 3 15 8 11; vgl. Hi 28 15-18). Denn die חכמה behütet und rettet den Menschen

---

[108] Deswegen beansprucht er, wie ein Prophet gehört zu werden (Hi 32 10), und glaubt in der verfahrenen Situation bessere Gründe als die Freunde Hiobs vorbringen zu können (32 14). Deswegen muß er als ein Gefäß des göttlichen Geistes unbedingt reden (32 18-20), da der Geist ihn wie einen Propheten zu sprechen drängt (vgl. Jer 20 9).

(Prov 2 8. 20), so daß er Anstöße vermeidet (Koh 2 14. 16) und manchen Schaden von sich abwendet (Prov 14 3), jeder Schwierigkeit Herr wird (Koh 8 5), den Fallstricken des Todes entgeht (Prov 13 14) und dem Unglück entrinnt (Prov 28 26). Positiv gewendet, kommt dem Menschen sein weises Verhalten zugute (Prov 9 12), so daß er Erfolg (Koh 9 11a) und »Gelingen in Fülle« erwarten darf (Hi 26 3; vgl. 5 12 6 13 11 6) und ans Ziel seines Weges gelangt (Prov 14 8). Er erlangt Ehre (Prov 3 35) und Heilung (Prov 12 18); denn die חכמה baut auf (Prov 14 1) und bringt Dauerhaftes zustande (Prov 24 3). Nicht bloßes Wissen, sondern praktisch angewandtes Klug- und Kundigsein ist Macht (Prov 21 22 Koh 7 19 9 15). Gelegentlich ist von dessen Wert für andere die Rede. Vor allem der Vater oder Lehrer freut sich über den »weise« Gewordenen (Prov 10 1 15 20 23 15. 24) und kann demjenigen, der ihn als schlechten Lehrer schmäht, die passende Antwort erteilen (Prov 27 11).

Es ist unübersehbar, daß diese Lebensauffassung einen gewissen utilitaristischen und eudämonistischen Zug aufweist. Nicht umsonst wird im Buche Hiob von den weisen Ratgebern mehrfach der Nutzen der Frömmigkeit erwogen (Hi 22 2f. 35 6-8) und seine Bestreitung dem Hiob unterstellt (34 9 35 3) bzw. durch diesen als Ansicht der Frevler vorgetragen (21 15)[109]. Jedes wie immer geartete Verhalten entspricht nicht nur einer bestimmten Grundhaltung, sondern erstrebt auch einen bestimmten Zweck und Erfolg. So verhält es sich nicht zuletzt bei חכם als einem Klug- und Kundigsein zum Zweck praktischer Gestaltung. Beides ist untrennbar miteinander verbunden; es handelt sich stets um ein auf praktischen Erfolg gerichtetes Klug- und Kundigsein. Allerdings ist gegenüber dem reinen Utilitarismus eine Einschränkung zu machen: Ein wesenhafter Unterschied oder Gegensatz zwischen dem im Handeln oder Verhalten selbst ruhenden »inneren« Wert des Tuns und dem »äußeren« Erfolg besteht nicht[110]. Beides ist ein und dasselbe, wenn der חכם sich um die Erkenntnis der Ordnungen in der Welt und im Leben bemüht, um sich der Welt zu bemächtigen und das Leben zu meistern. So fordern denn die Freunde Hiobs diesen immer wieder auf, sich dieser Ordnung zu unterwerfen und sich in sie einzuordnen; das ist die rechte innere Haltung mit dem daraus folgenden rechten Verhalten und verbürgt zugleich den äußeren Erfolg, so daß dann neues Heil winkt. Freilich stellt die Gottesrede von dieser Weltordnung (עֵצָה) fest, daß sie als göttliche Ordnung dem Menschen uneinsichtig ist und daher paradox erscheint, woraus Koh 3 1-15 die Folgerung zieht, daß keine Sicherheit hinsichtlich des Erfolges menschlichen Tuns gewährleistet ist.

---

[109] Vgl. auch die ethischen Finalsätze (ThW III 330).
[110] So mit Recht Gese a. a. O. 7—41.

Die Welt- und Lebensordnung ist nie von Gott gelöst, sondern durch ihn gesetzt und aufrechterhalten. Daher gefällt ihm die kluge, kundige oder fromme Einordnung in sie und mißfällt ihm der Verstoß gegen sie. Nach seiner vergeltenden Gerechtigkeit läßt er demgemäß dem חכם Glück und Erfolg als Segens- und Heilsgabe zuteil werden, dem Toren und Frevler dagegen Unheil. So bildet der zweiseitige Vergeltungsglaube eine tragende Säule der Lebensweisheit. Danach muß eine gute Tat stets einen guten Erfolg nach sich ziehen, eine Missetat dagegen Unheil. Mit der Gültigkeit des Satzes, daß Verhalten und Ergehen des Menschen einander entsprechen, steht und fällt die Weisheitslehre. Freilich beruht diese Entsprechung nicht auf einem Mechanismus, sondern geht auf Gott zurück, der nach seiner Gerechtigkeit so und nicht anders handeln kann[111]. Schien die Wirklichkeit dem zu widersprechen, so konnte man das Leid des Frommen damit erklären, daß er das Schicksal des von Natur unvollkommenen und unzulänglichen Menschen erleide (Hi 4 17-21) oder daß eine Erziehungsmaßnahme Gottes vorliege (Hi 5 17 33 13-24). Das Wohlergehen des Frevlers erklärte man als bloßes Scheinglück, da er in Wirklichkeit von Qualen geplagt sei (Hi 15 20-22). Für beide griff man auch über das Leben des einzelnen hinaus und wies auf die Vergeltung an den Kindern hin (Ps 37 25 Hi 5 4f. 18 19 20 10 27 14 Prov 13 22 20 7). Schließlich mündet die Auffassung in eine ausgesprochene Vergeltungslehre, in der jeder Sünde eine bestimmte Strafe zugeschrieben und vor allem von der Folge — Glück oder Unglück des Menschen — auf die Ursache — Frömmigkeit oder Sündhaftigkeit — zurückgeschlossen wird. Wert und Erfolg eines klugen und kundigen ethischen oder frommen Verhaltens liegen dann offen zutage.

2. Kritik

Richtet sich die frühe Kritik an der חכמה entweder gegen die heidnische Wahrsage- und Deutekunst (Gen 41 8 Jes 44 25) oder die sich klug dünkenden Politiker Jerusalems (Jes 5 21 29 14 31 1-3), so

---

[111] Die Wurzeln liegen in der urtümlichen Vorstellung, daß jede Tat eine Sphäre schafft, die den Menschen heil- oder unheilwirkend umgibt, so daß eine gute Tat ihrem Charakter gemäß glücken und gute Erfolge nach sich ziehen, eine schlechte dagegen Unheil schaffen muß. Entgegen der Ansicht von J. Pedersen, Israel, I—II 1926, 336—377 u. ö.; K. H. Fahlgren, Ṣedaqa nahestehende und entgegengesetzte Begriffe im Alten Testament, 1932, 4; K. Koch, Gibt es ein Vergeltungsdogma im Alten Testament?, ZThK 52 (1955), 1—42, ist diese Auffassung im Jahweglauben höchstens in Resten anzutreffen. Die fast magische und mechanische Gleichung von Guttat und Heil, Frevel und Unheil ist im Jahweglauben völlig dem personhaften Walten Jahwes und seiner vergeltenden Gerechtigkeit untergeordnet worden. Vgl. die Auseinandersetzung Gese 42—50; H. Graf Reventlow, Sein Blut komme über sein Haupt, VT 10 (1960), 311—327.

in der Spätzeit gegen das umfassende und in sich verfestigte Lehrsystem.

Gewiß räumt Kohelet der Schulweisheit einen relativen Wert ein (2 3. 14. 16 4 13 10 12), doch letztlich bringt sie seiner Ansicht nach keinen wirklichen Gewinn (2 15 9 11a), sondern ist nicht besser als die gleichfalls erfolglose Torheit (1 16f. 6 8). Sie ist nutzlos vom Besitz her gesehen, den man anderen hinterlassen muß, so daß man selbst nur die Mühe darum hat (2 21), nutzlos angesichts des Todes, der alle Menschen gleicherweise trifft (2 15f.; vgl. Ps 49 11) und — da er weder berechnet noch vermieden werden kann — eine unüberschreitbare Grenze der Schulweisheit bildet. Die zweite Grenze ist das Weib (nicht nur das fremde wie in Proverbia), das den Weisen umstrickt und verführt, so daß er seine Lebensgrundsätze vergißt und sein Bemühen um Lebensgestaltung illusorisch wird, wenn Gott es will (7 26). Das Geschick des Weisen hängt eben nicht — wie die Lehre behauptet — von seinem gerechten und frommen Verhalten ab, sondern ist in Gottes Hand unerforschlich und unerkennbar bereitgehalten (8 17 9 1). So bleibt nur übrig, den Anteil am Leben, der dem Menschen gewährt wird, in einer tätigen Existenz auszukosten (zusammenfassend in 9 7-10)[112].

Während Kohelet trotz solchen Tätigseins und Genießens auf eine aktive Lebensgestaltung verzichtet und ein Hinnehmen des Lebensanteils und vor allem eine starke Zurückhaltung im Leben empfiehlt, ringt der Hiobdichter in Auseinandersetzung mit dem Vergeltungsglauben gerade um eine neue Lebensgestaltung, die zum Eigentlichen der menschlichen Existenz jenseits des bloßen Lebensvollzugs führen kann. So wenig sie in der herkömmlichen Lehre der Freunde Hiobs erblickt werden darf, die von Hiob als falsch erwiesen[113] und von Gott als frevlerisch verurteilt wird (42 7f.)[114], so wenig in dem prometheisch-titanischen Aufbegehren Hiobs, der zunächst Gott sein Glück entreißen möchte und ihm im Bewußtsein seiner Tadellosigkeit

---

[112] Die Kritik an dieser Kritik liegt in Koh 12 12-14 vor, deren Verfasser in der Vielfalt der Bücher mit ihren vielfältigen Meinungen eine Gefahr für den Schüler erblickt. Daß er besonders Kohelet meint, zeigt sich an der Art, wie er dessen abweichende Meinung zusammenfassend interpretiert und korrigiert: Nach ihm vertritt Kohelet ein auf das göttliche Gebot gegründetes Ethos, verbunden mit dem Gedanken an das Vergeltungsgericht über die verborgenen Taten des Menschen.

[113] Wie sich in den Freundesreden die Lehre widerspiegelt, gegen die sich Hiob wendet, arbeitet E. Würthwein, Gott und Mensch in Dialog und Gottesreden des Buches Hiob, masch. schr. Habilitationsschrift Tübingen 1938, heraus.

[114] Die Freunde haben »Nicht-Wahres« geredet. Darin liegt zwar ein milder Ausdruck vor wie mehrfach in der Rahmenerzählung (Hi 1 5. 11. 22 2 5. 9); jedoch gilt in ihr unziemliches Reden über Gott als schlimmste und am meisten zu fürchtende Sünde (Hi 1 5. 22 2 10). Zur »Zungensünde« vgl. ThW I 720.

entgegentritt, um über ihn triumphieren zu wollen (31 35-37). Die wahre Einsicht folgt erst aus der persönlichen Begegnung mit Gott. Das rechte Verhalten besteht im demütigen und hingebungsvollen Schweigen aus dem Ruhen in Gott — aufgrund der Erfahrung, daß das Geschick des Menschen auf einem rätselvollen und undurchschaubaren, aber doch sinnvollen Handeln Gottes beruht, und aufgrund der Gewißheit der Gottesgemeinschaft, die alles andere überwiegt (40 4-5 42 2-3. 5-6). Ähnlich äußern sich Jes 51 7-8 Ps 73 25-28. Daher soll der Mensch sich nicht seiner »Weisheit« rühmen, sondern der »Erkenntnis« Jahwes, d. h. der Gemeinschaft mit dem Gott, der Welt und Menschen regiert, und des dadurch bestimmten Lebens (Jer 9 22-23).

σῴζω, σωτηρία, σωτήρ und σωτήριος im Alten Testament

I. Vorkommen und hebräische Äquivalente von σῴζω und σωτηρία

1. Vorkommen und Übersetzungsstatistik in der Septuaginta

σῴζω *bewahren, retten* begegnet in LXX zu den kanonischen Büchern des hebräischen Alten Testaments in fast drei Fünftel seiner Vorkommen als Wiedergabe des Verbs יָשַׁע, davon 143mal für hi. *retten, befreien, helfen, zu Hilfe kommen*, besonders in Jdc, I—II Reg, I Chr Ps Hos Hab Zeph Sach Jes 30ff. Jer 1—26 und 16mal für ni. *Hilfe empfangen, erfahren*. Je einmal umschreibt es die abgeleiteten Substantive יֵשַׁע (Hab 3 13), יְשׁוּעָה (Ps 80 3) und מוֹשָׁעוֹת (Ps 68 21) *Hilfeerweisungen*. — Ein weiteres Fünftel der Vorkommen dient der Wiedergabe der Stämme פלט und מלט: σῴζω steht viermal für פָּלִיט (Jes 45 20 Jer 42 17 44 14. 28) und einmal für פָּלִיט *Entronnener* (Jes 66 19), fünfmal für פְּלֵיטָה *Entronnenes, Entrinnen, Rettung* (Gen 32 9 Jes 10 20 37 32 Neh 1 2 II Chr 20 24) und für das einmalige מִפְלָט *Zufluchtsort* (Ps 55 9)[1], ferner für מלט 37mal im ni. *sich in Sicherheit bringen, entrinnen*[2], 11mal im pi. *retten, sich retten* und einmal im seltenen hi. *davonbringen, retten*. — Das letzte Fünftel der Vorkommen von σῴζω gibt eine Fülle verschiedener Ausdrücke wieder, die sonst auf andere Weise übersetzt werden, darunter 24mal נצל, dem überwiegend ῥύομαι und ἐξαιρέω entsprechen[3].

---

[1] Die einzige Wiedergabe des Verbs פלט pi. durch σῴζω in Ps 56 8 geht von einem verderbten MT aus, in dem gerade das Verb geändert werden muß.

[2] Als innergriechische Varianten finden sich in I Βας 30 17 διασῴζω und das nur an dieser Stelle vorkommende περισῴζω.

[3] Außerdem finden sich folgende innergriechische Varianten zu σῴζω: ἀνασῴζω Ιερ 31 19 Ob 21, διασῴζω Gen 19 20 Jos 10 40 I Sam 30 17 II Reg 19 37 Ιερ 48 15 Ez 17 15, ferner Dan 11 71 Θ, ἀποσῴζω Ιερ 41 3, σωτήρ Jdc 12 3. Umgekehrt findet sich einfaches σῴζω statt ἀνασῴζω Ιερ 51 14 Sach 8 7, statt διασῴζω I Sam 19 18, statt ὠθέω Ιερ 41 11, statt τίθημι II Chr 33 7. Durch ein ganz anderes Verb ist σῴζω ersetzt in I Sam 23 2 Jes 38 6 46 2 59 1 Ιερ 2 27 11 12 45 18 Ez 33 12 36 29 Sach 12 7 ψ 17 28 33 7 106 13, ferner Dan 3 95 6 21 Θ. — Zwischen MT und LXX sind verschiedene Textabweichungen festzustellen. MT ist mit Hilfe des σῴζω der LXX in I Sam 14 47 (ישׁע ni. für ירשׁיע) und Prov 19 7 (מלט ni. für המה) zu verbessern, in I Sam 10 1 I Reg 13 31 nach LXX zu ergänzen. LXX hat MT verlesen und fälschlich mit σῴζω übersetzt in Jes 15 7 Mi 6 9 Hi 27 8 Thr 2 13. Schließlich hat die LXX σῴζω in überschießendem Text in II Sam 14 4 Jes 12 2 Prov 10 25 Est 4 17b 10 3f. Dan 6 23. 28.

ἀνασῴζω *wieder erretten, für sich erretten* gibt außer dem nur einmal vorkommenden פלט (qal Ez 7 16) am häufigsten die von diesem Verb abgeleiteten Substantive wieder: zehnmal פָּלִיט, dreimal פָּלֵיט (Jer 44 14 50 28 51 50) und sechsmal פְּלֵיטָה (II Reg 19 31 Jer 50 29 Ez 14 22 Joel 2 3 3 5 II Chr 30 6). Dagegen steht es für מלט pi. nur einmal (Jer 51 6), für ni. zweimal (Jer 46 6 Sach 2 11) und für ישע hi. zweimal[4].

διασῴζω *glücklich durchbringen, retten* findet sich gleichfalls nur selten für ישע: zweimal ni. (Num 10 9 Jer 8 20), dreimal hi. (Dtn 20 4 Hos 13 10 Sach 8 13), statt dessen wieder häufiger für den Stamm פלט: zweimal für פלט pi. (Mi 6 14 Hi 21 10), einmal hi. (Mi 6 14), zweimal פָּלִיט (Jdc 12 4f.), einmal פָּלֵיט (Num 21 29) und fünfmal פְּלֵיטָה (Jdc 21 17 II Reg 19 30 Dan 11 42 Esr 9 14f.), sowie besonders für das Verb מלט: 20mal ni. *sich in Sicherheit bringen, entrinnen* und viermal pi. *retten, sich retten*. Außerdem gibt es siebenmal das פָּלִיט oft parallele und praktisch gleichbedeutende שָׂרִיד wieder und lediglich je einmal שרד, חיה pi. und עשת hitp.[5]

σωτηρία *Rettung, Erhaltung, Schutz, Wohlergehen, Heil* gibt 81mal und damit weitaus überwiegend den Stamm ישע wieder: fünfmal ישע hi. (II Sam 22 3 II Reg 13 5 Jes 38 20 47 15 63 8), 12mal יֵשַׁע (nach σωτήρ ein zweites Drittel der Vorkommen), 38mal יְשׁוּעָה und 26mal תְּשׁוּעָה *Rettung, Hilfe, Heil*. Demgegenüber steht das Wort sechsmal für פְּלֵיטָה (II Sam 15 14 Jer 25 35 Ob 17 Esr 9 8. 13 II Chr 12 7) und noch seltener für einige andere Ausdrücke: dreimal für שָׁלוֹם (Gen 26 31 28 21 44 17); zweimal für תּוּשִׁיָּה (Prov 2 7 Hi 30 22, wo aber ein Textfehler in MT vorliegt), je einmal für שֶׁלוּ (Hi 20 20, aber in MT verderbt), und מָנוֹס (Hi 11 20, in LXX mit umgestelltem Text)[6]. Öfters findet sich σωτηρία in einem Mehr an Text ohne Grundlage im MT: Ιερ 37 6 ψ 117 28 Hi 2 9a Est 4 17d 8 12 u[7].

Vereinzelt kommen als weitere Wortbildungen vor: II Εσδρ 9 8 in B¹ σωτήρισμα, in B³ σωτηρίαγμα für στήριγμα, Gen 45 7 bei ’Α ανασωσμός für פליטה und (Ps 66 9) bei ’ΑΘ διασωσμός für מפלט.

---

[4] Davon ist Ob 21 wahrscheinlich nach LXX-Varianten und Versionen in ישע ni. zu ändern, während Varianten zu Sach 8 7 einfaches σῴζω aufweisen.

[5] Als Varianten der LXX finden sich einfaches σῴζω in I Βας 19 18, andere Verben in 19 10 20 29. — Eine Änderung der LXX gegenüber MT liegt in Hi 36 12 vor, wo διασῴζω vielleicht aus ישמעו verlesen ist. Ohne Textgrundlage in MT steht διασῴξω in Gen 35 3 Jos 6 26.

[6] An Varianten innerhalb der LXX begegnen: σωτήρ in II Βας 22 47 Jes 25 9 I Chr 16 35 und σωτήριον in ψ 11 6. In Dan 11 42 hat Θ σωτηρία statt διασῴζω für פליטה.

[7] Zu σωτηρία im Buch Jesaja vgl. L. H. Brockington, The Greek Translator of Isaiah and his Interest in ΔΟΞΑ, VT 1 (1951), 30.

2. Vorkommen und Übersetzungsstatistik der hebräischen Äquivalente

Wie σῴζω und seine Ableitungen überwiegend für den Stamm יש״ע eintreten (abgesehen von der Wiedergabe von שָׁלֵם durch σωτήριον), so werden das Verb יש״ע und seine von ihm abgeleiteten Substantive mit verhältnismäßig wenigen Ausnahmen durch σῴζω usw. übersetzt: das Verb יש״ע hi. insgesamt 161mal gegenüber 22 abweichenden Übersetzungen (davon siebenmal ῥύομαι)[8], ni. 16mal gegenüber drei anderen, יֵשַׁע 33mal gegenüber drei anderen, יְשׁוּעָה 78mal ohne Abweichungen, תְּשׁוּעָה 31mal gegenüber drei anderen und מוֹשָׁעוֹת einmal. Während das Verb יש״ע mit 13 Ausnahmen durch entsprechende griechische Verbformen und seine Substantive besonders durch σωτηρία und σωτήριον wiedergegeben werden, wird יֵשַׁע in 12 Fällen mit σωτήρ *Retter* übersetzt[9].

Im Unterschied davon wird in LXX zur Wiedergabe des Stammes פלט in stärkerem Maße das um ἀνα- oder δια- erweiterte σῴζω verwendet, zwar selten für das meist anders übersetzte Verbum, wohl aber mit wenigen Ausnahmen für die abgeleiteten Substantive. Sie werden im Gegensatz zur Wiedergabe des Stammes יש״ע überwiegend mittels Verbformen übersetzt, nur פְּלֵיטָה auch sechsmal durch σωτηρία. So stehen σῴζω usw. lediglich fünfmal für פלט, das demgegenüber 22mal anders übersetzt wird, besonders durch ῥύομαι und in geringerem Maße durch ἐξαιρέω, dagegen 16mal für פָּלִיט (dreimal anders), fünfmal für פָּלֵיט, 22mal für פְּלֵיטָה (sechsmal anders) und einmal für מִפְלָט[10].

Das aus פלט entstandene Verb מלט[11] wird im Unterschied von den von פלט abgeleiteten Substantiven überwiegend durch σῴζω (zu-

---

[8] Besonderheiten weisen auf die Formen יְהוֹשִׁיעַ I Sam 17 47 Ps 116 6 mit beibehaltenem ה im impf. (W. Gesenius—E. Kautzsch, Hebräische Grammatik, 1909²⁸, § 53q) und וַיּוֹשִׁיעֵן Ex 2 17 mit Bindevokal a vor dem Suffix im impf.

[9] Mit יש״ע ist eine Reihe von Eigennamen gebildet worden, die z. T. aus יֵשַׁע und יהוה (יְשַׁעְיָהוּ) bzw. אֵל (אֱלִישָׁע) zusammengesetzt sind. LXX gibt die Namen, soweit sie nicht durch andere ersetzt sind, in Angleichung an den hebräischen Lautklang ohne Berücksichtigung des Sinns, d. h. ohne Verwendung von σῴζω, wieder. Neben יש״ע ist der Vollständigkeit halber auf שׁוע pi. *um Hilfe rufen* mit den Substantiven שֶׁוַע und שַׁוְעָה *Hilferuf* und den Namen יְהוֹשׁוּעַ bzw. יֵשׁוּעַ Ἰησοῦς hinzuweisen.

[10] Die Wichtigkeit des Ausdrucks zeigen die zahlreichen Eigennamen, die mit Hilfe des Stamms gebildet worden sind und für deren Wiedergabe in LXX das in Anm. 9 Gesagte gilt. Die Namen finden sich auch anderwärts im Alten Orient und sind nicht eigentümlich israelitisch, vgl. M. Lidzbarski, Handbuch der nordsemitischen Epigraphik, I 1898, 209; K. Tallqvist, Assyrian Personal Names, 1914, 179. 179a; Z. S. Harris, A Grammar of the Phoenician Language, 1936, 137; E. Littmann, Nabataean Inscriptions from Egypt, II 1954, 235.

[11] Zur Bildung aus פלט wird entweder auf arabisch *mlṭ* bzw. *mrṭ* (vgl. מרט) *glatt*,

sammen 49mal) und διασῴζω (20mal) übersetzt, während ἀνασῴζω stark zurücktritt (dreimal). Im einzelnen geben diese Verben מלט ni. in 55 Fällen (nur sechsmal anders übersetzt), pi. in 16 Fällen, davon 11mal ῥύομαι und ἐξαιρέω, und das zweimalige hi. in einem Fall wieder[12].

3. Verhältnis von Septuaginta und hebräischem Text

Mit der Übersetzung der Stämme ישע, פלט, und מלט durch σῴζω usw. ist kein grundlegender Bedeutungswandel vor sich gegangen. Dies ergibt sich daraus, daß σῴζω usw. noch eine Reihe anderer hebräischer Ausdrücke wiedergeben, die dem Sinn nach den genannten hebräischen Stämmen entsprechen[13]. Allerdings ist MT in LXX mittels σῴζω usw. mehrfach ziemlich frei, z. T. in bestimmter Deutung übertragen worden[14]. Manchmal ändert sich dadurch der Sinn gegenüber MT. In Jes 10 22 wird aus dem Rest, der sich bekehrt, der Rest, der gerettet wird. In Zeph 3 17 wird die Aussage, daß Gott ein גִּבּוֹר מוֹשִׁיעַ ist, dahin abgeschwächt, er sei δυνατὸς σώσει σε. In Hi 20 24 wird durch die Übertragung von ברח *fliehen* und in Est 8 6 durch die von ראה *anschauen* mit σῴζω der Sinn geändert. Stärker abgewandelt wird MT in Prov 10 5, wo die LXX vom Geschick statt vom Verhalten des Klugen spricht; ferner in den eschatologischen Umprägungen[15] von Prov 10 25, wo die LXX vom Gerechten, der in MT mit einem dauerhaften Fundament verglichen wird, sagt, daß er, der (dem

---

unbehaart sein (vgl. C. Landberg, Datîna, 1909/13, 1113, zu dem davon abgeleiteten südarabischen *entschlüpfen*) oder auf arabisch *mlḍ* (vgl. מרץ) *schlüpfrig sein, entschlüpfen* hingewiesen.

[12] Allerdings wird dieses Vorkommen in Jes 31 5 mit der Bedeutung *retten* in Frage gestellt, weil 1QJes^a statt dessen והפליט aufweist. Zwar bietet 1QJes^a 66 7 übereinstimmend mit MT מלט hi., das demnach auch außerhalb MT belegt ist, jedoch wie 1QH 3 9 in der Bedeutung (*davonbringen*) *gebären*; LXX hat sinngemäß ἐξέφυγεν καὶ ἔτεκεν. מלט hitp. findet sich nur in Hi 41 11 als *sich davonmachen* für das Sprühen von Feuerfunken.

[13] Die Verben stehen fünfmal für עזר *helfen* und einmal für שׂגב pu. *geschützt werden*, die bedeutungsmäßig ישע parallel sind; 14mal für שָׂרִיד *Entronnener* und einmal für שׂרד *entfliehen*, die besonders פלט parallel sind; sechsmal für verschiedene Formen von חיה *leben, leben lassen, das Leben retten* und zweimal für aramäisch שֵׁיזִב (hebräisch עזב) *retten* in engerer Parallele zu מלט; schließlich 24mal für נצל hi., das überwiegend durch ῥύομαι wiedergegeben wird. Je einmal liegen ידע *achten* (auf die Nöte eines Menschen) und עשׁת hitp. *gedenken* zugrunde, weil das Achten und Gedenken nach alter Vorstellung die Hilfe nach sich zieht. Da die hebräischen Ausdrücke außer der Hilfe und Rettung zugleich deren Folge und Wirkung bezeichnen, ist die dreimalige Wiedergabe von בְּשָׁלוֹם *in Frieden, wohlbehalten* mit σωτηρία verständlich.

[14] LXX übersetzt auf diese Weise פדה *loskaufen* Jes 1 27 Hi 33 28, חסה *Zuflucht finden* Jes 14 32 und סור (der Unterwelt) *entgehen* Prov 15 24. In Hi 21 20 wird MT *vom Grimm des Schaddaj trinken* in LXX zu: *nicht gerettet werden*, in Est 4 11: *daß nur ein Gesetz gilt, daß man ihn tötet* in LXX zu: *daß es für ihn keine Rettung gibt*.

[15] Vgl. G. Bertram, Die religiöse Umdeutung altorientalischer Lebensweisheit in der griechischen Übersetzung des ATs, ZAW 54 (1936), 166.

Sturm) ausweichen konnte, *in Ewigkeit gerettet* wird, und von Prov 11 31, wo MT: *Wenn dem Gerechten auf Erden vergolten wird, wieviel mehr dem Frevler und Sünder* in LXX lautet: *Wenn der Gerechte kaum gerettet wird, wo wird dann der Gottlose und Sünder bleiben?* Ebenso findet sich eine stärkere Abwandlung in Iεp 38 22, wo der unklare und wohl verderbte MT: *Jahwe schafft Neues im Lande: die Frau umschirmt (umgibt, umwirbt) den Mann* interpretierend umgewandelt wird in: *Der Herr schuf Heil zu einer neuen Pflanzung, in welchem Heil die Menschen wandeln werden*[16]. In Hi 35 14 übersetzt die LXX unter Verwendung von σῴζω ganz abweichend vom MT, der aber nicht danach geändert werden darf. Doch betrifft dies alles einzelne Stellen, ohne daß die allgemeine Verwendung der griechischen Ausdrücke dadurch berührt wird.

Eine leichte Änderung der Auffassung tritt aber für die von פלט abgeleiteten Substantive ein, die mit Ausnahme von sechs Fällen des Wortes פְּלֵיטָה durch Verbformen von σῴζω usw. übersetzt werden. Aus den *Flüchtlingen, Entronnenen* werden auf diese Weise *Gerettete*, aus dem *Entronnenen* wird *Gerettetes*. Dadurch wird einerseits das passive Verhalten unter Betonung der zuteil gewordenen Hilfe in den Vordergrund gestellt und andererseits darauf hingewiesen, daß einige nicht bloß übriggeblieben und entronnen, sondern absichtsvoll gerettet worden sind; darauf weisen auch die theologisch geprägten parallelen Ausdrücke für den »Rest« (Jes 10 20 37 32) hin[17]. Die sechsmalige Wiedergabe von פְּלֵיטָה mit σωτηρία ist in fünf Fällen sachgemäß, da das hebräische Wort *Entrinnen, Rettung* meint (II Sam 15 14 Jer 25 35 Ob 17 Esr 9 13 II Chr 12 7). Aber obgleich es in Joel 2 3 3 5 in der gleichen Bedeutung vorkommt, wird es dort mittels einer Verbform übersetzt. Umgekehrt findet sich II Εσδρ 9 8 σωτηρία, obwohl פְּלֵיטָה die Bedeutung *Entronnenes* hat, der eine Verbform besser entspräche[18]. Ein Grund für diese Verschiedenheit ist nicht ersichtlich.

II. *Der Stamm* ישע *im Alten Testament*

1. Wortbedeutung

Das Verbum ישע bedeutet nach arabischem *wasi'a* ursprünglich *geräumig, weit sein*[19], besonders im Gegensatz zur Drangsal, die eigentlich als *Engigkeit* צַר und nach צרר als *zusammenschnüren, umhüllen, einwickeln* und daher als *gehemmt, beengt, beklemmt sein* zu verstehen ist. Wie die Drangsal als eine Art räumliche Bedrängnis oder Gefangenschaft vorgestellt wird, so die Rettung daraus als eine Art räumliche

---

[16] Dagegen schließt sich C. Schedl, »Femina circumdabit virum« oder »via salutis«, ZKTh 83 (1961), 431—442, in seiner Rekonstruktion des Textes weitgehend an LXX an.

[17] שְׁאֵרִית selbst wird in IV Βας 19 31 durch κατάλειμμα, in II Εσδρ 9 14 durch ἐγκατάλειμμα, פְּלֵיטָה in IV Βας 19 31 durch ἀνασῴζω und in II Εσδρ 9 14 durch διασῴζω übersetzt.

[18] Außerdem hat Θ das Substantiv in Dan 11 42, wo LXX richtiger eine Verbform von διασῴζω aufweist.

[19] Das Wort findet sich auf der moabitischen Mesa-Inschrift Z. 3f., in den altsüdarabischen Namen *'ljt'* und *jt''l*, vgl. K. Conti-Rossini, Chrestomathia Arabica Meridionalis Epigraphica, 1931, und als aramäisch ויושע in 4QPsDan (J. T. Milik, »Prière de Nabonide« et autres écrits d'un cycle de Daniel, RB 63. 1956. 413).

Bewegung in die Weite[20]. Demgemäß besagt ישע hi., daß man es einem derart Beengten geräumig und weit macht, oder ישע ni., daß es ihm geräumig und weit gemacht wird. Da dies durch rettendes Eingreifen eines Dritten zugunsten des Beengten gegen dessen Bedränger geschieht, ergaben sich die Bedeutung *zur Rettung kommen* und *Rettung erfahren*. Die Rettung wird dem Schwachen oder dem in seinen Lebensrechten Bedrängten infolge eines Schutz- und Abhängigkeitsverhältnisses zuteil, in dem er zu einem Stärkeren oder Mächtigeren steht, der ihn aus seiner Zwangslage rettet. Es ist weder an Selbsthilfe noch gewöhnlich an Beihilfe unter Zusammenwirken mit dem Bedrängten, sondern an eine Hilfe gedacht, ohne die der Bedrängte verloren wäre. Dabei weist der Stamm ישע überwiegend personale Beziehungen auf. Rettung, Hilfe und Heil erfolgen einerseits zugunsten von Personen in Situationen, die oftmals durch den feindlichen Willen anderer Personen herbeigeführt worden sind, andererseits durch das Eingreifen von Personen und nur selten durch technische Mittel oder deren Einschaltung (Jes 26 1 60 18).

Von den abgeleiteten Substantiven ist יֵשַׁע aus dem einsilbigen, kurzvokaligen Stamm nach Art der Segolata, יְשׁוּעָה als f. nach Art der Nomina mit langem Vokal in der zweiten Silbe[21] und תְּשׁוּעָה nach Art der *taqtūl-* bzw. *taqtul*-Bildungen als der mittelhebräisch häufigen Formen der Stämme mediae ו gebildet[22], während מוֹשָׁעוֹת das pt. f. pl. von ישע hi. darstellt. Wie zahlreiche andere Ausdrücke umfassen die Substantive eine Ganzheit, indem sie sowohl die *Rettung*, *Hilfe* als auch das daraus folgende *Heil* bezeichnen, ohne daß die zeitliche Aufeinanderfolge von Vorher und Nachher, Ursache und Wirkung unterschieden wird; denn wirkendes Handeln und die erzielte Wirkung sind voneinander nicht zu trennen.

2. Rettung, Hilfe, Heil durch Menschen

Der Rettung bedarf derjenige, der ohne Kraft und Stärke ist (Hi 26 2) und daher in der Auseinandersetzung mit einem Gegner zu unterliegen droht. Diese Auseinandersetzung kann rechtlicher oder kriegerischer Art sein, so daß bei fehlender Hilfe die Kinder des plötzlich gestorbenen Toren aus ihrem Erbe verdrängt werden (Hi 5 4) oder die vom Feind bedrohte Stadt sich diesem bedingungslos ergeben muß (I Sam 11 3). Wird man in eine solche Streitsache (רִיב) verwickelt

---

[20] Chr. Barth, Die Errettung vom Tode in den individuellen Klage- und Dankliedern des Alten Testaments, 1947, 127.

[21] In Jon 2 10 Ps 3 3 80 3 findet sich die Form יְשׁוּעָתָה ohne Tonverschiebung.

[22] Vgl. C. Brockelmann, Grundriß der vergleichenden Grammatik der semitischen Sprachen, I 1908, 383; G. Beer—R. Meyer, Hebräische Grammatik, I 1952, 108. Es findet sich auch die Form תְּשָׁעָה.

und gerät als der schwächere Teil in Not (צָרָה), so tut man gut daran, den Zeterruf (זעק) über Unrecht und Gewalttat (חָמָס) auszustoßen (Jdc 10 12ff. 12 2f. II Sam 22 3 Hab 1 2 Ps 107 13. 19 II Chr 20 9) und einen Mächtigeren als den bedrängenden Gegner mit dem Ruf הוֹשִׁיעָה zur Rettung aufzufordern (II Sam 14 4 II Reg 6 26), damit er einem zum Recht verhilft (שפט Hos 13 10, דין Ps 54 3) oder seine Macht einsetzt (עֹז Ps 21 2), um den Bedrängten zu schützen (Jes 37 35) oder seine Kraft zu stärken (Sach 10 6 Ps 86 16). Aus diesem terminologischen Zusammenhang wird die Bedeutung des Stammes ישׁע ersichtlich. Gewöhnlich ist mit der Bitte um Rettung als selbstverständliche Voraussetzung verbunden, daß die Herrschaft und Verfügungsgewalt des Angerufenen anerkannt werden. Doch kann ein Abhängigkeitsverhältnis zugleich mit der Bitte um Rettung hergestellt werden, wie die Botschaft des Ahas an Tiglatpileser zeigt: »Ich bin dein Knecht und dein Sohn. Zieh herauf und rette mich ...« (II Reg 16 7); Ahas knüpft die Bitte an seine Unterwerfung als Vasall unter den Assyrerkönig an.

Die erbetene Errettung erfolgt einerseits mittels Kampf und Krieg. Hos 1 7 macht deutlich, daß man sie gewöhnlich durch Bogen und Schwert, Rosse und Reiter und also durch kämpferisches Eingreifen erwartet. So bringen die Richter als von Gott berufene Führer kriegerische Hilfe gegen die jeweiligen Feinde Israels (Jdc 2 16. 18 3 9. 15. 31 u. ö.), Saul gegen die Ammoniter (I Sam 11 9) und Philister (I Sam 9 16; vgl. I Sam 14 45 23 5). So versprechen zwei Abteilungen des Heeres, die gegen verschiedene Feinde kämpfen, einander im Notfall zu Hilfe zu kommen (II Sam 10 11), oder läßt ein dritter Staat dem einen von zwei kämpfenden anderen Staaten militärische Hilfe zuteil werden (II Sam 10 19). Gelegentlich hält man allerdings vergeblich Ausschau *nach dem Volk, das nicht rettet* (Thr 4 17), weil der angerufene Staat in Wirklichkeit gar nicht der mächtigere Dritte ist. Trifft diese Voraussetzung jedoch zu, so bringt das Eingreifen des Retters die erwünschte Wirkung: תְּשׁוּעָה *Sieg* (Jdc 15 18 II Sam 19 3).

Die Errettung erfolgt andererseits durch Beheben einer Rechtsnot. Hiob würde bereits in der Zulassung zu Gott den Sieg im Rechtsstreit erblicken (Hi 13 16). Vom Richter Tola heißt es, daß er Israel erretten sollte (Jdc 10 1), während sonst der Ausdruck שפט *richten, zum Recht verhelfen* gebraucht wird. Doch deckt sich ישׁע nicht mit שׁפט, weil es nicht *zum Recht verhelfen*, sondern ein *befreiendes Retten* aus der bedrängenden Rechtsnot meint. So erbittet man das persönliche Eingreifen des Königs, wenn die gesetzlichen Bestimmungen eigentlich eine Verurteilung erfordern (II Sam 14 4) oder in der völligen Verwirrung der Verhältnisse überhaupt nicht anwendbar sind (II Reg 6 26). Daher kann das rettende Eingreifen als Alternative zum Rechtsstreit erscheinen (Jdc 6 31).

Menschliche Rettungstaten erwartet man von kriegerischen Helden wie Richtern und Nasiräern (Jdc 13 5) oder Jonatan und David; ein solcher Held kann tatkräftig und wirkungsvoll eingreifen (vgl. Jer 14 9). Rettung erwartet man ferner von der Schutzmacht; darin liegt für den Vasallen die positive Seite der fremden Oberherrschaft (vgl. II Reg 16 7 Hos 14 4). Vor allem gehört die Hilfeleistung wie das Rechtschaffen überhaupt zu den Aufgaben des Königs (vgl. II Sam 14 4 II Reg 6 26), die als von Gott aufgetragen gelten und deren Erfüllung für das Volk ein glück- und heilvolles Leben bewirkt (Ps 72 3f. 13). Daher kann Hosea fragen: »'Wo' ist dein König, daß er dich rette, und all 'deine Beamten', daß 'sie dir Recht verschaffen'?« (Hos 13 10)[23]. Gehört das Retten zu den grundlegenden Aufgaben des Königs, so ist es verständlich, daß man einen Mann zum König zu wählen sucht, der bereits in solcher Weise gehandelt hat wie Gideon (Jdc 8 22) oder von dem es aufgrund eines Jahweorakels zu erwarten ist wie von David (II Sam 3 18).

3. Grenzen menschlichen Rettens

Mit starkem Nachdruck weist das Alte Testament auf die Grenzen hin, die allem nicht von Jahwe legitimierten Retten gesetzt sind. So ist es selbstverständlich, daß die hölzernen oder steinernen Götzen aus der Not nicht retten und kein Heil schaffen können (Jes 45 20b 46 7 Jer 2 27f. 3 23 11 12 Hos 14 4b), ebensowenig die Astrologen (Jes 47 13). Nicht ein Engel, der hauptsächlich als Bote dient, sondern Gott selbst hat Israel aus Ägypten gerettet (Jes 63 8f.). Israel hat nicht aus eigener Kraft die Landnahme erzwungen, sondern Gott hat diese Siegestaten vollbracht (Ps 44 4f.). Damit das Volk nicht behaupten kann, daß es sich selbst gerettet habe, dürfen nur 300 Mann gegen die Midianiter kämpfen (Jdc 7 2. 7). Demgemäß sind Hilfe und Sieg im Kampf überhaupt nicht von militärischer Macht (Hos 1 7 14 4 Ps 33 16f.), nicht von Fürsten und Menschen zu erhoffen (Ps 146 3), sondern vom stillen Warten und Vertrauen auf Gottes Eingreifen (Jes 30 15 Hos 14 4b). Infolgedessen bedeutet es nach I Sam 10 18f. eine schwere Sünde, daß Israel seinen wahren König Jahwe, der es aus Nöten und Drangsalen *gerettet* hat (מוֹשִׁיעַ, LXX: σωτήρ), verwirft und an seiner Stelle einen König aus den eigenen Reihen fordert; denn auf diese Weise will es letztlich sich selbst retten, anstatt sich retten zu lassen. Wenn aber ein Mensch sich selber mit eigener Hand hilft, muß er als der an sich schwächere oder rechtlich unterlegene Teil gegenüber dem Gegner zu unerlaubten Maßnahmen greifen, um sich dennoch durchzusetzen, und dadurch Blutschuld auf sich laden (I Sam 25 26. 31. 33).

---

[23] Es ist zu lesen אַיֵּה statt »ich will sein«, וְכָל־שָׂרֶיךָ statt »in all deinen Städten« und יִשְׁפְּטָךְ statt »und deine Richter«.

Nur Gott, der alle Macht und alles Recht besitzt, kann — ohne solche Gefahr zu laufen — sich selber helfen, sich Sieg und Heil schaffen (Ps 98 1-3); der Mensch könnte es nur, wenn er wie Gott wäre (Hi 40 9. 14). Helfendes und rettendes Eingreifen von Menschen (im Sinn des Stammes ישע) erfolgt in rechter Weise, wenn Gott in ihnen und durch sie wirkt[24].

So wird es in verschiedener Weise von den Richtern gesagt: Jahwe ließ sie erstehen (Jdc 2 16 3 9. 15) oder gab sie (Neh 9 27), und sie retteten Israel; oder er war mit den Richtern und rettete selber (Jdc 2 18) oder rettete durch die Hand der Richter (Jdc 6 36f.). In Übernahme und Abwandlung dessen ist anderwärts davon die Rede, daß Jahwe einen Retter sandte oder senden wird, der hilft (II Reg 13 5 Jes 19 20). Stets ist es Gott, der durch viel oder wenig hilft (I Sam 14 6; vgl. auch Jdc 13 5 I Sam 9 16 II Sam 3 18). Daher ist es verständlich, daß Gideon vor dem Kampf gegen die Midianiter als Helfer und Retter zurückschreckt, weil seine Sippe schwach und machtlos ist, und sich erst bereitwillig zeigt, als ihn das erbetene Zeichen dessen gewiß macht, daß Jahwe mit ihm sein wird (Jdc 6 14ff.).

4. Rettung, Hilfe, Heil durch Gott

Wie durch Menschen rettet und hilft Gott vor allem selber und unmittelbar als derjenige, der über alles Recht und alle Macht verfügt und daher am besten in Schutz und Fürsorge zugunsten des in eine Notlage geratenen Schwachen gegen dessen Bedränger eingreifen kann. Wie das Retten eine Hauptaufgabe des Helden und des Königs ist, so verbindet es sich mit der Vorstellung der göttlichen Heldenkraft (Ps 80 3) und Jahwes als des Königs (Jes 33 22 Ps 44 4f.), der seit dem Kampf gegen die chaotischen Mächte bei der Schöpfung immer wieder solche Siegestaten vollbringt (Ps 74 12ff.)[25]. Daher wendet sich der Beter an ihn wie der Hilfesuchende an seinen König mit dem Ruf: הושיעה *rette, hilf!*[26].

Israel kann auf so häufig erfahrene Hilfe durch göttliche Siege über seine Feinde zurückblicken, daß es geradezu als עם נושע ביהוה *ein Volk, siegreich durch Jahwe* (Dtn 33 29) bezeichnet werden kann. Seit der Rettung aus Ägypten (Ex 15 2 Ps 74 12 106 10. 21) hat Gott

---

[24] Dies geschieht, ohne daß sie dadurch zu Mittlern würden.

[25] Entgegen der Behauptung von E. Beaucamp, Le Psaume 21 (20), psaume messianique, in: Richesses et déficiences des anciens Psautiers latins, 1959, 41f., wird ישועה nicht als Heilskraft verliehen, sondern bezeichnet die einzelne rettende, heilvolle Tat oder den von Gott auf diese Weise herbeigeführten Heilszustand.

[26] Ps 12 2 20 10 28 9 60 7 86 16 108 7; mit dem Suffix der 1. pers. sg. Ps 3 8 6 5 7 2 22 22 31 17 54 3 59 3 69 2 71 2 109 26 119 94; mit dem Suffix der 1. pers. pl. Ps 106 47; mit dem verstärkenden נא *doch* Ps 118 25.

es immer wieder vor anderen Völkern gerettet und ihm geholfen (I Sam 11 13 14 23. 39 II Sam 8 6. 14 u. ö.). Auch die Anwesenheit der Lade, die die Gegenwart Gottes verbürgt, läßt den Sieg erhoffen (I Sam 4 3) — freilich vergeblich, wenn Gott nicht retten will, weil Israel ihn verlassen hat und zu anderen Göttern abgefallen ist, die doch nicht retten können (Jdc 10 12-14). Ist Israel aber treu, so kann ihm im Krieg die Hilfe Gottes vor dem Feind zugesagt werden (Num 10 9 Dtn 20 4[27] Hab 3 13). Diese Hilfe nimmt es am Morgen wahr (vgl. Jes 33 2) wie nach der Nacht am Schilfmeer und erkennt sie als Gottes Eingreifen, weil damals gewöhnlich kein Mensch irgendwelche Kampfhandlungen während der Nacht unternahm[28]. Daher kann Jahwe als *Held, der Sieg schafft* gefeiert (Zeph 3 17) oder als Israels *Retter in der Zeit der Not* im Volksklagelied angerufen werden (Jer 14 8).

Vor allem in den Psalmen wird der Stamm ישע verwendet, um die erbetene und erhoffte oder die erfahrene Hilfe Jahwes gegen die gemeinsamen oder persönlichen Feinde zu umschreiben; Jahwe möge vor ihnen retten, die den oder die Beter angreifen oder anklagen und sich dabei öfters die als vergeltende göttliche Strafe gedeutete Krankheit des Beters zunutze machen. Fast 80mal begegnet der Stamm ישע in dieser Weise als Ausdruck für das Helfen Jahwes vor dem Feind des Beters in den Psalmen (vgl. noch I Sam 2 1 Jer 15 20 17 14). Dabei handelt es sich mehrfach um den jeweiligen persönlichen Rechtsgegner, der den Beter bedrängt, anklagt und zu vernichten sucht, so daß die Hilfe in einer schwierigen und nahezu aussichtslosen Rechtslage gewünscht wird. Gott kann nicht nur im Kriege helfen und den Sieg schaffen, sondern auch vor Unrecht und Gewalttat (II Sam 22 3) oder aus dem Kerker retten (Ps 107 13ff.). »Er steht zur Rechten des Armen, um sein Leben vor 'seinen Richtern' zu *retten*« (Ps 109 31)[29]. Die Rettung erfolgt aus den Gefahren von Krankheit, Gefangenschaft oder Anfeindung — diese als alleinige Bedrängnis oder häufiger als Begleiterscheinung und Folge einer anderen Drangsal verstanden —, wobei die Gefahren eine Schwächung der Lebenskraft und damit eine Vorform des sich des Bedrängten bemächtigenden Todes bedeuten. Rettung ist deshalb Errettung vom Tode. Das Vertrauen auf solche Rettung und Hilfe durch Gott aus all den Nöten und Schrecken, denen der Mensch ausgesetzt ist und die ihn — wie die zahlreichen Ausdrücke zeigen — überall und ständig bedrängen, macht einen wesentlichen Zug des Selbstverständnisses des Glaubenden aus.

---

[27] Die priesterliche Kriegsansprache in Dtn 20 3f. beruht nicht auf einem tatsächlichen Brauch, sondern ist literarische Fiktion, zumal v. 2-4 ein späterer priesterlicher Einschub sind.

[28] Vgl. J. Ziegler, Die Hilfe Gottes »am Morgen«, in: Nötscher-Festschrift, 1950, 281—288.   [29] Es ist מִשְׁפָּטָיו statt »den Richtern« (seiner Seele) zu lesen.

Ohne Bezugnahme auf konkrete Nöte oder Feinde spricht das Alte Testament ferner von der allgemeinen und umfassenden *Rettung* und *Hilfe* oder dem *Heil*, die Gott zuteil werden läßt. Zwar hat Israel seinen rettenden und heilvollen Gott verstoßen, dem es seine Existenz verdankt (Dtn 32 15) und der es in der Wüste bewahrte (Ps 78 22), und verfällt darum dem Gericht (Jes 17 10). Doch der einzelne darf Gottes Hilfe aufgrund seiner Zugehörigkeit zum Volke Jahwes erhoffen (Ps 106 4). Wie Gott dem David und dem König alles zum Heil ausschlagen ließ (II Sam 23 5 Ps 18 51), so wünscht man später den Priestern, daß sie mit Heil angetan seien (Ps 132 16 II Chr 6 41)³⁰. Damit ist — wie auch für den einzelnen, der mit Kleidern des Heils bekleidet ist (Jes 61 10) — gemäß dem Vorgang Sach 3 4f. an Stelle der die Sünde symbolisierenden schmutzigen Kleidung eine die Sündenvergebung und Heilsbegnadung symbolisierende Kleidung gemeint. Ebenso kann der Begnadete den Heilsbecher als Symbol der göttlichen Heilsgnade (vgl. Ps 16 5) oder (nach dem Ritus des Trankopfers) des Dankes erheben (Ps 116 13).

Hilfe und Heil im allgemeinen Sinn zu gewähren, die das Lebensglück Hiobs ausgemacht haben (Hi 30 15), bestimmt Gottes Walten und Handeln auf Erden überhaupt (Ps 18 28 67 3 Hi 22 29). Freilich wird dies nicht dem hochmütigen Frevler, sondern dem Demütigen zuteil, der sich vor Gott gering weiß: der rein und lauter ist (Ps 24 5), Gott mit zerschlagenem Geist und zerbrochenem Herzen anruft (Ps 34 7. 19), auf seinen Wandel achtet (Ps 50 23), schwach und geistlich arm ist (Ps 116 6), den göttlichen Willen befolgt (Ps 119 155. 166. 174), Gott fürchtet und liebt (Ps 145 19f.) und schweigend auf sein Eingreifen harrt (Thr 3 26). Dann kann der Fromme ihn als *Hilfe seines Angesichts* und seinen Gott preisen (Ps 42 6. 12 43 5).

Obwohl Gott seine Hilfe dem Sünder gewöhnlich versagt, wird ישע doch einigemal dazu verwendet, die Rettung aus dem Gericht zu beschreiben. Dabei drückt der Stamm entsprechend seiner Verwendung in rechtlichen Zusammenhängen gemäß II Sam 14 4 aus, daß die Verurteilung an sich zu Recht besteht und das Gericht eigentlich erforderlich wäre. ישע meint also das entgegen der rechtlich einwandfreien Verdammung dennoch sich ereignende rettende Heilshandeln Gottes. So wird er dem schwachen, von der Oberschicht bedrückten Volksteil Israels wie ein Hirt seiner Herde helfen, obwohl die Bedrückten vor ihm nicht weniger schuldbeladen sind als die Bedrücker (Ez 34 22). Er wird Israel von allen Sünden *befreien* und ihm gegen diesen überlegenen Feind als der mächtigere Dritte *helfen* (Ez 36 29),

---

³⁰ II Chr 6 41-42a sind ein fast wörtliches Zitat aus Ps 132 8f. Während aber Ps 132 9 das Heil mit צֶ֫דֶק (und 132 16 mit יֶ֫שַׁע) umschreibt, hat II Chr 6 41 statt dessen תְּשׁוּעָה, so daß die Ausdrücke als austauschbar erscheinen.

um es neu zu schaffen und zu erlösen (vgl. Ez 36 24-28). Umgekehrt kann als Voraussetzung für die Rettung aus dem Gericht die Aufforderung ergehen: »Wasche dein Herz vom Bösen, Jerusalem, damit du *gerettet* wirst« (Jer 4 14).

Von da aus wird es verständlich, daß יֹשע auch in der eschatologischen Theologie als Ausdruck für *Rettung, Hilfe* und *Heil* der Endzeit begegnet. Dazu müssen die nach Babylonien Deportierten entsprechend der kriegerischen Verwendung von יֹשע wie Gefangene befreit (Jes 49 8f.) und damit zunächst für das Heil gerettet werden (Jes 45 17). Nur Jahwe vermag dies, außer dem es keinen Retter gibt (Jes 43 11 45 21) und der sich — nach dem späten Einschub Hos 13 4 — von Ägypten an als Israels Gott und Retter erwiesen hat. Bricht aber die eschatologische Heilszeit an, so ist sie als wirkliche »Erlösung« zu bezeichnen. Da גאל seit Deuterojesaja zum terminus technicus dafür wird, ist es nicht verwunderlich, daß יֹשע als einer der Ausdrücke für Rettung und Heil der Endzeit gelegentlich in Parallele dazu tritt (Jes 43 1-3 60 16 63 9)[31], ohne daß dies nachhaltig auf die Begriffsbildung eingewirkt hätte. Vielmehr bezeichnet der Stamm יֹשע in der Doppelheit von Vorher und Nachher, Ursache und Wirkung sowohl die zum Heil führende unverdiente *Rettung* als auch das dadurch ermöglichte *Heil* selbst; das gleiche gilt für צְדָקָה, mit dem es parallel stehen kann (Jes 46 13 51 6. 8). Die Rettung, die das Heil ermöglichen wird, ist die Bewahrung vor dem endzeitlichen Völkersturm (Sach 12 7) und vor allem das Sammeln und Heimbringen der Zerstreuten aus aller Welt (Jes 43 5-7 Jer 31 7 46 27 Zeph 3 19 Sach 8 7 Ps 106 47). So führt Gott durch sein helfendes Eingreifen (Jes 59 1 Sach 8 13) die Endzeit herbei (Jes 46 13 51 6. 8), sofern erneutes Sündigen ihn nicht davon abhält (Jes 59 11). Dann kann die endzeitliche Gemeinde aus den von Jerusalem ausgehenden Heilsquellen schöpfen (Jes 12 3), ja alle Welt an diesem Heil Anteil erlangen (Jes 45 22 49 6). Im Anschluß daran wird der messianische Herrscher, der auf Erden als Gottes Stellvertreter regiert, Israel retten und helfen, wie es Aufgabe eines Königs ist, so daß es in Sicherheit wohnen kann (Jer 23 6), wie der Messias selber von Gott durch dessen Sieg über den endzeitlichen Völkersturm gerettet worden ist (Sach 9 9).

III. Die Stämme פלט *und* מלט *im Alten Testament*

1. Die Substantive des Stammes פלט

Während das Verb פלט qal *entkommen*, pi. und hi. *in Sicherheit bringen, retten* bedeutet[32], bezeichnen פָּלִיט und das nur im pl. vor-

---

[31] Dagegen steht גאל als Parallele zu יֹשע in Ps 72 13f. 106 10 im rechtlichen Sinn in der Bedeutung *auslösen*.

[32] Vgl. akkadisch *balāṭu leben* (Barth a. a. O. 28—32; W. von Soden, Akkadisches

kommende פָּלִיט[33] sowohl denjenigen, der im Begriff ist zu entkommen, den *Flüchtling*[34], als auch denjenigen, der entkommen oder in Sicherheit gebracht worden ist, den *Entronnenen*[35]. פְּלֵיטָה[36] bezeichnet sowohl das *Entrinnen*, die *Errettung*[37] als auch und vor allem das *Entronnene* als Folge und Ergebnis des Entrinnens[38]. Wie bei den Substantiven des Stammes ישע wird ohne Unterscheidung der zeitlichen Aufeinanderfolge der gleiche Ausdruck für Vorher und Nachher, Ursache und Wirkung verwendet.

Überwiegend beziehen sich die Ausdrücke auf das Entrinnen aus einer tödlichen Gefahr[39]. Eine Ausnahme bildet Jdc 12 4 mit dem Vorwurf der Ephraimiten, daß die Gileaditer *entlaufene* Westisraeliten seien (vielleicht um sich den dortigen Verpflichtungen zu entziehen), in gewissem Sinn ferner die Beziehung auf die Gefangennahme in Gen 14 13 und auf die Unterwerfung eines Landes durch den Eroberer in Dan 11 42. Sonst aber handelt es sich bei den Vorkommen ohne religiösen Charakter stets um das Entrinnen aus der Gefahr eines gewaltsamen Todes. Man flieht vor dem überlegenen Feind, um nicht getötet zu werden (Num 21 29 II Sam 15 14 Jer 50 28), oder sucht wenigstens nach verlorenem Kampf zu entrinnen (Jdc 12 5 21 17). Ob der bei Ezechiel eintreffende Flüchtling (Ez 33 21) nach der Eroberung Jerusalems den Babyloniern entrinnen konnte oder nach der Ermordung Gedaljas aus Furcht vor Vergeltungsmaßnahmen geflohen ist, läßt sich nicht ersehen. Der kluge Jakob sucht der nach seiner Meinung von Esau drohenden Gefahr durch die Teilung seines Besitzes zu entgehen, so daß wenigstens eins der beiden Lager dem befürchteten Gemetzel entrinnen kann (Gen 32 9). Letztlich aber beruht es auf dem Eingreifen Gottes, wenn Israel vor dem Pharao Sisak

---

Handwörterbuch, Liefg. 2, 1959, 98f.); kanaanäisch *plṭ retten* (J. Aistleitner, Wörterbuch der ugaritischen Sprache, 1967³, 256; C. H. Gordon, Ugaritic Textbook, 1965, 468); Amarnabrief 185, 25. 33 (S. A. B. Mercer, The Tell-el-Amarna Tablets, II 1939) *paliṭmi ist entkommen, verschont geblieben*; arabisch *flt entkommen*; aramäisch *entfliehen*.

[33] Nach J. Barth, Die Nominalbildung in den semitischen Sprachen, 1894², 112, ist פָּלִיט aus *paliṭ entstanden, dagegen ist es nach J. Olshausen, Lehrbuch der hebräischen Sprache, 1861, 180, und P. de Lagarde, Übersicht über die im Aramäischen übliche Bildung der Nomina, 1889, 85, eine Diminutivform.

[34] Daher die Parallele נָס *Flüchtling* Jer 50 28 Am 9 1.

[35] Daher die Parallele שָׂרִיד *Entronnener* Jer 42 17 44 14 Ob 14 Thr 2 22.

[36] Die Form פְּלֵטָה findet sich Ex 10 5 Jer 50 29 Ez 14 22 I Chr 4 43.

[37] II Sam 15 14 Jer 25 35 Joel 2 3 3 5 Ob 17 Esr 9 13 II Chr 12 7.

[38] Gen 32 9 Jdc 21 17 II Reg 19 30f. (Jes 37 31f.) Jes 10 20 Jer 50 29 Ez 14 22 Dan 11 42 Esr 9 8. 14f. Neh 1 2 II Chr 20 24.

[39] Vgl. die akkadischen Beispiele bei Chr. Barth a. a. O. 62. Die Ausdrücke leben im deutschen Wort Pleite weiter; פָּלִיט ist der durch die Pleite Gegangene.

gerettet worden (II Chr 12 7) und aus der Assyrernot eine entronnene Schar übriggeblieben ist (II Reg 19 30f.) und wenn seine verbündeten Feinde sich gegenseitig umbringen, so daß aus diesem Kampf niemand entrinnt (II Chr 20 24).

Umgekehrt verkündigen die Propheten das göttliche Strafgericht über das sündige Israel als eine todbringende Gefahr, aus der es kein Entrinnen gibt. So schaut und hört es zuerst Amos: »Kein *Flüchtiger* נָס soll von ihnen entfliehen, kein *Entronnener* פָּלִיט von ihnen entrinnen« (Am 9 1). Wenn einige Jerusalemer sich doch aus Kampf und Belagerungsnöten retten sollten, sagt Ez 7 16, werden sie hilflos als Flüchtlinge in den Bergen umherirren, während Jer 42 17 den zur Flucht nach Ägypten Entschlossenen androht, daß niemand aus Schwert, Hunger und Pest entrinnen wird (vgl. 44 14). Am Tag Jahwes gibt es eben kein Entrinnen (Joel 2 3) — weder für Jerusalem (Thr 2 22) noch für die vom göttlichen Gericht ereilten Völker (Jer 25 35 50 29). Dennoch weiß man davon, daß im nordisraelitischen Gebiet einige Israeliten den Assyrern (II Chr 30 6) und daß die im Exil lebenden Judäer dem Schwerte Babels entronnen sind (Jer 51 50); daher darf man Gleiches für die in Ägypten Lebenden erwarten (Jer 44 28)[40]. Ezechiel zwar wandelt eine solche Erwartung in der Auseinandersetzung mit den Deportierten gründlich ab: Wenn in Jerusalem trotz aller Plagen eine gerettete Schar übrigbleibt, dann nur als Anschauungsmittel für die Deportierten, die an diesen Sündern erkennen sollen, daß das Gericht über die Stadt begründet war (Ez 14 12-23).

Ungeachtet dessen begegnen die Ausdrücke פָּלִיט und פְּלֵיטָה geradezu als terminus technicus für die dem göttlichen Strafgericht als einer tödlichen Gefahr *Entronnenen* (Jes 4 2 10 20 Ez 6 8f. Joel 3 5 Ob 17 Esr 9 8.13ff. Neh 1 2). Dazu will die am Anfang von Ez 6 8 eingefügte Glosse *und ich lasse übrig* betonen, daß es auf Gottes Wollen und Wirken beruht, wenn einige vom Gerichtsschwert verschont wurden. Erscheinen diese Entronnenen nahezu als eschatologische Größe, so gilt dies zweifellos für die *Entronnenen der* (heidnischen) *Völker*, die die durch die Siege des Kyros eingeleitete und den Beginn der endzeitlichen Geschehnisse bildende Welterschütterung überlebt haben, sich nun zu dem einen Gott bekehren und in das endzeitliche Heil retten lassen sollen (Jes 45 20-22). Den gleichen Ausdruck greift Jes 66 19 als Bezeichnung der bekehrten und daher dem Endgericht entrinnenden Nichtisraeliten auf, die zum Tempel Zutritt haben und von Jahwe missionierend in alle Welt gesandt werden.

---

[40] Diese nicht mehr von Jeremia stammende Verheißung hat bewirkt, daß zu der gegenteiligen Auffassung in Jer 44 14 (gleichfalls nicht von Jeremia) am Ende des Verses ein ausgleichender Zusatz hinzugefügt worden ist.

2. Das Verb מלט

Kennzeichnend für die Bedeutung des Verbs מלט ni. *entrinnen, sich in Sicherheit bringen* (aus tödlicher Gefahr) und pi. *entrinnen lassen, retten, sich retten* sind die parallelen Ausdrücke in dem Wort Jeremias an den Kuschiten, der ihm das Leben gerettet hat: nicht durchs Schwert fallen, das Leben zur Beute haben (Jer 39 18), der eine volle Niederlage des Feindes feststellende Ausdruck *niemand entrann* (Jdc 3 29 I Sam 30 17; vgl. die entsprechende Aufforderung Elias I Reg 18 40) und die Zusammenstellung mit einem das Fliehen bezeichnenden Verb (besonders נוס, ברח), wobei מלט als Ergebnis der Flucht vor todbringender Bedrohung angibt, daß sie gelungen ist und der Flüchtige sich *in Sicherheit gebracht* hat (I Sam 19 10. 12. 17f. 22 1 II Sam 1 3f. I Reg 20 20 Jer 48 6 51 6; vgl. 48 19)[41].

So bezieht sich מלט, ähnlich den von פלט abgeleiteten Substantiven überwiegend auf das Entrinnen vor dem drohenden Tod. Man entrinnt schon vor dem Eintritt einer Katastrophe (Gen 19 17-22)[42] oder entkommt aus ihr, so daß man über sie berichten kann (Hi 1 15ff.). David muß sein Leben immer wieder vor den Nachstellungen Sauls in Sicherheit bringen (I Sam 19 11 23 13 27 1) wie umgekehrt die Mörder vor ihren Verfolgern (Jdc 3 26 II Reg 19 37 Jer 41 15)[43]. Doch geht es nicht immer um Leben und Tod: Jesaja läßt die Einwohner der palästinischen Küstenebene erkennen, daß sie der Eroberung durch die Assyrer nicht entrinnen können (Jes 20 6)[44], und Hiob setzt voraus, daß man jemanden aus Feindesgewalt mit Geld retten kann (Hi 6 23). Ferner bezeichnet מלט das Entrinnen vor Strafe, so daß man *verschont* oder *gerettet* wird (Ez 17 15 Jer 48 8 Mal 3 15; vgl. Prov 11 21 19 5), vor Bewachung, so daß man durch ein Tor *durchschlüpft* (II Sam 4 6), und vom Hofdienst, so daß man *abkommen* und die Verwandten besuchen kann (I Sam 20 29)[45]. Schließlich gibt es allgemein die *Rettung* des Hilfsbedürftigen aus Bedrängnis an (Hi 29 12)[46].

Dementsprechend sind die Väter Israels, die auf Gott vertrauten, nicht zuschanden, sondern gerettet worden (Ps 22 6), wie überhaupt

---

[41] In umgekehrter Reihenfolge nur I Sam 22 20; Abjatar *entrann* מלט dem Blutbad und floh zu David.

[42] Die fünfmalige Verwendung von מלט ni. in diesen Versen enthält wohl ein Wortspiel mit dem Namen Lots, der entrinnen kann.

[43] מלט bedeutet *(das Leben) retten* ferner in II Sam 19 6 I Reg 1 12 Jer 51 45 Ps 41 2 89 49 107 20 116 4, ohne daß LXX die Wortgruppe σῴζω verwendet.

[44] Ähnlich II Sam 19 10: aus der Gewalt der Philister *retten* (LXX: ἐξαιρέω).

[45] Ferner II Reg 23 18: Gebeine der Vernichtung *entrinnen* lassen, d. h. unversehrt lassen (LXX: ῥύομαι); Koh 7 26: Nicht der Weise als solcher, sondern wer Gott gefällt, *entkommt* der Frau (LXX: ἐξαιρέω).

[46] In dieser Bedeutung ist מלט parallel mit נצל hi., das sich in dem in Hi 29 12 verwendeten Ps 72 12 findet.

der Schuldlose, der reine, unbefleckte Hände als Zeichen seiner Gerechtigkeit vorweisen kann, von Gott gerettet wird (Hi 22 30). Nicht entrinnen läßt dagegen das Vertrauen auf die Stärke des Rosses (Ps 33 17) oder die Macht eines anderen Staates (Jes 20 6), auf den Reichtum (Hi 20 20 Koh 8 8)[47] oder den eigenen Verstand (Prov 28 26). Während aber Prov 28 26 behauptet, daß derjenige dem Unglück entrinnt, der die weisen Lebensregeln befolgt, will Koh 9 15 die Nutzlosigkeit dieser Weisheit am Beispiel des armen Weisen zeigen, der die belagerte Stadt hätte retten können, aber nicht beachtet worden ist, weil seine Weisheit in wenig ansprechender Form und nicht in repräsentativer Vertretung auftrat. Wie Gott die Schuldlosen rettet, so vernichtet er die Frevler. Aus dem göttlichen Gericht über das schuldige Dasein gibt es kein Entrinnen für die Baalverehrer (I Reg 19 17), für ganz Israel (Am 2 14f. 9 1), für den König (Jer 32 4 u. ö.) oder für die babylonischen Götzenbilder (Jes 46 2). Nur wenn Gott sich, um die eschatologische Heilszeit heraufzuführen, der Verurteilten erbarmt, können die Gefangenen dank seiner befreienden Tat dem Gewalthaber wieder entrinnen (Jes 49 24f.)[48]. In der Endzeit werden diejenigen gerettet, die den Namen Jahwes anrufen (Joel 3 5) oder die im Buch des Lebens aufgezeichnet sind (Dan 12 1).

IV. σωτήρ im Alten Testament

Die LXX gibt mit σωτήρ zwar stets den Stamm ישׁע wieder[49]; aber das Wort findet sich lediglich siebenmal für dessen pt. hi. מוֹשִׁיעַ, für das man es hauptsächlich erwarten sollte, sonst für יֵשַׁע und יְשׁוּעָה. So treffen σωτήρ und מוֹשִׁיעַ nur selten zusammen (Jdc 3 9. 15 12 3 B I Sam 10 19 Jes 45 15. 21 Neh 9 27 [II Εσδρ 19 27]). Zudem läßt σωτήρ sich höchstens in Jdc 3 9. 15 als terminus technicus für die Richter verstehen, obschon zu bedenken ist, daß LXX in Jdc 2 16 und Neh 9 27 im Unterschied von MT, jedoch in Übereinstimmung mit diesem in Jdc 2 18 betont, daß nach der Einsetzung der Richter nicht diese, sondern Gott selbst Israel gerettet hat; so sollen die Richter jedenfalls nicht als Heilbringer verstanden werden. Ebenso scheint die LXX den Begriff σωτήρ für Könige zu vermeiden (vgl. IV Βασ 13 5). An den übrigen Stellen ist ganz entsprechend der Bedeutung des Stammes ישׁע an Menschen und besonders an Jahwe als *Helfer* und *Retter* aus irdischen Nöten gedacht. — Umgekehrt ist die Über-

---

[47] In Koh 8 8 ist עֹשֶׁר statt »Frevel« zu lesen.
[48] In Jes 49 24 ist wie in v. 25 עָרִיץ statt צַדִּיק zu lesen.
[49] Erst im nachchristlichen Judentum dient גּוֹאֵל dazu, den Messias in der Funktion des מוֹשִׁיעַ zu bezeichnen: als Vernichter der heidnischen Weltmächte und Befreier Israels aus der Knechtschaft; vgl. H. L. Strack—P. Billerbeck, Kommentar zum Neuen Testament aus Talmud und Midrasch, I 1956², 68f.

setzung des pt. hi. מוֹשִׁיעַ in der LXX sehr unregelmäßig. Außer dem siebenmaligen σωτήρ finden sich neunmal σῴζων, vielleicht um den Nachdruck auf das göttliche Handeln zu legen, zweimal andere Verbformen von σῴζω, viermal das unpersönliche σωτηρία, vielleicht zur Betonung der vom Retter gebrachten Hilfe, schließlich sogar viermal βοηθέω und einmal ῥύομαι.

Demnach ist σωτήρ in LXX durchweg kein terminus technicus. Dem widerspricht auch die Feststellung nicht, daß das Wort 12mal zur Wiedergabe von יֵשַׁע *Rettung, Befreiung, Hilfe, Heil*, d. h. in einem Drittel von dessen Vorkommen überhaupt, davon siebenmal in Psalmen, viermal in Prophetenbüchern und viermal zur Wiedergabe von יְשׁוּעָה *Hilfe, Heil* (Dtn 32 15 Jes 12 2 Ps 62 3. 7) gebraucht wird[50]. Denn darin handelt es sich um eine personale Wiedergabe von hebräischen Redewendungen, in denen Gott als *Hilfe* oder *Heil* des Menschen bezeichnet wird (vgl. ferner Jes 17 10 Ps 25 5 27 1. 9 65 6 79 9). Zudem ist die Übersetzung uneinheitlich. Während יְשׁוּעָה in Ps 62 3. 7 mit σωτήρ wiedergegeben wird, findet sich dafür in 62 2 ohne zwingenden Grund σωτήριον, und während יֵשַׁע in Hab 3 13 durch σωτηρία und σῴζω wiedergegeben wird, obwohl in zwei parallelen Halbversen stehend, begegnet dafür in 3 18 σωτήρ.

Demgemäß wird σωτήρ im griechischen Alten Testament nicht als Bezeichnung des Messias gebraucht. Eine Annäherung daran liegt an zwei anderen Stellen vor: In Sach 9 9 ist der Messias, der nach dem hebräischen Text von Gott gerettet worden ist, in Septuaginta ein König, der *rettet* (σῴζων), so daß ein wenig die frühjüdische Auffassung des Messias als des Heilbringers anklingt. In Jes 49 6, wo der hebräische Text vom Heil Jahwes redet, scheint in der Septuaginta der Knecht Jahwes als eine messianische Gestalt verstanden zu sein, der zum Heil (εἰς σωτηρίαν) für alle Welt werden soll[51]. Ebenso hat der neutestamentliche christologische Ausdruck σωτήρ zwar seine philologische Entsprechung im alttestamentlichen מוֹשִׁיעַ, jedoch weist kaum eine Spur darauf hin, daß Jesus im Anschluß an diese als σωτήρ bezeichnet worden ist[52].

---

[50] Als Varianten der LXX finden sich σῴζων Jdc 12 3, σωτηρία I Chr 16 35 II Εσδρ 19 27, dagegen σωτήρ Jes 25 9 Prov 29 25.

[51] Gegen G. Bertram, Praeparatio evangelica in der Septuaginta, VT 7 (1957), 242f., hat LXX Jes 62 11 nicht messianisch interpretiert, sondern in ihrer Vorlage statt יֵשַׁע das eigentlich zu erwartende מוֹשִׁיעַ vorgefunden. Anders dürfte die Sachlage in 1QJesᵃ überhaupt liegen, da sich darin mancherlei Textabweichungen von MT als messianische Deutung zumindest erklären lassen; vgl. J. V. Chamberlain, The Functions of God as Messianic Titles in the complete Qumran Isaiah Scroll, VT 5 (1955), 366—372.

[52] Dieser Beurteilung durch L. Köhler, Christus im Alten Testament und im Neuen Testament, ThZ 9 (1953), 242f., ist nach dem Befund in MT und LXX voll und ganz zuzustimmen.

V. σωτήριος im Alten Testament

Die Septuaginta gibt mit σωτήριον *Heilsames, Rettung* einerseits den Stamm ישע wieder: einmal ישע hi. (Jes 63 1), achtmal יֵשַׁע, 36mal יְשׁוּעָה und fünfmal תְּשׁוּעָה. Es ist dann mit σωτηρία praktisch bedeutungsgleich, so daß beide Ausdrücke füreinander eintreten können (vgl. die Vorkommen in Ps 42 6 43 5 mit 42 12 und Ps 119 41. 81. 123. 166. 174 mit 119 155). Außerdem findet sich σωτήριον in Gen 41 16 für שָׁלוֹם[53], Jes 33 20 für מוֹעֵד *Festzeit*, 38 11 wohl für eins der beiden יָהּ, das als Abkürzung von יְשׁוּעָה gedeutet worden ist, 40 5 an Stelle von יַחְדָּו in Parallele zu כָּבוֹד, 60 6 für תְּהִלַּת *Ruhm* entsprechend der Parallelisierung in v. 18[54].

Andererseits bezeichnet σωτήριον in 72 von 86 Vorkommen die Opferart שֶׁלֶם bzw. שְׁלָמִים (außer Am 5 22 stets im Plural: Ex 20 — Jdc 21 Ez 43—46 Am 5 22 I—II Chr, zusätzlich in der Aufzählung von Opfergaben Lev 17 4 Jos 22 29)[55]. LXX hat dieses Opfer demnach meist als *Heilsopfer, heilsames* oder *heilbringendes Opfer* verstanden. Dagegen erfolgt die Übersetzung in I Sam — II Reg regelmäßig unter verschiedenartiger Zusammensetzung mit εἰρηνικός in der Deutung als *Friedensopfer*; offensichtlich sind dort andere Übersetzer am Werk gewesen. In beiden Fällen bestimmt LXX das Opfer inhaltlich nach seinem vermuteten Ziel und Zweck, sicherlich durch seinen gelegentlich betonten freudigen Charakter (Dtn 27 7) gefördert, während das hebräische Wort wahrscheinlich eine formale Bestimmung trifft. Zwar ist das mit שֶׁלֶם oder שְׁלָמִים bezeichnete Opfer[56] infolge der Mehrdeutigkeit des Stammes שלם häufig im Anschluß an die beiden Auffassungen der LXX als *Heilsopfer* σωτήριον[57] oder *Friedensopfer*[58]

---

[53] Die zusagende Antwort Josephs, Gott (und nicht Joseph) werde dem Pharao שָׁלוֹם antworten, wird dahin eingeschränkt, daß ohne Gott keine heilvolle Antwort (σωτήριον) gegeben werden kann.

[54] Die Variante σωτηρία haben Jes 63 1 Jon 2 10 I Chr 16 23.

[55] An Varianten begegnen: σωτηρία Num 6 14, θυσιαστήριον Dtn 27 7, τελεῖαι Jdc 20 26, das Adjektiv σωτήριος Am 5 22.

[56] Vgl. auch phönizisch שלם als Opferart (Lidzbarski a. a. O. 376) und südarabisch משלם (F. Hommel, Die südarabischen Altertümer des Wiener Hofmuseums, Aufsätze und Abhandlungen arabistisch-semitologischen Inhalts, 1892, 138. 182).

[57] So z. B. G. Hölscher, Geschichte der israelitischen und jüdischen Religion, 1922, 77; F. Nötscher, Biblische Altertumskunde, 1940, 323; R. Schmid in: Bibel-Lexikon, 1968², 700.

[58] So z. B. B. Baentsch, Exodus-Leviticus, 1903, zu Ex 20 24; E. Meyer, Die Israeliten und ihre Nachbarstämme, 1906, 554; G. E. Wright, Biblische Archäologie, 1957, 111; E. L. Ehrlich, Kultsymbolik im Alten Testament und im nachbiblischen Judentum, 1959, 41 (mit Fragezeichen).

verstanden worden, gelegentlich in noch anderer Weise[59]. Aber am sachgemäßesten ist die Ableitung von שלם pi. in der freilich seltenen Bedeutung *vollenden* mit dem Sinn *Abschlußopfer*[60].

Dementsprechend wird das Abschlußopfer bei der Aufzählung in Reihen stets an letzter Stelle genannt (II Reg 16 13, in P: Num 15 8 29 39 Jos 22 27) und scheint ursprünglich den Abschluß einer aus Brandopfern bestehenden Feier gebildet zu haben (Ex 20 24 Jdc 20 26 21 4 I Sam 13 9 II Sam 6 17f. 24 25 I Reg 8 64), weil die mit ihm verbundene Opfermahlzeit (vgl. Dtn 27 7) eine enge Gemeinschaft der Opfernden untereinander und mit ihrem Gott stiftete[61]. Dieser Ritus war auch dem זֶבַח *Schlachtopfer* eigen und hat schon verhältnismäßig früh die Grundlage für die Zusammenfassung beider Opferarten geboten; in den 86 Vorkommen von שְׁלָמִים ist das Wort 49mal mit זֶבַח verbunden. Während שְׁלָמִים zunächst erläuternd zu זְבָחִים tritt (Ex 24 5 I Sam 11 15), also den Sinn hat: *Schlachtopfer, die Abschlußopfer sind* und der deuteronomischen Auffassung die Ausdrucksweise זבח שְׁלָמִים entspricht (Dtn 27 7 Jos 8 31), also: *Abschlußopfer* (als Schlachtopfer) *schlachten*, finden sich besonders in P engere Verknüpfungen mittels des Genitiv-Verhältnisses, die ein Zurücktreten des Schlachtopfers einschließen: זֶבַח שְׁלָמִים *ein Schlachtopfer, das in Abschlußopfern besteht* (Lev 3 1 u. ö.) und זִבְחֵי שְׁלָמִים *Schlachtopfer, die in Abschlußopfern bestehen* (Ex 29 28 u. ö.). Schließlich tritt bei der Aufzählung von Opferarten in Reihen שְׁלָמִים ganz an die Stelle des fehlenden זֶבַח (Lev 9 22 Num 29 39 Ez 45 15 u. ö.). So ist ersichtlich, daß das Schlachtopfer immer mehr an Bedeutung verliert und durch das im Ritus ähnliche Abschlußopfer zuerst neutralisiert und dann ersetzt wird[62].

---

[59] C. von Orelli in: RE³, XIV 392f.: Gemeinschaftsopfer; A. Wendel, Das Opfer in der altisraelitischen Religion, 1927, 96: Verbrüderungsopfer als eine Form des Gemeinschaftsopfers; G. B. Gray, Sacrifice in the Old Testament, 1925, 7: Bezahlungsopfer; R. Schmid, Das Bundesopfer in Israel, 1964: Bundesopfer.

[60] L. Köhler—W. Baumgartner, Lexicon in Veteris Testamenti Libros, 1958², s. v.; R. Rendtorff, Studien zur Geschichte des Opfers im alten Israel, 1967.

[61] Zum späteren Ritual von P vgl. Lev 3 und dazu R. Rendtorff, Die Gesetze in der Priesterschrift, 1954, 5—23.

[62] L. Köhler, Theologie des Alten Testaments, 1953³, 178f.

III. Geschichte

Die Vorgeschichte Israels im Lichte neuer Quellen

I.

Über keine andere Zeit der Geschichte des alten Israel besitzen wir so geringe und unzureichende Nachrichten wie über diejenige, die der Landnahme in Palästina und der Bildung Israels als eines Volkes vorangeht. Gewiß ist auch die spätere sog. Richterzeit zwischen der Landnahme und der Staatsbildung weithin ein dunkles und unbekanntes Gebiet, so daß die Historiker nur zu leicht verführt werden, alle möglichen und unmöglichen Hypothesen in dieser Epoche anzusiedeln. Immerhin enthalten die Erzählungen über die Richter eine ganze Reihe von Einzelnachrichten, die kaum angezweifelt worden sind und werden können. Doch selbst diese fehlen nach dem Urteil vieler Historiker für die Vorgeschichte der Israeliten vor der Landnahme.

Daher bewegen sich die Ansichten über diese älteste Zeit seit langem zwischen zwei Extremen. Einerseits findet sich eine konservativ-apologetische Auffassung, die mit Eifer darum bemüht ist, einen möglichst großen Teil der biblischen Überlieferung über jenen Zeitabschnitt als ursprünglich und historisch zu erweisen oder zumindest einen starken historischen Kern anzunehmen. Auch die gewagteste Annahme ist gut genug, um zu zeigen, daß die Bibel doch recht hat. Andererseits betrachtet man die biblische Überlieferung über diese Epoche mit größter Zurückhaltung und Skepsis. Die im Mittelpunkt stehenden Personen, die sogenannten Patriarchen Abraham, Isaak und Jakob, hat man als Gestalten einer ursprünglich babylonischen Mondreligion, als alte kanaanäische Gottheiten oder als Personifikationen von Sippen oder Stämmen, jedenfalls nicht als geschichtliche Einzelpersonen gedeutet.

Die Schwierigkeit, der sich der Historiker gegenübersieht, ist vor allem durch die Quellenlage bedingt. Es gibt keine außerbiblische Quelle, die die Frühisraeliten und ihre führenden Gestalten erwähnt. Nicht einmal von Mose und dem Auszug aus Ägypten ist die Rede, obwohl es sich bei letzterem nach der biblischen Darstellung um ein grundlegendes Ereignis gehandelt hat. Angesichts dessen sind wir auf die biblischen Quellen allein angewiesen. Wie es aber um sie bestellt ist, erscheint seit langem als die eigentliche Streitfrage. Es mag sein, daß sie manche alten Nachrichten enthalten und in manchen Einzelheiten etwas von den Lebensverhältnissen der Zeit widerspiegeln, in der sie spielen wollen. Das gilt, wie sich noch ergeben wird, auch für die Patriarchenerzählungen in Gen 12—50. Aber wie weit darf der Historiker solche Erzählungen über derartige Einzelheiten hinaus als historische Quellen betrachten? Es ist ja nicht mehr zu übersehen, daß gerade die Patriarchenerzählungen eine Fülle von ursprünglich fremdem, nichtisraelitischem Gut enthalten, das im Lauf der Jahrhunderte in sie aufgenommen worden ist. Da gibt es aufzählende Listen wie das Verzeichnis der Könige von Edom (Gen 36 31-39), kanaanäische Natursagen wie diejenigen vom Untergang Sodoms (Gen 19), stammes- und volksgeschichtliche Notizen oder Erzählungen wie diejenigen von der Entstehung der Moabiter und Ammoniter (Gen 19 30ff.) und die große Novelle der Josephgeschichte. Vor allem finden sich immer wieder ursprünglich kanaanäische Heiligtums- und Kultlegenden, die den Ursprung bestimmter Kultstätten oder Kultbräuche angeben wollen und die die Israeliten übernommen haben. Dazu gehören die Erzählungen über die Offenbarung des El Roi in Beer Lachaj Roi (Gen 16), über den Ersatz des Menschenopfers durch ein Tieropfer an einem nicht mit Sicherheit zu lokalisierenden Heiligtum (Gen 22), über die Entdeckung der heiligen Stätten von Betel (Gen 28 10ff.) und Penuel am Jabbok (Gen 32 25ff.). Zieht man all das fremde, nichtisraelitische Gut von der uns vorliegenden Überlieferung ab, so schrumpfen die Patriarchentraditionen sogleich auf wenige Notizen und Erzählungen zusammen, so daß man in der Tat fragen kann, worin denn nun noch historische Erinnerungen vorliegen sollen und können.

Dennoch haben Funde altorientalischer Texte in den letzten drei Jahrzehnten manche Einzelheiten und allgemeine Züge der Vorgeschichte Israels neu beleuchtet. Davon soll im Folgenden die Rede sein. Von vornherein ist allerdings zu vermerken, daß die Funde lediglich Einzelheiten oder allgemeine Züge betreffen. Wir sind nach wie vor nicht in der Lage, ein in sich geschlossenes und zusammenhängendes Bild der Vorgeschichte Israels entwerfen zu können. Höchstens einige Grundzüge des Geschehens lassen sich rekonstruieren.

II.

In dem schmalen Streifen des Kulturlandes entlang dem mittleren Euphrat liegt der *tell ḥarīri*. Es ist ein ausgedehnter, aber flacher Ruinenhügel, der in der Landschaft so wenig auffällt, daß er viele Jahrzehnte unbeachtet blieb. Erst aufgrund eines Zufallsfundes begann man ihn vom Winter 1933/34 an auszugraben, identifizierte die Stätte als die Stadt Mari, im 19.—18. Jh. v. Chr. der Mittelpunkt eines bedeutenden Staatswesens, und stieß bei der Ausgrabung bald auf den Königspalast, in dem man ein Archiv von etwa 20 000 Keilschrifttafeln fand. Abgesehen von ihrer Wichtigkeit für die Geschichte Mesopotamiens — unter anderem für eine von der bisherigen abweichenden Datierung des bekannten Königs Hammurabi — werfen sie einiges für die Frage nach dem Ursprung der Israeliten ab[1]. Schon lange kannte man aus mesopotamischen Texten der ersten Hälfte des 2. Jt. eine Reihe von Personennamen, die zwar semitisch waren, aber nicht zu dem Typ der dort gebräuchlichen akkadischen Namen gehörten. Sie ähneln vielmehr dem Typ der ältesten israelitischen Personennamen. Vor allem sind es Satznamen, die aus dem semitischen Imperfekt eines Verbs und einer Gottesbezeichnung bestehen wie der Name »Israel« selber, oder Kurznamen, die die Gottesbezeichnung nicht aufweisen wie »Isaak«. Tatsächlich sind Namen wie Abraham und Jakob für jene Zeit und nur für sie mehrfach belegt. Nun ergibt sich aus den Texten von Mari, daß das Königshaus und die Herrenschicht der Stadt zu den Trägern dieser nichtakkadischen Gruppe von Personennamen gehören und daß außerdem manche ihrer Einrichtungen und Bräuche denjenigen des alten Israel entsprachen. Daher sind einige Vergleiche und Rückschlüsse möglich.

Eine erste Reihe von Übereinstimmungen in Worten und Redensarten stammt aus dem Bereich des Wanderhirtentums mit seiner Stammesorganisation und seinen eigentümlichen Institutionen. Sie können zum Vergleich herangezogen werden, weil die nomadische oder halbnomadische Lebensweise dieses Wanderhirtentums für die israelitischen Patriarchen ebenso wie für einen beachtlich großen Teil der Mari-Leute — trotz ihres Staates — charakteristisch war. Die Himmelsrichtungen werden mit nichtakkadischen Worten oder Wortformen nach der Orientierung zum Sonnenaufgang im Osten bezeichnet, so daß der Osten auf der »Vorderseite« (*aqdamātum*) und der Westen auf der »Rückseite« (*aḫarātum*), der Norden »links« (*sim[ḫ]al*) und der Süden »rechts« (*jamin[a]*) liegt. Auf diese Weise hat man in Mari zwei große Stämmegruppen bezeichnet: die *banū-sim'al* und die *banū-jamin*, wie noch in Palästina ein israelitischer Stamm die *bᵉnê jᵉmînî* »Benjaminiten« genannt wurde, ohne daß er freilich mit dem Stamm im Reich von Mari verwandt gewesen wäre. In diesem Zusammenhang gehören ferner Ausdrücke für größere oder kleinere

---

[1] Darauf hat vor allem M. Noth, Die Ursprünge des alten Israel im Lichte neuer Quellen, 1961, unter Auswertung der Texte von Mari hingewiesen. Vgl. ferner H. Cazelles, Mari et l'Ancien Testament, in: XVᵉ Rencontre Assyriologique Internationale, 1967, 73—90; J. M. Holt, The Patriarchs of Israel, 1964; H. B. Huffmon, Amorite Personal Names in the Mari Texts, 1965; A. Malamat, Aspects of Tribal Societies in Mari and Israel, in: XVᵉ Rencontre Assyriologique Internationale, 1967, 129—138; Mari and the Bible: Some Patterns of Tribal Organization and Institutions, JAOS 82 (1962), 143—150; The Ban in Mari and in the Bible, in: Biblical Essays, 1967, 40—49; A. Parrot, Abraham et son temps, 1962; R. de Vaux, Die hebräischen Patriarchen und die modernen Entdeckungen, 1959; Die Patriarchenerzählungen und die Geschichte, 1965.

Stammeseinheiten: das Wort *gājum* (*gāwum*), das wahrscheinlich die Bedeutung »Schar, Gruppe, Gemeinschaft« besitzt und in den semitischen Sprachen nur noch im Alten Testament und in der von ihm abhängigen Literatur in der Form *gôj* mit der verallgemeinerten und abgeblaßten Bedeutung »Volk, Nation« vorkommt; *ummatum*, das große Stammesorganisationen im Gebiet des mittleren Euphrat bezeichnet und im Alten Testament in der Form *'ummā* als besonderer Ausdruck für nichtisraelitische, nomadische Stämme begegnet (Gen 25 16 Num 25 15 Ps 177 1); und das Wort *ḫibrum* für eine engere Vereinigung mehrerer gemeinsam wandernder Familien innerhalb der größeren Einheit des Stammes, dem das hebräische Wort *hæbær* »Verbindung, Gemeinschaft« entspricht. Dazu treten schließlich Ausdrücke für die Aufenthaltsorte der Wanderhirten: *nawūm*, das die »Steppe« als das »Lager« der nicht fest angesiedelten Wanderhirten benennt (auch: *ḫibrum ša nawīm* für die Familiengruppe des Steppenlagers) und dem hebräischen Wort *nawǣ* »Weideplatz, Stätte« entspricht; das Wort *ḫaṣarum* für die unbefestigte zeitweilige Niederlassung einer Stammesgruppe, also für eine Art von Zeltdorf, wie auch das Alte Testament solche unbefestigten Ortschaften (Lev 25 31) als Niederlassungen in der Nähe einer Stadt (Jos 19 8) oder als Wohnorte von nomadischen oder halbnomadischen Stämmen *hᵃṣerīm* nennt (Gen 25 16 Dtn 2 23 Jes 13 11); und das Wort *kaprum* für die Vorratshäuser der Wanderhirten, das im Hebräischen zu *kapar* »Dorf« geworden ist.

Eine zweite Reihe von Übereinstimmungen findet sich im Bereich der Rechtsanschauungen und -bräuche. In Mari und in Israel gab es die Zuweisung eines Stückes vom Landeigentum des Stammes an einen Stammesangehörigen als persönliches Erbeigentum (*niḫlatum-nǎhᵃlā*), das unveräußerlich sein und dessen Übergang in den Besitz eines anderen Stammes durch besondere Bestimmungen verhindert werden sollte (Num 36 7). Den Rechtsakt der Zuweisung konnte man durch ein gemeinsames Mahl und die Salbung mit Öl besiegeln (Gen 26 30 31 54). In Mari und in Israel gab es eine Eheform, bei der die Frau im Elternhaus blieb und von ihrem Ehemann, der vielleicht sogar in einer anderen Ortschaft wohnte, besucht zu werden pflegte. Diese Eheform, die keine Beziehungen zur sonstigen mesopotamischen Tradition aufweist, begegnet in der Ehe Gideons mit einer Sichemitin und Simsons mit einer Philisterin. Ebenso ist für die Erbteilung in Mari und in Israel eigentümlich, daß der Erstgeborene bevorzugt wurde und zwei Drittel des Erbes erhielt (Dtn 21 17; vgl. II Reg 2 9).

Weitere Übereinstimmungen mit Israel liegen in Mari in dem Auftreten prophetenartiger Gestalten, in einer Form der sakralen Verpflichtung durch das »Eseltöten« analog dem Zerteilen von Tieren Gen 15 9f. Jer 34 18 und in der Redewendung »die Hand (jemandes) füllen« für die Einsetzung in ein Amt vor.

Dies alles ist sicherlich kein Zufall. Freilich ist auch zu beachten, daß die in Mari lebende Bevölkerungsgruppe mit nichtakkadischen Namen zwar den Schwerpunkt ihrer Ansiedlung am mittleren Euphrat und seinen Nebenflüssen Balichu und Chabur gehabt hat, jedoch gleichzeitig an anderen Orten begegnet, darunter in Syrien-Palästina, wie das Vorkommen ihrer Namen in den sogenannten ägyptischen Ächtungstexten aus dem 18. Jh. zeigt. Es handelt sich offensichtlich um eine größere Wanderungsbewegung, die vom 20.—18. Jh. in die Kulturländer besonders des Nordteils des »fruchtbaren Halbmonds« zahlreiche Einwanderer geführt hat, die teils kleinere oder größere Staatengebilde schufen, teils ihre bisherige nomadische oder halbnomadische Lebensweise beibehielten. Man hat sie als Westsemiten, Amoriter, Ostkanaanäer oder Protoaramäer bezeichnet; doch ist dem auch entschieden widersprochen worden, weil die philologische Prüfung der angeführten Beispiele ergebe, daß sie es nicht zulassen, die Sprache der nichtakkadischen semitischen Bevölkerung als protoaramäisch zu bezeichnen[2]. Doch ungeachtet dessen weiß die alttestamentliche Überlieferung um die Herkunft israelitischer Gruppen aus Mesopotamien, betont die aramäische Verwandtschaft und Verschwägerung der Patriarchen und bezeichnet in Gen 24 10 als ihr Heimatland »Aram-Naharaim«: das Aramäerland an den beiden Flüssen, d. h. am Euphrat und einem seiner Nebenflüsse (vielleicht dem Balichu). In diese Gegend weist die Nennung der Stadt Harran, von der aus Abraham nach Palästina aufgebrochen sein soll und die Jakob auf der Flucht vor Esau aufsucht. Dorthin führen ebenso die Namen von angeblichen Verwandten Abrahams: Nachor entspricht dem Namen der Stadt Naḫur im Bezirk von Harran, Serug dem Namen der Stadt Sarūgi zwischen Harran und dem Euphrat und Terach dem Til Turaḫi im Becken des Balichu.

Wird damit der mesopotamische und vielleicht aramäische Ursprung eines großen Teiles der Israeliten klar — nur eines großen Teils, weil später noch andere Volkselemente hinzugekommen sind —, so darf man deswegen nicht gleich die Patriarchen im 18. Jh. ansetzen wollen. Denn die Zuwanderung nach Palästina ist ein langer geschichtlicher Vorgang gewesen. Und daß die Ahnen Israels auch nach dem 18. Jh. im nordmesopotamischen Gebiet gelebt haben, zeigen andere Texte.

III.

Zu Beginn des 2. Jt. wanderten nicht nur die Aramäer in das mesopotamische Kulturland ein. Sein Reichtum lockte auch die in

---

[2] D. O. Edzard, Mari und Aramäer?, ZA NF 22 (56) (1964), 142—149.

seinen Randgebirgen hausenden nichtsemitischen Hurriter an, die sich schon im 18. Jh. in kleineren Gruppen von Alalach in Nordsyrien bis nach Mari finden. Bald darauf ergriffen sie, verstärkt durch indoiranische Elemente, die Macht, die sie vielfach noch im 16./15. Jh. innehatten. Das gilt auch für das schon genannte altaramäische Gebiet des mittleren Euphrat mit seinen Nebenflüssen.

Für die Rechtsverhältnisse dieser Hurriter besitzen wir eine Reihe von Zeugnissen aus der Zeit um 1500 v. Chr. Sie stammen aus der alten Stadt Nuzu bei Kerkuk, östlich des mittleren Tigris (etwa 300 km ostnordöstlich von Mari). Sie wurden dort in den Jahren 1925—1931 gefunden, aber erst etwa ein Jahrzehnt später ausgewertet. Die gleichen Rechtssitten und -bräuche, die sich dort finden, können und müssen wir bei den Hurritern überall, auch im Euphratgebiet, voraussetzen. Sie sind für uns deshalb wichtig, weil eine Reihe von Patriarchenerzählungen diese Rechtsformen widerspiegeln. Und da sie in palästinischen Erzählungen und Gesetzen nicht vorkommen und außerhalb der Patriarchenerzählungen nicht mehr wiederkehren, liegen darin doch wohl alte Erinnerungen an das Leben im mittleren Euphratgebiet etwa im 16. Jh. vor.

So gab es die Adoption von Freien oder Sklaven durch einen kinderlosen Mann, wobei die Adoptierten ihn im Alter zu versorgen und nach dem Tode zu beerdigen hatten und dafür seine Erben wurden. Dem entspricht die Absicht Abrahams, seinen hausgeborenen Sklaven Elieser zu seinem Erben zu machen, als er keine eigenen Kinder mehr erhoffte. Dann aber lehnt Jahwe diese Regelung ab und verheißt dem Abraham einen leiblichen Sohn (Gen 15 1ff.). Genauso ist in den Nuzu-Texten vorgesehen, daß der Adoptierte von seinem Erbrecht zurücktreten mußte, wenn der Adoptivvater doch noch einen Sohn bekam.

Sara gab nach Gen 16 ihrem Mann die Sklavin Hagar, als sie keine Kinder zu bekommen glaubte, damit sie durch die stellvertretende Sklavin dazu käme. Ähnliches wird von Rahel und Lea erzählt (Gen 30). Dem entsprechen Heiratsverträge in Nuzu, nach denen eine kinderlos bleibende Frau ihrem Mann eine Sklavin zuführen sollte: »wenn Gilimninu nicht gebiert, wird sie Schennima eine Frau aus dem Lande der Lullu vermählen«, woher sehr viele Sklaven kamen.

Nach der Geburt Isaaks verlangt Sara dann die Forttreibung der Hagar mit ihrem Sohn, Abraham aber weigert sich, dem nachzukommen, bis ein Gebot Jahwes ihn dazu nötigt (Gen 21 8ff.). Dabei handelt Abraham zunächst wieder nach dem Nuzu-Vertrag, der festlegt, daß die Kinder der stellvertretenden Sklavin nicht fortgetrieben werden sollten: »die Abkömmlinge (der Sklavin) wird Gilimninu (die Gattin) nicht forttreiben«.

Bei der Werbung um Rebekka fragen ihr Bruder Laban und seine Mutter sie um ihr Einverständnis (Gen 24 57f.) — ein für den semitischen Alten Orient eigentlich unerhörter Vorgang. Aber Verträge aus Nuzu, nach denen ein Bruder seine Schwester verheiratet, weisen solche Zustimmungsvermerke auf: »Mit meiner Einwilligung hat mein Bruder mich dem oder dem zur Frau gegeben«. Darin begegnen wir einer Rechtsanschauung, nach der innerhalb der patriarchalischen Familie die Brüder eine Art von fratriarchalischer Autorität über ihre Geschwister ausüben. Im Alten Testament bilden Gen 34 5-18 über die Verhandlungen nach der Schandtat Sichems an der Dina und vielleicht Gen 37 27f. über den Verkauf Josephs an die Ismaeliter durch seine Brüder weitere Beispiele. In allen Fällen handeln die Brüder — in Mari und in Israel in erster Linie bei der Verheiratung weiblicher Familienangehöriger — zu Lebzeiten der Eltern in eigener Autorität, die sie unabhängig von derjenigen des Vaters in bestimmten Rechtslagen zu besitzen scheinen.

Außerdem konnte man in Nuzu das Erstgeburtsrecht verkaufen, wie Esau es dem Jakob verkaufte (Gen 25 27ff.). Einmal erhält der Verzichtende drei Schafe als Gegenleistung — immerhin mehr als ein Linsengericht. Noch eine andere Erbsache: Als Jakob mit seinem Besitz von Laban flieht, stiehlt Rahel die Teraphim, den Hausgott, ihres Vaters (Gen 31 19). Nach dem Gesetz von Nuzu gingen solche Idole auf den Haupterben über, und demzufolge verlieh ihr Besitz eine Anwartschaft auf das Erbe. Daher der Versuch Rahels, sich in den Besitz des Hausgottes zu setzen, und daher das Bemühen Labans, diesen Gegenstand zurückzuerhalten[3].

All diese Rechtssitten, die sich durchweg auf das Familienrecht beziehen, begegnen uns im Alten Testament nur in den Patriarchenerzählungen, sonst nicht mehr. Sie entsprechen den späteren Rechtsverhältnissen der Israeliten in Palästina nicht, sondern spiegeln die Verhältnisse im hurritischen Mesopotamien um die Mitte des 2. Jt. wider. Natürlich darf man daraus nicht folgern, daß die Erzählungen der Genesis, in denen sie erwähnt werden, historische Berichte seien. Aber sie sind unter Verwertung der Erinnerungen daran, die lebendig geblieben sind, entstanden. Das bedeutet aber, daß wenigstens ein Teil der Ahnen Israels sie im 16. Jh. in Mesopotamien kennengelernt haben muß. Haben wir sie also zunächst als eine Gruppe gesehen, die zu den im 20./19. Jh. ins Kulturland Eingewanderten gehörte und im 18. Jh. in Nordmesopotamien lebte, so zeigen die Erinnerungen an hurritische Rechtssitten, daß sie offenbar noch im 16. Jh. dort weilte und erst danach allmählich nach Palästina gekommen ist.

---

[3] Anders M. Greenberg, Another Look at Rachel's Theft of the Teraphim, JBL 81 (1962), 239—248.

IV.

Auf die Verhältnisse dieser von Nordmesopotamien nach Palästina wandernden Hirten wirft ein altorientalischer Begriff ein wenig Licht. Die Amarnabriefe, meist aus dem 14. Jh., enthalten oft Hilferufe palästinischer Stadtkönige an den ägyptischen Pharao gegen Eindringlinge, die als Chapiru bezeichnet werden. Man hat diesen Ausdruck gern mit dem Wort *'ibrî* »Hebräer« gleichgesetzt und manchmal außerdem gemeint, daß die Amarnabriefe sich auf das Eindringen der Israeliten unter der Führung Josuas bezögen. Das Letztere trifft freilich ganz bestimmt nicht zu. Auch das Alte Testament gebraucht den Ausdruck »Hebräer« nie für diejenigen Israeliten, die unter Mose aus Ägypten ausgezogen und unter Josua in Palästina eingedrungen sein sollen. Zudem kann die Haupteinwanderung erst im Laufe des 13. Jh. stattgefunden haben. Dagegen ist die Gleichsetzung Chapiru — *'ibrî* möglich.

Inzwischen gibt es eine Fülle weiterer Belege für solche Chapiru oder 'Apiru; sie reichen von Ägypten über Syrien bis nach Nordmesopotamien und Nuzu. Überall erscheinen sie als landlose und landfremde Söldner und Beutemacher, Gefangene und Sklaven. Die Ansicht geht heute dahin, daß es sich nicht um einen ethnischen, sondern um einen soziologischen Begriff handelt. Er bezeichnet »Personen ohne Familienzugehörigkeit«, wie auch *'ibrî* im Alten Testament für den nicht vollfreien Mann verwendet werden kann (Ex 21 2 Dtn 15 12). Da aber diese Menschen vornehmlich Ausländer waren, vollzog sich allmählich eine Bedeutungswandlung oder -ausweitung des Begriffs Chapiru. Er wurde auf die Ausländer im Bereich eines Staates überhaupt angewendet und bezeichnete sie als die minderberechtigten Fremden.

Leitet man *'ibrî* von Chapiru ab, vielleicht von einer adjektivischen Form, so ergibt sich, da eine einfache Gleichsetzung ausscheidet, daß die Frühisraeliten eine Gruppe in dem Ganzen der Chapiru gebildet haben können. Von anderen wurden auch sie so genannt, weil sie als Wanderhirten viel herumzogen und also zu den minderberechtigten Fremden zählten. Dem entspricht ja durchweg die Art, wie sie in den Erzählungen der Genesis geschildert werden. Wenn man also nicht auf die Volkszugehörigkeit, sondern auf die Lebensweise sieht, ist wohl anzunehmen, daß Gruppen der Frühisraeliten — unter ihnen die Patriarchen — zu denen gehörten, die man damals Chapiru-'Apiru nannte. Als solche sind sie in Palästina erschienen — sicher erst im 15. oder 14. Jh., also gewiß gleichzeitig mit den Chapiru der Amarnabriefe, aber nicht identisch mit ihnen. Denn einmal sind diejenigen Chapiru, die die kleinen Stadtkönige Palästinas bedrängen, viel zahlreicher als die Sippen der israelitischen Patriarchen. Ferner werden diese als Wanderhirten wohl mit Recht als durchweg friedlich und keineswegs kriegerisch geschildert — ein Zug, der sie von den späteren israelitischen Stämmen und dem Volke Israel deutlich unterscheidet und der darum schwerlich erdichtet ist. Und schließlich liegt es im Wesen dieses Wanderhirtentums, daß es vertragliche Übereinkommen mit den Kulturlandbewohnern sucht, um im Zuge des Weidewechsels jedes Jahr nach Ablauf der Regenzeit und des Frühjahrs aus der Steppe ins Kulturland zu ziehen und die Herden auf den abgeernteten Äckern weiden zu können.

V.

Man könnte sagen, daß dem die Erzählung in Gen 14 von dem Kampf Abrahams gegen die vier Ostkönige, denen er die in Palästina gemachte Beute wieder abjagt, widerspricht. Man hat diese Erzählung gern für die Datierung Abrahams ins Feld geführt — vor allem, indem man den einen der Ostkönige, Amraphel, mit dem König Hammurabi von Babylon gleichsetzte, so daß Abraham nach der alten Chronologie um 1900 v. Chr. gelebt hätte. Aber diese Gleichsetzung hat in eigentümlicher Weise an Beifall verloren, seitdem infolge der durch die Mari-Texte veränderten Chronologie Hammurabi gegen 1700 v. Chr. anzusetzen ist. In der Tat läßt der Name Amraphel sich nicht auf Hammurabi zurückführen, sondern eher auf ein »Amar-pi-el« = »der Mund des Gottes hat gesprochen«. Der zweite König Ariok könnte auf ein Arriwuk zurückgehen (so hieß der Sohn des Königs Zimrilim von Mari); er wäre dann von hurritischer Prägung. Der dritte Name Tidʻal entspricht der Form Tudḫalia, die mehrere der hetitischen Könige in Kleinasien tragen. Der vierte Name Kedor-Laʻomer hat seine Entsprechung in dem elamitischen Namen Kuter-Lagamar, obschon die elamitischen Königslisten den Namen nicht enthalten.

So überaus historisch scheint Gen 14 demnach gar nicht zu sein. Eine literar- und überlieferungsgeschichtliche Analyse ergibt denn auch, daß der Abschnitt einer der jüngsten des Pentateuchs ist. Zwar enthält er einige alte, sozusagen gelehrt-antiquarische Notizen, die der Verfasser verwertet hat, aber Abraham ist mit ihnen erst sekundär verknüpft worden. Geschichtliche Aufschlüsse über ihn gibt der Text überhaupt nicht. Damit wird zugleich die neuerdings vertretene Annahme hinfällig, daß Abraham und seine Nachkommen fürstenähnliche Kaufleute aus der kleinasiatischen Stadt Ura im 14. Jh. gewesen seien.

Außer einer alten Notiz mit den Namen von Königen oder Heerführern verwertet der Text noch eine zweite über das vorisraelitische Jerusalem: über den kanaanäischen Stadtkönig Melchisedek, der —wie damals üblich — auch priesterliche Rechte hatte, und den kanaanäischen Gott El, der in Jerusalem den Beinamen Äljon »der Höchste« erhalten hat. Damit treffen wir auf die Religion, die die frühisraelitischen Patriarchensippen in Palästina vorfanden und die sie in mehr oder weniger starkem Maße übernommen haben — vor allem seit ihrer Seßhaftwerdung und bis zu der Neueinführung des Jahweglaubens durch die aus Ägypten kommende Moseschar.

Diese kanaanäische Religion, über die wir früher nur aus den polemischen Äußerungen des Alten Testaments und den Bemerkungen einiger späten griechischen Schriftsteller etwas wußten, ist in vieler Hinsicht klarer und eindrücklicher geworden, seitdem von 1929 an in Ras Schamra, dem alten Ugarit, die ersten kanaanäisch-religiösen Texte gefunden worden sind. Noch heute lassen die Stadtanlage von Ugarit, soweit sie schon ausgegraben ist, und noch mehr die zahlreichen kostbaren Fundstücke in den Museen von Damaskus und Aleppo etwas von dem Glanz und der Pracht dieser Kultur erkennen. Es ist wohl auch kein Zufall, daß gerade in diesen phönizischen Handels-Stadtstaaten die alphabetische Schrift entwickelt worden ist.

Nun war die kanaanäische Religion im bäuerlichen Palästina sicher von einer anderen Art als im Norden an der Küste. Soweit wir sie erfassen können, handelt es sich um einen Vegetationskult, in dem es um die Fruchtbarkeit des Ackers, des Viehs und auch des Menschen ging. Wenn man sich näher mit dieser Religion befaßt, versteht man die Anziehungskraft, die sie jahrhundertelang auf Israel ausgeübt hat — und das gewiß schon in der Frühzeit. Sofort nach ihrer jeweiligen Landnahme und Seßhaftwerdung scheinen alle israelitischen Gruppen dem Zauber dieser Religion erlegen zu sein — zumindest so, daß sie sie mit ihrer bisherigen Religion verschmolzen haben.

VI.

Vor ihrer Landnahme waren die Frühisraeliten keine Vollnomaden oder Beduinen. Deren Heimat- und Lebensbedingungen sind durch die Kamelzucht bedingt. Die Frühisraeliten waren jedoch keine Kamelzüchter. Die gründlich untersuchten Belege aus dem Alten Orient zeigen, daß das Kamel gewiß schon recht früh bekannt war, aber erst vom 12. Jh. an domestiziert und als Haustier verwendet wurde. Bis dahin und als zweiten Typ auch weiterhin gab es die Kleinviehnomaden mit dem Esel als Reittier. Sie wechseln nur langsam den Standort und sind an Gegenden und Marschrouten gebunden, an denen die Wasserstellen nahe beieinander liegen und die Weiden ergiebig genug sind, so daß die eigentliche Wüste ausscheidet. Sie wechseln von den Steppen am Rande des Kulturlandes immer wieder in dieses hinein und stehen zum besiedelten Land und seinen Ortschaften in reger Beziehung. Vielfach tragen diese Beziehungen dazu bei, daß sie allmählich seßhaft werden.

Diese Existenz, die bis in unsere Zeit auch halbnomadische Sippen der Wüste Juda und des Negeb geführt haben, ist offenbar auch die der Frühisraeliten gewesen. In der Tat werden die Patriarchen in den Genesiserzählungen fast ganz in dieser Art geschildert — als hin- und herziehende Kleinviehbesitzer, die am Recht auf die Brunnen interessiert sind, sich gelegentlich schon Besitztum an Grund und Boden sichern und hier und da eine gewisse Ackerkultur mit der Viehzucht verbinden. Die Patriarchen in Palästina sind keine reinen Nomaden und keine Karawanenführer im Negeb, aber auch noch keine festangesiedelten Bauern, sondern lediglich dem Einfluß des seßhaften Lebens ausgesetzt, daher Halbnomaden auf dem Wege zum Seßhaftwerden.

Wie steht es mit ihrer ursprünglichen Religion? Die starke Bearbeitung der alttestamentlichen Überlieferung hat den Eindruck nicht verwischen können, daß Sippengötter die entscheidende Stelle eingenommen haben, ob man sie nun als Vätergötter oder als die nomadische Form einer El-Religion bezeichnen will. Sie wurden aufgrund einer Offenbarung, die der Sippengründer oder -führer erhielt, angenommen und in einem darauf folgenden Kultus verehrt. Was sie aber den Sippen gaben, waren die Verheißungen von Nachkommenschaft und Landbesitz, die zum Urgestein der Patriarchenerzählungen gehören. Die Empfänger der Offenbarungen und Verheißungen und die Kultstifter sind die sogenannten Patriarchen, die in der noch ungeteilten und nichtspezialisierten nomadischen Kultur als die Führer ihrer Sippen zu verstehen sind — und zwar verschiedener Sippen, weil die literarische Untersuchung der Quellen lehrt, daß die verwandtschaftlichen Beziehungen zwischen ihnen erst später hergestellt worden sind.

So legen die in der Genesis verarbeiteten Überlieferungen der Abraham-, der Isaak- und der Jakobsippe deren religiös-rechtlich begründeten Ansprüche auf das Kulturland dar, wobei wohl der Stammvater einer ostjordanischen Gruppe mit demjenigen der westjordanischen Jakobsippe gleichgesetzt wurde. Und da die Überlieferungen die Patriarchensippen in verschiedenartigen Stadien im Verhältnis zum Kulturland zeigen — von der flüchtigen Berührung bis zur beginnenden Seßhaftigkeit und im Jakob-Esau-Laban-Kreis mit dem Anspruch auf ein ganz bestimmtes ostjordanisches Gebiet, vielleicht auch schon in Beziehungen zu bestimmten Heiligtümern im Lande —, handelt es sich zugleich um Überlieferungen über die Landnahme der ersten israelitischen Gruppen in Palästina. In ihrem Kern sind die Patriarchenerzählungen die Landanspruchs- und Landnahmeerzählungen mehrerer israelitischer Gruppen, die — aus dem Bevölkerungsstock Nordmesopotamiens nach dessen hurritischer Überwanderung kommend — sich in Palästina festsetzen wollten und festsetzten. Abraham,

Isaak und Jakob sind die Sippengründer und -führer, jedenfalls geschichtliche Gestalten, die zu ihren Lebzeiten in ihrer Sippe oder Gruppe die ausschlaggebende Rolle gespielt und ihr die entscheidende Ausrichtung gegeben haben.

Joseph darf man in diese Reihe freilich nicht hineinnehmen. Denn aus der neueren Untersuchung der Joseph-Novelle in Gen 37—50 geht eine solch enge Verflechtung mit Ägypten hervor, daß man annehmen muß, es handle sich um die allmähliche Umarbeitung einer ursprünglich ägyptischen Erzählung. Jedenfalls sind die Israeliten, die die Moseüberlieferung in Ägypten voraussetzt, nicht die Ahnen der späteren israelitischen Stämme oder ihre ersten Nachkommen, sondern eine von ihnen zu unterscheidende israelitische Gruppe, die man am besten als Moseschar bezeichnet. Analysiert man das, was von ihr erzählt wird, so trifft man auf die gleichen Elemente wie in den Patriarchenerzählungen. Wieder liegt eine Erzählung von dem auf göttliche Zusage gegründeten Landanspruch einer nomadischen oder halbnomadischen Gruppe und von der im Zug nach Palästina beginnenden Verwirklichung der beabsichtigten Landnahme vor. Und schließlich stellen die Josuaerzählungen nochmals die Landnahmeüberlieferungen eines israelitischen Stammes dar.

VII.

Überblicken wir das Ganze, so können wir mit der gebotenen Vorsicht und Zurückhaltung wenigstens einige Grundzüge der Vorgeschichte Israels erfassen. Ein gewisser Teil der Frühisraeliten stammt aus einer vielleicht aramäischen Bevölkerungsschicht vor allem in Nordmesopotamien, obschon später mannigfache andere Volkselemente hinzugekommen sind. In Nordmesopotamien haben jene Frühisraeliten sich wenigstens bis zum 16. Jh. aufgehalten, sind dann allmählich nach Palästina gewandert, wobei sie überall als minderberechtigte Fremde betrachtet und behandelt worden sind, und haben im weiteren Verlauf in mehreren kleinen Gruppen in Palästina, in dem weite Teile dünn oder gar nicht besiedelt waren, einsickern können. Dort kamen sie mit den Bewohnern des Kulturlandes in Berührung, wurden unter Berufung auf die göttliche Landzusage allmählich seßhaft und gliederten sich in die palästinische Ackerbaukultur und -religion ein, bis der von der Moseschar mitgebrachte Jahweglaube religiös revolutionierend wirkte und ein neues Zeitalter heraufführte.

Israels Staatsordnung im Rahmen des Alten Orients

Zu Eric Voegelin, Israel and Revelation

I.

In seinem umfassenden Werk »Order and History« will E. Voegelin die hauptsächlichen Formen der staatlich-gesellschaftlichen Ordnung mitsamt den Symbolen, in denen sie sich Ausdruck verschafft haben, herausarbeiten. Dabei stellt sich zugleich das Problem der Auseinandersetzung zwischen den symbolischen Formen und ihrer gegenseitigen Einwirkung, da die älteren Formen durch jeweils neue nicht einfach abgetan werden, sondern ihre Geltung innerhalb der Bereiche behalten, die von den neuen Einsichten nicht erfaßt werden.

Der umfangreiche erste Band des Werkes, »Israel and Revelation« (1956) ist zwei Ordnungstypen und Symbolformen gewidmet: den staatlichen Organisationen des Alten Orients mit ihrer Existenz in der Form des kosmologischen Mythos und dem Volke Israel mit seiner Existenz in geschichtlicher Form. Da der Nachdruck auf der Ordnung Israels liegt, das sich aus der Umwelt der kosmologisch gegründeten Staaten des Alten Orients erhebt, wird die kosmologische Ordnung nur als Hintergrund für den Aufbruch der Geschichte betrachtet, die die auf die göttliche Offenbarung antwortende Existenzform bildet und durch den Exodus Israels aus der kosmologisch bestimmten Kultur erlangt wurde.

1. Im Alten Orient sind nach dieser Darstellung die verschiedenen Gesellschaften und Kulturen in der Form des kosmologischen Mythos geordnet, der sich auch sonst als typische Erscheinung der Frühzeit findet.

Die älteste bekannte politische Form in Mesopotamien ist der Stadtstaat — eine Ansammlung von Tempeln mit großem Landbesitz. Jeder Stadtstaat gilt als einem Gott gehörig und wird von dessen irdischem Statthalter politisch und geistlich verwaltet. Als kraftvolle Eroberer die Stadtstaaten zusammenfassen und darüber hinaus weitere Gebiete an sich ziehen, wird ihre Herrschaft der kosmischen Regierung der Gottheit parallel gesetzt und ein entsprechender Symbolismus entwickelt. Die Begründung der Herrschaft wird als ein Ereignis in der kosmischen Ordnung der Götter aufgefaßt, für das das irdische Geschehen den analogen Ausdruck bildet. Der Sonnengott Marduk wird zum Herrscher über die Völker ernannt, und der babylonische König als seine irdische Analogie steigt wie die Sonne über dem Volk auf und erhellt das Land. Das babylonische Reich ist der Mikrokosmos, der immer nur als einziger existieren kann.

Diese kosmologische Symbolik, die sich bis in die persische Zeit (Achämeniden) gehalten hat, ist weder eine Theorie noch eine Allegorie, sondern der mythische Ausdruck der realen Teilnahme der Gesellschaftsordnung am göttlichen Sein, das auch den Kosmos ordnet. Die politische Ordnung wird mit Hilfe kosmischer Analogien symbolisiert. Und wie die politische Ordnung kosmologisch verstanden wird, so die kosmische Ordnung politisch. Wie der Staat eine Analogie des Kosmos ist, so spielen sich in der himmlischen Sphäre politische Ereignisse ab. Der Staat ist ein Teil des Kosmos, der Kosmos aber wiederum ein Reich, zu dem die menschliche Herrschaft als ein Teil gehört.

Obwohl die Auffassung in Ägypten vom gleichen Typ wie die mesopotamische ist, ergibt sich dort doch eine eigene kulturelle Form. Das Pharaonenreich entsteht plötzlich und ohne eine der mesopotamischen vergleichbare Vorgeschichte. Die Symbolik des Nils und der Sonne werden ausschlaggebend. Besonders die Umwandlung des sichtbaren Sonnengottes in den unsichtbaren, transzendenten Schöpfergott, also die Gleichzeitigkeit von kosmischer Sichtbarkeit und transzendenter Unsichtbarkeit, hat die eigentliche politische Gottheit Ägyptens geschaffen und die Staatsordnung beeinflußt.

Die Gottheit offenbart sich nicht dem Volke unmittelbar, sondern ist bei ihm durch ihre Manifestation im Herrscher gegenwärtig. Der Pharao ist zwar kein Gott, wohl aber die Manifestation eines Gottes; und infolge der göttlichen Gegenwart in ihm ist der König der Mittler göttlicher Hilfe für das Volk. Die Göttlichkeit des Pharao strahlt über die Gesellschaft aus und macht sie zu einem Gottesvolk; durch die Vermittlung des Königs wirkt die Ordnung des Kosmos ein. Die Gesellschaftsordnung hat daher an der Substanz der Weltordnung teil, die der Gott geschaffen hat. In der pharaonischen Ordnung wird die ewige kosmische Ordnung ständig erneuert und in Kraft gesetzt.

Allerdings ist diese Ordnung in den beiden »Zwischenzeiten« der ägyptischen Geschichte gebrochen und auch sonst kleineren Erschütterungen ausgesetzt worden. Während die grundlegende Erfahrung der Konsubstantialität bleibt und im kosmogonischen Mythos ihren Ausdruck findet, macht sie doch einen Prozeß der Differenzierung durch, der infolge neuer und unterschiedlicher Erfahrungen zur Zersetzung führen kann. Das zeigen im einzelnen die memphitische Theologie, die sich mit Auflösungserscheinungen befassende Literatur und die revolutionären Jahre des Königs Echnaton.

Weder Aufstieg und Fall der mesopotamischen Großreiche noch die wiederholten ägyptischen Krisen haben den Glauben an eine göttlich-kosmische Ordnung, von der die menschliche Gesellschaft einen Teil bildet, brechen können. Man hat zwar den Gegensatz zwischen der dauernden kosmischen und der wechselnden irdischen Ordnung bemerkt, ist jedoch nicht zu neuen Einsichten gelangt. Politische Katastrophen sind weiterhin als von den Göttern bestimmte kosmische Ereignisse verstanden worden.

2. Im israelitischen Volk erstand eine neue Art von Gesellschaft. Israel konstituierte sich, indem es seine Volkwerdung durch die göttliche Erwählung als ein Ereignis von besonderer Bedeutung in der Geschichte berichtete. Geschichte dient nun als symbolische Form der Existenz, und die beispielhafte Erzählung in geschichtlicher Form ist ein Äquivalent des kosmologischen Mythos. Diese geschichtliche Auffassung tritt an die Stelle der kosmischen Ordnung.

Ursprung und Schlüssel für das Werden und Verstehen des israelitischen Geschichtsverständnisses liegen im Kultus: in alten Riten und Liturgien. Erst aufgrund dieser von Kultlegenden bestimmten Traditionen beginnt im 9. Jh. v. Chr. die Geschichtsschreibung. Ein Strom von Motivationen fließt von den ursprünglichen Erfahrungen über die Feste, Riten und Kultlegenden in die spekulative Konstruktion der Erzählung, ohne an Substanz zu verlieren. So kommt es schließlich zur Darstellung einer Weltgeschichte, die von dem Drama der göttlichen Schöpfung ausgeht; in der Geschichte setzt Gott sein Schöpfungswerk fort, wie die Weltschöpfung das erste geschichtliche Ereignis ist.

Diese Auffassung ist diejenige der jüngsten Erzählungs- oder Interpretationsschicht, von denen sich nacheinander mehrere über die ursprünglichen Traditionen und Berichte gelegt haben. Ihre Symbole und Motivationen haben dem Ganzen das letzte Gepräge verliehen.

3. Nunmehr kann die Spur der Symbole durch die Jahrhunderte der israelitischen Geschichte verfolgt werden — von den Abraham-Traditionen bis zum Ende des israelitischen Nordreiches.

Zunächst beschreiben Gen 14—15 die Situation, in der bei Abraham die Erfahrung des »Bundes« mit Jahwe im Gegensatz zur kosmologischen Ordnung der Kanaanäer ihren Ursprung hat, und den Inhalt dieser Erfahrung. Diese jahwistische Erfahrung wird bis zur Zeit Moses weitergereicht, ohne daß wir Genaueres darüber wissen.

Das Israel der biblischen Erzählungen begegnet uns dann als ein amphiktyonischer Verband auf der Grundlage des Jahweglaubens mit dem Heiligtum von Silo als Mittelpunkt, jedoch ohne politische Organisation, da die Sippe (»clan«) die grundlegende Einheit bildet. Nach der wichtigen alten Quelle des Deboraliedes (Jdc 5) versteht sich Israel in dem besungenen kriegerischen Ereignis erstmalig als ein Volk, das in einer politischen Handlung unter Jahwe geeint ist. Es zeigt sich der Bruch mit der kosmologischen Ordnung, weil Jahwe als ein Gott geglaubt wird, der sich in einem geschichtlichen Handeln als Schöpfer einer wahrhaften Ordnung enthüllt. Freilich brauchte die weitere Entwicklung nicht unbedingt zu einem organisierten Volk zu führen, das seine politischen Angelegenheiten unter der wirksamen Leitung seines Gottes betrieb, sondern konnte ebenso eine »pacifist« Gemeinschaft entstehen lassen, die ohne eigene militärische Anstrengungen alles vom göttlichen Eingreifen erwartete. Tatsächlich sind beide Wege gegangen worden; und die Erkenntnis dieser Doppelheit ist der Schlüssel zum Verständnis der israelitischen Geschichte.

Der nächste Schritt war das erste Königtum des Gideon über Ophra und seine Umgebung — eine Übergangsform vom nationalen Führertum im Jahwekrieg zum nationalen Königtum Sauls (Jdc 6—8). Gideon errichtet einen Tempel als kultisches Zentrum seiner Herrschaft und schafft so ein neues Symbol politischer Ordnung. Damit setzt die Wandlung Jahwes zu einem begrenzten nationalen Gott ein; Jahwe wird zum transzendenten Repräsentanten der Nation. Es zeigte sich, daß der ursprüngliche Jahweglaube keine bestimmte politische Form festlegte, sondern Jahwe jeder politischen und sozialen Situation angepaßt werden konnte, die ein Verständnis als Manifestation der göttlichen Macht erforderte.

Infolge der Bedrängnis durch die Philister wird Saul der erste nationale König. Die Ereignisse werden in wenigstens zwei Versionen erzählt, in einer königsfreundlichen und einer königsfeindlichen. Nach der königsfreundlichen Version ist das Königtum von Jahwe errichtet und der König durch das Sakrament der Salbung in eine unmittelbare Beziehung zu Gott versetzt worden. Das Königtum verbindet sich mit dem von den Prophetengenossenschaften vertretenen populären Jahweglauben und der orgiastischen Religiosität des Volkes, was später den Protest der großen Einzelpropheten hervorruft. Es führt aber auch zu Spannungen mit der Rationalität staatlicher Einrichtungen. Die königsfeindliche Version, die im Königtum einen Bruch mit der königlichen Herrschaft Jahwes über Israel erblickt, hat eine bedeutsame politische Symbolik geschaffen: Die Beziehung zwischen Samuel und Saul ist das Paradigma der geistlichen Aufsicht und Gewalt über zeitliche Herrschaft und der Gedanke der theokratischen Ordnung das Symbol für die Spannung zwischen göttlicher und menschlicher Gesellschaftsordnung.

Das folgende Großreich Davids stellt eine neue Reichsbildung dar, die der Eroberer mit seinem Heer und seiner Sippe den Territorien und Völkerschaften von Israel, Juda und kanaanäischen Stadtstaaten aufzwang. Die Erzählung von David und Batseba enthüllt die dadurch hervorgerufene ernste Krise der Jahweordnung; insbesondere zeigt die Parabel Natans (II Sam 12) die Lebensführung des Königs als Ordnungsproblem in der neuen Situation. Obwohl das davidische Königtum seinen eigenen Gesetzen der Symbolbildung folgte, die grundsätzlich von denen des Alten Orients nicht verschieden waren, kam es infolge der Einwirkung des Jahweglaubens in Israel nicht zu einer rein kosmologischen Ordnung, sondern nur zu einer synkretistischen Verbindung beider Elemente. Immerhin ist die Reichsymbolik der kosmologischen Kulturen deutlich in den Psalmen erkennbar, die als »Imperial Psalms« verstanden werden müssen. Jahwe erscheint als der summus deus eines Großreiches, während Israel in einem Reichsvolk unter einem pharaonischen Mittler aus dem Davidsgeschlecht aufgeht. Und der salomonische Tempel stellt nach Bauart und Ausstattung eher die Sammlung eines Kenners der altorientalischen kosmologischen Symbole als das Heiligtum Jahwes dar.

Das Großreich endet mit der Revolte gegen Salomos Nachfolger. Der Nordteil organisiert sich als Königreich Israel, das bis 721 v. Chr. besteht, ohne daß die gewonnene Unabhängigkeit eine große politische Form geschaffen hat. Der Süden bildet das Königreich Juda unter der davidischen Dynastie, ohne daß in der Beibehaltung der davidischen Symbolik bemerkenswerte Entwicklungen stattgefunden haben.

Am bemerkenswertesten ist die durch die Dynastie Omri im Nordreich heraufgeführte Krise (9. Jh. v. Chr.). Hatte Israel im davidischen Großreich der Verlust seiner volklichen Identität gedroht, so drohte ihm nunmehr infolge der Einführung des Gottes Baal von Tyrus der Verlust seiner geistigen Identität. Die Antwort Israels darauf bestand zunächst im Bemühen um die Kodifizierung des Gesetzes in schriftlicher Form im sogenannten Bundesbuch (Ex 20 23— 23 19). Es ist ein vielschichtiger Versuch, den Sinn und die Absicht der knappen Gebote und Verbote aus der Frühzeit in konkrete Verordnungen über die soziale Ordnung zu fassen. Ferner findet die Bewegung gegen die Dynastie Omri die Unterstützung einer Gruppe von Einzelpropheten, unter denen Elia die wichtigste Gestalt ist. Der prophetische Protest in diesem für die Geschichte der Eschatologie entscheidenden Jahrhundert findet seinen Ausdruck in dem antiköniglichen Symbol des schrecklichen Gerichtstages Jahwes gegenüber der freudigen Erwartung, in der das Volk trotz seines Abfalls von Jahwe verharrt.

4. Als das Reich Israel untergegangen war, verschob sich das Interesse in Juda während des 8. Jh. auf die Klärung der Frage nach der rechten Ordnung im Licht der Sinaioffenbarung. Daher geht es nun um die Symbolik Moses und der Propheten, deren eigentliche Aufgabe es war, das Volk zu seinen Aufgaben zurückzurufen und seine innere Form wiederherzustellen. Eine besondere Stellung nimmt das Buch Deuteronomium ein, auf das zwar der prophetische Geist eingewirkt hat, in dem aber auch die Existenz in der Gegenwart unter Gott in eine solche unter der Tora (dem »Gesetz«) verderbt wird. Ein mythisches Element dringt ein, indem die unmittelbare Existenz

unter Gott durch die Mittlerschaft Moses als des fiktiven Verfassers der Tora gebrochen wird. Dadurch bildet das Deuteronomium den Ausgangspunkt für das spätere Judentum.

Demgegenüber muß man nach dem geschichtlichen Mose fragen. Die alten Quellen sind allerdings von mehreren Schichten überlagert worden, während die geschichtliche Substanz in dem Zusammenstoß der jahwistischen Erfahrung Moses mit der kosmologischen Ordnung des ägyptischen Reiches liegt, wie es die von den biblischen Erzählern verwendete Formel ausdrücken will: Jahwe brachte Israel durch Mose aus Ägypten! Die israelitischen Sippen, die den Sinai-»Bund« schließen, werden infolge ihrer Antwort auf die Offenbarung zu einem neuen Volk; ihre Existenz als die einer Gottesherrschaft wird durch grundlegende Gebote geordnet. Der Dekalog ist kein religiöser und ethischer Katechismus, sondern die Proklamation des Gottkönigs, der die Regeln für die Ordnung der neuen Herrschaft niederlegt.

Ohne Mose und die Ereignisse seiner Zeit hätte es keine Propheten gegeben; so aber waren sie erforderlich, um für das von Gott erwählte Volk die Gegenwart unter Gott wiederzugewinnen, die es zu verlieren drohte. Dabei bildeten sie zugleich die Symbole des Jahwekönigtums der Mosezeit um.

Am deutlichsten bemerkt man bei Jeremia den Konflikt zwischen der geschichtlichen Ordnung der Gesellschaft und der göttlich geoffenbarten Ordnung. Aber die Propheten überhaupt gewinnen die Einsicht, daß Existenz unter Gott vor allem Liebe, Demut und gerechtes Handeln bedeutet. Daraus ergeben sich sowohl ihre Anklagen gegen Staat, Religion und Kultur des Volkes als auch die in verschiedenem Maße erlangte Erkenntnis, daß Ermahnungen erfolglos, ja vielleicht sogar stumpfe Waffen seien. Daraus erwuchs eine ganze Reihe von Versuchen, die rauhe Wirklichkeit der Welt dennoch durch eine Umwandlung in Übereinstimmung mit den Erfordernissen des Jahwekönigtums zu bringen.

Drei solcher Versuche sind zu beobachten. Zunächst entsprach bei Amos und Hosea der Kritik an der gegenwärtigen Ordnung die Erwartung einer vollkommenen künftigen Ordnung, die — von der Ausmerzung aller Unvollkommenheiten abgesehen — der institutionellen gegenwärtigen Ordnung entsprechen würde. Dann beginnt mit Jesaja die metastatische und mit Jeremia die existentielle Phase. Jesaja verließ die konkrete Ordnung Israels zugunsten einer Zukunft, in der die wahrhafte Ordnung eines »Restes« den Mittelpunkt einer friedvollen Menschheit bilden sollte. Jeremia bezog die »Völker« ein; während sie alle in Unordnung waren und die Jahweordnung sich im Augenblick in der Person des Propheten konzentrierte, erwartete er, daß »Israel« in der Zukunft der heilige Mittelpunkt bleiben, die neue Gemeinschaft aber alle Völker umfassen werde. Beide Propheten entfernen sich vom konkreten Israel ihrer Zeit und blicken auf eine Gemeinschaft, die zwar in gewisser Weise vom gegenwärtigen Israel abgeleitet, aber nicht mit ihm identisch sein wird. Sie denken dabei nicht an eine konkrete Gemeinschaft oder an eine bestimmte neue Ordnung; es handelt sich um Ordnungsprobleme jenseits der Existenz einer konkreten Gemeinschaft und ihrer Einrichtungen. So erfährt Jesaja den Abstand jeder konkreten Gesellschaftsordnung von der wahren Ordnung; Jeremia erfährt, daß die Existenz einer konkreten Gesellschaft in einer bestimmten Form das Problem der Ordnung in der Geschichte nicht löst. Mit alledem beginnt ein neuer schöpferischer Akt göttlicher Ordnung in der Geschichte: der Exodus Israels von sich selbst.

Die Qual dieses Exodus wurde von dem unbekannten exilischen Propheten durchlebt, den man Deuterojesaja nennt. Das Geheimnis dieses Exodus aus der konkreten Ordnung wird durch den leidenden Gottesknecht symbolisiert. Der Exodus aus der Ordnung der konkreten Gesellschaft führt zur Erlösungsordnung, die freilich noch nicht vollendet wird. Der Gottesknecht bildet einen neuen Typus in der Geschichte der Ordnung — geschaffen vom Propheten in und für Israel, damit er von anderen verkörpert wird, bis die Aufgabe erfüllt ist. Das Knechtssymbol geht von Israel als dem Knecht Jahwes über den Propheten selbst als den Repräsentanten Israels bis zu dem ungenannten Nachfolger, der das Werk vollendet. »The Servant who suffers many a death to live, who is humiliated to be exalted, who bears the guilt of the many to see them saved as his offspring, is the King above the kings, the representative of divine above imperial order. And the history of Israel as the people under God is consummated in the vision of the unknown genius, for as the representative sufferer Israel has gone beyond itself and become the light of salvation to mankind« (515).

II.

Zweifellos ist das Buch Voegelins, von dessen reichhaltigem Inhalt auch eine noch eingehendere Darstellung nur einen schwachen Eindruck vermitteln kann, eine äußerst beachtliche Leistung, insbesondere hinsichtlich der israelitischen Probleme. Der Verfasser besitzt eine tief eindringende Kenntnis des Stoffs, hat die neuere wissenschaftliche Literatur in großem Umfange durchgearbeitet und herangezogen und befaßt sich in mehreren, teilweise langen Exkursen mit der wissenschaftlichen Situation, um seine Stellungnahme daraus zu begründen. In alledem könnte man durchaus vermuten, in ihm einen Vertreter der alttestamentlichen Wissenschaft selbst zu begegnen. Außerdem hat er dieses Ganze von neuen Gesichtspunkten aus betrachtet, für die er wiederum erst die Grundlagen schaffen mußte, die er in kleineren

Exkursen darlegt. Im Vordergrund steht dabei das Bemühen um eine Philosophie der symbolischen Formen der Staats- und Gesellschaftsordnung.

Angesichts dieser großartigen Leistung sieht sich der Kritiker in einer mißlichen Lage. Ist es nicht ein kleinliches und rechthaberisches Bemühen, an einer derartigen Arbeit etwas beanstanden zu wollen? Die Situation wird noch dadurch verwickelter, daß Voegelin sich weitgehend der neueren skandinavischen Forschung am Alten Orient und Alten Testament angeschlossen hat, neben der es wenigstens zwei andere Forschungsrichtungen gibt: von diesen erwähnt Voegelin die konservative, archäologisch orientierte so gut wie gar nicht, während er die kritischere, literarisch-historisch interessierte weithin scharf ablehnt. Infolgedessen wird jede Kritik an seinem Buch zugleich zu einer Auseinandersetzung über Forschungsmethoden innerhalb der alttestamentlichen Wissenschaft.

1. Zunächst handelt es sich um die Fragen, die durch die weitgehende Zustimmung Voegelins zur skandinavischen Forschung entstehen. Er folgt ihr in der schroffen Ablehnung der literarkritischen Analyse der alttestamentlichen Bücher, die sich — wie üblich — in dem Namen Wellhausens symbolisch darstellt, und in ihrer Ersetzung durch die traditionshistorische Erklärung. Damit steht und fällt ein nicht unbeträchtlicher Teil der Ausführungen Voegelins. Die traditionshistorische Erklärung rechnet für die vorexilische Zeit Israels noch nicht mit schriftlicher Niederlegung der einzelnen Erzählungen, Erzählungskränze oder Quellenschichten, sondern mit der mündlichen Weitergabe der Stoffe in bestimmten Traditionskreisen. In ihnen hätten die Stoffe schon eine feste Form erlangt, die ihnen auch die in exilischer oder nachexilischer Zeit erfolgte Niederschrift innerhalb eines jüngeren vorherrschenden Traditionskreises belassen hätte, so daß sich an dem überlieferten Stoff kaum Veränderungen vollzogen haben. Hält man sich dann aber — wie auch Voegelin — an die Darstellung jenes letzten Traditionskreises, so muß notwendig ein falsches Bild vom israelitischen Geschichtsverständnis entstehen, weil die älteren Traditionen in je ihrer Eigenart nicht mehr berücksichtigt werden. Ferner ist die Voraussetzung der traditionshistorischen Methode — die Annahme, daß auch die älteren Stücke des Alten Testaments erst in exilischer oder nachexilischer Zeit niedergeschrieben wurden — völlig unverständlich angesichts der Beobachtung, daß der Gebrauch der Schrift in Syrien-Palästina viel älter als früher angenommen ist (»Erfindung« des Alphabets im kanaanäisch-phönizischen Raum um die Mitte des 2. Jt.) und die israelitische Königszeit ein ausgesprochen »schreibseliges« Zeitalter war. Außerdem müßte man, wenn die mündlich weitergegebenen Stoffe schon eine feste Form erlangt und diese bei der Niederschrift beibehalten hätten, auf sie immer

noch die gleiche analytische Methode anwenden, die die Literarkritik unter der Annahme einer frühen schriftlichen Festlegung entwickelt hat. Denn ob die Stoffe in einer mündlichen Tradition oder in einem literarischen Vorgang zu ihrer jetzigen Gestalt zusammengefügt worden sind — einheitliche Gebilde stellen sie keinesfalls dar und müssen daher analysiert werden, wenn nach ihrem Wachsen und Entstehen gefragt wird. Schließlich liegt der traditionshistorischen Methode der Fehler zugrunde, daß sie gegenüber der Literarkritik mit der literarischen Frage sogleich andere Probleme vermischt, die getrennt behandelt werden müssen, und sich »on a much more thorough understanding of the contents of the narrative than the source-critical conception« stützt (159). Zweifellos sind die in den Erzählungen verwendeten Stoffe oft sehr alt und stammen aus verschiedener Zeit und Umgebung. Aber um dem nachgehen zu können, muß zuerst die literarische Analyse der jetzt vorliegenden Gestalt der alttestamentlichen Bücher vorgenommen werden; danach ist die formgeschichtliche, überlieferungsgeschichtliche und motivgeschichtliche Untersuchung an der Reihe. Der Pentateuch (oder Hexateuch) ist nach wie vor zunächst in Längsschnitten auf die verschiedenen Erzählungs- oder Quellenschichten aufzugliedern, die jeweils in sich geschlossene Darstellungen waren — vom Anfang der Menschheit oder Israels bis zur Landnahme in Palästina — und im Laufe der Jahrhunderte zu dem vorliegenden großen Werk zusammengewachsen sind; danach ist jede dieser Quellenschichten weiter zu untersuchen[1]. Man kann Voegelin darin zustimmen, daß sich daraus keine pragmatische Historie Israels, sondern eine paradigmatische Geschichte ergibt; jedoch stellt sich bei der Annahme von drei oder vier Quellenschichten ein wesentlich vielgestaltigeres Bild als bei der alleinigen Berücksichtigung der jüngsten Schicht heraus.

Ähnlich bedenklich ist die Auslegung der Psalmen, die Voegelin im Gefolge der skandinavischen Forschung mit dem Königtum in Verbindung bringt. Alle Psalmen waren danach ursprünglich Königspsalmen oder — wie Voegelin sagt — »Imperial Psalms«. Während freilich die skandinavische Forschung einfach von dem darin zu beobachtenden Eindringen altorientalischer Elemente (der »Königsideologie«) in Israel spricht, handelt Voegelin davon als von einer Ergänzung und Ausfüllung des Vakuums, das im Jahweglauben der vorstaatlichen Zeit notwendig bestehen mußte. Ungeachtet dieser Modifizierung geht es aber um das Grundverständnis der Psalmen. Unter ihnen gibt es zweifellos einige, die sich auf den König beziehen (vor allem Ps 2 18 20 21 45 72 101 110 132 144 1-10); bei einigen anderen ist

---

[1] Vgl. im einzelnen E. Sellin — G. Fohrer, Einleitung in das Alte Testament, 1969[11], § 16—28.

die Sachlage nicht so eindeutig. Jedenfalls aber ist es unmöglich, alle Psalmen als ursprüngliche Königslieder zu verstehen. Dagegen spricht schon die stilistische und motivgeschichtliche Untersuchung, die deutlich ergibt, daß zahlreiche Psalmen erst in exilischer oder nachexilischer Zeit gedichtet worden sein können, in der es kein israelitisches Königtum mehr gab. Zudem handeln viele Psalmen von Gebet oder Lobpreis einer Gemeinschaft, die teilweise gar nicht politischer Art ist, oder von den Anliegen eines einzelnen Menschen, bei dem es sich um jeden beliebigen Israeliten und nicht um den König handelt. Jede genauere Untersuchung der Psalmen enthüllt die oberflächliche Art, in der man manchmal in ihnen die Königsgestalt erblickt.

Ähnliches gilt für die Psalmen, die als sogenannte Thronbesteigungslieder ihren Platz im Rahmen des Neujahrsfestes gehabt haben sollen und das heilige Drama der jährlichen Thronbesteigung Gottes, verkörpert durch den König, feierten. Außer mehreren Gesichtspunkten, die in diesem Rahmen nicht noch zusätzlich behandelt werden können, ist einfach auf die fragwürdige philologische Grundlage dieser Annahmen hinzuweisen. Man gelangte zu ihnen, weil mehrere Psalmen mit den Worten *jhwh malăk* beginnen, übersetzte dies mit »Jahwe ist König geworden« und schloß daraus auf die sonst nicht erwähnte Feier der Thronbesteigung. Jedoch die Übersetzung trifft nicht den Sinn der hebräischen Worte, so daß die ganze Theorie zusammenbricht. Die im Hebräischen ungewöhnliche Satzfolge Subjekt-Prädikat soll das vorangestellte Subjekt betonen, und das verwendete Verb bedeutet »als König herrschen, Königsmacht ausüben«[2]. *jhwh malăk* heißt »Es ist Jahwe (und kein anderer Gott), der Königsherrschaft ausübt«. Es handelt sich in den betreffenden Psalmen um monotheistische Hymnen, die die Wirksamkeit des Propheten Deuterojesaja voraussetzen und spätexilischer oder nachexilischer Herkunft sind; sie haben weder mit dem Königtum noch mit einem Fest zu tun.

Damit sind wir beim Kernpunkt der skandinavischen Forschung angelangt; der Annahme, daß im ganzen Alten Orient ein einheitliches Kultschema bestanden habe, dessen zentrale Gestalt der Gottkönig als Verkörperung des Volkes und zugleich der Gottheit gewesen sei. Die gleiche Anschauung soll auch in Israel geherrscht haben. Sowohl gegen die Allgemeingültigkeit dieser Anschauung für die außerbiblischen Kulturen als auch gegen ihre Anwendung auf Israel, die den Panbabylonismus unseligen Angedenkens durch einen umfassenderen Panorientalismus ersetzt, sind schwerwiegende Bedenken erhoben worden[3]. Tatsächlich ist die Annahme eines altorientalischen

---

[2] Vgl. L. Köhler in: VT 3 (1953), 188f.; D. Michel ebd. 6 (1956), 40—68.

[3] Vgl. z. B. M. Noth, Gott, König und Volk im Alten Testament, ZThK 47 (1950),

Kultschemas unhaltbar. Selbst wenn die psychologische Grundstruktur vieler altorientalischer Völker infolge ihrer gemeinsamen semitischen Herkunft einander ähnlich war, berechtigt dies noch nicht zur Konstruktion religionsphänomenologischer oder -geschichtlicher Zusammenhänge, die sich nicht ausdrücklich nachweisen lassen. Deshalb beruht die Annahme eines Kultschemas auf falschen Voraussetzungen und einem methodischen Fehler. Das Schema ist denn auch nirgends geschlossen belegt, wie man bei seiner angeblich zentralen Stellung doch vermuten müßte; vielmehr werden seine einzelnen Motive aus Texten entnommen, die zeitlich und räumlich zum Teil sehr weit voneinander entfernt sind, und dann mosaikartig zum Ganzen zusammengesetzt.

Von wem sollten die Israeliten das Gottkönigtum übernommen haben? Bevor sie sich in Palästina niederließen — zum größeren Teil unmittelbar aus der Steppe ohne vorherigen Aufenthalt in Ägypten —, waren sie Nomaden oder Halbnomaden, denen jede Voraussetzung dafür fehlte. Der Scheich des Stammes verdankt seine führende Stellung seinem Erfolg und Ansehen, die als Wirkung des göttlichen Geistes betrachtet werden, der aber wieder schwinden kann. Zudem ist er nur der primus inter pares in der Versammlung der Sippenältesten und ohne Befehlsgewalt[4]. Ebensowenig fanden die Israeliten in Palästina ein Gottkönigtum vor. Die dynastische Ordnung, die es voraussetzt, läßt sich für diesen Zeitraum nur in wenigen der kanaanäischen Stadtstaaten nachweisen; teilweise sind die Fürsten auch Nachkommen früherer nichtsemitischer (u. a. indo-arischer) Geschlechter, bei denen wiederum die psychologischen Grundlagen für jene altorientalische Vorstellung fehlen. Die politische Schwäche und Zersplitterung des Stadtstaaten-Systems läßt schließlich jede wirkliche Grundlage für ein Gottkönigtum vermissen, nicht zuletzt dadurch, daß neben oder an Stelle des Königs manchmal die Oligarchie der Kriegergeschlechter oder Grundbesitzer die Macht ausübt (vgl. z. B. Jos 9 3f. Jdc 8 5 9 2).

Später haben David und Salomo allerdings versucht, dem Königtum eine überragende Stellung zu verschaffen, die sich in der praktischen Auswirkung dem altorientalischen Königtum nähert; sie haben dabei wohl vor allem das ägyptische Vorbild benutzt. Es ist eine synkretistische Mischung zwischen dem israelitischen Volkskönigtum und dem altorientalischen absoluten Königtum. Dabei bleibt das

---

157—191 (= Gesammelte Studien zum Alten Testament, 1957, 188—229); J. Gray, Canaanite Kingship in Theory and Practice, VT 2 (1952), 193—220; J. de Fraine, L'aspect religieux de la royauté israélite, 1954; K.-H. Bernhardt, Das Problem der altorientalischen Königsideologie im Alten Testament, 1961.

[4] Vgl. im einzelnen S. Nyström, Beduinentum und Jahwismus, 1946.

Element des Volkskönigtums in dem Vertrag zwischen König und Volk vor Gott bestehen, das Element der Geistbegabung in seiner Übertragung auf die Dynastie[5]. Ansonsten übernahm man hauptsächlich die äußeren »Errungenschaften« des altorientalischen Königtums: Berufsheer, Beamtentum, Steuererhebung und Frondienst; alles das blieb den nunmehr als »Untertanen« behandelten freien Bürgern stets fremd und verhaßt. Auch der Tempelbau Salomos, der nach kanaanäischem und nicht nach babylonisch-ägyptischem Muster erfolgte, beweist kein Gottkönigtum. Der Tempel war Hofkapelle und königlicher Eigentempel, in dem der König die Rechte des Stifters und Patrons ausübte. Es darf nicht vergessen werden, daß die Darbringung von Opfern oder die Erteilung des Segens damals kein priesterliches Monopol war, sondern jedem Laien — auch dem König — offen stand. Es mag sein, daß die davidische Dynastie die Anerkennung eines Gottkönigtums erstrebt hat; sie hat sie unter den Israeliten nie erreicht. Man kann höchstens an ein Gottkönigtum innerhalb des selbständigen Stadtstaates Jerusalem denken, in dem aber neben der einheimischen kanaanäischen Bevölkerung und Ausländern nur sehr wenige Angehörige des israelitisch-judäischen Volkes gelebt haben.

Noch deutlicher hebt sich das Königtum im Nordreich Israel vom Gedanken des Gottkönigtums ab. Während wir in Juda immerhin ein grundsätzlich dynastisches Königtum bemerken, allerdings mit Einbeziehung von Elementen des Volkskönigtums und mit Übertragung der Geistbegabung auf die Dynastie, hat das Königtum des Nordreiches in viel stärkerem Maße den ursprünglichen spontanen Charakter bewahrt — sogar in völlig säkularisierter Form — und daher nie besondere Festigkeit und religiöse Bedeutung gewonnen. Eigentlich machte nur Ahab den Versuch, ein von der Bevölkerung unabhängiges, dynastisches und absolutes Königtum durchzusetzen und das in der Umwelt geltende Staatsrecht einzuführen[6] — doch ohne Erfolg. Die dadurch entfachte Revolution Jehus hat seine Dynastie hinweggefegt.

Insgesamt steht die skandinavische Auffassung von Kultschema und »Königsideologie« mitsamt dem daraus abgeleiteten »Messianismus« (der göttliche König als gegenwärtiger Heilbringer) ebenso wie ihre Auslegungsmethoden auf tönernen Füßen.

2. Der Übernahme der skandinavischen Forschung ist es wohl vor allem zuzuschreiben, daß bei Voegelin an die Stelle einer geschichtlich gegründeten oft eine phänomenologische Betrachtung tritt. Dies zeigt sich deutlich, wenn man seine Darstellung der ägyptischen Situation

---

[5] Vgl. A. Alt, Das Königtum in den Reichen Israel und Juda, VT 1 (1951), 2—22 (= Kleine Schriften zur Geschichte des Volkes Israel, II 1953, 116—134); G. Fohrer, Der Vertrag zwischen König und Volk in Israel, s. u. 330—351.

[6] Vgl. im einzelnen G. Fohrer, Elia, 1968².

mit einer wirklichen Geschichte Ägyptens[7] vergleicht und dann der reichen Differenzierung nicht nur innerhalb der einzelnen Perioden, sondern sogar innerhalb der verschiedenen Dynastien gewahr wird. Ähnliches gilt von der Beurteilung Israels als »set off from the civilisations of the age by the divine choice«, als eines Volkes »that moved on the historical scene while living toward a goal beyond history« (113). Richtiger hätte es heißen müssen, daß gewisse religiöse Kreise Israels es als Volk göttlicher Erwählung verstanden und daß man es in spätjüdischer und christlicher Zeit als »living toward a goal beyond history« gedeutet hat. Aber solche Aussagen werden nicht aus der Geschichte und als geschichtlich bedingte Deutungen verstanden, sondern die Deutungen werden phänomenologisch als Fakten hingenommen. Das gleiche gilt für die Verwendung des Gottessohngedankens. Daß das israelitische Volk manchmal als »Sohn Jahwes« bezeichnet wird wie der König als »Sohn Gottes«, läßt sich schwerlich — unter Einbeziehung von Mose und Jesus — derart spielerisch-phänomenologisch anwenden, wie es geschieht (390. 397f.). Diese Bezeichnungen sind geschichtlich einfach als bildliche Ausdrücke zu verstehen, die das persönliche, ethisch bestimmte Verhältnis zwischen zwei Partnern umschreiben, d. h. zwischen Jahwe und dem Volk oder dem König.

So aber führt die Betrachtungsweise Voegelins zu geschichtlich unhaltbaren Ergebnissen. Der Abrahamerzählung von Gen 14 kann kein für Abraham authentischer Sinn entnommen werden, denn die Gestalt Abrahams ist erst nachträglich mit einigen selbständigen Traditionsresten (Feldzug von Ostkönigen, Melchisedek) verbunden worden[8]. Die für die Zeit Ahabs aufgezeigte Gefährdung Israels beruht nicht auf der Einführung des tyrischen Baal, die nur ein Zeichen des Bündnisses zwischen Israel und Tyrus war, sondern auf der innenpolitischen Situation. Dem alten und spannungsreichen Nebeneinander von Israeliten und Kanaanäern im Staatsgefüge suchte Ahab durch eine neutrale und paritätische Politik gerecht zu werden, die angesichts des vorherigen Zurückdrängens der Kanaanäer einer Förderung der kanaanäischen Minderheit und ihrer Religion gleichkam. Eine sorgfältig geschichtliche Untersuchung müßte das von Voegelin entworfene Bild an vielen Stellen ändern.

Ein zweiter Grundsatz, den Voegelin befolgt, ist die Ersetzung des Begriffs »Fortschritt« in der Entfaltung der Probleme durch die Vorstellung von »Compactness« und »Differentiation«. Eine ursprünglich

---

[7] Vgl. z. B. E. Otto, Ägypten, 1953.
[8] Daß es sich um eine sehr junge Komposition handelt, zeigt sich u. a. an der Verwendung der Gematrie: Die 318 Knechte Abrahams sind aus den Zahlwerten der Buchstaben des Namens seines angeblichen Knechtes Elieser errechnet worden.

»kompakte«, noch verdichtete Symbolik wird demnach allmählich »differenziert«, in ihre einzelnen Bestandteile auseinandergelegt. Diese Auffassung schließt ein, daß jede spätere Auslegung eine Einzelheit einer Tradition hervorhebt und in zutreffender Weise aus ihr folgert, weil alles schon im alten Symbol enthalten ist (vgl. z. B. 410f.). Daß eine kompakte Symbolik auch falsch differenziert werden kann, wird dabei übersehen; vor allem werden die Dinge auf den Kopf gestellt. Das jeweils Neue ist nicht von vornherein schon in der alten Vorstellung enthalten, so daß es aus ihr abgeleitet werden könnte, sondern wird gewöhnlich aus einer unmittelbaren existentiellen Erfahrung gewonnen und vor der altehrwürdigen Tradition mittels deren Neuinterpretation gerechtfertigt. Das uns begegnende Problem ist dasjenige von Tradition und Interpretation, wobei die entscheidenden Gesichtspunkte in der neuen Interpretation und ihrem Unterschied zur Tradition zutage treten. Wenn Amos und Jesaja die volkstümliche Tradition vom Tage Jahwes aufgreifen und aus der freudigen Erwartung des mit Hilfe Jahwes errungenen Sieges über alle Feinde Israels in die schreckliche Androhung des Untergangs Israels durch das göttliche Gericht umwandeln, interpretieren sie den alten Begriff so, daß nur der bekannte Ausdruck bleibt, während sein Inhalt sich völlig ändert. So verhält es sich grundsätzlich überall im Alten Testament; stets werden alte Traditionen neu interpretiert — im einzelnen natürlich in sehr verschiedener Weise und keineswegs derart scharf akzentuiert wie im obigen Beispiel[9].

III.

Daß sich schließlich aus dem Alten Testament mancherlei andere Gesichtspunkte ergeben, die Voegelin gar nicht oder bloß am Rande streift, soll an wenigen Punkten gezeigt werden.

1. Das israelitische Volk als Gemeinschaft der freien und rechtsfähigen Vollbürger hat stets eine bedeutende Rolle gespielt. Schon Saul wird, ungeachtet der geheimen Designation durch den Seher Samuel, vom »ganzen Volk« am Heiligtum von Gilgal »zum König gemacht« (I Sam 11 15), nachdem er sein Charisma durch den Sieg über die Ammoniter erwiesen hat. Das Volk ist es, das als Versammlung der Vollbürger oder vertreten durch die Sippenältesten den König erwählt. Auch David bedurfte der Zustimmung der Judäer, um König von Juda zu werden (II Sam 2 4); und die Ältesten von Israel kommen zu ihm und salben ihn zum König auch von Israel, nachdem er sich mit ihnen über die beiderseitigen Verpflichtungen geeinigt hatte

---

[9] An jeweils einem ganzen alttestamentlichen Buch durchgeführt von G. Fohrer — K. Galling, Ezechiel, 1955; G. Fohrer, Das Buch Hiob, 1963; zum Grundsätzlichen vgl. Tradition und Interpretation im Alten Testament, s. o. 54—83.

(II Sam 5 3). Als aber Salomos Nachfolger den Nordisraeliten nicht genug Zugeständnisse macht, schließen sie sich ihm nicht an, sondern sagen sich von der davidischen Dynastie los (I Reg 12).

Damit begegnet uns ein zweites wichtiges Merkmal des israelitischen Königtums: der Vertrag, den der König vor Jahwe mit dem Volke schließt[10]. In der Zeit des Königs Josia hat dies nebst weiteren Einflüssen und Gegebenheiten nahezu zu einer konstitutionellen Monarchie mit einer Staatsverfassung geführt. Diese Verfassung ist das deuteronomische Gesetz in seiner Urform, das aufgrund eines Vertrages von König und Volk angenommen wird (II Reg 23 1ff.). Während die Befugnisse des Königtums eingeengt werden, ruft das deuteronomische Gesetz zugleich das politische Gemeinschaftsbewußtsein und die tätige Mitverantwortung der Staatsbürger wach, die gemeinsam als die »Brüder« handeln sollen. Der Staatsgedanke ruht auf einer religiösethischen Entscheidung für den göttlichen Willen. Wer sie getroffen hat, trägt das Gesetz in sich und handelt aus seiner Absicht und Gesinnung heraus. Wenn vom Glauben das Leben nicht getrennt werden darf, sondern geheiligt werden soll, gilt dies auch vom staatlichen Leben und vom öffentlichen Handeln des einzelnen Menschen. So lehrt das deuteronomische Gesetz, daß die rechte innere Haltung des Menschen die lebendige Kraft einer Staatsverfassung ist. Ob sich das im täglichen Leben bewährt hätte, wissen wir freilich nicht; denn bald danach ist der Staat Juda untergegangen. Was aber das Gesetz wollte, als es von den »Brüdern« redete, kann für das moderne Staatsleben wichtig sein. Es bedeutet, daß der Staatsbürger sich nicht als Untertan, sondern als Teilhaber der Herrschaft versteht, und daß die Träger der staatlichen Funktionen von dem Bewußtsein erfüllt sind, nicht eine abstrakte und absolute Staatsallmacht zu verkörpern, sondern Beauftragte im Dienste aller zu sein.

2. In stärkerem Maße als auf der Ebene des Staates sah sich der israelitische Vollbürger in seinem Wohnort in das öffentliche Leben hineingezogen. Es ist die untere Ebene der Rechtsgemeinde, in der er lebt[11]. Die örtliche Rechtsgemeinde greift ein, wenn ein Streit zwischen zwei Bürgern das Leben der Gemeinschaft berührt oder gar gefährdet. In diesem Falle will sie befrieden, den Streit schlichten und das Wohl der Gemeinschaft wahren, indem sie nach Möglichkeit die Anliegen aller Beteiligten gütlich ausgleicht. Tatsächlich hat diese Rechtsgemeinde die Streitigkeiten geschlichtet und mit Erfolg wirken können, solange sie die Versammlung freier, unabhängiger und mit ziemlich gleichem Besitztum versehener Bauern bildete. Jedoch nach der Ver-

---

[10] S. u. 330—351.
[11] Vgl. im einzelnen L. Köhler, Die hebräische Rechtsgemeinde, in: Der hebräische Mensch, 1953, 143—171.

schiebung der Besitzverhältnisse durch den Übergang von der Naturalzur Geldwirtschaft wurde das Recht nur zu leicht zugunsten der wirtschaftlich Mächtigen gebeugt. Die Rechtsgemeinde versagte nunmehr.

Wiederum sucht das deuteronomische Gesetz nach Abhilfe. Es schränkt die Befugnisse der örtlichen Rechtsgemeinde ein und löst den Schiedsspruch von der lokalen Befangenheit und Unfreiheit, um die soziale Ungerechtigkeit zu mindern, die sich eingeschlichen hatte. Am Tempel in Jerusalem wird deshalb ein oberstes Gericht eingesetzt, an das man sich in schwierigen Fällen wenden soll, besonders bei Eigentumsfragen, Blutvergießen und tödlichen Mißhandlungen (Dtn 17 8-13). Dieses Gericht kann unbeeinflußt von örtlichen Verhältnissen und unbefangen gegenüber dem abweichenden Gewohnheitsrecht der verschiedenen Landschaften, aber in tiefer Verpflichtung gegenüber dem göttlichen Rechtswillen urteilen. Auch in diesem Fall wissen wir nicht, ob die Neuordnung sich bewährt hätte, weil der Staat Juda bald danach zusammengebrochen ist.

Ungeachtet dessen lehrt die Rechtsgemeinde, daß alles menschliche Zusammenleben, besonders im staatlichen Bereich, auf der Grundlage des Rechts beruht und daß stets das von Gott gewollte Recht verwirklicht werden soll. Gott ist ein Gott des Rechts und der Gerechtigkeit. Er fordert die Befolgung seines Rechtswillens und die Bewährung in einem Verhalten, das die eigenen Ansprüche mit den Anrechten des Mitmenschen ausgleicht. Wer sein eigenes Recht sucht, muß zugleich dem anderen das seine zukommen lassen.

3. Wie das deuteronomische Gesetz zeigt, hat Israel sich nicht leichthin mit den Zuständen abgefunden, die im öffentlichen Leben zu beobachten waren, sondern immer wieder nach der rechten Ordnung für Staat und Gesellschaft gesucht. Auch an kritischen Stimmen hat es nicht gefehlt (vgl. z. B. Jdc 9 8-15).

Die eigentliche Kritik am Staate aber findet sich bei den Propheten. Sie richten scharfe Angriffe gegen das Königtum, das der Repräsentant des Staates und der Exponent seiner Politik ist. Da ist keinerlei Unterwürfigkeit, vielmehr ist der Prophet von seiner Überlegenheit gegenüber den Regierenden erfüllt. Groß ist Gott allein. Der König und seine Regierung sind nur Beauftragte und Diener Gottes und besonders strenge Rechenschaft schuldig. Wehe ihnen, wenn sie sich vergehen! Der Prophet sieht, daß das Unheil nicht nur von unten, sondern auch von oben ausgehen kann. Daher richtet er seine Anklage nicht nur gegen die Masse des Volkes, sondern auch gegen seine herrschende Schicht. Der eigentliche Beitrag des Alten Testaments zu den Problemen der Staatsordnung liegt in dieser prophetischen Kritik und in den Folgerungen, die aus ihr zu ziehen sind.

Die Gründe für die scharfe prophetische Kritik sind zunächst in der Politik der Staatsführung zu suchen. Die Propheten verurteilen manchmal die Methoden der Innenpolitik (z. B. Jes 3 12-15 Jer 22 13-17), insbesondere der Religionspolitik. Sie haben dem Versuch, den alten Gottesglauben zur Staatsreligion zu erheben, ablehnend gegenübergestanden. Ihr Kampf gegen Heiligtümer und Priester und ihre Verachtung des ganzen Kultus sind zu einem Teil darauf zurückzuführen, daß all dies eifrig und gehorsam zur Stützung der Staatsreligion und der mit ihrer Hilfe betriebenen Politik ausgenutzt worden ist. Daher protestieren sie gegen die unheilige Allianz von Thron und Altar. Ebenso scharf wird die Außenpolitik verurteilt. Am liebsten möchten die Propheten diese treulose und ränkevolle Politik, mit deren Hilfe Israel zwischen den Großmächten eine Rolle spielen will, ganz beseitigt wissen. Denn letztlich zeigt sich in ihr die abgrundtiefe Dummheit und Verdorbenheit der Staatsmänner, die dabei Gottes Willen doch nicht entgehen können (Hos 7 11-12). Jede Politik, die in eitlem Machtstreben auf der Weltbühne eine Rolle spielen will, aber Gott außer acht läßt, ist von vornherein zum Scheitern verurteilt.

Der Staat bietet der Prophetie zahlreiche Angriffspunkte für ihre Kritik. Freilich richtet sich diese nicht gegen die Staatsordnung überhaupt. In ihrem Niedergang, in der Anarchie, kann Jesaja gerade das vernichtende Gericht beginnen sehen (Jes 3 1-9). Der Staat wird als geordnete Form menschlichen Zusammenlebens durchaus anerkannt und bejaht. Aber die naive Selbstverständlichkeit wird bezweifelt, mit der man im Handeln des Königs und in der Politik seiner Regierung das Walten Gottes erblickt. Nicht nur jeder Anklang an ein Gottkönigtum, sondern auch das Element der Geistbegabung wird ausgeschieden. Der Wille von Staat und König ist nicht einfach und leichthin als der Wille Gottes zu bezeichnen. Die Propheten tragen vielmehr die Spannung zwischen dem göttlichen und dem menschlichen Willen in das öffentliche Leben hinein. Sie zeigen in aller Deutlichkeit die Doppelseite des Staates, die das Nebeneinander der Überlieferungen von der Einsetzung Sauls zum König nur andeutet. Der Staat hat im menschlichen Zusammenleben eine wichtige Aufgabe zu erfüllen. Indem er es tut, ist er an sich weder göttlich noch widergöttlich. Aber die Erfahrung lehrt, daß er nur zu leicht und immer wieder von dem von Gott gewollten Recht abweicht und sich selbst gottähnliche Vollmacht und letztgültige Entscheidungen anmaßt. Wenn dies eintritt, muß man ihm widerstehen und ihn in seine Schranken zurückweisen. Aus diesem Grunde rügen und bekämpfen die Propheten den Staat. Sie wenden sich gegen ihn, sofern und soweit er sich auf seine Heeresmacht und seine Bündnisse verläßt, um damit eine Politik zu treiben, die den wahren Herrn der Welt völlig aus den Augen verliert. Gewiß bedeutet das nicht, daß die Propheten eine jede mit den Tatsachen rechnende Staatsordnung ablehnen. Sie tun es nicht mehr oder weniger, als sie umgekehrt jede religiöse Utopie vermeiden. Sie rechnen durchaus mit den Tatsachen, aber <u>wissen Gott darüber erhaben</u>. Sie könnten auch große Zukunftspläne entwickeln, sind sich aber darüber klar, daß Gott allein über die Zukunft verfügt und seine eigenen Wege geht.

Die prophetische Haltung gegenüber der Staatsordnung begegnet weitgehend in negativen Formulierungen. In ihnen verurteilen die Propheten vor allem die Gewalt als Gegenteil des Rechts, das die Vergewaltigung der Kleinen und Schwachen gerade verhindern will. In der Verwerfung der Gewalt betonen die Propheten das Recht und verteidigen es gegen das Unrecht. Sie setzen sich für den Rechtsstaat ein, den Gott will. Gott ist ein Gott des Rechts und der Gerechtigkeit; das Recht ist ein Ausdruck seines Willens. <u>Alle Sünde zieht den Verfall der Rechtsordnung nach sich.</u> Solches Recht ist aber nicht einfach das staatlich-juristische Recht; Staatsrecht und Staatsgesetz ist nicht dem göttlichen Recht gleich. Denn es dient oft genug dem Unrecht, so daß die Propheten ihm leidenschaftlich entgegentreten müssen. Dem Satze »fiat justitia, pereat mundus« halten sie das gottgewollte und gottgegebene Recht des Menschen entgegen. Die Propheten sind die Hüter der Rechte des Menschen gewesen, längst bevor diese Rechte für das Staatsleben entdeckt wurden. Aus diesen Rechten spricht Gott; wer sie verletzt, greift Gott selbst an. Von da aus ist es wohl deutlich, daß das so bedeutsame deuteronomische Gesetz ohne den vorhergehenden prophetischen Einfluß nicht denkbar ist; es stellt wenigstens teilweise einen Versuch dar, die prophetische Haltung für die Lösung der konkreten Probleme nutzbar zu machen.

Aber noch eins ist zu beachten, wenn wir die Propheten und das Alte Testament überhaupt verstehen wollen. Was ist das Eigentliche des Menschen und wie verhält sich die Staatsordnung dazu? Das Ziel allen Menschenlebens, auch der menschlichen Gemeinschaften, soll sein, daß Gott im Leben und durch das Leben der Glaubenden auf Erden herrscht und daß die Glaubenden in Gemeinschaft mit ihm leben. Die Aufgabe des glaubenden Menschen besteht darin, diese Herrschaft und diese Gemeinschaft zu verwirklichen — in seinem eigenen Leben und in den Gemeinschaften, denen er angehört. Demgemäß ist es Aufgabe des Staates als einer Form menschlicher Gemeinschaft, einen Raum zu schaffen, in denen jene Herrschaft und Gemeinschaft sich durch das Leben der Menschen entfalten kann. Damit erhält er seine Aufgabe, sein Ziel und seine Grenze gesetzt. Er ist etwas Behelfsmäßiges; er hat seinen Wert nicht aus und in sich selbst, sondern soll dienenden Charakter tragen. Er ist nicht um seiner selbst willen da, sondern nur erforderlich, um den Raum und die geordneten Verhältnisse zu schaffen, in denen sich das Eigentliche des menschlichen Daseins abspielen und entfalten kann: die Gottesgemeinschaft des Menschen und die Gottesherrschaft auf Erden im menschlichen Leben.

Daraus ergibt sich eine wichtige praktische Folge. Der Gedanke des Rechts und der Gerechtigkeit ist zwar die eigentliche Grundlage der Rechtsgemeinde gewesen und auch für die Staatsordnung immer wieder gefordert worden. Aber seine Geltung ist nur zu oft durch andere Einflüsse und Mächte beschränkt worden; daraus rühren die Unzuträglichkeiten her, die die Propheten rügen. Es muß eben noch ein zweiter Grundsatz hinzutreten, den die Propheten hervorheben und den das deuteronomische Gesetz in die Waagschale wirft, als es einen Neubau von Staat und Rechtsgemeinde anordnet. Dieser Grundsatz ist das Gebot der Liebe, das stets zur Gottesgemeinschaft und -herrschaft hinzugehört. Nicht das Recht allein kann und soll herrschen, sondern Recht und Liebe müssen gemeinsam das menschliche Zusammenleben bestimmen und formen. Die volle Botschaft des Alten Testaments erhalten wir, wenn wir die beiden Grundsätze des Rechts und der Liebe zusammennehmen.

4. Dem Staat kommt gegenüber der für das menschliche Leben grundlegenden Familiengemeinschaft nur zweitrangige Bedeutung zu, so daß er nicht das Recht zu störenden oder zerstörenden Eingriffen in die Familie besitzt. Außerdem darf die Freiheit des einzelnen Menschen als des von Gott zu ihr Berufenen nicht beeinträchtigt werden. So gewiß also die Notwendigkeit des Staates gesehen und anerkannt wird, geht es doch angesichts des ständig zu beobachtenden Strebens des Staates auf Ausdehnung seiner Befugnisse darum, ihn zu beschränken und in seine Grenzen zu weisen. Die glaubensmäßig bedingte kritische Haltung, die das Alte Testament durchweg dem Staat gegenüber einnimmt, ist theologisch allein gerechtfertigt. Die manchmal auffällige Staatsfreudigkeit in Theologie und Kirche weicht bedenklich von dieser Linie ab. Die Gleichsetzung des staatlich Gegebenen mit der Ordnung Gottes ist jener Abfall vom göttlichen Willen, den die Propheten gegeißelt haben. Es ist gänzlich ausgeschlossen, den Staat als Schöpfungs- oder Erhaltungsordnung Gottes zu verstehen: er ist in keinem höheren Sinn von Gott gewollt als jede beliebige andere menschliche Einrichtung.

5. In vielen Staatslehren begegnet eine Absolutheitsforderung des Staates und des Staatsdenkens, die den Staat — den jeweils bestehenden Staat! — zum absoluten Prinzip und höchsten Wert erhebt. Während der alttestamentliche Mensch aus einem ganzheitlichen Verhältnis zu Gott lebt und aus dieser Ganzheit heraus dem Staat das Seine geben kann, bis die zumutbare Grenze erreicht ist, haben sich in diesen Staatslehren die Verhältnisse umgekehrt. Der Mensch soll zum Staat in solch einer ganzheitlichen Beziehung stehen und dann — wenn es ihm persönlich so paßt — Gott das Seine geben, soweit die Grenzen des staatlichen Verpflichtetseins dadurch nicht über-

schritten werden. Es hängt damit zusammen, wenn man sich bemüht, das politische Prinzip überall in den Mittelpunkt zu stellen und den Menschen in erster Linie zu einem staatlich gebundenen und politisch bedingten Wesen zu machen.

Die Folgen sind deutlich. Menschen, deren persönliches Leben unangreifbar ist, lügen und betrügen, foltern und töten im Dienst des Staates oder der politischen Gruppe, die ihnen befehlen. Denn diese beiden glauben über das zu verfügen, was man sonst von Gott erhofft: die Möglichkeit der Vergebung alles dessen, was in ihrem Namen an Unmenschlichkeiten getan wird. Jede eigene Überlegung und Entscheidung ist überflüssig. Die Staats- oder Parteiethik gebietet, was man tun und lassen soll. Der einzelne hat dem zu folgen, ohne daß er sich im Konflikt mit einer allgemein-menschlichen oder gar göttlich gebotenen Ethik fühlen soll.

Es ist keine Frage, daß derartige Anschauungen in ausschließendem Gegensatz zum biblischen Denken stehen. Ihnen gegenüber gibt es nur ein Entweder-Oder! Freilich sollte die Wahl nicht schwer fallen, wenn das Alte Testament mit seinem nüchternen Blick für die tatsächlichen Gegebenheiten einem die Augen öffnet.

6. Wir stehen schließlich vor der Frage nach der Pflicht zum Gehorsam und dem Recht zum Widerstand im Staat. Nun zeigt das Alte Testament, daß es zweifellos ein ethisches Recht zum Widerstand gegen das Böse im staatlich-politischen Bereich gibt. An dem Verhalten der Propheten gegenüber dem Königtum erkennen wir zudem, daß dieses Recht auch dann in Anspruch genommen werden darf, wenn diejenigen, gegen die sich der religiös-ethisch begründete Widerstand richtet, nicht nur im tatsächlichen Besitz der Macht, sondern, formal gesehen, sogar im Recht sind und die Legalität für sich haben.

Freilich kann nicht jeder nach seinem freien Belieben und seiner bloßen Meinung solches Widerstandsrecht in Anspruch nehmen, sondern nur derjenige, den sein Gewissen treibt. Dennoch ergibt sich eine Schwierigkeit. Ist nicht jedes geordnete Leben im Staat durch die Freiheit der persönlichen Entscheidung bedroht oder unmöglich gemacht? Kann sich nicht eine grundsätzlich gemeinschaftsfeindliche und anarchistische Haltung herausbilden, die sich gewöhnlich mit mangelnder Kritik am eigenen Urteil verbindet? Kann man sich nicht gegen jede Ordnung auflehnen und dabei noch ein gutes Gewissen zu haben glauben? Eine solche anarchistische Haltung wird vom Alten Testament allerdings ebenfalls verurteilt, weil das Moment der gerechten Ordnung in ihm eine große Rolle spielt. Eben dies Beharren auf dem gottgewollten Recht und der Existenz des gerechten Menschen ist entscheidend. Es besagt, daß denen kein Widerstandsrecht zusteht, die sich nicht an ethische Grundlagen binden. Nur dort ist es anzuerkennen, wo es mit dem verbunden ist, was das Leben des Menschen in der Gemeinschaft nicht entbehren darf: Wahrung der Menschenwürde, Sicherung der menschlichen Freiheit und Herrschaft des Rechts.

Ein solches Widerstandsrecht, das im ethisch-religiösen Verhalten gründet, läßt sich freilich juristisch nicht festlegen. Es setzt seiner Art nach einen besonderen Notstand voraus, den die Staatsführung in ihre Überlegungen nicht aufnehmen kann. Wird dieses Recht in Anspruch genommen, so erfordert es einen revolutionären Akt — wie in der Revolution Jehus im Nordreich Israel —, der vorübergehend ein bestimmtes Recht außer Kraft setzt, um Unrecht zu beseitigen und neues Recht zu schaffen.

Wenn nicht das Widerstandsrecht, so muß doch ein anderer Grundsatz verankert werden: das Recht auf Verweigerung des Gehorsams gegenüber Anordnungen und Befehlen, die unsittlich sind und höhere Rechte als die des augenblicklichen Befehls verletzen. Ebenso muß die Staatsführung willens sein oder dazu aufgefordert werden, alle staatlichen Ordnungen so aufzubauen und alle Handlungen ihrer Beauftragten so vornehmen zu lassen, daß eine Gehorsamsverweigerung unnötig und ein aktiver Widerstand überflüssig wird.

7. Die Propheten erstreben keine Abhängigkeit des Glaubens von der Politik, aber ebensowenig wünschen sie die Bevormundung des staatlich-politischen Handelns durch den Glauben. Statt dessen fordern sie glaubende Staatsmänner, die in eigener Verantwortung ihre Entscheidungen zu treffen wagen, weil sie — wie in ihrem ganzen Dasein — auch in staatlich-politischen Fragen als Glaubende handeln.

Das Alte Testament erteilt keine genauen Anweisungen für die staatliche Ordnung und das politische Handeln. Auch die Propheten nehmen niemandem die eigene Entscheidung ab, sondern legen sie ihm gerade auf. Diese Notwendigkeit, sich selbst entscheiden zu müssen, ist gewiß schwer und oft eine Last; doch sie macht zugleich die Freiheit des Menschen aus. Wie in allen Fragen wird der Mensch auch in derjenigen der staatlichen Ordnung und des politischen Handelns nicht durch eine Autorität eingeschränkt und genötigt, sondern vor die Entscheidung gestellt, ob und wie er als Glaubender handeln will.

Dabei ist er nun nicht auf seine Einsichten und Kräfte allein angewiesen. Als Wegweiser hat er die prophetische Grundeinsicht, wie sie sich aus den einzelnen Entscheidungen ergibt, die sie selbst in ihrer eigenen Lage haben treffen müssen. Wenn er von dieser Grundeinsicht ausgeht — wiederum nicht in sklavischer Übernahme, sondern weil er sich in freier Entscheidung zu ihr bekennt —, wird er in der Lage sein, in verantwortungsbewußter Weise politisch zu handeln und an einer rechten Staatsordnung für seine Zeit mitzubauen.

Der Vertrag zwischen König und Volk in Israel

Während Art und Stellung des israelitischen Königtums in den letzten Jahren Gegenstand zahlreicher Untersuchungen und teilweise grundlegender Auseinandersetzungen geworden und gerade auch die den Zusammenhang mit dem Kultus berührenden Fragen vielfach erörtert worden sind, ist ein für das Gesamtverständnis nicht unwichtiger Einzelzug nur am Rande erwähnt worden: die Verpflichtung des einzusetzenden Königs gegenüber dem Volke oder die gegenseitige Verpflichtung beider, die ihren Niederschlag in einem mündlichen oder schriftlichen Vertrage fand. Man hat gelegentlich darauf hingewiesen[1], doch gewährt eine zusammenfassende Betrachtung des Materials größere Einblicke und Rückschlüsse[2].

I.

1. Von einem Übereinkommen, das der ausersehene König vor oder bei seiner Einsetzung eingeht, ist ausdrücklich bei David die Rede. Nachdem er zum König über Juda gesalbt worden war, suchte der israelitische Heerführer Abner die Verbindung mit ihm aufzunehmen. Er hatte mit den Führern der Israeliten und Benjaminiten hinter dem Rücken des Saulssohnes Ischbaal längst Verhandlungen mit dem Ziel gepflogen, sie für ein Königtum Davids zu gewinnen (II Sam 3 17-19). Er schlug David vor, daß dieser mit ihm eine gegenseitige Verpflichtung eingehen möge, um Israel auf Davids Seite zu bringen (3 12). David ging nach der geforderten Vorleistung der Rückgabe der Michal, durch die er als Sauls Schwiegersohn auch legitime Ansprüche erheben konnte, auf diesen Vorschlag ein (3 13-16). Und Abner verpflichtete sich, ganz Israel dahin zu bringen, daß es mit

---

[1] Vgl. J. Pedersen, Der Eid bei den Semiten, 1914, 60—63 (mit Hinweis auf den eidlichen Charakter des Vertragsschlusses 40—44); C. R. North, The Religious Aspects of Hebrew Kingship, ZAW 50 (1932), 37; M. Noth, Die Gesetze im Pentateuch, 1940, 11f. (= Gesammelte Studien zum Alten Testament, 1957, 26f.); J. de Fraine, L'aspect religieux de la royauté israélite, 1954, 206f.; R. Hentschke, Die sakrale Stellung des Königs in Israel, ELKZ 9 (1955), 69—74; R. de Vaux, Das Alte Testament und seine Lebensordnungen, 1964², 163ff.; Le roi d'Israël, vassal de Yahvé, in: Mélanges Tisserant, I 1964, 119—133 (= Bible et Orient, 1967, 287—301).

[2] Vgl. E. Kutsch, Gesetz und Gnade, ZAW 79 (1967), 18—35; Der Begriff בְּרִית in vordeuteronomischer Zeit, in: Rost-Festschrift, 1967, 133—143; J. A. Soggin, Das Königtum in Israel, 1967.

David eine Verpflichtung eingehe, der diesem weitgehende Königsrechte zubilligen und möglichst geringe Einschränkungen gegenüber dem schwächeren Teil abnötigen sollte:

»Ich will mich auf den Weg machen und ganz Israel um meinen Herrn König versammeln, damit sie eine Verpflichtung mit dir eingehen. Dann kannst du ganz so, wie du es begehrst, als König herrschen.« (3 21)

Dabei stand nicht die Verpflichtung selbst, sondern die weitgehende Fassung der darin für David festzulegenden Rechte im Mittelpunkt. Daß eine Verpflichtung eingegangen werden sollte, schien selbstverständlich; entscheidend war, daß Abner eine für David günstige Verpflichtung zu erreichen hoffte. Jedenfalls aber hätte Davids Königtum über Israel auf einem Vertrag beruht, den er aufgrund der Verpflichtung mit Abner oder anderen Vertretern des Volkes geschlossen hätte. Daß es vorerst nicht dazu kam, ist bekanntlich der Blutrache Joabs an Abner zuzuschreiben (3 22ff.).

Als aber auch Ischbaal ermordet worden war, kam der Plan ohne die Vermittlung Abners zustande. In II Sam 5 1-3 sind zwei wichtige Motive miteinander verbunden: der Hinweis auf die schon erfolgte Designation Davids zum König durch Jahwe, die für das israelitische Königtum kennzeichnend ist[3], und die Erwähnung der Verpflichtung, die die israelitischen Ältesten als Vertreter der Stämme mit David eingingen. Diese fand am Heiligtum statt, anschließend erfolgte die Salbung:

»Da kamen alle Ältesten Israels zum König nach Hebron, und der König David ging in Hebron vor Jahwe eine Verpflichtung mit ihnen ein. Dann salbten sie David zum König über Israel.« (5 3)

Einzelheiten des Vertragsschlusses, insbesondere über die Art des Vertrages, sind nicht ersichtlich. Doch kommen nach der Sachlage nur zwei verschiedenen Formen des Vertrages[4] in Frage: entweder der zweiseitige Vertrag, der das Verhältnis der Zusammengehörigkeit zweier gleichwertiger Partner mit ihren Rechten und Pflichten regelt, oder der einseitige Vertrag mit alleiniger Bindung des Mächtigeren (Davids), der einen weniger Mächtigeren (das Volk) in ein bestimmtes Verhältnis zu sich setzt und bestimmte Verpflichtungen auf sich nimmt[5]. Da es David anscheinend von vornherein darum ging, mög-

---

[3] Ein derartiges Jahweorakel zugunsten Davids wird auch I Sam 20 15f. 24 5. 21f. 25 28. 30 II Sam 3 18 als allgemein bekannt vorausgesetzt. Es muß wohl wirklich bestanden haben und dürfte am ehesten auf die in I Sam 22 13 erwähnte Jahwebefragung in Nob zurückzuführen sein.

[4] Vgl. dazu im einzelnen J. Hempel in RGG³, I 1513—1516.

[5] Auf diese Form hat vor allem J. Begrich, Berit, ZAW 60 (1944), 1—11 (= Gesam-

lichst geringe einschränkende Verpflichtungen zu übernehmen, ist am ehesten an die letztgenannte Form zu denken.

Freilich wird demgegenüber in II Sam 2 4 nur erzählt, daß die Männer von Juda David zum König gesalbt haben, ohne daß von Verpflichtung und Vertrag die Rede ist. Hat David also lediglich mit den Vertretern der schon zum Königtum Sauls gehörigen Stämme einen Vertrag für nötig befunden, mit dem sich erstmalig einem König unterstellenden Großjuda (Juda mitsamt den ihm angeschlossenen Gruppen) dagegen nicht? Eine derartige Schlußfolgerung aus der Nichterwähnung eines Vertrages wäre voreilig, wie die Erzählungen über die Erhebung Sauls zum König erkennen lassen. Denn die jüngere, dem Königtum kritisch gegenüberstehende Version der Königwerdung Sauls (I Sam 8 10 17ff.) berichtet ebenfalls nichts von einer Verpflichtung und einem Vertragsschluß, erwähnt aber die Vertragsurkunde. Sie wird in I Sam 10 25 als »Recht des Königtums« bezeichnet, das Samuel vorgetragen, schriftlich festgehalten und dann an heiliger Stätte niedergelegt haben soll. Inhaltlich ist im jetzigen Zusammenhang das schon in 8 11ff. warnend aufgeführte Königsrecht gemeint, das deutlich die tatsächlichen Verhältnisse der späteren Königszeit voraussetzt und seine Herkunft aus der deuteronomischen Theologie nicht verleugnen kann[6]. Dagegen liegt in 10 21bβ-27a das Fragment einer älteren Erzählung vor, nach der Saul als der durch seine körperliche Größe vor allem Volke Ausgezeichnete durch göttliches Orakel zum König bestimmt wurde[7]. Diesem Erzählungsfragment ist das Motiv des »Rechtes des Königtums« entnommen und vorgreifend in 8 11ff. als Verkündigung des »Königsrechts« behandelt worden. Immerhin zeigt aber das Erzählungsfragment, daß schon die ältere Erzählung einen Vertragsschluß voraussetzt[8]. Ebenso ergibt sich, daß in der

---

melte Studien zum Alten Testament, 1964, 55—66) hingewiesen. Für den zweiseitigen Vertrag vgl. schon J. Pedersen a. a. O.

[6] Daran ändert sich auch nichts durch die Untersuchung von I. Mendelsohn, Samuel's Denunciation of Kingship in the Light of the Accadian Documents from Ugarit, BASOR 143 (1956), 17—22, der das Königsrecht als Beschreibung der halbfeudalen kanaanäischen Gesellschaftsordnung betrachtet. Denn eben diese hat auf die Gestaltung der späteren israelitischen Verhältnisse stark eingewirkt.

[7] O. Eißfeldt, Die Komposition der Samuelisbücher, 1931, 7f.; M. Noth, Überlieferungsgeschichtliche Studien I, 1957², 58.

[8] I. Hylander, Der literarische Samuel-Saul-Komplex, 1932, 153f., und M. Buber, Die Erzählung von Sauls Königswahl, VT 6 (1956), 129f., erblicken in dem Opfermahl von I Sam 9 22-25 die Versammlung des Ältestenrates von Israel; dieser hätte also gewisse Vorverhandlungen über die Königswahl gepflogen, sich den von Samuel ausersehenen Anwärter vorstellen lassen und vielleicht auch mit ihm ein Übereinkommen getroffen. Doch fragt es sich, ob damit nicht zuviel in den Text hineingelesen wird.

Zeit der Erzählung der Vertrag zwischen König und Volk, der ursprünglich die Existenz des Königtums ermöglichen und die Rechte des Volkes durch die Verpflichtung des Königs soweit wie möglich sichern sollte, zu einem Instrument für das Recht des Königtums geworden war. Anscheinend ist an einen einseitigen Vertrag gedacht, der aber nicht der alleinigen Bindung des Mächtigeren, sondern der überwiegenden Verpflichtung des Volkes als des schwächeren Empfängers dienen sollte[9].

Ungeachtet dieses Einblicks in den späteren Wandel des Wesens des Vertrages zwischen König und Volk läßt I Sam 10 21bβ-27a den Schluß zu, daß auch dort eine Verpflichtung eingegangen und ein Vertrag geschlossen worden sein kann, wo der Abschluß nicht ausdrücklich erwähnt wird. Vielleicht spielen die Worte des Dornstrauchs in der Jotamsfabel parodistisch auf den Inhalt eines solchen Königsvertrages an:

»Wenn ihr mich im Ernst
zum König über euch salben wollt,
kommt und bergt euch in meinem Schatten!
Wenn nicht, wird Feuer vom Dornstrauch ausgehen
und die Zedern des Libanon verzehren!« (Jdc 9 15)

Bei der Belagerung von Jabes in Gilead bitten die Einwohner den Ammoniterkönig um eine Zusicherung, die er ihnen gewähren soll:

»Gib uns die Zusicherung, daß wir deine Untertanen werden!« (I Sam 11 1)

Sie sind also bereit, den Ammoniter als ihren König anzuerkennen, um der geplanten Verstümmelung, Hinrichtung, Versklavung oder Vertreibung zu entgehen. Wäre diese Vereinbarung zustande gekommen, so hätte sie sich deutlich von der in Jos 9 gemeinten Zusicherung unterschieden, die das friedliche Beisammenleben von Israeliten und Kanaanäern begründen sollte[10].

Nach alledem dürfte es sich wahrscheinlich so verhalten, daß die Judäer mit David ebenfalls einen Vertrag ausgehandelt haben. Der Initiative Davids, der sich mit seinen Söldnern in Hebron festsetzte, entsprach die Initiative der Männer von Juda, die dorthin kamen,

---

[9] H. Wildberger, Samuel und die Entstehung des israelitischen Königtums, ThZ 13 (1957), 442—469, weist ebenfalls darauf hin, daß bei der Einführung des Königtums eine rechtliche Regelung getroffen werden mußte und Saul Bedingungen gestellt zu haben scheint, die in einem zu erlassenden Königsrecht ihren Niederschlag fanden.

[10] Jos 24 25 erzählt vom Vertragsschluß Josuas mit Israel und von dem Gesetz und Recht, das dabei gesetzt worden ist. Ungeachtet der sich stellenden geschichtlichen Fragen, auf die in III, 1 eingegangen wird, ist die Vorstellung vom Vertragsschluß und der sich daraus ergebenden Verpflichtung als solche bedeutsam.

um ihn zum König zu erheben. Beide zusammen ergaben die gegenseitige Bindung, auf der das Staatswesen beruhte[11].

2. Von diesen Gesichtspunkten aus scheint es, daß später das Bemühen Absaloms um die nach Jerusalem kommenden Israeliten einen zweifachen Zweck verfolgte. Er machte David die Herzen der Israeliten nicht nur abspenstig (II Sam 15 6), um sich Anhänger für seine Umsturzpläne zu sichern. Vielmehr zeigen die Worte: »Wenn man doch mich zum Richter im Lande bestellte ...!« (15 4), daß er die Leute zu gewinnen suchte, weil er mit ihnen einmal einen Königsvertrag zu schließen hoffte.

Nachdem freilich der Aufstand ausgebrochen und David zunächst geflohen war, ging Achitofel einen anderen Weg, um die Rechte des Königtums sofort und ohne Verzögerung für Absalom zu sichern. Er ließ ihn sich den in Jerusalem zurückgebliebenen Teil des königlichen Harems aneignen (16 21ff.). Seine Besitznahme bekundete symbolisch die Übernahme der Herrschaft und den Eintritt in die königlichen Hoheitsrechte. Daher vollzog sie sich in der Form eines Hoheitsaktes — in diesem Fall in einem Zelt auf dem Palastdach, in das sich der neue König in voller Öffentlichkeit zu begeben hatte (16 22).

Daß es sich darin um eine auch sonst vorkommende Rechtssitte handelte, ist bekannt. Sie wurde von Ischbaal hinter dem Vorgehen Abners (II Sam 3 7) und von Salomo hinter dem Verlangen Adonias (I Reg 2 22) geargwöhnt — ob zu Recht oder nicht, wird nicht mehr zu entscheiden sein. Von David selbst wird die Befolgung dieser Rechtssitte behauptet (II Sam 12 8). Er beanspruchte ebenfalls den von Absalom übernommenen Teil seines Harems wieder, versorgte die Frauen aber nur, ohne sich ihnen noch zu nähern (II Sam 20 3).

Die Rechtssitte kann also allein schon die Übernahme der Königsmacht vom Vorgänger auf dem Thron symbolisieren, ebenso neben einem Vertragsschluß zusätzlich zur weiteren Sicherung der Macht erfolgen. Sicherlich war der sexuelle Gebrauch damit nicht unabweisbar verbunden. Daher haben gewöhnlich die späteren judäischen Könige jeweils den Harem ihres Vorgängers offiziell in Besitz genommen und — wie David nach dem Aufstand Absaloms — sozusagen aufs Altenteil gesetzt. Sie bekundeten auf diese Weise ihre Herrschaft. Von da aus erklärt sich die hohe Bedeutung der Königsmutter in Juda; sie als wichtigste Person des früheren Harems legitimierte die Hoheitsrechte ihres Sohnes, in dessen Besitz sie sich offiziell befand. Einen wieder anderen Schritt tat der Benjaminit Seba in dem aus einer augenblicklichen Erregung entstandenen und sich mehr gegen

---

[11] A. Alt, Die Staatenbildung der Israeliten in Palästina, 1930, 51 (= Kleine Schriften zur Geschichte des Volkes Israel, II 1953, 41).

Juda als gegen David persönlich richtenden Aufstand. Wenn er erklärte:

»Wir haben kein Teil an David
und kein Erbe am Sohne Isais!« (II Sam 20 1),

dann proklamierte er die Aufhebung der seinerzeit von den Vertretern Israels mit David eingegangenen Verpflichtung. Der Königsvertrag sollte von einem der beiden Partner, vom Volke, annulliert werden. Aber da der König seine Söldner zur Verfügung hatte, die er einsetzen konnte, ließ sich die Auflösung des Vertrages nicht mehr erzwingen. Die unter David schon anhebende Umwandlung des israelitischen Königtums aus einem Wahl- und Vertragskönigtum zu einem absoluten Königtum begann das Volk als Vertragspartner zu entmündigen. Wenn die Auflösung des Vertrages mit Gewalt unmöglich gemacht wird, kann von einer echten gegenseitigen Bindung unter Übernahme einschränkender Verpflichtungen seitens des Königs als Grundlage des Staatswesens keine Rede mehr sein.

Es ist für beide Aufstände bezeichnend, daß Israel sich frei fühlte, den mit David eingegangenen Vertrag von sich aus zu lösen, als es der Meinung war, daß der König die übernommenen Verpflichtungen nicht einhielt oder die ihm übertragenen Vollmachten überschritt, um ein absolutes Großkönigtum durchzusetzen. Der Unterschied zwischen den beiden Versuchen liegt darin, daß durch den ersten, sorgfältig geplanten und vorbereiteten des Absalom nur die Person des Königs gewechselt und dadurch die Stellung Israels im Reich verbessert werden sollte, während der zweite die Auflösung des Vertrages mit David überhaupt bezweckte, also die volle Selbständigkeit Israels und die Aufhebung des davidischen Großreiches erreichen wollte[12].

3. Es war nur folgerichtig, daß David seine tiefere Schuld an den beiden Umsturzplänen nicht einsah, sondern in der Furcht vor einem neuen Aufruhr Adonias einfach zum Mittel des Staatsstreiches griff. Zwar hatte sich Adonia tatsächlich noch nicht zum König ausrufen lassen, wie man David meldete, sondern befand sich erst in den entscheidenden Stadien seiner Verhandlungen; aber zum Abschluß eines Vertrages mit Juda und Israel zugunsten Salomos hatte David in dieser Lage keinesfalls mehr genügend Zeit. So beging er einen Staatsstreich von oben, indem er den neuen König vom Hofpriester salben ließ — ohne Teilnahme von Vertretern der Reichsteile und ohne Vertrag mit ihnen —, ihn noch zu Lebzeiten in seine Mitherrschaft aufnahm und ihm auf diese Weise die Thronfolge sicherte (I Reg 1). Diese Maßnahme hätte im ungünstigen Fall dazu führen können, daß Salomo allein in Jerusalem — dem Eigenbesitz der Davidsfamilie —

---

[12] Vgl. A. Alt a. a. O. 58.

und in unterworfenen Gebieten anerkannt worden wäre, während Juda und Israel sich gegen die getroffene Entscheidung hätten auflehnen können. Denn sie entsprach der israelitischen Rechtsanschauung nicht. Daß sie trotzdem hingenommen wurde, hat seine Gründe im Überraschungsmoment, im Ansehen Davids zumindest in Juda und in der Aussichtslosigkeit der Empörung gegen die militärische Macht des Königs, der zwei zugunsten Israels unternommene Aufstände niedergeschlagen hatte. Hinzu kam, daß der einzige andere ernsthafte Thronanwärter Adonia anscheinend nur die Unterstützung judäischer Kreise genoß und von Salomo zunächst zeitweilig und dann durch seine Ermordung endgültig aus dem politischen Leben ausgeschaltet wurde.

Es ist verständlich, daß die Erzählung von der Thronnachfolge Davids die getroffenen Maßnahmen wenigstens nachträglich zu rechtfertigen sucht. Sie ist ja wahrscheinlich am Hofe Salomos unter einem politischen Gesichtspunkt und mit einem politischen Ziel entstanden. Sie sollte nachweisen, daß Salomo der rechtmäßige Nachfolger Davids war, und erklären, wie es zu dieser Nachfolgeregelung kommen mußte. Sie wollte die Ereignisse aus dem Gang der Geschichte rechtfertigen.

Dennoch hat Salomo das Ungute der Nachfolgeregelung gespürt und zu spüren bekommen. Als er es bemerkte, hat er den seinem Königtum anhaftenden Mangel des Staatsstreiches ohne Wahl und Vertrag dadurch zu beheben gesucht, daß er seine Legitimation im Rahmen einer dem ägyptischen Vorbild entlehnten »Königsnovelle«[13] von Jahwe selbst herleitete. Die Erzählung I Reg 3 4-15 geht von dem Augenblick der ägyptischen Königsnovelle aus, in dem am Krönungstage dem neuen Herrscher in einer Gottesbegegnung die Titel und Namen seines Königtums verliehen werden. Die göttliche Legitimation tritt bei Salomo damit an die Stelle des irdischen Königsvertrags und gleicht sein Fehlen aus. Daher ist sie an den Anfang der Darstellung der Regierung Salomos gestellt und sind die vorher erzählten politischen Morde mitsamt der Verbannung des Priesters Abjatar noch zu den Folgen des Staatsstreiches gerechnet worden. Seine eigentliche Einsetzung zum König hat Salomo mit I Reg 3 4-15 begründen lassen. Diese Form hatte den Vorzug, das Fehlen des irdischen Vertrages mit dem Hinweis auf den ausdrücklichen göttlichen Willen übertrumpfen zu können, zugleich allerdings den Nachteil, daß die Lösung des Problems nur für die Person Salomos selbst zutraf. Zumindest bei seinem Nachfolger mußte es wieder wach werden.

Noch Salomo selbst bekam die Schwierigkeiten zu spüren. Es mag fraglich sein, wie der Bericht über die symbolische Handlung des Pro-

---

[13] Vgl. S. Herrmann, Die Königsnovelle in Ägypten und in Israel, WZ Leipzig 3 (1953/4), 51—62.

pheten Ahia von Silo (I Reg 11 29-39) einzugliedern und zu bewerten ist; manches spricht für die von der Septuaginta vollzogene Einordnung nach der Rückkehr Jerobeams aus Ägypten[14]. Jedenfalls aber lassen die andeutenden Verse über die Erhebung Jerobeams gegen Salomo (11 26-28. 40) noch etwas vom Widerstand nordisraelitischer Kreise erkennen. Für sie war Salomo eben ein König ohne hinreichende Legitimation durch das Volk, weil kein Vertrag geschlossen worden war. Sie konnten mit dem statt dessen erfolgenden Hinweis auf die Gotteserscheinung schwerlich besänftigt werden.

4. In dieser Situation wird nach dem Tode Salomos die Forderung der Israeliten in Sichem verständlich. Sie wollten nun endlich wieder einen Königsvertrag — und zwar einen Vertrag mit günstigeren Bedingungen, als sie ihnen in der vertragslosen Zeit unter Salomo aufgenötigt worden waren (I Reg 12 1-4). Wir erhalten einen kleinen Einblick in die Verhandlungen, die geführt worden sind. Es ging um die Milderung der absoluten Gewalt und Verfügungsmacht des Königs, und der Königsvertrag schien das richtige Mittel, die Befugnisse des Herrschers klar zu umreißen und zu begrenzen. Aus den vorgetragenen Wünschen hätte sich als Form des erstrebten Vertrages diejenige der freiwilligen Selbstbeschränkung des Machthabers ergeben.

Da Rehabeam jedes Zugeständnis und vielleicht den Abschluß eines Vertrages überhaupt ablehnte, kündigten die Israeliten jede weitere Gemeinschaft mit der Dynastie Davids auf. Sie verwendeten dabei die etwas erweiterte Auflösungsformel aus der Zeit Sebas (I Reg 12 16). Nicht einmal militärische Gewalt konnte sie diesmal bezwingen (14 30)[15]. Wie das davidische Reich mit Hilfe des Königsvertrages zustande gekommen war, so zerbrach es an dessen Nichterneuerung. Andererseits haben die Israeliten von Jerobeam, den sie zum Könige erhoben (12 20), zweifellos ähnliche Garantien wie von Rehabeam verlangt und auch erhalten. Obwohl es nicht berichtet wird, muß ein Vertrag zwischen Jerobeam und den israelitischen Stämmen am Heiligtum von Sichem als selbstverständlich angenommen werden.

II.

1. Wie legitimierten die Davididen weiterhin ihr Königtum in Juda? Sie konnten sich zunächst auf die Rechtssitte der Übernahme des Harems vom Vorgänger als einer immer neuen Betrauung mit den Hoheitsrechten berufen. Die Rolle der Königsmutter in Juda

---

[14] Zur Frage der Geschichtlichkeit und späteren Überarbeitung vgl. G. Fohrer, Die symbolischen Handlungen der Propheten, 1968², 75.
[15] Der Prophetenspruch in I Reg 12 21-24 sollte später den Mißerfolg der kriegerischen Versuche Rehabeams verdecken.

zeigt, daß wohl auch so verfahren worden ist. Das genügte jedenfalls zur Legitimation in der im Eigenbesitz der Dynastie befindlichen Hauptstadt Jerusalem.

Die davidischen Könige konnten ferner den Eindruck erwecken, als hätten die Judäer mit David zugleich seiner ganzen Dynastie zugestimmt. Den Vertrag, der ja vermutlich geschlossen worden war, bezogen sie nicht auf die Person Davids, sondern auf die Dynastie; daher waren nicht bei jedem Thronwechsel eine neue Verpflichtung ein neuer Vertrag erforderlich. Infolgedessen bildete der Vertrag mit David rechtlich die Grundlage für das Königtum in Juda bis zu seinem Untergang im Jahre 586 v. Chr. Nachdem David selbst »einen seiner Söhne als seinen Nachfolger durchgesetzt hatte, hat man in diesem Staate an der Erbfolge innerhalb der davidischen Dynastie unentwegt festgehalten, wobei sich wohl einfach das Schwergewicht der einmal geschaffenen Institution als entscheidend erwies«[16].

Vor allem aber hielt man eine göttliche Legitimation zur Begründung des dynastischen Königtums für wünschenswert und fand sie in jener ewigen Zusicherung, die Jahwe selbst für die Dynastie gegeben und schon dem David habe mitteilen lassen. Sie garantierte den unerschütterlichen Fortbestand von Davids Thron und Dynastie (II Sam 23 5) und die Annahme des jeweiligen Thronfolgers an Sohnes Statt durch Jahwe (II Sam 7 8ff.). Daraus folgt an sich ein einseitiger Vertrag mit einer Verpflichtung des Mächtigeren, doch wird die Zweiseitigkeit in der Betonung des doppelseitigen Vater-Sohn-Verhältnisses angebahnt (7 14). Mit Hilfe dieser Vorstellung wurden sowohl der dynastische Grundsatz als auch der jeweilige einzelne König als Abkömmling der Dynastie legitimiert (vgl. auch Jer 33 21 Ps 89 4. 29f. 40 132 12)[17].

---

[16] M. Noth, Die Gesetze im Pentateuch, 1940, 12 (= Gesammelte Studien zum Alten Testament, 1957, 27), der allerdings fälschlich den nach II Sam 5 3 mit Israel geschlossenen Vertrag als Grundlage für Juda anführt.

[17] Ps 89 40 beruft sich auf die Zusicherung (ברית) an David, die Jahwe entweiht habe, geradezu als einen Rechtstitel, aus dem man einen Anspruch auf die Hilfe Jahwes ableitet. Ein wichtiger Hinweis könnte auch in Gen 14 17-20 vorliegen, falls die Verbindung des sicherlich alten Überlieferungselementes von Melchisedek mit der Gestalt Abrahams schon in der Königszeit erfolgt sein sollte. Dann läge darin der Versuch vor, den königlichen Anspruch der davidischen Dynastie auf die Herrschaft über Gesamtisrael in der Vorzeit zu gründen: Abraham, der Ahnherr des Volkes, hat Melchisedek gezehntet und in ihrem Vorgänger eigentlich schon den Davididen gehuldigt, umgekehrt schon den Segen des Vorläufers Davids empfangen und sich dadurch wiederum dem Ort und dem König von Jerusalem verpflichtet (vgl. G. von Rad, Das erste Buch Mose, 1952, 152). Allerdings fehlt eine wirkliche Handhabe für eine derartige Festlegung in vorexilischer Zeit; nur Ps 110 4 bietet einen gewissen Anhaltspunkt. Sicherlich aber hat die Melchisedek-Episode in nachexilischer Zeit dazu gedient, den Anspruch des Jerusalemer Tempels und Hohen-

Es kann wohl kein Zweifel darüber herrschen, daß II Sam 7 keinen einheitlichen und in sich geschlossenen Abschnitt bildet, sondern aus einem älteren Grundbestand und späteren Erweiterungen zusammengesetzt ist[18]. Ursprünglich hat die Erzählung lediglich von der Verhinderung des von David geplanten Tempelbaus berichtet und den Abschluß der Ladeerzählung gebildet (I Sam 4—6 II Sam 6); dazu gehören 7 1-7. 17. Diese Erzählung ist durch 7 8-16. 18-29 erweitert worden, wobei es dahingestellt sein mag, ob diese Verse im Laufe der Zeit nicht selbst noch Erweiterungen und Umbildungen erfahren haben. Jedenfalls zeigt die Einleitungsformel in 7 8 den neuen Einsatz; im Anschluß an ihn stehen nicht mehr die Lade oder der Tempel, sondern allein David im Mittelpunkt. Die Einfügung wurde durch das mehrdeutige Wort בַּיִת ermöglicht, dessen Bedeutung sich vom »Haus« als Wohnung für Jahwe zum »Haus« als Königtum oder Dynastie wandelt. Sobald vom »Haus« im letzteren Sinn die Rede ist, wird die Lade nicht mehr erwähnt. Zur Einfügung trug ferner die Bekanntschaft mit der ägyptischen Königsnovelle bei, die Salomo erstmalig zur Begründung seines Königtums verwendet hatte. Denn »Tempelbau und Königstheologie sind die Hauptthemen der ägyptischen Königsnovelle«[19]. So bilden 7 8-16 eine Sachparallele zur Legitimation Salomos

---

priesters gegenüber dem sich manchmal regenden Widerstand, der am deutlichsten in der Trennung der Samaritaner zum Ausdruck kommt, zu rechtfertigen.

[18] Vgl. vor allem L. Rost, Die Überlieferung von der Thronnachfolge Davids, 1926 (= Das kleine Credo und andere Studien zum Alten Testament, 1965, 119—253); ferner S. Mowinckel, Natanforjettelsen 2. Sam Kap. 7, SEA 12 (1947), 220—229; J. L. McKenzie, The Dynastic Oracle: II Sam. 7, ThSt 8 (1947), 187—218; H. van den Bussche, Le Texte de la Prophétie de Nathan sur la Dynastie Davidique, ALBO II, 7, 1948 (aus: EThL 24, 1948, 354—394); H. J. Kraus, Die Königsherrschaft Gottes im Alten Testament, 1951, 35ff.; M. Simon, La prophétie de Nathan et le Temple, RHPhR 32 (1952), 41—58; G. Widengren, Sakrales Königtum im Alten Testament und im Judentum, 1955, 59—61; M. Noth, David und Israel in 2 Samuel 7, in: Mélanges A. Robert, 1957, 122—130 (= Gesammelte Studien zum Alten Testament, 1960², 334—345); G. Ahlström, Der Prophet Nathan und der Tempelbau, VT 11 (1961), 113—127; E. Kutsch, Die Dynastie von Gottes Gnaden, ZThK 58 (1961), 137—153; A. Caquot, La prophétie de Nathan et ses échos lyriques, VTSuppl IX, 1963, 213—224; M. Tsevat, Studies in the Book of Samuel III, HUCA 34 (1963), 71—82; H. Gese, Der Davidsbund und die Zionserwählung, ZThK 61 (1964), 10—26.

[19] S. Herrmann a. a. O. 58, der allerdings das ganze Kapitel durch die Merkmale der Königsnovelle und den jeweils dominierenden Begriff »Haus« zusammengehalten sieht. Damit überschätzt er allerdings die Tragweite der formgeschichtlichen Untersuchung, die nicht auf eine ursprüngliche Einheit hinweisen muß, da die Zusammenfügung ebensogut sekundär und aufgrund der Bekanntschaft mit der Königsnovelle und des Begriffes »Haus« erfolgt sein kann. Welche dieser Möglichkeiten zutrifft, muß auf andere Weise entschieden werden.

in I Reg 3 4-15; nach dem Vorbild der Königsnovelle ist sie in 7 18-29 um ein Gebet bereichert worden[20].

Ein Vergleich mit der Legitimation Salomos ergibt zugleich, daß die Erzählung von der Davidszusicherung jünger als I Reg 3 4-15 sein muß. Nach einer Legitimation der ganzen Dynastie, wie sie in II Sam 7 8-16. 18-29 erfolgt, wäre ja eine gesonderte Begründung des Königtums Salomos nicht mehr erforderlich gewesen; dergleichen hat sich denn auch in späterer Zeit nicht wiederholt. Was in I Reg 3 4-15 die Person Salomos allein betraf, wurde durch die Davidszusicherung vielmehr auf die ganze Dynastie ausgedehnt: die göttliche Legitimation. Ob dies noch in einem späteren Stadium der Regierung Salomos erfolgt ist, läßt sich nicht entscheiden. Doch hat der Hof sicherlich in der Zeit Rehabeams diesen Schritt tun können und müssen, der eine letzte Folgerung aus dem Staatsstreich Davids darstellt. Die Zusicherung Jahwes an David ist jedenfalls keine Parallele zum Vertrag des Königs mit dem Volk (II Sam 5 3)[21]. Vielmehr wurde der irdische Königsvertrag mit dem Volk, der den Nachfolgern Davids fehlte oder der bei der Erweiterung des von David geschlossenen Vertrages auf die Dynastie lückenhaft schien, durch die von Gott selbst gesetzte Zusicherung übertrumpft[22]. Daß dies die Zustimmung der Judäer hat gewinnen können, erweist die stete Treue der freien Vollbürger zur Dynastie[23].

Dennoch war der Gedanke des Königsvertrages in Juda nicht ganz erstorben. Zunächst ist darauf hinzuweisen, daß andere mit ihm zusammenhängende Elemente lebendig blieben. So ist trotz des Bestehens der Dynastie ein gewisser Einfluß der freien Vollbürger auf die Auswahl des Königs aus den Angehörigen der Königsfamilie ersichtlich. Noch in später Zeit ist das Volk am »Königmachen« (vgl. I Sam 11 15 II Sam 2 4 5 3 I Reg 12 1. 20) entscheidend beteiligt. Auf diese Weise werden Asarja (II Reg 14 21), Josia (21 24) und Joahas (23 30) auf den Thron erhoben, zumindest teilweise unter Übergehen des eigentlichen Thronerben. Meinungsverschiedenheiten zwischen den Vollbürgern Judas und den Jerusalemern haben anscheinend zur Wahl Ahasjas durch die Letzteren geführt (II Chr 22 1).

---

[20] Belegstellen bei S. Herrmann a. a. O. 60 Anm. 4.
[21] So G. Widengren, King and Covenant, JSS 2 (1957), 21f.
[22] Dadurch wird die Ausbildung eines Rituals für den Regierungsantritt des neuen Königs erforderlich. In ihm mußten Jahwe die entscheidenden Maßnahmen vorbehalten sein, um den jeweiligen Thronfolger als von ihm ausersehen zu bezeichnen und ihm die für die Herrschaft notwendigen Vollmachten und Fähigkeiten zu verleihen. Vgl. A. Alt, Das Königtum in den Reichen Israel und Juda, VT 1 (1951), 2—22 (= Kleine Schriften zur Geschichte des Volkes Israel, II 1953, 116—134).
[23] Über das Verhältnis zu den älteren Traditionen Israels vgl. L. Rost, Sinaibund und Davidsbund, ThLZ 72 (1947), 129—134.

Ferner aber hat der Gedanke des Königsvertrages in wenigstens zwei geschichtlich wichtigen Situationen unmittelbar nachgewirkt. Dies läßt doch wieder seine grundlegende Bedeutung für das judäische Königtum erkennen.

2. Zum erstenmal begegnet der Königsvertrag wieder bei jener Palastrevolution gegen die Atalja, durch die der siebenjährige Joas auf den Thron erhoben wurde. Der erste Teil des Krönungsrituals, dessen wichtigste Phasen in II Reg 11 12ff. genannt werden, fand im Heiligtum statt. Der Königssohn wurde aus dem Tempel, in dem er verborgen gehalten war, herausgeführt (11 12) und — wie es Brauch war — an den für den König bestimmten Platz gestellt (11 14). Dort wurde er gesalbt, nachdem er vom Oberpriester das Diadem und עֵדוּת »das Mahnzeichen« erhalten hatte (11 12). Man hat dieses letzte Wort oft ändern wollen, doch schwerlich mit Recht. Es ist an ein geschriebenes Dokument zu denken; und da das ganze Ritual weithin ägyptischen Vorbildern entlehnt ist[24], legen diese Parallelen die Vermutung nahe, daß das »Königsprotokoll« gemeint ist. Es wurde in Ägypten bei der Krönung verlesen und im Tempel niedergelegt. Gewöhnlich enthielt es die Proklamation der Gottessohnschaft des Königs und seiner sogenannten »guten Namen«, wie die von der Gottheit verliehene Herrschertitulatur bezeichnet wird. Analog kann das jerusalemische Königsprotokoll die Adoption des neuen Königs durch Jahwe (vgl. Ps 2 7) und seine Titulatur — den »großen Namen«, den Jahwe verleihen will (vgl. II Sam 7 9 I Reg 1 47) — enthalten haben[25]. Dieser Teil des Rituals schloß mit der Akklamation durch das Volk (11 12). Der zweite Teil wurde im Königspalast begangen, in den man den neuen Herrscher geleitete: die Thronbesteigung mit Proklamation und Huldigung (11 19).

Im Falle des Joas wurde nun zwischen beiden Teilen die bisherige Königin Atalja getötet und der Ablauf durch eine weitere Zeremonie unterbrochen, die der Oberpriester vornahm:

»Dann legte Jojada die Zusicherung zwischen Jahwe, dem König und dem Volk (daß sie Jahwes Volk sein wollten) und die Verpflichtung zwischen dem König und dem Volk fest.« (11 17)

---

[24] Zur Anlehnung der äußeren Formen an das ägyptische Vorbild vgl. G. von Rad, Das judäische Königsritual, ThLZ 72 (1947), 211—216 (= Gesammelte Studien zum Alten Testament, 1958, 205—213). Auch der besondere Platz des Königs im Tempel geht auf ein ägyptisches Vorbild zurück, vgl. S. Herrmann a. a. O. 55.

[25] Das Königsprotokoll ist ebenfalls mit dem Begriff עֵדוּת in Ps 132 12 gemeint. Wahrscheinlich sind die Angaben des Königsprotokolls auch in I Reg 3 4-15 verarbeitet, vgl. im einzelnen S. Herrmann a. a. O. 55. Die Gleichsetzung von עֵדוּת mit dem »Gesetz« durch G. Widengren a. a. O. 5—7 ist daher unwahrscheinlich.

In dieser Bemerkung sind die beiden Motive einer Zusicherung Jahwes und einer Verpflichtung zwischen König und Volk miteinander verbunden. Zugleich findet sich eine andere Form als bisher. Der Oberpriester Jojada legt als Dritter die Verpflichtung zwischen den jeweiligen zwei Partnern fest, sowohl die Zusicherung Jahwes als auch die Verpflichtung im innermenschlichen Bereich[26]. Von ihnen hat zunächst die zweite in der Thronerhebung des Joas ihren geschichtlichen Ort. Denn nach der Herrschaft der ausländischen — nichtjudäischen und nichtdavidischen — Königin mußte die angestammte Dynastie mit Hilfe einer Verpflichtung und eines Vertrages von Juda wieder anerkannt werden. Dabei wird die Reihenfolge der vorgenommenen Handlungen gegenüber II Sam 5 3 umgekehrt; zuerst erfolgt die Erhebung zum König mitsamt der Salbung, danach erst die Verpflichtung. Daran wird die feste Stellung des längst konsolidierten Königtums erkenntlich. Daß es sich aber doch um einen wirklichen Königsvertrag gehandelt hat, geht noch aus der chronistischen Erzählung hervor, die Zusicherung und Verpflichtung voneinander trennt. Sie spricht in II Chr 23 3 zunächst von einer Verpflichtung zwischen den Vertretern des Volkes und Joas. Seinen eigenen Ansichten entsprechend hat der Chronist dabei die Leviten einbezogen und die Vertreter des Volkes zum »ganzen Volk« (23 5b) und zu »ganz Juda« (23 8) ausgeweitet. Trotzdem ist der ursprüngliche Sinn deutlich zu erkennen.

Doch auch die Bemerkung über die Zusicherung zwischen Jahwe, dem König und dem Volk, die in II Chr 23 16 aufgenommen worden ist, hat ihre Berechtigung. Zwar scheint erst der deuteronomische Verfasser der Königsbücher den jetzigen Wortlaut formuliert zu haben, um den Satz auf die Bekehrung zu Jahwe nach dem Abfall der vorhergehenden Zeit zu deuten; aber eine neue Zusicherung Jahwes an den König durch die Vermittlung Jojadas, vielleicht mit der rechtlichen Anerkennung durch das Volk verbunden, ist durchaus denkbar. Nach dem Bruch in der Linie der Dynastie, der in II Sam 7 8-16. 18-29 eine ewige Herrschaft zugesagt war, mußte die göttliche Legitimation erneuert oder bekräftigt werden. Daher diente die in II Reg 11 17 an erster Stelle genannte Zusicherung Jahwes einer derartigen Erneuerung oder Bekräftigung der Davidszusicherung.

3. Zum zweitenmal begegnet der Königsvertrag bei Josia im Zuge der Annahme des deuteronomischen Gesetzes. Nach II Reg 23 1-3 ist der König mit dem Volk durch seine nach Jerusalem ent-

---

[26] Zu dieser Form des Bundes oder Vertrages vgl. M. Noth, Das alttestamentliche Bundschließen im Lichte eines Mari-Textes, Annuaire de l'Institut de Philologie et d'Histoire Orientales et Slaves 13 (1953), Mélanges Isidore Lévy, 1955, 433—444 (= Gesammelte Studien zum Alten Testament, 1957, 142—154).

botenen Vertreter eine Verpflichtung eingegangen, durch die sich beide Teile gleicherweise auf das neue Gesetz verpflichteten:

»Da ließ der König alle Ältesten von Juda und Jerusalem bei sich zusammenkommen. Dann ging der König zum Jahwetempel hinauf und alle Männer Judas und alle Bewohner Jerusalems mit ihm (die Priester und die Propheten und das ganze Volk, klein und groß), und er las ihnen den ganzen Inhalt des Gesetzbuches vor, das im Jahwetempel aufgefunden worden war. Dann trat der König an die Säule und legte vor Jahwe die Verpflichtung fest, daß sie Jahwe folgen und seine Gebote, Befehle und Vorschriften von ganzem Herzen und von ganzer Seele halten wollten, um so alle Worte dieses Gesetzes, die in jenem Buche geschrieben standen, auszuführen. Das ganze Volk trat der Verpflichtung bei.«

In diesem Falle schloß demnach der König einen Vertrag an heiliger Stätte. Weder handelte es sich um eine Verpflichtung gegenüber Jahwe, da der Ausdruck »vor Jahwe« lediglich angibt, daß die Handlung im Heiligtum als der Stätte der göttlichen Gegenwart stattfand, noch legte Josia als Dritter eine Verpflichtung zwischen Jahwe und dem Volk fest, da er selber ebenfalls einbezogen war. Diese Auffassungen beruhen auf der Verwendung des geläufigen, aber zumindest an dieser Stelle sachlich mißverständlichen Verbs כרת. Tatsächlich schlug der König den Abschluß der Verpflichtung vor, so daß ein zweiseitiger Vertrag zustande gekommen wäre, oder legte die Verpflichtung fest, so daß es sich um einen einseitigen Vertrag mit überwiegender Verpflichtung des Volkes als des schwächeren Teils gehandelt hätte. Im letzteren Falle wäre die בְּרִית eine »Verpflichtung«, auf die das Volk eingeht, weil der König auf sie einzugehen befiehlt[27]. Berücksichtigt man jedoch die Beschränkung der königlichen Macht und die erweiterten Befugnisse des Volkes im deuteronomischen Gesetz, auf das sich der Vertrag bezog, so dürfte eher der erstere Fall zutreffen und ein zweiseitiger Vertrag abgeschlossen worden sein. Jedenfalls handelte es sich um eine Verpflichtung und einen Vertrag zwischen König und Volk. Daher wurden »alle Ältesten von Juda und Jerusalem« als Vertreter und Sprecher des Staatsvolkes des judäischen Reiches versammelt und als Vertragspartner hinzugezogen.

Fragt man also nach dem Sinn der deuteronomischen Formulierung in 23 3, die mehr umschreibt und verhüllt als klar aussagt, so erklärte der Vertrag, daß nunmehr dem Königtum und dem Verhältnis zwischen König und Volk — d. h. dem Staat — das neue deuteronomische Gesetz zugrunde gelegt werden sollte. Staat und Königtum erhielten eine neue Grundlage, daher war ein neuer Vertrag erforderlich, der die bisherige Regelung ersetzen sollte. Damit wurde das deuteronomische Gesetz zum Staatsgrundgesetz erhoben. Als solches hat

---

[27] J. Pedersen a. a. O. 62.

Josia es denn auch behandelt und zur Grundlage staatlicher Maßnahmen auf kultischem Gebiet gemacht.

Freilich hat er seine Nachfolger durch diesen Vertrag nicht binden können. Daher brauchte Jojakim das deuteronomische Gesetz gar nicht förmlich außer Kraft zu setzen, sondern bei seiner Betrauung mit dem Königtum nur auf die vorjosianischen Formen zurückzugreifen und sie zu benutzen.

4. In zwei der verhältnismäßig wenigen Königspsalmen liegen Berührungen mit dem Königsvertrag vor. Ps 72, der als Gebet des Königs an Jahwe formuliert ist, spricht als eigentlichen Wunsch aus, daß Recht und Gerechtigkeit im Lande blühen mögen, und gibt damit den wesentlichen Inhalt der vertraglich festgelegten Verpflichtung des Königs in Gebetsform wieder. Ps 101 umschreibt gleichfalls den Inhalt des Vertrages, soweit er Pflichten für den König enthält, und legt ihn dem König selbst als Gelöbnis in den Mund; der König gelobt die Beachtung des Vertrages.

III.

1. Daß im Nordreich Israel nach der Zeit Davids und Rehabeams weiterhin Verträge zwischen König und Volk geschlossen worden sind, zeigen zunächst die Verhandlungen Jehus mit der im Eigenbesitz der bisherigen Dynastie Omri befindlichen Hauptstadt Samaria. Er setzte sich mit den Vertretern der Stadt auf brieflichem Wege zu Verhandlungen in Verbindung (II Reg 10 1ff.) und stellte sie vor die Frage, ob sie ihm einen König aus den in ihrer Mitte lebenden Angehörigen der bisherigen Dynastie entgegenstellen und es damit auf eine kriegerische Auseinandersetzung mit ihm ankommen lassen oder ob sie es vorziehen wollten, die letzten Angehörigen der bisherigen Dynastie umzubringen und ihn als ihren König anzuerkennen. Diese Verhandlungen hätten folgerichtig zu einem wirklichen Vertrag führen können und müssen. Daß es nicht mehr dazu kam, hat seinen Grund in der radikalen Säuberung Samarias von allen Baalverehrern durch die Gewaltmaßnahmen Jehus. Ihnen waren gewiß auch die vorher genannten Vertreter der Stadt restlos zum Opfer gefallen, so daß Jehu sich die Stadt ohne weiteres aneignen konnte.

Statt dessen ist ein Vertrag zwischen Jehu und den Vertretern der israelitischen Stämme anzunehmen, der die politische und kulturell-religiöse Gleichstellung und praktische Bevorzugung des kanaanäischen Elements, für die besonders Ahab verantwortlich war, wieder aufhob. An die Stelle einer fehlenden unmittelbaren Bezeugung dessen ist wohl die Überlieferung vom Sichem-Vertrag in Jos 24 zu setzen[28]. Sie eilt zumindest in der Beziehung auf ganz Israel und wohl

---

[28] So K. Galling, Die israelitische Staatsverfassung in ihrer vorderorientalischen Umwelt, 1929, 55.

auch in der Fragestellung »Jahwe oder Baal« der Zeit Josuas voraus, muß jedoch wiederum älter als Dtn 27 sein. Daher dürfte die Überlieferung ihren Ausgangspunkt in der Tat im Königsvertrag Jehus besitzen, der vor allem den Jahweglauben als Staatsreligion bestimmte.

2. Deutlich setzen zwei Worte Hoseas die Sitte voraus, daß zwischen König und Volk Verpflichtungen bestehen müssen. Zunächst ist auf 6 7—11a zu verweisen[29]:

> »'In' Adam brachen sie die Verpflichtung,
>   dort wurden sie mir untreu.
> Gilead ist eine Stadt von Übeltätern,
>   'deren Fußspuren' blutig sind.
> Und wie 'gewalttätige' Räuber verfährt
>   die Bande von Priestern,
> die an dem Weg nach Sichem morden
>   und Schandtaten verüben.
> In 'Betel' sah ich Gräßliches [ ]:
>   Es hat 'sich Götzenbilder' aufgestellt!«

Hosea spielt in diesem Wort nicht auf Frevel der Vergangenheit an, sondern auf solche, die den Zeitgenossen aus ihrer Gegenwart unmittelbar bekannt sein müssen, so daß die allgemeinen Hinweise genügen. Auch das Imperfekt »sie morden« (v. 9) und der Ausdruck »ich sah« (v. 10) weisen auf die Gegenwart des Propheten. Von den genannten Orten sind nur Sichem und Betel israelitische Heiligtümer gewesen, nicht alle genannten. Der Gedanke einer Wallfahrt vom Ostjordanland nach Betel paßt weder zu Hosea selbst noch zum Text. Insgesamt ist also die Rede von der Gegenwart Hoseas, einer Verbindungslinie zwischen dem Ostjordanland und dem Herzen von Ephraim und dazu von allerlei Gewalttat und Frevel. Das läßt darauf schließen, daß es sich um eine der Revolutionen aus der Zeit des Propheten und um ihren Verlauf von Gilead bis Sichem und Betel handelt[30]. Damals sind ja mehrere Umwälzungen von Gilead vor sich gegangen; gegen eine von ihnen richtet sich das Scheltwort

---

[29] In v. 7 dl »Und sie« als redaktionelle Glosse; 1 בְּ pr »Wie ...«, da das folgende שָׁם einen Ort voraussetzt. — V. 8 1 עִקְבֵיהֶם דָּם da מ von דם heranzuziehen ist, pr »schwierig von (Blut)«. — V. 9 1 וּכְכֹחַ »Und (gemäß) der Gewalt (eines Räubers)« pr »Wartende«. — V. 10 1 בֵּית־אֵל pr »Haus Israel«; dl »dort ist Hurerei für Ephraim, es verunreinigte sich Israel« als erläuternde Glosse; dl »Auch Juda!« als vervollständigende Glosse. — V. 11 1 שָׁת שִׁקּוּצִים לוֹ pr »eine Ernte ist dir gesetzt«.

[30] So auch A. Alt, Hosea 5 8—6 6, Ein Krieg und seine Folgen in prophetischer Beleuchtung, NkZ 30 (1919), 537—568 (= Kleine Schriften zur Geschichte des Volkes Israel, II 1953, 163—187). Wenn 6 7—11a allerdings in den Zusammenhang der Spruchsammlung 5 8ff. gehört, die sich auf den syrisch-ephramitischen Krieg bezieht, kommen nur die Revolutionen Pekachs oder Hoseas in Frage, nicht aber die von Alt genannten Revolutionen Sallums oder Menachems. Vgl. auch W. Ru-

Hoseas. Im einzelnen kämen die Revolutionen Sallums, Menachems, Pekachs oder Hoseas in Frage; bekannt ist aber nur, daß Sallum vielleicht aus Gilead stammte, während Pekach über die aktive Hilfe von 50 Gileaditern verfügte (II Reg 15 25).

Für die Frage des Königsvertrages ist nur der erste Langvers wichtig. In ihm schilt Hosea den Treubruch in Adam, einer Ortschaft im Lande Gilead in der Nähe der Mündung des Jabbok in den Jordan. Angesichts dieser örtlichen Begrenzung ist schwerlich an den Bruch zwischen Jahwe und Israel zu denken. Vielmehr haben die Leute dort den Vertrag mit dem zuletzt regierenden König gelöst — der Aufstand ist ausgebrochen. Und da der Vertrag einst an heiliger Stätte geschlossen und die Urkunde in einem Heiligtum niedergelegt worden war, bedeutet der Aufstand für Hosea gleichzeitig Untreue gegen den Gott, vor dessen Angesicht der Vertrag feierlich beschworen worden ist. So setzt das Wort Hoseas auch dort einen bestehenden Königsvertrag voraus, wo die Königsbücher keinerlei Hinweis darauf enthalten.

Noch allgemeiner spricht Hos 10 3-4 davon[31]:

» Jetzt sagen sie:
   Wir haben keinen König,
     denn Jahwe fürchten wir nicht,
        und was soll uns der König tun?
   Sie machen Worte,
     schwören Meineide
        und legen Verpflichtungen fest;
   und 'Blutvergießen' blüht wie eine Giftpflanze
     an den Ackerfurchen.«

In diesem aus der Diskussion hervorgegangenen Scheltwort weist Hosea den Einwand zurück, als beruhe die herrschende Gesetzlosigkeit darauf, daß das Volk im Augenblick keinen König habe. Dabei hat der Prophet im Zitieren den Einwand schon umgeformt und in ihn den Hinweis auf die fehlende Gottesfurcht als Ursache der gegenwärtigen Not hineingelegt. In den folgenden, von ihm selbst formulierten Scheltsätzen legt er dar, daß die üblen Folgen der revolutionären Verhältnisse in eben diesem revolutionären Treiben selbst begründet sind. Man setzt zwar immer wieder einen neuen König ein, mit dem man Verpflichtungen festlegt — doch man hält diese nicht ein! Man gibt Loyalitätsversicherungen und schwört Huldigungseide — doch sind es leere Worte und Meineide! Deswegen schießt der politische Mord wie Unkraut empor. So setzt dieses Wort Hoseas

---

dolph, Hosea, 1966, 145f. (Eine andere Auffassung des Hoseawortes vertritt neuerdings H. W. Wolff, Dodekapropheton, 1, Hosea, 1965², 154—156.)

[31] In v. 4 1 מִשְׁפָּט pr »Recht«.

ebenfalls den Abschluß von Verträgen zwischen König und Volk als selbstverständliche Übung voraus. Dergleichen scheint also im Nordreich Israel viel häufiger vorgekommen zu sein, als die spärlichen Mitteilungen der erzählenden Bücher des Alten Testaments mit ihrer judäisch gefärbten Geschichtsbetrachtung erkennen lassen.

IV.

1. Das israelitische Volk als Gemeinschaft der freien und rechtsfähigen Vollbürger hat demnach bei der Einsetzung des Königs wenigstens grundsätzlich und staatsrechtlich und oft genug in der Wirklichkeit eine bedeutende Rolle gespielt. Das Volk ist es, das als Versammlung der Vollbürger oder vertreten durch die Ältesten den König erwählt — mögen auch die Designation des Geistbegabten durch einen von Jahwe Beauftragten und der Erweis der Geistbegabung in der Schlacht voraufgegangen sein. In Zusammenhang mit der Wahl wird ferner aufgrund einseitiger oder gegenseitiger Verpflichtungen ein Vertrag zwischen König und Volk vor Jahwe geschlossen. Außer den für die Inthronisierung vorgesehenen Riten, zu denen wie sonst im Alten Orient die Akklamation des Volkes gehört, war grundsätzlich ein derartiger Vertrag unter göttlicher Autorität erforderlich, selbst wenn er nicht regelmäßig zustande kam. Es handelte sich um einen staatsrechtlichen Akt innenpolitischer Art[32], zu dem die »Salbung« des Königs ursprünglich in Beziehung zu stehen scheint[33]. Während aber der Vertrag in Juda von Salomo an gewöhnlich durch die göttliche Legitimation als ersetzt galt und nur noch in ganz besonderen Fällen angewandt wurde, dürfte er in Israel die Regel geblieben sein, wenn ein neuer Revolutionär oder Usurpator den Thron bestieg. Er zeigte, daß der Staat auf einer verfassungsmäßigen

---

[32] Auch der Eroberer, der einen König von seinen Gnaden einsetzte, konnte mit ihm einen Vertrag schließen, der eidlich besiegelt wurde (Ez 17 13) und an die Stelle des Vertrags mit dem Staatsvolk oder der Jahwezusicherung trat.

[33] Von der Salbung des Königs wird oft so geredet, als führe sie eine Mehrheit — das Volk — aus. Praktisch wird sie allerdings wohl von einer einzigen Person vollzogen, die jedoch als Vertreter und Repräsentant der Gesamtheit handelt (anders J. Wellhausen, Zwei Rechtsriten bei den Hebräern, ARW 7, 1904, 33—41). Die Salbung soll eine besonders enge Beziehung herstellen oder ausdrücken, in diesem Falle diejenige zwischen dem König und Jahwe — zunächst durch das Volk, später unmittelbar vermittelt. Sie dient also der Herstellung einer sakral begründeten Communio neben der rechtlichen des Königsvertrages. Beide bewirken nach alter Vorstellung eine wirkliche Gemeinschaft des »Segens« und des »Lebens«, in der der Schwächere einen Anteil an der »Macht« des Stärkeren gewinnt oder beide Partner einander gegenseitig Anteil an ihrer »Macht« gewähren (J. Hempel a. a. O. 1514). Zur Salbung vgl. vor allem E. Kutsch, Salbung als Rechtsakt im Alten Testament und im Alten Orient, 1963.

Grundlage stand und bildete die eigentliche Rechtsgrundlage der königlichen Herrschaft. Daher bedeutete der Bruch oder die Auflösung des Vertrages von seiten des Volkes die Infragestellung der Königsgewalt mittels eines Aufstandes oder die versuchte Auflösung des Staatswesens überhaupt.

Der Königsvertrag hat in der älteren Zeit vornehmlich die Form eines dem Mächtigeren abgenötigten Vertrages gehabt, durch den er sich binden sollte. Später trat er unter anderen Formen auf: als Bindung des Schwächeren (Saul-Erzählung), Stiftung durch einen Dritten (II Reg 11 17) und zweiseitiger Vertrag (II Reg 23 3). Ungeachtet dieser verschiedenen Formen, die wenigstens teilweise durch die jeweilige geschichtliche Situation und die Machtstellung des Königtums bedingt waren, wirft er ein bezeichnendes Licht auf das Wesen israelitischen Königtums. Er macht deutlich, daß es keinesfalls als Gottkönigtum und Element einer zeitlos gültigen göttlichen Weltordnung zu verstehen ist, sondern zwar eine göttliche Beauftragung voraussetzt, praktisch und rechtlich aber auf menschlichen Abmachungen mit den Vertretern der israelitischen Stämme beruht, die außer in Königswahl und -salbung vor allem in einem derartigen Vertrag zum Ausdruck kommen. Gewiß ist dieser keine profane Angelegenheit gewesen, sondern »vor Jahwe« geschlossen worden. Doch besagt dies nicht mehr, als daß er religiös begründet ist und seine Geltung unter göttlicher Autorität steht, während er bestimmte politische Verhältnisse rechtfertigt. Sogar die Davidszusicherung, die doch auf fremden, ägyptischen Vorbildern beruhte, ist letztlich ein dem irdischen Königsvertrag analoger Vorgang, bei dem Jahwe an die Stelle der Stammesvertreter tritt. Dadurch ist in ihm die Vorstellung von der göttlichen Herkunft oder dem göttlichen Wesen des Königs grundlegend abgewandelt worden. Zur Legitimation des jeweiligen Königs genügte seine Ernennung zum adoptierten Sohn Gottes.

Die Ursprünge des Königsvertrages liegen in den nomadisch-beduinischen Vorstellungen, die in Israel lange und kräftig nachgewirkt haben[34]. Aus ihnen ist auch das ursprünglich geistbegabte

---

[34] Besonders deutlich ist der Unterschied gegenüber den Verhältnissen des hetitischen Staates, die auf den Anschauungen der indogermanischen Herrenschicht beruhen. A. Goetze, Kleinasien, 1957², 86 (mit weiterer Literatur), weist darauf hin, daß das hetitische Königtum anfänglich ein Wahlkönigtum gewesen zu sein scheint. Die Könige der ältesten Zeit bedurften der Anerkennung durch die Angehörigen ihrer Sippe und den Adel. Zwar designierte der regierende König dann seinen Nachfolger, machte damit jedoch nur einen Vorschlag an den Adel, der ihm zustimmen mußte, damit er rechtswirksam wurde. Diese Designationsurkunde war eine Art Vertrag. Der Adel garantierte die Thronfolge des Designierten, dieser verpflichtete sich, die Vorrechte des Adels unangetastet zu lassen. Erwies sich der Designierte als un-

Königtum erwachsen. Denn der als König anerkannte Anführer handelt nicht aufgrund einer vom Stamm oder Stammesverband erteilten Vollmacht, sondern aus der überraschend auftretenden Begeisterung heraus, die als göttliche Gabe verstanden und anerkannt wird. Doch ist diese Vorstellung vom geistbegabten Königtum angesichts des Königsvertrages etwas einzuschränken: In Israel handelt es sich um ein durch die Geistbegabung bedingtes Wahl- und Vertragskönigtum. Denn im Vertrag suchte man zwar einerseits die Geistbegabung festzuhalten und als Grundlage eines Amtes, einer Institution festzulegen, um so den Übergang von der in der Geistbegabung begründeten Einzeltat zur institutionell verfestigten Dauerregierung zu gewährleisten. Andererseits aber ging es darum, die Befugnisse des unberechenbaren Geistbegabten zu umgrenzen und die unantastbaren Rechte des Volkes zu sichern, damit das Freiheits- und Unabhängigkeitsstreben keine Einbuße erlitt. Das gleiche galt später für die Wiedererringung einiger Rechte der inzwischen zu »Untertanen« degradierten freien Vollbürger gegenüber dem absoluten Königtum, wie David und Salomo es weithin durchgesetzt hatten.

Die dem Saul erteilte Vollmacht erstreckte sich nur auf den Aufruf und die Führung des Heerbanns der Stämme zur Abwehr feindlicher Nachbarn, während es nicht sehr viel später unter Rehabeam um den verzweifelten Versuch ging, die grobe Bedrückung der Untertanen durch den Herrscher zu verhindern. Zur Zeit Jehus war nicht einmal mehr daran zu denken; man wollte vielmehr das kanaanäische Element zurückdrängen und den Jahweglauben zur Staatsreligion erheben. Nur Josia hat aufgrund des deuteronomischen Gesetzes noch einmal einen neuen Anfang machen wollen. Das Staatsgesetz, das von König und Volk angenommen wurde, setzte dem Königtum einige Schranken, die jede absolutistische und imperialistische Politik ausschließen sollten (Dtn 17 14-20). Der König sollte daran gehindert werden, das Volk in willkürlich begonnene Kriege zu führen, fremde Einflüsse in seiner Regierung walten zu lassen und die Steuerlasten zu erhöhen. Berücksichtigt man weiterhin die Einsetzung der Richter durch das Volk, die Errichtung eines obersten Gerichts am Heiligtum statt am Königshof und die Sozialgesetzgebung (Dtn 16 18-20 17 8-13 20—25), so erkennt man die Absicht, den Staat in bestimmter Weise zu gestalten. Während unter Eingrenzung der königlichen Befugnisse eine Art konstitutioneller Monarchie geplant war, wurden zugleich das politische Gemeinschaftsbewußtsein und die tätige Mitverant-

---

fähig oder unwürdig, so konnte er wieder enthoben werden. Es ging also stets um das Verhältnis zwischen König und Adel, in dem der König primus inter pares war. Wie sehr das ganze Staatswesen der Hetiter auf Staatsverträgen beruhte, zeigt A. Goetze a. a. O. 95ff.

wortung der Staatsbürger wachgerufen. Denn sie sollten gemeinsam als die »Brüder« handeln. In dem Gedanken, daß vom König bis zum Sklaven alle Israeliten »Brüder« seien, wurde auf einer vertieften religiös-ethischen Grundlage nochmals das Pathos der Frühzeit wachgerufen und das staatliche Leben über die geschichtlich gewordenen Abgründe hinweg auf der Entscheidung für den göttlichen Willen aufzubauen versucht. Wie das Leben des einzelnen vom Glauben nicht getrennt, sondern in ihm geheiligt werden sollte, so galt dies ebenfalls vom staatlichen Leben und politischen Handeln. Der Staatsbürger sollte sich letztlich nicht mehr als Untertan, sondern als Teilhaber der Herrschaft verstehen. Ob sich diese Auffassung auf die Dauer im täglichen Leben bewährt hätte, wissen wir freilich nicht; denn mit dem Leben Josias hat zugleich dieser Versuch ein frühes Ende gefunden. Immerhin zeugt er für die Kraft, die in der Rechtsordnung des Königsvertrages wirksam war.

2. Angesichts dieser Sachlage erhebt sich die Frage, ob und wie weit die בְּרִית Jahwes unter dem gleichen Gesichtspunkt wie die Verpflichtung zwischen König und Volk zu betrachten ist. Wie er als Landeseigentümer oder Eheherr in einem bestimmten Verhältnis zu Israel steht, so ja auch als König. Daher fragt es sich, ob nicht schon der Vorstellung von der Sinaiverpflichtung, die doch ursprünglich bei einer vorwiegend nomadischen Schar von Israeliten beheimatet war, mit einem auf die religiösen Verhältnisse übertragenen Vertrag mit dem König oder dem charismatischen Anführer zusammenhängt. Vor allem wäre zu untersuchen, wie weit die spätere theologische בְּרִית-Vorstellung vom Gedanken des Königsvertrages getragen oder beeinflußt worden ist. Jedenfalls ist doch der »Gedanke der Theokratie: Jahwe ist König (vgl. Jdc 8 33: יהוה יִמְשֹׁל בָּכֶם) ... dem des Gottesbundes nahe verwandt, so daß man den mit Gott geschlossenen Bund als einen Königsbund deuten darf«[35].

In diesem Rahmen können zu dieser Frage, die nur in einem größeren Zusammenhang betrachtet werden kann, lediglich einige Hinweise gegeben werden. Der Abschluß der Gesetzesmitteilung in Dtn 26 16-19 geht zur Kennzeichnung des Verhältnisses zu Gott geradezu vom Königsvertrag aus: Israel einerseits hat Jahwe veranlaßt, die Zusicherung zu erteilen, daß er sein Gott sein werde — unter der Bedingung, daß Israel ihm gehorcht und seine Anordnungen befolgt. Jahwe andererseits hat Israel zu der Erklärung veranlaßt, daß es sein Eigentumsvolk sei und alle seine Befehle einhalten werde — unter der Bedingung, daß er es zum ersten aller Völker machen und es ein ihm geheiligtes Volk sein wird. So haben beide Partner miteinander verhandelt, ihre Angebote gemacht und ihre Bedingungen

---

[35] G. Quell in: ThW II 123.

gestellt. Nachdem sie sich darüber geeinigt haben, gibt jeder Partner seine Erklärung und Zusicherung ab, die ihn selbst und den anderen verpflichtet. Diese Erklärungen werden beiderseitig angenommen; damit ist der Vertrag geschlossen. Es zeigt sich von da aus, daß die Formel »Ihr sollt mein Volk sein, und ich will euer Gott sein« auf einer Nachahmung des vom König gegebenen Vertrages beruht.

Einen anderen Inhalt erhält die in Ps 105 10 genannte Verpflichtung in 105 11: die Zusicherung der Verleihung des Landes Kanaan als erblichen Besitz. Ebenso gehen Jer 14 21 und Ps 44 18 von der Vorstellung des Königsvertrages aus: Jahwe (als König) möge die Zusicherung nicht aufheben oder für ungültig erklären, da das Volk seinerseits seine Verpflichtung nicht gebrochen hat.

Zum Vertrag gehört der Schwur; so leistet man Jahwe den Schwur, wie man dem König schwört (Jes 19 18 45 23 II Chr 15 14). Als Verpflichtungs- oder Vertragsurkunde werden die Gesetze betrachtet. Daher begegnet בְּרִית als Wechselausdruck für חֹק, מִשְׁפָּט und עֵדוּת (vgl. Dtn 4 13f. II Reg 17 15 Ps 105 10). Urkunden wurden in verschiedenen Behältern, darunter auch tönernen oder anderen Kisten aufbewahrt[36]. Gleiches gilt nach Dtn 10 2 für die Tafeln des Dekalogs, für die zu diesem Zweck die Lade angefertigt wird. Aus dieser Auffassung der Lade als Aufbewahrungsort für die als Verpflichtungs- oder Vertragsurkunde geltenden Gesetzestafeln ergibt sich ihre Bezeichnung als אֲרוֹן (הַ)בְּרִית oder אֲרוֹן הָעֵדוּת.

Schließlich gehen anscheinend die Erwartungen einer »neuen Verpflichtung« (Jer 31 31-34) oder einer künftigen »Heilszusicherung« (Ez 34 25 37 26), die Jahwe geben wird, auf die Vorstellung des Königsvertrages zurück. Insbesondere erwartet Ezechiel für das neue Israel zuletzt nicht mehr einen eigenständigen König, sondern einen נָשִׂיא, der von Jahwe abhängig und niederen Ranges ist. Er wird nur als Unterhirt unter und nicht neben dem göttlichen Oberhirten tätig sein, der als eigentlicher König mit seinem Volk zur Begründung seiner Herrschaft eine neue Zusicherung und Verpflichtung eingegangen ist.

---

[36] E. Weidner, Amts- und Privatarchive aus mittelassyrischer Zeit, in: Christian-Festschrift, 1956, 111—118, zeigt an Hand von Ausgrabungen und inschriftlichen Belegen, daß es in Mesopotamien mindestens seit Beginn des 2. Jt. üblich war, private oder amtliche Keilschrifttexte in Tongefäßen verschiedener Form aufzubewahren.

Eisenzeitliche Anlagen im Raume südlich von *nāʿūr* und die Südwestgrenze von Ammon

I.

In den Jahren 1957 und 1959 konnte der hauptsächliche Verlauf der Westgrenze des ammonitischen Reiches aufgrund der alten Grenzfestungen vom *wādi es-sīr* bis wenig südlich von *nāʿūr* geklärt werden[1]. So lag es nahe, die Arbeit fortzusetzen, zumal es ohnehin nicht wenige Jahre dauern dürfte, bis auf diese Weise der Verlauf der gesamten ammonitischen Grenze festgestellt und die zahlreichen weiteren Festungsanlagen im Inneren des Landes aufgenommen sein können. Praktisch bedeutete dies, daß die südwestliche Ecke der Grenze von dem zuletzt erreichten Punkt *šaǧarat bilʿās* aus (1 km südöstlich von *nāʿūr*) bis zum vermutlichen Ansatzpunkt für die in allgemein westöstlicher Richtung zu erwartende Südgrenze zu erkunden war. Dies erfolgte vom 5. bis 6. 9. und teilweise noch am 8. 9. 1960.

Die Erkundung begegnete einigen Schwierigkeiten. Für den Grenzverlauf südlich von *nāʿūr* fehlte so gut wie jeder Anhaltspunkt, so daß das ganze Gelände zwischen dem zuletzt erreichten Punkt und dem wahrscheinlich moabitischen *es-sāmik* abgesucht werden mußte. Dies hatte zudem in einem verhältnismäßig breiten Geländestreifen zu geschehen, da die alten Wehranlagen in diesem Gebiet meist bis auf die Grundmauern abgetragen waren, so daß trotz der einst zwischen ihnen bestehenden Sichtverbindung jetzt von einer Stelle aus die Lage der nächsten Befestigung nur ganz selten auszumachen war, und da die vorhandenen Landkarten sich als wenig ausreichend erwiesen. Die Gleichförmigkeit des Berg- und Hügellandes, das keine hervorstechenden Merkpunkte besitzt, erschwerte die Übersicht und Orientierung. Schließlich schienen für die Lage der in Abschnitt IV beschriebenen Befestigungen zunächst unbekannte Faktoren eine Rolle zu spielen, die sich erst infolge anderer Untersuchungen zu einem späteren Zeitpunkt klärten. Dennoch dürfte es gelungen sein, die Kette der Befestigungen südlich von *nāʿūr* weiter zu verfolgen und in Zusammenhang

---

[1] Vgl. H. Gese, Ammonitische Grenzfestungen zwischen *wādi eṣ-ṣīr* und *nāʿūr*, ZDPV 74 (1958), 55—64; R. Hentschke, Ammonitische Grenzfestungen südwestlich von *ʿammān*, ZDPV 76 (1960), 103—123.

Eisenzeitliche Anlagen im Raume südlich von *nā'ūr* 353

damit den annähernden Verlauf der südwestlichen Grenze des ammonitischen Reiches zu bestimmen[2].

Im folgenden Bericht sollen zuerst die ammonitischen Befestigungen beschrieben werden, die in Grenznähe die vermutliche Hauptlinie gebildet haben (II.), danach die sich aus der Lage zweier weiterer Gruppen ergebenden Sonderfragen erörtert werden (III.—IV.). Die

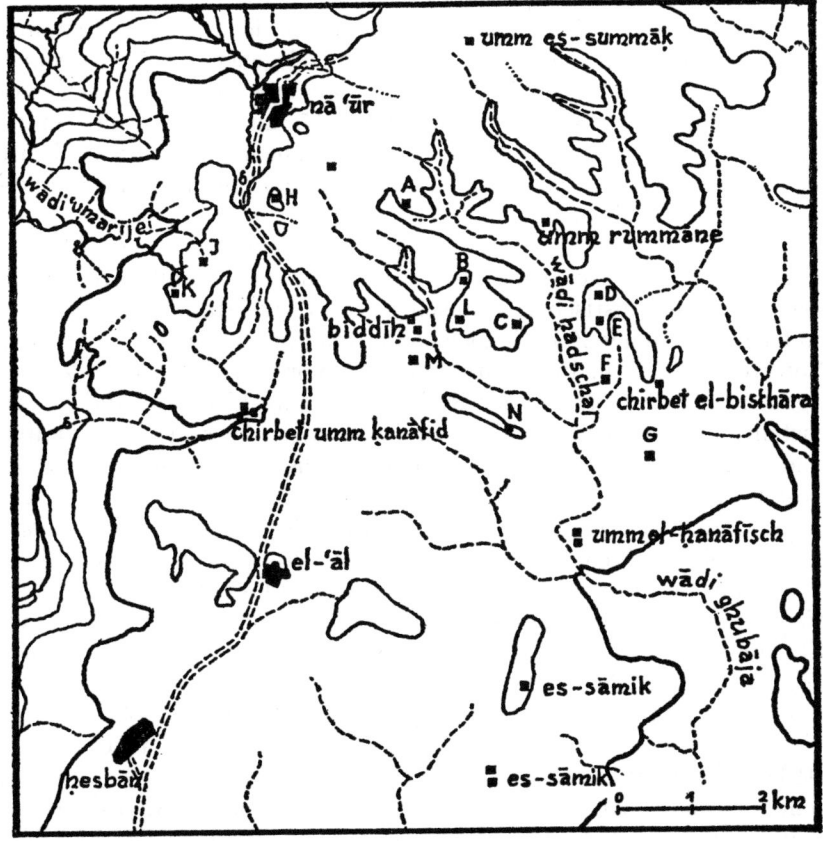

Die Umschrift der ursprünglichen Abbildung ist beibehalten worden; sie weicht von der im Aufsatz verwendeten geringfügig ab.

Wehranlagen werden dabei mit den Buchstaben A bis N bezeichnet (vgl. auch die Skizze), besonders da sie nicht sämtlich durch Gelände- oder Ortsnamen zu charakterisieren sind.

---

[2] Für die Fortsetzung vgl. H. Graf Reventlow, Das Ende der ammonitischen Grenzbefestigungskette?, ZDPV 79 (1963), 127—132.

II.

1. Geht man von den beiden Befestigungen aus, die über dem Südrand von *nāʿūr* und südöstlich davon an der *šaǧarat bilʿās* schon früher festgestellt worden sind[3], so schließt sich als nächstes Glied, etwa 900 m von der letzteren entfernt und in Sichtverbindung damit, in ostsüdöstlicher Richtung das auf der Kartenskizze mit A bezeichnete *bilʿās* an. Es liegt oberhalb eines kurzen Seitenarms des *wādi ḥaǧal* mit Blick in das *wādi*[4]. Von A aus besteht wieder Sichtverbindung zu B und D sowie zu dem nordöstlich gelegenen *umm es-summāq* mit einem großen *ruǧm malfūf* und zu *umm rummāne*, das fast genau in Fortsetzung der Linie von *šaǧarat bilʿās* zu A liegt; die beiden letztgenannten Stellen müssen noch untersucht werden; doch ist nicht daran zu zweifeln, daß sie zum ammonitischen Stützpunktsystem gehört haben.

Nach Ausweis der Keramik ist *bilʿās* eisenzeitlich besiedelt gewesen. Es finden sich sehr viele eisenzeitliche Keramikreste, ferner solche aus hellenistischer, römischer (terra sigillata), byzantinischer und früharabischer Zeit, jedoch keine mamlukischen mehr. Auf der Nordwestseite, d. h. in Richtung zu der nordwestlich von *bilʿās* gelegenen *šaǧarat bilʿās*, ist der Rest eines rechteckigen Gebäudes festzustellen. Die Mauern, die bis zu drei Steinlagen übereinander erhalten sind und eine Stärke von etwa 1,5 m aufweisen, verlaufen von Nordwesten nach Südosten in einer Länge von 12,3 m und von Nordosten nach Südwesten in einer Länge von 11,75 m. Nach Stein- und Mauerart sind die oberen Lagen wahrscheinlich als byzantinisch anzusprechen, jedoch auf der Grundlage eines älteren Gebäudes errichtet, das bis in die Eisenzeit zurückreichen kann. Das Gebäude und seine unmittelbare Umgebung weisen eisenzeitliche, römische und byzantinische Keramikreste auf. Auf der Nordostseite von *bilʿās* befinden sich die Fundamentreste eines weiteren, fast quadratischen Gebäudes, das jedoch so stark abgetragen ist, daß sich keine näheren Feststellungen machen lassen. Daß es sich in *bilʿās* lediglich um eine ammonitische Einzelbefestigung gehandelt haben sollte, wird der Sachlage, insbesondere angesichts der weit verstreuten Keramik, nicht voll gerecht. Vielmehr ist eine, dem Umfang nach nicht bestimmbare, ammonitische Siedlung anzunehmen, die befestigt und in das Stützpunktsystem einbezogen war.

2. Etwa 1,3 km in Luftlinie südöstlich von A befindet sich B, das in Sichtverbindung sowohl mit *šaǧarat bilʿās* und A als auch mit D steht[5]. Der in der älteren deutschen Karte angegebene Name *ḫirbet*

---

[3] Vgl. R. Hentschke a. a. O. 119 ff.
[4] Nach der Karte 1:100000 South Levant Series, Sheet N. H. 36 F. 2 Amman: 23041413.
[5] Lage nach der Karte: 23111401.

ḫešrūm wurde unabhängig davon durch Bewohner der Gegend genannt und bestätigt. B liegt am westlichen Hang des Höhenzugs zwischen dem _wādi ḥaǧal_ und dem westlich folgenden breiten Tal, das den östlichen Oberlauf des _wādi el-ġubāja_ (nördlich von _umm el-ḥanāfīš_) bildet.

Wie in _bilʿās_ finden sich auch in _ḫirbet ḫešrūm_ die Reste einer diesmal größeren und als solcher zu erkennenden Ortslage in der Größe von 100 zu 100 m, wobei unentscheidbar bleibt, ob sie quadratische, rechteckige oder ovale Form besessen hat. Die Keramikreste sind vornehmlich eisenzeitlich und mamlukisch, in wesentlich geringerem Maße römisch, byzantinisch und arabisch. Aufgrund der Keramik, der Lage und der Sichtverbindung zu anderen Punkten dürfte wie bei _bilʿās_ ein in Grenznähe gelegener, befestigter ammonitischer Ort anzunehmen sein.

3. Von _ḫirbet ḫešrūm_ (B) aus liegt in mehr ostsüdöstlicher Richtung und etwa 1 km in Luftlinie entfernt, zugleich etwa 600 m östlich von _sabbāḥ_ (vgl. L in III, 1), der Punkt C[6]. Er hat Sichtverbindung zu _šaǧarat bilʿās_, D und von der ursprünglichen Mauerhöhe aus auch zu L. Die Lage auf dem Höhenzug zwischen dem _wādi ḥaǧal_ und dem östlichen Oberlauf des _wādi el-ġubāja_ ist durch die Ausrichtung auf das erstgenannte _wādi_ bestimmt. Die wahrscheinliche Sichtverbindung zu L stellt aber zugleich die Verbindung zu der vorgelagerten Gruppe L—N her.

Als Ganzes handelt es sich um eine römisch-byzantinische Ortslage. Jedoch sind am Rande die Reste eines runden Gebäudes mit etwa 8 m Durchmesser festzustellen, die immer noch über das allgemeine Niveau hinausragen und bei denen es sich nach ähnlichen Funden um einen Turm gehandelt hat. Auffällig ist, daß sich gerade und ausschließlich an und um diesen Turm viele eisenzeitliche Keramikreste finden, wie sie anderswo in der Umgebung nicht vorkommen; hingegen weist die Turmumgebung im Unterschied von der eigentlichen Ortslage nur wenig römische und byzantinische Keramik auf. Weitere ähnliche Reste, die eine Ortsbefestigung aus jüngerer Zeit vermuten lassen könnten, sind nirgendwo zu beobachten. Nach alledem legt sich der Schluß nahe, daß in diesem Fall der Überrest einer ammonitischen Wehranlage vorliegt, die lediglich aus einem _ruǧm malfūf_ bestanden hat, falls das quadratische oder rechteckige Hauptgebäude nicht ursprünglich auch vorhanden war und erst in römisch-byzantinischer Zeit überbaut worden ist. Handelt es sich aber bei C und den im Folgenden zu nennenden Anlagen um ammonitische Befestigungen, so wird rückblickend die Annahme bekräftigt, daß A und B in dieses System einbezogen waren und die Verbindung von _šaǧarat bilʿās_ zu C und den weiteren Wehranlagen herstellten.

---

[6] Lage nach der Karte: 23191397.

4. Mit D wechseln wir von der Westseite des *wādi ḥaǧal*, auf der nunmehr der Höhenzug nach Süden hin abfällt und für weitere Anlagen nicht mehr geeignet war, auf die Ostseite hinüber. D liegt etwa 1,1 km ostnordöstlich gegenüber C auf dem nördlichen Teil von *umm el-qubūr* und hat Sichtverbindung zu C und E[7].

Die Stelle weist den Rest eines großen rechteckigen Gebäudes auf; die Stärke der bis zu zwei Steinlagen erhaltenen Mauern beträgt etwa 1,5 m und läßt auf eine Wehranlage schließen. Die Mauern verlaufen von Norden nach Süden in einer Länge von 23,5 m und von Osten nach Westen in einer Länge von 21 m. An der Westseite, d. h. zum *wādi ḥaǧal* hin, scheint ein rechteckiger Turm in das Gebäude eingebaut gewesen zu sein. In der Mitte, ein wenig zur Ostseite hin, findet sich eine Vertiefung, die eher eine Art Zisterne als eine Höhle gewesen sein dürfte. Es sind viele eisenzeitliche Keramikreste, danach auch solche aus römischer, byzantinischer und ganz junger Zeit festzustellen. Mit aller Wahrscheinlichkeit ist eine ammonitische Befestigung anzunehmen.

5. Auf dem südlichen Teil von *umm el-qubūr*, etwa 500 m südlich von D, liegt E, das Sichtverbindung mit D und F hat[8].

Außer byzantinischer und arabischer Keramik, die überwiegend zu finden ist, weist die Stelle auch eisenzeitliche auf. Zu erkennen ist ein ehemaliges Turmrund von 6,5—7 m Durchmesser. Das genaue Maß ist schwer feststellbar, da das Fundament zerstört und der frühere Verlauf nur in groben Umrissen auszumachen ist. Statt dessen sind in der Mitte der Rundung die schweren Steine des Bauwerks angehäuft. Es ist eine lediglich aus einem *ruǧm malfūf* bestehende ammonitische Wehranlage anzunehmen.

6. Etwa weitere 600 m südlich liegt F auf dem Sporn westlich der Höhe 905 und *ḫirbet el-bišāra*[9]. Sichtverbindung besteht einerseits zu den beiden Befestigungen südlich und südöstlich von *nāʿūr*, andererseits zu den benachbarten Punkten E und G.

Die Stelle weist zunächst zahlreiche schwere Steine auf. Aus ihnen lassen sich die Umrisse eines rechteckigen Gebäudes erschließen, dessen Ausmaße allerdings nicht mit Sicherheit zu ermitteln sind. Südwestlich vorgelagert befinden sich die Reste eines runden Turms, dessen eines Halbrund im Fundament erkennbar ist. Nordöstlich des rechteckigen Gebäudes ist eine runde Tretkelter von mindestens 3 m Durchmesser ausgehauen, von der ein Abfluß in ein rechteckiges Sammelbecken führt; in der Nähe liegt noch eine Zisterne. Die Keramikreste sind eisenzeitlich, römisch, byzantinisch und arabisch. Wird man also

---

[7] Lage nach der Karte: 23301400.
[8] Lage nach der Karte: 23311395.
[9] Lage nach der Karte: 23321389.

auf jeden Fall eine ammonitische Anlage annehmen müssen, so könnte diese wie in anderen Fällen aus einem rechteckigen Gebäude und einem runden Turm bestanden haben. Eine gewisse Unsicherheit in dieser Hinsicht bleibt bestehen, da das rechteckige Gebäude nur in Umrissen zu erschließen und nicht ganz eindeutig nachzuweisen ist.

7. Etwa 1,2 km südöstlich von F und südsüdwestlich von *ḫirbet el-bišāra* liegt die mit G bezeichnete Stelle auf dem südlichen Sporn der Höhe 905[10]. Es besteht Sichtverbindung zu F und vielleicht zu N.

Die Keramik ist überwiegend eisenzeitlicher, daneben in viel geringerem Maße römischer Herkunft. Ist demnach eine ammonitische Benutzung und Anlage als sicher anzunehmen, so fehlt jetzt doch jede Spur von Gebäuden, die es dort wohl einmal gegeben hat und deren Reste den Beweis für eine Befestigungsanlage erbringen könnten. Allein angesichts der beherrschenden Lage über dem südlichen Eingang in das *wādi ḥaǧal* von *umm el-ḥanāfīš* aus und angesichts des Anschlusses an die nördlicheren Wehranlagen D—F darf G als deren Fortsetzung und zugleich Abschluß vor dem gleich südlich davon beginnenden welligen Gelände, das zur moabitischen Hochebene überleitet, bezeichnet werden.

Insgesamt ergibt sich eine zusammenhängende Linie von sieben Anlagen. Nimmt man die beiden weiteren südlich und südöstlich von *nāʿūr* hinzu, so ist eine allgemeine Richtung von Nordwesten nach Südosten unverkennbar. Von den beschriebenen Anlagen sind A und C—G auf das *wādi ḥaǧal* ausgerichtet, B auf den westlich davon gelegenen östlichen Oberlauf des *wādi el-ǧubāja*. Daß mit dieser Linie jedoch nicht der unmittelbare Grenzverlauf gekennzeichnet ist, machen zwei weitere Gruppen von Anlagen deutlich, die dieser Hauptlinie westlich vorgelagert sind.

III.

Aus praktischen Gründen empfiehlt es sich, zuerst die südlichere Gruppe der vor der Hauptlinie gelegenen Anlagen L—N darzustellen und die mit ihr gestellten Fragen zu erörtern, weil sie wie die Anlagen der Hauptlinie mit dem südlichen Talsystem in Zusammenhang stehen und — wie sich zeigen wird — eine ähnliche Aufgabe wie B gehabt haben.

1. L liegt am Rande von *sabbāḥ*[11]. Es hat Sichtverbindung zu dem etwa 600 m östlich gelegenen C besessen, wenn man die ursprüngliche Mauerhöhe der heute zerstörten Anlagen berücksichtigt. Daher bildet C den Ausgangspunkt für L, das von den Anlagen der Haupt-

---

[10] Lage nach der Karte: 23381380.
[11] Lage nach der Karte: 23131397.

linie nur mit C in Sichtverbindung steht und sich zunächst als eine Art Vorposten von C nach Westen hin darstellt. Sichtverbindung besteht ferner mit M und N.

Am Hang zu der Straße, die den bei *umm el-ḥanāfīš* mündenden östlichen Oberlauf des *wādi el-ġubāja* durchzieht, finden sich die Reste eines rechteckigen Gebäudes. Die Mauern, deren Stärke nicht mehr auszumachen ist, messen in westöstlicher Richtung 8,3 m und in nordsüdlicher Richtung 8,8 m. Die Keramikreste sind eisenzeitlich, römisch, byzantinisch und mamlukisch. Die Gebäudereste lassen ihrer Art nach in Verbindung mit der Keramik auf eine ammonitische Anlage schließen.

2. Auf der westlichen Talseite gegenüber *sabbāḥ*, d. h. etwa 900 m in Luftlinie in südwestlicher Richtung, liegt M, das den Namen *ḫirbet abu ġurūš* trägt[12]. Sichtverbindung besteht zu L und wohl auch zu N und zu K, wenn dies auch wegen der stark eingeebneten Bauten nicht mit Sicherheit zu ermitteln ist.

Es scheint bei *ḫirbet abu ġurūš* um eine größere Anlage zu handeln, die nach Ausweis der Keramik in eisenzeitlicher, vielleicht in hellenistischer, sicher aber wieder in römischer und byzantinischer Zeit benutzt worden ist. Die eisenzeitliche Keramik ist zwar schwächer als die römisch-byzantinische, aber doch eindeutig vertreten. In die älteste Zeit scheint eine rechteckige Umwallung zu gehören, die auf der nordöstlichen und südwestlichen Seite etwa 35 m, auf der nordwestlichen und südöstlichen Seite etwa 25 m mißt. Auf der Südostseite findet sich das vorgelagerte und offenbar tiefer als das römisch-byzantinische Niveau gelegene Fundament eines runden Gebäudes, doch wohl eines Turms, von dem ein Halbkreis sichtbar ist. Im Querschnitt durch das Turmrund verläuft eine gerade Mauer von vermutlich byzantinischer Herkunft, durch die der nicht mehr sichtbare Halbkreis überbaut worden ist. Nach alledem legt sich die Annahme einer ursprünglich ammonitischen Anlage nahe, die dann die Fortsetzung von L bildete und in Verbindung damit das Tal hätte verteidigen oder sperren können, wie ja auch B für dieses Tal angelegt worden ist (vgl. II, 2). Jedoch ist wegen der geringen und schwer bestimmbaren Reste von *ḫirbet abu ġurūš* keine Sicherheit zu gewinnen.

3. Etwa 500 m südwestlich von *ḫirbet abu ġurūš* und 2 km nordwestlich von *umm el-ḥanāfīš* liegt ein langgestreckter Höhenrücken, der eine Längsausdehnung von etwas mehr als 1,2 km hat und den zwei Sättel in drei Abschnitte gliedern[13]. Der Name dieser als N bezeichneten Erhebung lautet nach der deutschen Karte *ed-ǧumle*, nach den Angaben von Beduinen dagegen *ǧamʿān* oder *ǧimʿān*.

---

[12] Lage nach der Karte: 23051393.
[13] Lage nach der Karte: 23101388—23201382.

Als Gesamtanlage hat auf dem Höhenrücken eine große, über 1 km ausgedehnte römisch-byzantinische Siedlung bestanden, die aber auf älteren Vorläufern und Fundamenten errichtet worden ist. Wenigstens auf der nordwestlichen und nordöstlichen Seite ist ein großer Wall zu bemerken, der vielleicht einmal die ganze Anlage umgeben hat. Für ihn wie für die noch zu erwähnenden Mauern sind in auffällig großem Ausmaß Feuersteine verwendet worden. Die Untersuchung des nordwestlichen Abschnitts ergab eine Reihe von römischen oder byzantinischen Bebauungsspuren: mehrere Säulenbasen, die in drei Reihen angeordnet sind und zwar am ehesten römischer Herkunft sein dürften, bei denen sich aber auch byzantinische Mosaiksteine finden; seitlich davon, nahe dem südwestlichen Rand der Höhe, ein Rundturm, der für eine ammonitische Grenzfestung jedoch zu klein ist und zudem auf dem gleichen Niveau wie die Säulenbasen steht; schließlich geringe Mauerreste, teilweise mit Randschlag und Bosse. Geht man über den ersten Sattel zum mittleren Abschnitt, so stößt man zunächst auf geringe und nicht näher bestimmbare Mauerreste in der Mitte zwischen den Abhängen der Höhe, danach auf der Südwestseite auf ein römisches Schachtgrab; kurz vor dem zweiten Sattel ist der Fels in römischer Zeit als Steinbruch benutzt worden. Die wichtigsten Beobachtungen sind im südöstlichen Abschnitt zu machen. Dort findet sich bald nach dem zweiten Sattel gegen den südwestlichen Hang hin ein etwa rechteckiges Areal von etwa 100 m Durchmesser mit Resten einer äußeren Umgrenzung oder Umwallung. Innerhalb dieser ḫirbe, nahe der südwestlichen Seite der Umwallung am Hang der Höhe, sind Mauerreste eines quadratischen Gebäudes mit 6 m Seitenlänge zu erkennen, das am ehesten als ehemaliger Turm zu verstehen ist. Seine Mauern laufen nicht parallel zur Umgrenzung, sondern im Winkel zu ihr, so daß eine Ecke des vermutlichen Turms fast auf die Umwallung trifft. Die Keramik ist überwiegend eisenzeitlich und nur in geringem Maße römisch und byzantinisch, so daß die umgrenzte Anlage mit Turm als eisenzeitlich bezeichnet werden darf. Südöstlich von ihr ist in etwa 200 m Entfernung eindeutig ein *ruǧm malfūf* von 12 m Durchmesser zu erkennen; wieder ergeben sich überwiegend eisenzeitliche und nur wenig römische und byzantinische Keramikreste. Jeweils weitere 50 m südlich und südöstlich dieses Turms und voneinander 30 m entfernt, liegen zwei mit Feldsteinen zugeworfene und bedeckte Steinhaufen in runder Form, die dem Durchmesser bzw. Umfang nach die Überreste ehemaliger Befestigungstürme darstellen. Sie bilden mit dem zuvor genannten die Endpunkte eines spitzwinkligen Dreiecks mit der Basis nach Süden und eine der Umwallung mit Turm südlich bis südöstlich vorgelagerte verhältnismäßig starke Befestigung. Während diese offensichtlich dem Schutz der Süd- bis Südwestseite des Höhenrückens diente, liegt ein weiterer Steinhaufen der gleichen Art etwa 100 m in nahezu östlicher Richtung von der Umwallung entfernt, also mehr zur Nordostseite des Höhenrückens hin. In allen Fällen weisen die Keramikreste in die Eisenzeit. Schließlich findet sich am nordöstlichen Hang, ziemlich am Südostende der Höhe, ein letzter Turm, der in Hanglage über dem nach *umm el-ḥanāfīš* verlaufenden östlichen Oberlauf des *wādi el-ġubāja* errichtet worden ist. Er weist überwiegend eisenzeitliche und nur vereinzelt römisch-byzantinische Keramikreste auf.

Es stellt sich die Frage, ob diese große eisenzeitliche Anlage, die jene Umwallung mitsamt quadratischem Turm und fünf runde Türme auf engem Raum aufweist, als ammonitisch bezeichnet und in Verbindung mit den kleinen Anlagen L und (vielleicht) M, über diese dann aber mit der Hauptlinie beiderseits des *wādi ḥaǧal* gesehen werden darf. Ist dies zu bejahen, so bildet die stark befestigte Höhe den südwestlichen Eckpunkt des ammonitischen Befestigungssystems und ist sicherlich in unmittelbarer Grenznähe zu denken. Denn das weitere wellige Gelände mit dem südlich emporragenden *es-sāmik* hebt sich deutlich von dem Bergland nördlich und östlich des Höhenrückens ab und ist zweifellos zu Moab und nicht mehr zu Ammon zu rechnen. Wäre die Anlage dagegen nicht eine ammonitische, sondern eine moabitische gewesen, so müßte die Grenze zwischen beiden Staaten durch den Oberlauf des *wādi el-ġubāja* nördlich von *umm-el-ḥanāfīš* in Richtung auf *nāʿūr* verlaufen sein. Die moabitische Anlage wäre dann unmittelbar hinter der Grenze errichtet worden, die Lage der Turmgruppe am Südostende der Höhe müßte daraus erklärt werden, daß die Höhe an dieser Stelle, d. h. von *umm el-ḥanāfīš* aus, am leichtesten erreichbar ist, und das Ganze hätte die Bedeutung einer vorgeschobenen Bastion vor der rückwärtigen Stellung *es-sāmik*. Freilich müßte bei dieser Annahme die ammonitisch-moabitische Grenze nördlich des Höhenrückens scharf nach Westen und bald wieder nach Süden abgebogen sein, da sich weiter nordwestlich die vorgelagerte ammonitische Gruppe H—K befindet. Der Höhenrücken in moabitischer Hand hätte demnach einen einzelnen moabitischen Vorsprung in einer entsprechenden Einbuchtung des ammonitischen Gebiets gebildet. Um ihn behaupten zu können, wären jedoch von moabitischer Seite ganz unzweckmäßige Verteidigungsmaßnahmen getroffen worden. Denn die Hauptbefestigung der Höhe läge an der rückwärtigen Seite, dem eigenen Lande zugekehrt und dennoch ohne Sichtverbindung mit der nächsten Stellung in *es-sāmik* (vgl. III, 4), während an dem der ammonitischen Seite zugewandten Hang lediglich ein einziger Turm errichtet worden wäre. Dies dürfte gegen die Annahme einer moabitischen und für diejenige einer ammonitischen Anlage sprechen, die somit der vorgelagerten Gruppe L und (vielleicht) M zuzurechnen ist. Sie hatte als Südwestpfeiler des ammonitischen Stützpunktsystems den Zweck, die

Besetzung der an der Südseite leichter zugänglichen Höhe — der letzten vor dem in die moabitische Hochebene übergehenden welligen Gelände mit nur einzelnen isolierten Erhebungen — und damit den Einbruch in den östlichen Oberlauf des *wādi el-ġubāja* zu verhindern. Und mittels des am nordöstlichen Hang errichteten einzelnen Turms sollte — gemeinsam mit L, (vielleicht) M und B — ein unmittelbarer Durchzug durch das Tal abgewehrt werden.

4. Südlich von G und N findet sich keine ammonitische Anlage mehr. Westlich der jetzigen Ortschaft *umm el-ḥanāfīš*[14] hat zwar eine ausgedehnte römische Siedlung gelegen, von der am aufsteigenden Hang zunächst Säulenreste, weiter hinauf Mauerreste und eine liegende Säule festzustellen sind. Aber für eine eisenzeitliche Siedlung war die Lage unmittelbar unterhalb von N ungünstig. Eine moabitische Siedlung hätte nur bestehen können, wenn N in moabitischem Besitz gewesen wäre, eine ammonitische war in dem sich abflachenden Vorgelände selbst dann unvorteilhaft, wenn N eine ammonitische Anlage war. So sind denn dort auch keine Spuren einer eisenzeitlichen Besiedlung anzutreffen.

Von dort aus gelangt man durch das *wādi el-ġubāja* zu dem hochgelegenen Höhenrücken von *es-sāmik*[15], der sich in zwei durch einen Sattel unterschiedene Kuppen gliedert. Auf dem nördlichen Teil, der nur römische, byzantinische und mamlukische Keramikreste aufweist, findet sich eine ausgedehnte *ḫirbe* mit Hausruinen (byzantinisch oder arabisch), Mauerresten, Wohnhöhlen und Zisternen. Der 250 m entfernte südliche Teil, der mehr Siedlungsschutt als die ammonitischen Grenzfestungen aufweist und an der Südostseite Zisternen besitzt, ist von einer Ringmauer mit etwa 200 m Durchmesser umgeben. Innerhalb dieser ist zunächst ein quadratisches Gebäude zu erkennen, dessen Mauern in nordsüdlicher und westöstlicher Richtung verlaufen. Darin sind undeutlich weitere Mauerzüge (Stärke 1 m) festzustellen, die das Gebäude in der Mitte in nordsüdlicher Richtung in zwei annähernd gleich große Räume und den östlichen Raum nochmals geteilt haben. An der Südmauer haftet teilweise römischer Verputz. In Verlängerung der Nordmauer ist östlich ein kleineres, ebenfalls quadratisches Gebäude mit 6,5 m Seitenlänge vorgelagert. Wie sich bei beiden Gebäuden große Mengen eisenzeitlicher Keramikreste, dagegen nur wenig römische und byzantinische finden, so weisen die Größe und Schwere der Mauersteine gleichfalls am ehesten in die Eisenzeit. Doch ist der Befund nicht von vornherein eindeutig. Es handelt sich entweder um eine eisenzeitliche Ortslage mit Ringwall samt einer inmitten darin gelegenen, durch die Gebäudereste aufgewiesenen Befestigung, die in

---

[14] Lage nach der Karte: 23281369.
[15] Lage nach der Karte: 23171346—23231359.

römischer Zeit instandgesetzt und erneut benutzt worden ist (Verputz), oder um eine nur durch den Ringwall geschützte Ortslage, auf deren Trümmern und aus deren Steinen in römischer Zeit in Zusammenhang mit der gleichzeitigen Besiedlung des nördlichen Höhenteils ein Kastell errichtet worden ist. Am ehesten trifft die zweite Annahme zu. Denn eine bereits eisenzeitliche Befestigung mit Kastell setzt eigentlich voraus, daß sie das südlich anschließende moabitische Hochland bedrohen sollte und müßte dann wohl ammonitisch sein. Jedoch besteht keinerlei Verbindung zu den ammonitischen Grenzbefestigungen, da der nördliche Teil des Rückens, der in der Eisenzeit noch nicht besiedelt war, den Blick vom südlichen Teil nach Norden zum ammonitischen Gebiet hin versperrt, während der Blick nach allen anderen Seiten hin frei ist und insbesondere Sichtverbindung zu eindeutig moabitischen Siedlungen wie *el-ʿāl* und *ḥesbān* besteht. So ist denn *es-sāmik* als eine ursprünglich moabitische Ortslage auf einem isolierten Höhenrücken anzusprechen, der von dem ammonitischen Grenzpunkt N und dessen sanft abfallendem Bergzug durch das *wādi el-ġubāja* getrennt ist.

Daraus ergibt sich, daß der westliche Oberlauf des *wādi el-ġubāja*, der von *umm el-ḥanāfīš* aus zunächst südlich und danach westlich am Höhenrücken N vorbeiführt, die Grenzlinie zwischen Ammon und Moab gebildet hat, nicht aber der östliche Oberlauf des *wādi el-ġubāja* oder gar das noch östlicher gelegene *wādi ḥaǧal*. Diese Grenzlinie hat sich weiter nördlich in der Gegend des vielleicht ammonitischen Stützpunkts M in den Ausläufern der Berge westlich von M und nördlich von *umm el-qanāfid* fortgesetzt, um über die vorgelagerte Gruppe H—K den Anschluß an die Hauptlinie bei *nāʿūr* zu erreichen.

IV.

1. Die der Hauptlinie vorgelagerte nördliche Gruppe von Befestigungen beginnt mit dem etwa 1 km südlich des Ortsendes von *nāʿūr* und etwa 1,8 km westlich von *bilʿās* (A) am Kopf des westlich von *nāʿūr* nach Süden führenden *wādi* gelegenen Punkt H[16]. Sichtverbindung besteht nur mit *šaǧarat bilʿās* und dem weiter südwestlich vorgelagerten I, nicht aber mit der Befestigung über dem Südrand von *nāʿūr* oder anderen Befestigungen der Hauptlinie. Daraus ergibt sich, daß H—K eine von *šaǧarat bilʿās* aus besonderen Gründen nach Südwesten vorgeschobenen Gruppe von Wehranlagen darstellen. Der Platz von H trägt keinen eigenen Namen; nach Angaben von Ortskundigen wird der Landstrich westlich von A gleichfalls noch *bilʿās* genannt.

H weist ein rechteckiges Gebäude auf, dessen Mauern sich 8 m in nordsüdlicher und 8,5 m in westöstlicher Richtung erstrecken. Doch

---
[16] Lage nach der Karte: 22871413.

sind nur geringe Reste erhalten, da es am Rand des Kulturlandes und unmittelbar neben einem Weinberg liegt. Auf der Westseite ist die unterste Steinlage deutlich erkennbar, während alles übrige verfallen oder an anderer Stelle wiederverwendet worden ist. Außer der erhaltenen Steinlage weist die eisenzeitliche Keramik, neben der sich noch römische findet, die Stelle als ursprünglich eisenzeitliche Anlage und nach allen Analogien als eine ammonitische Befestigung aus. Ihre Lage auf der Nordseite des Hügels zeigt, daß sie im Unterschied von den bisher genannten Anlagen nicht Eindringlinge aus südlicher, sondern solche aus nördlicher oder nordwestlicher Richtung abwehren sollte. Man könnte erwägen, ob H gemeinsam mit den beiden Befestigungen südlich und südöstlich von *nāʿūr* dem Schutz dieses Ortes dienen sollte, wenn er in ammonitischer Hand war, oder der Abwehr von dort aus vorstoßender Eindringlinge, wenn es sich um einen israelitischen Ort handelte. Jedoch erweisen sich diese Erwägungen als unzutreffend, weil zwischen H und der Befestigung unmittelbar über dem Südrand von *nāʿūr* keine Sichtverbindung besteht und vor allem sich in und bei *nāʿūr* keine Spur einer eisenzeitlichen Siedlung nachweisen läßt. Statt dessen hat die Befestigung H dem Zweck gedient, ein Vordringen in das ammonitische Gebiet durch das westlich von *nāʿūr* nach Süden führende *wādi* zu verhindern.

2. Auf der etwa 400 m südlich von H gelegenen Kuppe[17] finden sich lediglich ein paar größere zusammenliegende Steine. Sie könnten auf einen ehemaligen *ruǧm malfūf* schließen lassen, der dann den gleichen Zweck wie H gehabt hätte, doch ist dies nicht mehr zu entscheiden und muß als unsicher außer Betracht bleiben.

3. Etwa 1 km südwestlich von H und 2,5 km südsüdwestlich von *nāʿūr* liegt auf einer beherrschenden Höhe mit freiem Blick nach allen Seiten der Punkt I, dessen Name nach den Angaben von Ortskundigen *ruǧm ʿarqūb* lautet[18]. Sichtverbindung besteht mit H, K und *šaǧarat bilʿās*.

Die Stelle weist etwas eisenzeitliche, römische und byzantinische, vielleicht auch früharabische und mamlukische Keramikreste auf[19]. Die Befestigung scheint lediglich aus einem *ruǧm malfūf* bestanden zu haben, der jedoch vor allem infolge der Anlage einer kleinen Nekropole aus junger Zeit mit einem größeren Grab in der Mitte fast völlig abgetragen worden ist. Nur an der nordwestlichen Seite ist der Rest der alten Mauer erkennbar.

4. Wiederum etwa 900 m südwestlich von I liegt K mit dem Namen *ʿarqūb umm quttēn* am Kopf des *wādi menšīje*, dem südlichen

---

[17] Lage nach der Karte: 22881411.
[18] Lage nach der Karte: 22781409, durch ein Grabzeichen gekennzeichnet.
[19] Das Vorhandensein früharabischer und mamlukischer Keramik bleibt unsicher, da die gefundenen Bruchstücke zu wenig charakteristisch waren.

Oberlauf des *wādi ʿumarīje*[20]. Es hat Sichtverbindung zu I und zu dem Punkt M, der freilich nicht mit Sicherheit als ammonitischer Stützpunkt bestimmt werden konnte (vgl. III, 2).

An dieser Stelle finden sich ausschließlich eisenzeitliche Keramikreste. Von der Wehranlage sind lediglich die Fundamente erhalten, die eine runde Form der Anlage mit etwa 10 m Durchmesser und einer Mauerstärke von etwa 1,5 m, also wieder nur einen *ruǵm malfūf*, erschließen lassen. Alle anderen Steine sind von Anwohnern der Gegend erst in jüngster Zeit abgetragen und neu verwendet worden.

5. Im südlich anschließenden Gelände ließen sich keinerlei Spuren weiterer eisenzeitlicher Anlagen feststellen. Weder *ḫirbet umm qanāfid*, das zahlreiche Reste römischer Besiedlung aufweist[21], noch *biddīḫ*[22] noch die drei südlichen Ausläufer des Berglandes zwischen K und *biddīḫ* bzw. M ergeben irgendwelche Anhaltspunkte, wenn man nicht annehmen will, daß frühere Befestigungen völlig überbaut oder restlos abgetragen und zugleich damit die Keramikreste beseitigt worden oder verschwunden sind. Näher liegt wohl die Annahme, daß H—K eine von *šaǵarat bilʿās* nach Südwesten vorgeschobene Gruppe gebildet haben, die außer zu ihrem Ausgangspunkt keine weitere Verbindung zur Hauptlinie oder zu der weiter südlich vorgelagerten Gruppe L—N aufweist, weil das Gelände zwischen K und N von Süden her nicht bedroht oder durch die Gruppe L—N hinreichend geschützt schien. Jedenfalls aber verläuft die ammonitische Grenze in Fortsetzung des westlichen Arms des *wādi el-ǵubāja* südlich der drei erwähnten Ausläufer des Berglandes zu K und von dort über I und H in den Raum von *nāʿūr*.

Es bleibt die Frage zu beantworten, welche Aufgabe den vorgelagerten Befestigungen H—K zugedacht war. Offensichtlich sollten sie wie die unmittelbar nördlich folgenden Befestigungen von *nāʿūr* bis *wādi es-sīr* ein Eindringen in ammonitisches Gebiet aus nordwestlicher bis westlicher Richtung verhindern, insbesondere ein Vordringen durch das westlich von *nāʿūr* nach Süden führende *wādi* (H und die vielleicht auf der 400 m südlich gelegene Kuppe anzunehmende Befestigung) und durch das *wādi ʿumarīje* mit seinen Verästelungen (I und K). Hatte demnach H letztlich eine ähnliche Aufgabe wie die Befestigungen bei *nāʿūr*, so sind I und K in erster Linie nach Westen orientiert. Dort aber kann das von ihnen kontrollierte *wādi ʿumarīje* vom weiter westlich gelegenen *wādi abu ʿanēze* aus erreicht werden; und in diesem Tal bestand auf dem *tell abu ʿanēze* eine größere, eindeutig eisenzeitliche Siedlung, die als ein nicht unbedeutender israelitischer Ort anzu-

---

[20] Lage nach der Karte: 22721403.
[21] Lage nach der Karte: 22821386.
[22] Lage nach der Karte: 23061398.

sprechen ist²³. Demnach sollten die Grenzanlagen I und K ein israelitisches Vordringen in ammonitisches Gebiet durch die Täler *wādi abu 'anēze* und *wādi 'umarīje* ausschließen.

V.

Die Untersuchung der eisenzeitlichen Anlagen im Raume südlich von *nāʿūr*, über die in den vorhergehenden Abschnitten berichtet wurde, zeitigt mehrere Ergebnisse:

1. Es ist zwischen der Hauptlinie der Wehranlagen und den vorgelagerten Gruppen zu unterscheiden. Die Hauptlinie schließt sich an die beiden Anlagen südlich und südöstlich von *nāʿūr* an und verläuft von A—G in allgemein südöstlicher Richtung beiderseits des *wādi ḥaǧal*, wobei B nicht auf dieses *wādi*, sondern auf den östlichen Oberlauf des *wādi el-ġubāja* ausgerichtet ist. Wegen der darin einbezogenen befestigten Ortslagen (A und B) und wegen der westlich vorgelagerten Gruppen bezeichnet die Hauptlinie noch nicht die Grenze, sondern befindet sich in einem Abstand von mindestens 2 km hinter dieser. Dagegen reichen die vorgelagerten Gruppen H—K und L—N bis in unmittelbare Nähe der Grenze heran. Sie sind an zwei besonders wichtigen Stellen von einer der Wehranlagen der Hauptlinie aus, mit der sie Sichtverbindung haben, vorgeschoben worden.

2. Der kleinere Teil der Wehranlagen ist am Kopf von *widjān* errichtet worden, um Einblick in sie zu erhalten und sich nähernde Eindringlinge aufhalten zu können. Dies gilt für die Anlagen A und H—K. Dagegen ist die Mehrzahl der Befestigungen auf den Höhenzügen oder Kuppen zu beiden Seiten der von Süden nach Norden in das ammonitische Bergland führenden *widjān* angelegt worden. Die ammonitischen Wehranlagen müssen also nicht immer am Kopf eines *wādi* liegen, sondern können auch — hintereinander gestaffelt — längs des Verlaufes eines *wādi* auf dessen beiden Seiten errichtet werden, um es zu sperren. Die Art der Anlage hängt allein von der Form des Geländes ab. Ferner zeigen die Punkte E, I, K und vielleicht auch C, bei denen sich keinerlei Spuren eines quadratischen oder rechteckigen Gebäudes finden, daß die Befestigungen manchmal lediglich aus einem *ruǧm malfūf* bestanden haben²⁴.

3. Das untersuchte Gebiet südlich von *nāʿūr* ist dadurch gekennzeichnet, daß das ammonitische Bergland nach Süden hin in ein welliges Gelände vor der moabitischen Hochebene ausläuft, das nur noch einzelne isolierte Erhebungen aufweist (*es-sāmik*). Die meisten ammonitischen Wehranlagen sind auf den auslaufenden Höhenzügen

---

²³ Vgl. W. Schmidt, Zwei Untersuchungen im *wādi nāʿūr*, ZDPV 77 (1961), über den *tell abu 'anēze*.
²⁴ Vgl. dazu die Auseinandersetzung bei H. Gese a. a. O. 56 Anm. 11.

errichtet worden, um die dazwischen in nördlicher Richtung in das eigene Gebiet führenden *widjān* zu sperren. So dienten die Anlagen A und C—G der Sperrung des *wādi ḥaǧal* und die Anlagen B und L—N (vielleicht mit weiterer Unterstützung durch G) der Sperrung des östlichen Oberlaufs des *wādi el-ǧubāja* gegenüber möglichen Eindringlingen aus dem moabitischen Gebiet. Sind sie also nach Süden und Südwesten ausgerichtet, so H—K nach Westen oder Nordwesten. Diese Wehranlagen hängen ihrer Aufgabe nach mit den weiter nördlich festgestellten zusammen. Sie dienten dem Schutz gegen ein israelitisches Vordringen aus westlicher Richtung, wobei für J und K an das *wādi abu ʿanēze* als Ausgangspunkt für ein solches Vordringen gedacht war.

4. Aus der Lage der Befestigungen läßt sich der Verlauf der ammonitischen Südwestgrenze annähernd bestimmen. Vom Raum um *nāʿūr* zog sie sich in südlicher bis südwestlicher Richtung bis K hin, bog danach in eine südöstliche Richtung ein und führte südlich der — östlich von K gelegenen — Bergausläufer durch den westlichen Oberlauf des *wādi el-ǧubāja* bis in die Gegend von *umm el-ḥanāfīš* südlich des Stützpunktes G [25].

5. Bemerkenswert sind schließlich die Rückschlüsse auf die Siedlungsgeschichte des Gebiets. Für die Eisenzeit haben sich nur drei ammonitische Ortslagen an den Punkten A, B und N ergeben, wobei zu fragen bleibt, ob es sich in N wirklich um eine Siedlung und nicht vielmehr um ein größeres Wehr- und Grenzlager an der eigentlichen Südwestecke der Grenze gehandelt hat. In allen anderen Fällen liegen militärische Befestigungen ohne benachbarte Siedlungen vor. Demgegenüber ergibt sich für die römische und byzantinische Zeit ein ganz anderes Bild. Keramik der römischen Zeit findet sich außer bei E und K mehr oder weniger zahlreich an allen anderen Punkten, ferner in *ḫirbet umm qanāfid*, *umm el-ḥanāfīš* und *es-sāmik*, Keramik der byzantinischen Zeit außer bei G, H und K an allen anderen Punkten, ferner in *es-sāmik*. Häufig bezeugt sie zusammen mit anderen Überresten nicht einen kleinen Stützpunkt, sondern eine größere Siedlung der römisch-byzantinischen Zeit (A, C, E, F, L, M, N, *ḫirbet umm qanāfid*, *umm el-ḥanāfīš* und *es-sāmik*), die manchmal in frütharabischer und mamlukischer Zeit weiterbestanden hat (A, B, E, F, L und *es-sāmik*). Diese zeitweilige starke Besiedlung und enge Nachbarschaft einer größeren Zahl von Ortslagen verdient festgehalten zu werden. Zeigt sich daran doch, daß das Land weitaus mehr Menschen ernähren kann, als die offensichtlich schwächere ammonitische Besiedlung und erst recht die heutige Siedlungs- und Menschenleere der Landschaft zunächst vermuten lassen.

---

[25] Damit korrigieren sich die andersartigen Vermutungen von R. Hentschke a. a. O. 122 f.

Quellenverzeichnis

Die Beiträge des vorliegenden Bandes erschienen erstmals in folgenden Zeitschriften und Sammelwerken:

Die wiederentdeckte kanaanäische Religion,
    in: ThLZ 78 (1953), 193—200.
Universale Vorstellungen in der kanaanäischen und der israelitischen Religion,
    in: Parliament of Religions, 1965, 59—67 (Universal Ideas in the Ancient Canaanite and Biblical Israelite Religions).
Die zeitliche und überzeitliche Bedeutung des Alten Testaments,
    in: EvTh 9 (1949/50), 447—460.
Die Judenfrage und der Zionismus,
    in: Judaica 7 (1951), 45—64.
Tradition und Interpretation im Alten Testament,
    in: ZAW 73 (1961), 1—30.
Altes Testament — »Amphiktyonie« und »Bund«?,
    in: ThLZ 91 (1966), 801—816. 893—904.
Das sogenannte apodiktisch formulierte Recht und der Dekalog,
    in: KuD 11 (1965), 49—74.
»Priesterliches Königtum« (Ex 19 6),
    in: ThZ 19 (1963), 359—362.
4QOrNab, 11QTgJob und die Hioblegende,
    in: ZAW 75 (1963), 93—97.
Das Gottesbild des Alten Testaments,
    in: Das Wort im evangelischen Religionsunterricht 1960/61, Nr. 1, 8—16.
Theologische Züge des Menschenbildes im Alten Testament,
    in: Das Wort im evangelischen Religionsunterricht 1959/60, Nr. 1, 9—21.
Zion-Jerusalem im Alten Testament,
    in: ThW VII 291—318.
Die Weisheit im Alten Testament,
    in: ThW VII 476—496.
σῴζω, σωτηρία, σωτήρ und σωτήριος im Alten Testament,
    in: ThW VII 970—981. 1013. 1022f.
Die Vorgeschichte Israels im Lichte neuer Quellen,
    in: Das Wort im evangelischen Religionsunterricht 1965/66, Nr. 2, 2—10.
Israels Staatsordnung im Rahmen des Alten Orients,
    in: Österr. Zeitschrift für Öffentliches Recht 8 (1957), 129—148.
Der Vertrag zwischen König und Volk in Israel,
    in: ZAW 71 (1959), 1—22.
Eisenzeitliche Anlagen im Raume südlich von nāʿūr und die Südwestgrenze von Ammon,
    in: ZDPV 77 (1961), 56—71.

Register der Bibelstellen

(mit Ausnahme der ursprünglich in ThW erschienenen Studien)

Genesis

Stelle	Seite
1—11	176
1—10	66
1—3	177
1 1—2 4a	133, 177
1 27	170, 177
1 28	178
1 29	178
2—3	180
2 4b—3 25	179
2 1-4a	138
3 14-19	179
3 20-24	180
5 1.3	178
6 1-4	180
6 5—8 22	180
6 5-7	66, 181
8 21-22	181
9 1-7	178
9 6	178
12—50	182, 298
10	55
11 1-9	180
11 10-26.27	55
12 1-9	182
12 3	18
12 7	182
12 10-20	182
13 1-13	184
14	67, 111, 185, 305, 321
14 2	183
14 17-20	338
15	66, 111f.
15 1ff.	302
15 1b-2.7-12.17-18	183
15 6	184
15 9f.	300
16	67, 186, 188, 302
16 13	59
17	60
17 6	150
17 9-14	184
17 17	187
18 12ff.	187
18 12	187
18 16—19 29	183
18 22b-33	183
19	298
20 1-18	184, 185
21	67
21 8ff.	302
21 6	187
21 8-21	188
21 22-34	185
21 25-26.28-30.32	186
21 27.31	186
22	67, 298
22 1-19	187, 188
22 20-24	55, 93
24	188
24 10	301
24 12	169
24 57f.	303
25 2-4.13-16	55
25 2	93
25 13-16	93
25 16	300
25 27ff.	303
25 29-34	189
26 1-11	188
26 3	188
26 12-17	188
26 18-22	189
26 23-33	189
26 30	300
27 1-45	189
28 10ff.	67, 298
28 10-22	189
28 16.19	59
28 18	60
29 29ff.	67
29 31ff.	100
29 31—30 24	55
30	67, 302
30 37ff.	189
31	67
31 7	123
31 19	303
31 45	60
31 54	300
32 25ff.	67, 298
32 25-33	190
32 29	103
34	95
34 5-18	303
35 1ff.	95
35 1-4.6b-7	190
35 1-5	96
35 6a.9-13.15	190
35 11	150
35 20	60
36 10-14	93
36 20-28	93
36 31-39	298
37—50	308
37 1-11	191
37 27f.	303
48 22	95
49	55, 87, 100
50 20	191

Exodus

Stelle	Seite
3 7.10	112
3 13ff.	60
3 14f.	128
3 14	166
4 23-26	60
5 1. 23	112
6 3	60
7 16	112
8 16ff.	112
9 1. 13	112
10 3	112
15 21	173
19 3b-8	69, 110, 152
19 5	152
19 6a	149
20	107f., 137ff., 143ff.
20 1-17	124, 127, 141
20 1	135, 140
20 2	108, 130f., 140
20 3	136, 163
20 4aβ-6	131
20 4	136
20 5a	134
20 9-11	135
20 11	133
20 18-21	141
21 2	304
21 12. 15-17	146
21 17	134, 139
22—23	87
22 17-20f. 27	147
22 18f.	146
22 20-23	79
23	148
23 9	145
23 10-19	144
23 32	110
24 3-8	140
24 7f.	112
24 9-11	112
31 15	146
32	94, 115
33 18ff.	166
34	107, 135, 138f., 145f., 148
34 6	168
34 7	132
34 10-13	141
34 10. 27f.	112
34 14ff.	136
34 14-26	128, 141, 143
34 14	131
34 17	136
34 27-28	141
34 27f.	112

Leviticus

Stelle	Seite
17—26	87, 152
18	126, 139f., 146ff.
18 7ff.	125
18 7-17a	124
18 7-16	135
19	148
19 3ff.	137
19 3-12	138, 141, 144
19 11	137
19 13-18	145
19 18	28
19 26	152
20 2. 9-13.15-16.27	146
20 26	152
23 9ff.	142
24 16	146
24 17	147
25 31	300
26 26	123
27 29	146

Numeri

Stelle	Seite
1	100f.
1 5-15	55
10 33	110
12	67
12 8	131
14 18	132
14 22	123
14 44	110

15 38ff. 60	27 13 121	17—18 70	I. Könige
16 .... 67f.	27 14 121	19—21 ..... 70, 98f.	1—2 71
21 4-9 60	27 15-26 147	20 27f. 96	1 335
25 12f. 110	27 19 79	21 3 87	2 22 334
25 15 300	28 20-57 115		3 4ff. 114
26 ...... 55, 100f.	28 35 155	I. Samuel	3 4-15 113, 336, 340f.
36 7 300	29f. 107	2 27b-30 87	3 6 169
	29 23 183	5 4f. 60	5 1 151
Deuteronomium	31 10f. 121	8 .... 119, 332	9 4 .... 71, 110
2 23 300	33 ...... 55, 87, 100	8 11ff. 332	10 20 151
4 .... 107, 131		9 1—10 16 118	11 26-28. 40 337
4 8 110	Josua	9 22-25 332	11 29-39 337
4 12. 15 131	2 1 98	10 17ff. 332	11 33. 38 71
4 13f. 351	3—4 .... 97f.	10 17-27* 119	11 41f. 118
4 16. 23. 25 131	3 3. 6 110	10 18 151	12 323
5 6-22 127	5 2ff. 60	10 21bβ-27a ...... 332f.	12 1-4 337
6 4 174	6 97	11 118	12 1. 20 340
6 21-23 69	7 11 137	11 1 333	12 16 337
7 10 132	7 11. 15 110	11 15 .... 322, 340	12 20 337
10 2 351	8 30 95	13 1 118	12 21-24 337
10 18 79	9 333	20 15f. 331	14 30 337
12—26 87	9 3f. 319	22 13 331	18 10 150
14 22 68	9 7-20 81	24 5. 21f. 331	19 10. 14 113
14 23. 27 68	10 1-15 95	25 28. 30 331	22 30
14 24-26 68	11 1-9 95		
15 12 304	13 1—19 160	II. Samuel	II. Könige
15 19 68	19 8 300	2 4 ... 322, 332, 340	2 9 300
15 20-23 68	21 24 340	2 6 169	10 1ff. 344
16 1 59	24 .. 69, 88, 91, 95f.	3 7 334	11 12ff. 341
16 18-20 349	102, 107, 344	3 12 330	11 17 .... 342, 348
17 8-13 ...... 324, 349	24 25 ...... 110, 333	3 13-16 330	14 21 340
17 14-20 349		3 17-19 330	15 25 346
17 16f. 147	Richter	3 18 331	17 7-23 71
19 16b. 17. 19b ... 128	2 1b-5a 110	3 21 331	17 15 351
20—25 349	2 20 113	3 22ff. 331	18 3 71
20 5-8 ...... 60, 147	4 4a.5*.6-10.12-16 98	5 1-3 331	18 4 60
20 5b-6 132	5 .. 87, 94, 98f., 173	5a 323, 338, 340, 342	22 2 71
20 7b 131	5 13 113	6 2 61	23 1ff. 323
20 9-10 131	6—8 118	7 .... 113, 339	23 1-3 ...... 115, 342
20 12b 131	8 5 319	7 5b-7 87	23 3 348
20 17b 131	8 22f. 118	7 8ff. 114, 338	23 30 340
20 18-21 128	8 33 350	7 8-16.18-29 340, 342	
20 22ff. 128	9 118	7 9 341	Jesaja
21 17 300	9 2 319	9—20 71	1—11 64
21 22f. 60	9 8-15 324	11 25 171	1 64
22 12 60	9 15 333	12 8 334	1 2f. 80
24 16 132	10 1-2 117	15 4 334	1 16b-17 .... 78f.
24 17 79	10 3-5 117	15 6 334	1 19f. 63
24 19-21 60	10 6—12 7 118	15 20 169	1 21 81
26 5-9 69	12 8-10 118	16 21ff. 334	2 1 64
26 16-19 .... 115, 350	12 11-12 118	20 1 335	2 2-4 19, 33, 64, 71
27 .... 120f.	12 13-15 118	20 3 334	2 6—4 1 64
27 4 95		23 5 ...... 113f., 338	2 12-17 63
			3 1-9 325